Cultural Foods

Traditions and Trends

Pamela Goyan Kittler, M.S.
Cultural Nutrition Consultant

Kathryn P. Sucher, Sc.D., R.D.
Department of Food and Nutrition
San Jose State University

NO LONGER PROPERTY OF
THE QUEENS LIBRARY.
SALE OF THIS ITEM
SUPPORTED THE LIBRARY

Wadsworth
Thomson Learning™

Australia • Canada • Denmark • Japan • Mexico • New Zealand • Philippines • Puerto Rico
Singapore • South Africa • Spain • United Kingdom • United States

Publisher: Peter Marshall
Development Editor: Laura Graham
Marketing Manager: Becky Tollerson
Project Editor: Sandra Craig
Print Buyer: Barbara Britton
Permissions Editor: Robert Kauser
Production Service: The Book Company

Text and Cover Designer: Devenish Design
Photo Researcher/Illustrator: EmSpace Artwork
Copy Editor: Ellen Silge
Compositor: Parkwood Composition
   Service, Inc.
Printer: Custom Printing Co.

COPYRIGHT © 2000 by Wadsworth,
A division of Thomson Learning

All rights reserved. No part of this work covered by the copyright hereon may be reproduced or used in any form or by any means—graphic, electronic, or mechanical, including photocopying, recording, taping, or information storage and retrieval systems—without the written permission of the publisher.

Printed in the United States of America
3 4 5 6 03

For permission to use material from this text, contact us by
   web: www.thomsonrights.com
   fax: 1-800-730-2215
   phone: 1-800-730-2214

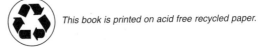 This book is printed on acid free recycled paper.

Wadsworth/Thomson Learning
10 Davis Drive
Belmont, CA 94002-3098
USA
www.wadsworth.com

International Headquarters
Thomson Learning
290 Harbor Drive, 2nd Floor
Stamford, CT 06902-7477
USA

UK/Europe/Middle East
Thomson Learning
Berkshire House
168-173 High Holborn
London WC1V 7AA
United Kingdom

Asia
Thomson Learning
60 Albert Street #15-01
Albert Complex
Singapore 189969

Canada
Nelson/Thomson Learning
1120 Birchmount Road
Scarborough, Ontario M1K 5G4
Canada

Library of Congress
Cataloging-in-Publication Data
Kittler, Pamela Goyan, 1953-
   Cultural foods / Pamela Goyan Kittler, Kathryn P. Sucher.
      p. cm.
   Includes bibliographical references (p.   ).
   ISBN 0-534-57339-8
   1. Cookery, International.   2. Food habits Cross-cultural studies.
   I. Sucher, Kathryn, II. Title.
   TX725.A1K545 2000
   641.59—dc21   99-28961

Contents

PREFACE

The population of the United States is increasingly heterogeneous, moving toward a plurality of diverse ethnic and religious groups. When we look around us, we see faces that differ from our own. Regardless of our cultural heritage, we overhear conversations in unfamiliar languages, notice traditional ethnic or religious clothing that is unlike the t-shirts and jeans advertised on television, and find new foods appearing in our restaurants and grocery aisles.

Each ethnic and religious group in the United States has its own traditional cultural foods, some of which vary tremendously from the so-called typical North American diet. The introduction of new ingredients and ideas about how dishes should be prepared and served has stimulated exciting changes in American eating from the widespread acceptance of salsas to the creation of unique styles that meld many influences, such as Pacific Rim cooking. Conversely, most immigrants to the United States quickly add the abundant meats and sweets of American fare into their daily meals.

The foodservice industry stands at the crossroads of this culinary interchange. Whether developing meals designed to appeal to a new clientele, creating items marketed toward up-scale consumers seeking novel taste adventures, or learning to work with persons from diverse ethnic and religious backgrounds, foodservice professionals experience the challenges and opportunities of diversity every day.

This book is written for foodservice professionals, students of cultural diversity interested in the role of food, and readers curious about traditions and trends in Ameriican fare. We present the information needed to become familiar with the food practices of U.S. ethnic and religious groups as understood within the context of culture. Our goal is to provide the cultural overview necessary to avoid ethnocentric assumptions about a particular cuisine, while at the same time offering specific data on ingredients, dishes, and meals for each group discussed—a combination of the conceptual with the practical.

Chapter 1 is an introduction to the study of cultural foods. Chapter 2 describes the major western and eastern religions, with a review of their dietary practices. Chapter 3 through 10 profile American ethnic groups and their cuisines. We have included cultural groups with significant pop-ulations in the United States, as well as smaller groups who maintain homogeneous cultural communities. Other groups with low numbers of immigrants but with notable influence on American cooking, including South Americans and Thais, are described only by their traditional cuisines. The order of presentation is determined by the approximate arrival sequence of the various groups in the United States.

The first section of each cultural group chapter includes the history of the nation or region of origin, the history of the group in the United States, and current demographics. Worldview (outlook on life) is exam-ined, including religion, family structure, and the communication style of each group. This background information illuminates the context from which cultural foods emerge and evolve. The second section of each chapter describes the traditional diet, including ingredients and some common dishes, meal patterns, special-occasion items, the role of food in the society, and the therapeutic uses of foods. The third section explains the contemporary diet of the group, such as adaptations made by the group after arrival in the United States and changes made in the American diet due to the influences of the group.

One or more "Cultural Foods Group" tables are found in each of the cultural group chapters. The emphasis is on ingredients common to the populations of each region. Important variations within regions and unique food habits are listed under the "Comments" column of the tables. Known adaptations in the United States are also noted.

Chapter 11 considers the regional American fare of the Northeast, the Midwest, the South, and the West. Each section includes demographics data and an examination of the foods common in the region, followed by state-by-state descriptions. This chapter brings the study of American cul-tural foods full circle, discussing the significant influence of different eth-nic and religious groups on the development of cuisine in each U.S. region. Canadian regional cooking is also briefly considered. Chapter 12 introduces multicultural communication techniques useful in the food-service workplace. The book concludes with a glossary of ethnic ingredi-ents and a list of additional resources.

Each cuisine covered is worthy of a book in itself. We have chosen breadth over depth, including an overview of numerous ethnic and reli-gious groups rather than the singular examination each group warrants. We encourage readers to study groups of interest in more detail.

We recognize that any definition of cultural foods implies homogene-ity in the described group. In daily life, however, each member of a group has a distinctive diet, practicing traditional food habits to an individual degree. We do not want to stereotype the fare of minority groups. Rather, we hope to generalize common U.S. cultural food trends as a basis for understanding the personal preferences of individual Americans.

One final note on terminology used in the text: We have attempted to be sensitive to the designations used by each cultural group, although sometimes there is no consensus among group members regarding the proper name for the group. Also, there may be some confusion about dates in the book. Nearly all religious traditions adhere to their own calendar of events based on solar or lunar months. These calendars frequently differ from the Gregorian calendar used throughout most of the world in business and government. Religious ceremonies frequently move around according to Gregorian calendar dates, yet usually are calculated to occur in the correct season each year. Historical events in the text are listed according to the Gregorian calendar, using the terms *before common era* (BCE) and *common era* (CE).

We believe that this book will do more than introduce the concepts of American cultural foods. It should also encourage self-examination and individual cultural identification by the reader. If it sparks a gustatory interest in the foods of other cultures, we will be personally pleased.

Acknowledgments

There are many people who have contributed, over the years, to the development of this book. The authors would like to thank our colleagues who have graciously provided their expert review and advice: Dileep Bal, MD; Stella Cash, MEd, MS, RD; Roy E. Costa, RS, MS; Chuck Darrah, MPH; Norma Jean Downes, MS; Lillian Estrada-Castillo, RD; Caroline Fee, MS; James Freeman, PhD; Francine Genta, MS, RD; Joan Giampaoli, MS, RD; K.C. Kraven, PhD; Shiriki Kumanyika, PhD; Louise Little, PhD; Jessica Lower; David Newman, MA; Fadesh Palakurthi, PhD; Melinda Poliarco, MS RD; Audrey Spindler, PhD, RD; Christine Tompson, PhD; Tar Toyafuda; Rose Tseng, PhD, RD; Irene Tupper; Cathy Williamson, MA, RD; and Virginia Ziegler, MS, RD. We are especially grateful for the continuing patience of our family members, Peter, Richard, Erika, Adrienne, and Alexander, who support and indulge our passion for food and culture.

1

Cultural Foods

What do Americans eat? Meat and potatoes, according to popular myth. There's no denying that more beef is consumed than any other protein food in the United States and that franchise restaurants sell more than $5 billion worth of hamburgers and french fries each year. Yet the American diet cannot be so simply described. Just as the population of the United States contains many different ethnic and cultural groups, so are the foods and food habits of Americans equally diverse. It can no more be said that the typical U.S. citizen is white, Anglo-Saxon, and Protestant than it can be stated that meat and potatoes are what this typical citizen eats.

Data from the 1990 U.S. census and other demographic data show that one in every four Americans is of non-European heritage. These figures greatly underestimate the number and diversity of American cultural groups, however. For instance, data do not list members of white ethnic or religious groups, nor do they account for mixed ancestry. Census terminology, such as the category "Hispanics" (which may be defined as persons who were born in Latin America, whose parents were born in Latin America, who have a Spanish surname, or who speak Spanish), is sometimes ambiguous and confusing to census respondents. Furthermore, the census does not survey the millions of U.S. residents who are not citizens (it is estimated 200,000 arrive in America each year). Thus the proportion of American ethnic group members is larger than statistics indicate, and, more important, it is rapidly increasing.

Asians are the fastest growing ethnic group in America. Their population more than doubled between 1980 and 1990; four out of every ten immigrants to the United States in 1993 were born in Asia. African Americans are numerically the largest ethnic group (approximately

As suggested by their names, not even hamburgers and french fries are American in origin. Chopped beef steaks were introduced to the United States from the German city of Hamburg in the late nineteenth century and were popularized at the St. Louis World's Fair. Although the potato is a New World vegetable, it was brought to America by the Irish in 1719. The term *french fried potatoes* first appeared in the 1860s and may have come from the way the potatoes were cut or cooked. Other foods considered typically American also have foreign origins, such as hot dogs (*frankfurters*), apple pie, and ice cream.

Due to differences in definitions of race and ethnicity for birth certificates, statistical surveys, and death certificates, it is possible to be born one ethnicity, to be counted as another in census data, and to die as a member of yet a third ethnic group (Hahn, 1992).

Data from the 1996 Canadian census indicate that 15 percent of the population is of non-European heritage. The largest ethnic group is Native Americans (called Aboriginals in the report), followed by the Chinese and South Asians (mostly Asian Indians and Sri Lankans). Asians and Middle Easterners are the fastest growing minorities.

The term *majority* describes the culture shared by the dominant white, Anglo-Saxon, Protestant population in the United States.

Americans collectively consume approximately 900 billion calories each day.

12% of the total U.S. population), although Latinos, with a growth rate of more than 50 percent between 1980 and 1990, are expected to surpass blacks by the middle of the twenty-first century.

Each American ethnic group has its own culturally based foods and food habits. Many of these traditions have been influenced and modified through contact with the majority culture. The foods and food habits of the majority culture have, in turn, been affected by those of the many diverse ethnic groups. Today a fast-food restaurant or street stand is just as likely to offer pizza, tacos, egg rolls, or falafels as it is to offer hamburgers. The American diet encompasses the numerous varied cuisines of the U.S. population. To understand this diet fully, one must study not only the traditional foods and food habits of the many ethnic groups but also the interactions between these traditions and those of the majority culture.

Food and Culture

What Is Food?

Feeding versus Eating

Food, as defined in the dictionary, is any substance that provides the nutrients necessary to maintain life and growth when ingested. When animals feed, they repeatedly consume those foods necessary for their well-being, and they do so in a similar manner at each feeding.

Humans create complex rules, commonly called manners, as to how food is actually eaten. (© Mary Kate Denny/PhotoEdit.)

Humans, however, do not feed. They eat. Eating is distinguished from feeding by the ways in which humans use food. Humans not only gather or hunt food, but they also cultivate plants and raise livestock. Food is thus regularly available to most humans, permitting the development of food habits, such as the setting of mealtimes. In addition, humans cook food, which greatly expands the number and variety of edible substances available. Choice of what to eat follows. Humans use utensils to eat food and create complex rules, commonly called manners, about how food is actually ingested. Humans share food. Standards for who may dine with whom in each eating situation are well defined.

Development of Food Habits

The term *food habits* refers to the ways in which humans use food, including how food is obtained and stored, how it is prepared, how it is served and to whom, and how it is consumed. A. H. Maslow's theory of human maturation as applied to food habits (Lowenberg, 1970) explains how food use progresses from eating for existence to eating for self-actualization:

1. *Physical needs for survival:* This is the most basic use of food, nearly equivalent to feeding. Daily nutrient needs must be met before more complex food use can occur.

2. *Social needs for security:* Once the immediate need for food is satisfied, future needs can be considered. The storage of food, in a granary or in a refrigerator, represents security.

3. *Belongingness:* This use of food shows that an individual belongs to a group. The need to belong is satisfied by consuming the foods that are eaten by the social group as a whole. These foods represent comfort and happiness for many people; during periods of stress or illness, people often want the foods they ate during childhood.

   Sometimes people adopt a special diet to demonstrate belongingness. For example, African Americans who live outside the South may choose to eat what is called *soul food* (typically Southern black cuisine, such as pork ribs and greens) on certain occasions as an expression of ethnic identity.

   Etiquette, the appropriate use of food, is also a way of demonstrating belonging. Entirely different manners are required when lunching with business associates at an expensive restaurant, when attending a tea, when eating in the school cafeteria, when drinking with friends at a bar, or when picnicking with a lover.

4. *Status:* Food can be used to define social position. Champagne and caviar imply wealth; mesquite-grilled foods and goat cheese suggest upward mobility; beans or potatoes are traditionally associated with the poor. Status foods are used for social

Drinking rituals, such as making a toast and participating in the round of drinks, date back to ancient magical rites of communal inebriation.

The status of food can change over time. In the early years of the United States, lobster was so plentiful it was considered fit only for the poor (Root & deRochemont, 1976).

interaction. When a man picks up his date, he brings her chocolates, not broccoli. Wine is considered an appropriate gift to a hostess—a gallon of milk is not.

In general, eating with someone connotes social equality with that person. Many societies regulate who can dine together as a means of establishing class relationships. Women and children may eat separately from men, or servants may eat in the kitchen, away from their employers. This attempted separation by class was also seen in some U.S. restaurants that excluded blacks before the civil rights legislation of the 1960s.

5. *Self-realization:* This stage of food use occurs when all previous stages have been achieved to the individual's satisfaction. Personal preference takes precedence, and the individual may experiment with the foods of different ethnic or economic groups.

Food as Self-Expression

The correlation between what people eat, how others perceive them, and how they characterize themselves is striking. In one study, researchers listed foods typical of five diets: vegetarian (broccoli quiche, brown rice, avocado and bean sprout sandwich), gourmet (oysters, caviar, French roast coffee), health food (protein shake, wheat germ, yogurt), fast food (Kentucky Fried Chicken, Big Mac, pizza), and synthetic food (Carnation Instant Breakfast, Cheez Whiz). It was found that each category was associated with a certain personality type. Vegetarians were considered to be pacifists, drug users, and likely to drive foreign cars. Gourmets were also believed to be drug users, liberal, and sophisticated. Health food fans were described as drug users, antinuclear activists, and Democrats. Fast-food and synthetic food eaters were believed to be religious, conservative, and wearers of polyester clothing. These stereotypes were confirmed by self-description and personality tests completed by persons whose diets fell within the five categories (Sadella & Burroughs, 1981).

Another study asked college students to rate profiles of people based on their diets. The persons who ate "good" foods were judged thinner, more fit, and more active than persons with the identical physical characteristics and exercise habits who ate "bad" foods. Further, the people who ate good foods were perceived by some students as being more attractive, likable, practical, methodical, quiet, and analytical than people who ate bad foods. The researchers attribute the strong morality–food effect to several factors, including the concept that "you are what you eat" and a prevailing Puritan ethic that espouses self-discipline (Stein & Nemeroff, 1995).

Food as self-expression is especially evident in the experience of dining out. Researchers suggest that restaurants often serve more than food; they also meet emotional needs such as belongingness, sta-

In a study of the morality–food effect, researchers found consistent agreement among subjects that "good" foods were healthy and unfattening, especially fruit, salad, home-made whole wheat bread, chicken, and potatoes. "Bad" foods were identified as unhealthy and fattening, in particular, steak, hamburgers, french fries, doughnuts, and double-fudge ice cream sundaes (Stein & Nemeroff, 1995).

The term *restaurant* comes from the French for "restorative" and was first used in the 1800s.

tus, and self-realization. In Japan, for example, homes are private; therefore, guests are entertained in the homelike environment of a restaurant. The host chooses and pays for the meal ahead of time, the guests are all served the same dishes, and the servers are expected to be part of the conversation. Although some segments of the American restaurant business also cater to the family meal experience (i.e., those that offer playgrounds or children's entertainment), others emphasize other dining functions—the business club for financial transactions, or the candlelit neighborhood restaurant for romantic interactions (Wood, 1995). The newest restaurant, with an acclaimed chef and a need to make reservations a month in advance, represents status to some people. Ethnic restaurants appeal to those individuals seeking authenticity in the foods of their homeland or are a novelty to those interested in culinary adventure. Conversely, exposure to different foods in restaurants is sometimes the first step in adopting new food items at home (McComber & Postel, 1992).

Symbolic Use of Food

It is clear from the various uses of food that, for humans, food is more than simply nutrients. Humans use foods symbolically. A *symbol* is something that suggests something else due to relationship, association, or convention. Bread is an excellent example of food symbolism. Bread is the "staff" of life; one "breaks bread" with friends; bread represents the body of Christ in the Christian sacrament of communion. White bread was traditionally eaten by the upper classes, dark bread by the poor. A person of wealth has a lot of "bread," and whole wheat bread is eaten by people in the United States who are concerned more with health than with status. It is the symbolic use of food that is important to each cultural group. The foods and food habits of each group are often associated with religious beliefs or ethnic behaviors. Eating, like dressing in traditional clothing or speaking in a native language, is a daily reaffirmation of cultural identity (Figure 1.1).

The symbolic importance of bread can be seen in some of the superstitions associated with it: Greek soldiers took a piece from home to ensure their safe, victorious return; English midwives placed a loaf at the foot of the mother's bed to prevent the woman and her baby from being stolen.

Role of Culture in Food Habits

Definition of Culture

Culture is broadly defined as the values, beliefs, attitudes, and practices accepted by a community of individuals. Cultural behavior patterns are reinforced when a group is isolated by geography or segregated by socioeconomic status. Culture is learned, not inherited; it is passed from generation to generation through a process called *enculturation* (Plawecki, 1992).

Cultural membership is defined by the term *ethnicity.* Unlike national origin or race (which may include numerous ethnic groups), it is a social identity associated with shared behavior patterns, including

FIGURE 1.1

An edible map—food-related names of cities and towns in the United States. Food often means more than simply nutrients.

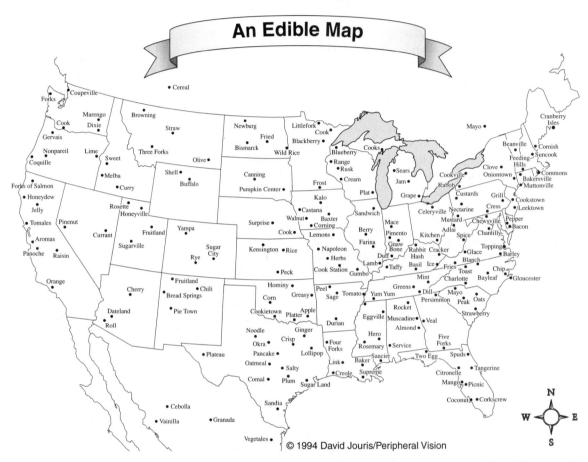

Source: Excerpted from *All Over the Map,* copyright 1994 by David Jouris, with permission from Ten Speed Press, P.O. Box 7123, Berkeley, CA 94707. Reprinted with permission.

food habits, dress, language, family structure, and often religious affiliation. Members of the same ethnic group usually have a common heritage through locality or history and participate together with other cultural groups in a larger social system. As part of this greater community, each ethnic group may have different status or positions of power. Diversity within each cultural group, called *intraethnic variation,* is also common due to racial, regional, or economic divisions as well as differing rates of acculturation to the majority culture (Harwood, 1981).

When people from one cultural group move to an area with different cultural norms, adaptation to the new majority society begins. This process is known as *acculturation,* and it takes place along a continuum of behavior patterns. Typically, first-generation immigrants remain emotionally connected to their culture of origin. They integrate into their new society by adopting some majority culture values and practices, but generally surround themselves with a reference group of family and friends who are from their ethnic background. For example, Asian Indians living in the United States who consider themselves to be "mostly or very Asian Indian" may encourage their children to speak English and allow them to celebrate American holidays, but they do not permit them to date non-Asian Indian peers (Sodowsky & Carey, 1988). Other immigrants become *bicultural,* which happens when the new majority culture is seen as complementing, rather than competing with, an individual's ethnicity. The positive aspects of both societies are embraced and the individual develops the skills needed to operate within either culture (Brookins, 1993). Asian Indians who call themselves Indo-Americans or Asian Americans fall into this category, eating equal amounts of Indian and American foods, thinking and reading equally in an Indian language and in English (Sodowsky & Carey, 1988).

Assimilation occurs when people from one cultural group shed their ethnic identity and fully merge into the majority culture. Although some first-generation immigrants strive toward assimilation due perhaps to personal determination to survive in a foreign country or to take advantage of opportunities, most often assimilation takes place in subsequent generations. Asian Indians who identify themselves as being "mostly American" do not consider Asian Indian culture superior to American culture, and they are willing to let their children date non-Indians. It is believed that ethnic pride is reawakened in some immigrants if they become disillusioned with life in America, particularly if the disappointment is attributed to prejudice from the majority society (Sodowsky & Carey, 1988). A few immigrants exist at the edges of the acculturation process, either maintaining total ethnic identity or rejecting both their culture of origin and that of the majority culture (Meleis et al., 1992).

Culturally based food habits are often one of the last traditions people change through acculturation. Unlike speaking a foreign language or wearing traditional clothing, eating is usually done in the privacy of the home, hidden from observation by majority culture members. Adoption of new food items does not generally develop linearly as a steady progression from traditional diet to diet of the majority culture. Instead, research indicates that consumption of new items is often independent of traditional food habits (Pelto et al., 1981; Dewey et al., 1984; Szathmary et al., 1987). The lack of available native ingredients may force immediate acculturation, or convenience or cost factors may speed change. Samoans may be unable to find the

Typically, first-generation immigrants remain emotionally connected to their ethnicity, surrounding themselves with a reference group of family and friends who share their cultural background. (© Peter Mengel/Stock, Boston.)

The concept *conservatism of cuisine* suggests that most people are reluctant to try new foods. Acceptance occurs if, after being introduced to the item, a person determines that it is tasty, is nontoxic and nutritive, and that it is compatible with other food habits (Rozin, 1991).

coconut cream needed to prepare favorite dishes, for instance. Foods that are tasty are easily accepted, such as pastries, candies, and soft drinks; conversely, unpopular traditional foods may be the first to go. Mexican children living in America quickly reject the variety cuts of meat, such as tripe, that their parents still enjoy. It is the foods that are most associated with ethnic identity that are most resistant to acculturation. Muslims will probably never eat pork, regardless of where they live. People from China may insist on eating rice with every meal, even if it is the only Asian food on the table.

Worldview

Each cultural group has a unique outlook on life based on the beliefs, attitudes, values, and practices they share. These standards typically express what is worthy in a life well lived and are the measures through which one assesses personal behavior and that of others. It defines the expectations of each individual in a society. This outlook, or *worldview*, is observed in numerous cultural variables, including religious affiliation, how the family is structured, and communication style (see Chapter 12 on intercultural communication). Food habits are also indicative of worldview (Schilling & Brannon, 1986; Randall-David, 1989).

Majority, white American values, which are shared to some degree by many other ethnic groups in the United States, emphasize individuality and control over fate (Table 1.1). Personal responsibility and self-help are considered cultural cornerstones. Most other cultures worldwide believe that fate, including the will of God, the actions of supernatural agents, or birthright (i.e., astrological alignment or cosmic karma), is a primary influence in life matters. Majority Americans try to control certain physical conditions through diet, especially weight and health. They may also use what they eat to influence the opinions others have about their social status or even their moral characteristics, such as self-discipline (Stein & Nemeroff, 1995). In other cultures, diet is more often used to express identity with the group or to achieve harmony in body and soul.

The significance of fate often coincides with differences in perceptions of time. Many Americans place great value on promptness and schedules; they are also future-oriented, meaning that they are willing to work toward long-term goals or make sacrifices so that they or their children will reap rewards in the future. A person may be willing to give up favorite foods to prevent future illness and enhance longevity. The majority members in the United States are also monochronistic, with a preference for concentrating on one issue or task at a time sequentially. Eating is an interruption in the daily schedule of some majority Americans, a chore to be completed as quickly as possible. Others adhere to precise mealtime schedules. Many cultural groups live in the present and are often polychronistic, or comfort-

A story about industrialist Henry Ford tells how he liked to take potential employees out to dinner to observe their eating habits. Those who salted their food without tasting it first weren't hired because they lacked the analytical skills needed in the auto business.

TABLE 1.1
Comparison of Common Values

Majority, White American Culture	Other Cultural Groups
Mastery over nature	Harmony with nature
Personal control over the environment	Fate
Doing—activity	Being
Time dominates	Personal interaction dominates
Human equality	Hierarchy/rank/status
Individualism/privacy	Group welfare
Youth	Elders
Self-help	Birthright inheritance
Competition	Cooperation
Future orientation	Past or present orientation
Informality	Formality
Directness/openness/honesty	Indirect/ritual/"face"
Practicality/efficiency	Idealism
Materialism	Spiritualism/detachment

Source: Adapted from Randall-David, E. *Strategies for Working with Culturally Diverse Communities*. Association for the Care of Children's Health, 19 Mantua Rd. Mt. Royal, NJ 08061. Copyright 1989. Reprinted with permission.

able doing many things at once. Immediate interests and responsibilities, including interpersonal relationships, are more important than being on time. A few cultures, such as certain Native American nations, are past-oriented, living according to historical direction. When one is present- or past-oriented, there may be no connection between what is eaten today and health tomorrow—who can know the future? In polychronistic societies, meals are leisurely events in and of themselves, a chance to enjoy the blessings of food with family and friends.

Most majority, white Americans emphasize "doing." They are task-oriented, like to keep busy, and prefer direct involvement in decisions that affect them. Work, or other accomplishment, may define their existence. Other cultures place a greater value on "being" and feel comfortable with inactivity. Self-worth in these cultures is based on personal relationships. Often the welfare of the family outweighs that of the individual. Decision making may be a group process, or the head of the household may make choices on behalf of all family members. Responsibility for choices about what is eaten, and when, differs among cultures.

Most Americans consider honest, open dialogue essential to effective communication, and informality is usually a sign of cordiality. Many other cultures prefer indirect communication techniques and expect a formal relationship with everyone but intimate family

Majority Americans say clocks *run*. The Spanish say clocks *walk*. Native Americans say clocks *tick* (Henderson & Primeaux, 1981).

members. In cultures in which identity with a group is more significant than individuality, social rank and hierarchy are respected. Mealtime behavior, especially etiquette, is frequently dictated by these communication constructs, including type and tone of conversation permitted at the table. The status of guests, elders, men, women, children, and persons who prepare or serve food in a culture is often reflected in how they are treated at meals.

Majority, white Americans tend toward materialism and acquisitiveness. Social pundits have noted that the more meals are eaten outside the home, the more kitchen gadgets and specialty food preparation equipment is purchased. Abundance has also impacted rates of obesity in the United States. In contrast, many cultures make do with minimal provisions and preparation tools. Sacrifice, through fasting or limited food intake, is often deemed necessary to spirituality.

In developing stereotypes, it is believed that people typically recall the positive traits of their own culture and tend to remember the negative traits of other ethnic groups (Gudykunst & Nishida, 1994).

One cannot assume that every member of a cultural group will subscribe to the collective values, beliefs, attitudes, and practices of the group. Acculturation, for example, can blur the distinctive traits attributed to a group. *Stereotyping* results from overestimating the association between group membership and individual behavior (Gudykunst & Nishida, 1994). Worldview is helpful as a starting point for understanding culturally based food habits, but many other factors typically affect the dietary choices each person makes.

Factors That Influence Food Habits

There are numerous factors that affect the food habits of each person within a culture (Figure 1.2). Many operational models have been developed to describe these influences, including the lifestyle model of dietary habits (Pelto, 1981), which attempts to explain how these factors interact to result in specific food behaviors.

Societal Factors

The governments in most developed nations often manipulate food pricing to meet agricultural objectives but are more reluctant to use food prices to meet nutrition goals (Josling & Ritson, 1986).

The food production and distribution system is responsible for the availability of foods, which differs from region to region and country to country. Individuals may have access only to homegrown food, or they may be able to purchase exotic products from around the world. Food availability influences, and in turn is influenced by, the socioeconomic and political systems. These serve to control the production and distribution of food in the culture. In the public sector, for example, farm subsidies both in the United States and in Europe promote the production of dairy and grain foods far in excess of what can be used by their populations, while deprivations during wartime required that food be strictly rationed. Government policy may also be involved with the purchasing power of consumers through pro-

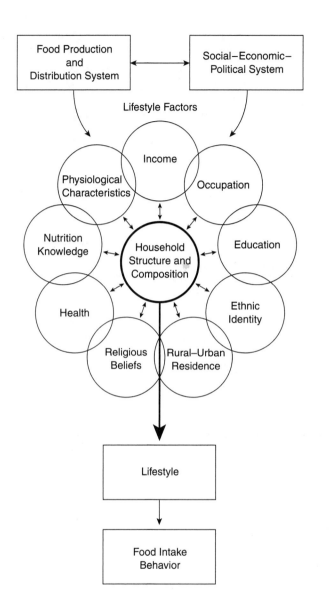

FIGURE 1.2

Factors that influence food habits.

Source: From G. H. Pelto, 1981, "Anthropological contributions to nutrition education research," *Journal of Nutrition Education,* 13 (suppl.), S4. Copyright 1994. Reprinted with permission.

grams such as food subsidies for the poor, as well as the oversight of food quality through safety standards, nutrition labeling requirements, and other production programs (Josling & Ritson, 1986).

In the private sector, advertising is another form of control, greatly influencing some food habits, such as cereal, snack, and beverage preferences. Research indicates that, in blind taste tests, people often have difficulty discriminating between different brands of the same food item. Consumer loyalty to a particular brand is believed to be more related to the sensual and emotional appeal of the name and packaging (Lannon, 1986); after all, purchase of food is a form of self-expression.

Consumer preference is a powerful factor in both the public sector as well as the private sector. The U.S. Congress, responding to extensive public outcry opposing the 1977 Food and Drug Administration (FDA) decision to ban saccharin when it was found to cause cancer in animals, exempted the sugar substitute from food safety laws.

For example, similar-tasting flake cereals such as Wheaties ("breakfast of champions"), Special K, and Total target sports enthusiasts, dieters, and the health-conscious, respectively. Mass media images have increasing influence; television programming models nutrition beliefs and behaviors, as well as provides general health information. There is often substantial distortion. In content studies, snacking was found to be as prevalent as eating meals, and only 2 to 6 percent of television characters were overweight as compared to approximately 33 percent of the total American adult population (Neuendorf, 1990).

Lifestyle Factors

Both availability and control of food at the societal level affect the lifestyle factors of individuals. These factors include income, which limits what foods can be purchased. Even when nutritious food is abundantly available, the prestige of certain food items, such as lobster or truffles, is often linked to affordability. Occupation influences food habits in several ways. The amount of activity involved in a job affects the actual number of calories a person requires each day, for example. The location of the job also influences meal patterns. In some cultures everyone's job is near home and the whole family joins in a leisurely midday lunch. In urbanized societies, people often work far from home; therefore, lunch is eaten with fellow employees. Instead of a large, home-cooked meal, employees may eat a quick, light, fast-food meal. Furthermore, who is employed is also important. In the United States the greater the number of hours a woman spends working outside the home each day, the fewer the hours she spends in meal preparation.

Income is directly affected by occupation, and occupation is in turn affected by education. The status and self-realization phases of food use are usually, though not always, dependent on higher levels of education. Educational attainment may also influence other lifestyle factors that affect food habits, such as nutrition knowledge. Nutrition knowledge, however, may or may not translate into knowledge-based behavior. Other lifestyle factors often exert greater influence over what someone eats than what he or she knows about nutrition.

In 1991 the Ford Institute discovered the following regional food preferences: People in the Northeast eat more frozen vegetables and doughnuts and drink 66 percent more tea than the national average; southerners eat more fish and fruit jellies; people in the north central states eat more ice cream and 25 percent more candy and potato chips; and westerners eat more fresh fruits, vegetables, and cheese and eat 100 percent more whole wheat bread than the national average.

Ethnic identity may be immediate, as in persons who have recently arrived in the United States, or it may be remote, a distant heritage that has been modified or lost over the generations through acculturation. The degree of ethnic identity directly influences food habits. An individual who has just immigrated from Japan, for example, is more likely to prefer traditional Japanese cuisine than is a third- or fourth-generation Japanese American. Place of residence (rural versus urban) may also affect which foods people eat. A poor farmer, for example, may have access to more fresh ingredients than a person with the same income who lives in a city apartment.

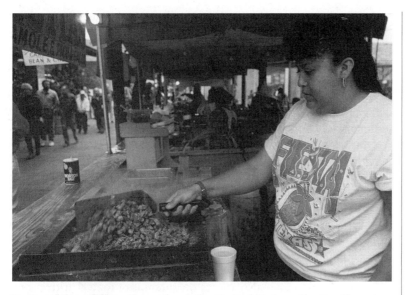

Regional fare differs throughout the United States—the Southwestern foods at this Texas fair are uncommon in many other parts of the nation. (Phil Schermeister/Corbis.)

Regional differences are evident as well. The foods of New England differ from those of the Midwest, and local specialties such as Pennsylvania Dutch, Cajun, and Tex-Mex influence the cooking of all residents in those areas.

Religious beliefs are similar to ethnic identity in that they may have a great impact on food habits or they may have no influence at all. It depends both on what religion is followed and on the degree of adherence (see Chapter 2, "Food and Religion," for details on specific religions). Many Christian religions have no food restrictions, but some, such as the Seventh-Day Adventists, have strict guidelines about what church members may eat. Judaism requires that only certain foods be consumed, in certain combinations, yet most Jews in the United States do not follow these rules strictly. Health beliefs also influence food habits in varying ways. Specific foods are often credited with health-promoting qualities, such as ginseng in Asia, chicken soup in Eastern Europe, and corn in Native American culture. A balance of hot and cold or yin and yang foods may be consumed (see the section on the therapeutic use of foods later in this chapter for more information). Vegetarianism is another way in which health beliefs can affect food habits.

One of the lifestyle factors most influential on food habits is physiological characteristics. This term includes age, gender, body image, and state of health. Food preferences and the ability to eat and digest foods vary in the life cycle. Pregnant and lactating women commonly

Old age is a cultural concept; among some Native Americans and Southeast Asians a person becomes an elder in their 40s (Wray, 1992).

Anthropologists note that malnutrition rates among women and children are higher than among men in many societies, because men are given the choicest and largest portions of food so that they can maintain the strength needed to provide for the family.

In the United States, men are infrequently involved in meal planning (23%), shopping (36%), or preparation (27%). Men who are heads of households in small families, those whose wives work full-time, and those who are younger are more likely to be involved in these activities (Harnack et al., 1998).

Health food advocate Sylvester Graham, of graham cracker fame, was among the first in the mid-nineteenth century to associate obesity with moral weakness, calling gluttony the greatest of all causes of evil (Cassell, 1995).

In a survey of fifty-eight cultures, it was found that 81 percent consider plumpness to be the female ideal (Raymond, 1986).

eat differently than other adults. In the United States, women are urged to consume more food when they are pregnant, especially dairy products. They are also believed to crave unusual food combinations, such as pickles and ice cream. They may avoid certain foods, such as strawberries, because they are believed to cause red birthmarks. In some societies with subsistence economies, pregnant women may be allowed to eat more meat than other people; in others, pregnant women avoid beef because it is feared that the cow's cloven hoof may cause a cleft palate in the child. Most cultures also have rules regarding what foods are appropriate for infants; milk is generally considered wholesome, and frequently any liquid resembling milk, such as nut "milk," is also believed to be nourishing.

Puberty is a time for special food rites in many cultures. In America, adolescents are especially susceptible to advertising and peer pressure at this time in their lives. They tend to eat quite differently from both children and adults, rejecting those foods typically served at home and consuming more fast foods and soft drinks. A rapid rate of growth at this time also affects the amount of food that teenagers consume. The opposite is true of older adults. As their metabolism slows, their caloric needs decrease. In addition, they may find that their tolerance for fatty foods or highly spiced foods decreases. Elders often face other eating problems related to age, such as the inability to chew certain foods or a disinterest in cooking and dining alone.

Gender has also been found to influence what a person eats. In some cultures, women are prohibited from eating specific foods or are expected to serve the best pieces of food to the men. In other societies, food preference is related to gender. Some people in the United States consider steak to be a masculine food and salad to be a feminine one; men drink beer, and women drink white wine.

Body image is an area of significant cultural variation. Perceptions of weight, health, and beauty differ worldwide. In the United States there is significant societal pressure to be thin. Although there is no scientific concurrence on the definition of ideal or even healthy weight for individuals, being overweight is usually believed to be a character flaw in the majority American culture. Many people, even health care professionals, reportedly make moral judgments about obesity, depicting overweight persons as weak-willed, ugly, and self-indulgent (Cassell, 1995). Yet thinness has historically been associated with a poor diet and disease. In many cultures today, including those of some Africans, Caribbean islanders, Filipinos, Latinos, Middle Easterners, Native Americans, and Pacific Islanders, being overweight is a protective factor that is indicative of health as well as an attribute of beauty.

A person's state of health has an impact on what is eaten. A chronic disease such as diabetes requires an individual to restrict or omit certain foods. An individual who is sick may not be hungry or may find it difficult to eat. Even minor illnesses may result in dietary changes, such as drinking ginger ale for an upset stomach or hot tea for a cold. Those who are exceptionally fit, such as student or professional athletes, may practice other food habits, including carbohydrate loading or consumption of high-protein bars.

Finally, at the center of all the lifestyle factors are household structure and composition. Lifestyle is defined by and organized around the family unit, which may be a nuclear family, an extended family, a single-parent family, a couple with no children, a group of unrelated adults with or without children, or an adult living alone. In each household, food behavior develops from the complex interaction of lifestyle factors. Although the lifestyle of each family is unique, similar household composition, influenced by similar societal and lifestyle factors, results in similar food habits.

In many homes, few meals are eaten together as a family. The term *grazing* refers to individuals who eat throughout the day, consuming a doughnut here and a hot dog there, usually on the go.

The Complexity of Cuisine

The Pelto model details the many connections between diet and culture. One example of the complexity of food habits within a society can be seen in the impact that house porches had on nutrition in Mississippi during the 1930s (Camp, 1991). Researchers were stumped as to why farm families who moved into low-income housing units reduced their consumption of vegetables during the winter, even though annual supplies were unaltered. What was discovered was that the new homes did not have front porches and that the residents no longer spent evenings outside shelling peas and breaking beans as they socialized with their family and neighbors. Canning activity therefore also dwindled, and those families who could not afford to buy commercially prepared vegetables simply did without.

In some ways, food can be likened to the chemical spark that bridges the gap (*synapse*) between nerve cells. In this synaptic model, food is the link between biological impulses for sustenance and social needs for fellowship, demonstrated in the way food is served at both festive and solemn occasions (Camp, 1989). Food habits are social constructs integral to human interaction. As stated by one sociologist,

> the system which they form cannot be understood apart from the ways in which it interrelates with other social institutions, in the process of historical development. At one and the same time, the system provides a communicative resource, a language, which both expresses the main themes and values of the society and enables individuals to pursue their individual projects and purposes. Every occasion of usage is, then, both a reaffirmation of a world view and a subtle modification of its shape as the individual interprets and restates it.
>
> (Gofton, 1986, p. 131)

The Study of Cultural Foods

As can be seen by considering the numerous factors that influence food habits, learning about a particular cuisine requires more than a glossary of ingredients and recipes for traditional dishes. What a person eats must be examined within a cultural context. Researchers from the fields of anthropology, nutrition, and psychology have all contributed methods and approaches to the study of food habits.

Cultural Perspective

Everyone is so intimately involved with his or her own culture that it is nearly impossible to study another culture objectively. There are two different theoretical ways in which a culture may be viewed. The first and most common method is the *etic* approach, which is the viewpoint of an outsider to the culture. The other method is the *emic* approach, which is the viewpoint of an insider to the culture. Anthropologists generally live in a cultural group for months or years to gain an insider's perspective.

Food habits that appear illogical to an outsider usually make sense to insiders. Complex symbolic, economic, sociological, ecological, or even physiological reasons for how a culture uses food often escape an outsider's recognition. A frequently cited example of well-meaning, but misguided, outsider viewpoint was the U.S. Agency for International Development's provision of powdered milk to undernourished populations in developing nations after World War II. Complaints by recipients that drinking the milk caused stomachaches, bloating, gas, and diarrhea were attributed to eating the powder without mixing it with water, improper dilution, or impure water sources. It was assumed that if milk was a nutritious food for most Americans, it was a nutritious food for hungry people elsewhere in the world. It was not discovered until 1965 that most adults in the world cannot digest milk, a condition called *lactose intolerance.*

The assumption that powdered milk was a beneficial food for any malnourished person also illustrates another aspect of cultural perspective, the concept of *cultural relativity.* This refers to understanding a culture within the context of that culture, avoiding the biases of one's own culture. The bias in favor of milk was so strong that it prevented the donors from recognizing that the milk was causing illness, not alleviating hunger, even after the clinical discovery of lactose intolerance was made.

The study of culturally based food habits is not an exact science; further, there are no absolute right or wrong ways to use food. It is sometimes difficult not to apply value judgments to other peoples' food habits, especially those that are repugnant within the context of one's own culture. The use of dog meat in some Asian cultures is an

Lactose intolerance, the inability to digest the milk sugar lactose, develops as a person matures. It is believed that only 15 percent of the adult population in the world (those of northern European heritage) can drink milk without some digestive discomfort.

example. It is tempting to label such food habits as immoral or disgusting, yet this is cultural bias. Most Asians do not share the Americans' adoration of dogs as pets. Instead, within the context of their cultures, dogs are considered an acceptable food source. *Ethnocentric* is the term applied to a person who does not practice cultural relativity and who believes that his or her own habits are superior in some way to those of another culture.

Methodology

Given the appropriately sensitive cultural perspective, the next step in studying culturally based food habits is to describe observations systematically for further analysis. In the United States, food has typically been classified by food group (as in the Basic Four Food Groups: protein, dairy, cereal and grain, fruit and vegetables), by percentage of important nutrients (as identified in the Recommended Dietary Allowances [RDA] for energy, protein, vitamins, and minerals), or according to recommendations for health (the U.S. Department of Agriculture [USDA] Food Guide Pyramid). The way in which food is classified is also a matter of culture. For instance, the Basic Four Food Groups, which include a category for dairy foods, is useful only in cultures whose members consume significant amounts of milk and milk products. Such categories are also limited in the types of information they provide about food use in different cultures. Although they list what foods people eat, they reveal nothing about how, when, or why foods are consumed.

Researchers have suggested many other ways of categorizing foods and food habits. Some models have been developed based on intercultural uses of food, such as the culinary triangle (Levi-Strauss, 1969) of raw, cooked, and rotten food. In this universal approach, it is postulated that all raw food is transformed culturally by cooking or naturally by decomposition. Other categories, found in both developing and industrialized societies, include cultural superfoods, usually staples that have a dominant role in the diet; prestige foods, often protein foods, usually expensive or rare; body image foods, those believed to influence health and well-being; sympathetic magic foods, which by their form or color are associated with specific effects on the body; and physiologic group foods (those that are reserved for, or forbidden to, groups with certain physiologic status, such as sex, age, or health condition) (Jelliffe, 1967).

Foods and food habits can also be classified according to their symbols (content) or their meanings (context). Content includes the observable practices of food use, such as ingredients, preparation methods, equipment, and food-handling roles. All content has meaning within context. Context can be connotative (physical and economic properties of food, such as appearance, aroma, flavor,

The same food practice (content) often has different implications interculturally (context): Consuming a small portion of food may mean that more food is unaffordable; it may connote characteristics of self-control or health-consciousness; it may be due to concerns about body image (dieting); it may reflect gender role within the family (saving larger amounts for the husband or children); or it may be adherence to religious proscriptions regarding moderation of intake.

convenience, and availability) and image-based self-expression (communicating cultural or social identity). The complexity of food habits can be ranked in both content and context categories (Fewster et al., 1973; Hertzler et al., 1982). Some classification approaches that are helpful in understanding the food habits of a culture include (1) which foods are considered edible and (2) how often those foods are consumed. The daily, weekly, and yearly use of food in a culture can be characterized through meal patterns and meal cycles. Further, most cultures also use food therapeutically to promote health and prevent illness.

Edible or Inedible?

One approach (National Research Council, 1945) describes the process each person uses to determine what is considered food.

1. *Inedible foods:* These foods are poisonous or are not eaten because of strong beliefs or taboos. Which foods are defined as inedible varies culturally. Examples of foods that are frequently prohibited (*taboo*) include animals that are useful to the cultural group, such as cattle in India; animals that are dangerous to catch; animals that have died of unknown reasons or of disease; animals that consume garbage or excrement; and plants or animals that resemble a human ailment (i.e., strawberries or beef during pregnancy, as described previously). The reasons behind food taboos are often unknown.
2. *Edible by animals, but not by me:* These foods are items such as locusts, ants, and termites in the United States or corn in France (where it is used only as a feed grain). Again, the foods in this category vary widely by culture.
3. *Edible by humans, but not by my kind:* These foods are recognized as acceptable in some societies, but not in one's own culture. Examples of unacceptable foods in the United States that are acceptable elsewhere include giant snails in Africa, dog meat in Asia (as discussed previously), iguana in the Caribbean, horse meat or blood sausage in Europe, and bear paw in Mongolia.
4. *Edible by humans, but not by me:* These foods include all those that are accepted by a person's cultural group but not by the individual, due to factors such as preference (e.g., tripe, raw oysters), expense, or health reasons (a low-sodium or low-cholesterol diet may eliminate many traditional American foods). Other factors, such as religious restrictions, may also influence food choices.
5. *Edible by me:* These are all foodstuffs accepted as part of an individual's diet.

There are always exceptions to the ways in which foods are categorized. It is assumed, for instance, that poisonous plants and animals would always be avoided. In Japan, however, *fugu* (blowfish or globe-

Taboo is Polynesian, from the Tongan term *tabu*, meaning "marked as Holy."

Children younger than the age of 2 will eat anything and everything. Children between 3 and 6 years of age begin to reject culturally unacceptable food items. By age 7, children are completely repulsed by foods that their culture categorizes as repugnant (Rozin et al., 1985).

Insects, such as termites and ants, provide 10 percent of the protein consumed worldwide.

According to a 1987 Roper poll, the foods Americans like least are tofu, liver, and yogurt. Brussels sprouts, lamb, and prunes also were frequently mentioned.

fish) is considered a delicacy despite the deadly toxin contained in the liver, intestines, testes, and ovaries. These organs must be deftly removed by a certified chef as the last step of cleaning (if they are accidentally damaged, the poison spreads rapidly through the flesh). Eating the fish supposedly provides a tingle in the mouth prized by the Japanese. Several people die each year from fugu poisoning.

Core Foods

Those foods that are defined as edible within a culture can be grouped according to frequency of consumption. Passim and Bennett's (1943) expanded concept of *core foods* states that the staples regularly included in a person's diet, in unmodified form, are at the core of food habits. Foods that are widely but less frequently eaten are termed *secondary core foods*. Foods that are eaten only sporadically are called *peripheral foods*. These foods are characteristic of individual food preference, not cultural or group habit. It is hypothesized that changes in food behaviors happen most often with peripheral foods and least often with core foods. A Mexican American who is adapting to life in the United States, for example, is much more likely to give up some peripheral food item such as *nopalitos* (cactus) than to eliminate core foods, such as tortillas or beans.

Meals and Meal Cycles

A more comprehensive method of categorizing food habits has been developed through the structural analysis of eating patterns (Douglas, 1972). Food can be considered a code that transmits messages about social relations and events in a culture by means of meals and meal cycles.

The first step in decoding eating patterns is to determine what constitutes a meal. In each culture a meal is made up of certain elements. In the United States, for instance, cocktails and appetizers, or coffee and dessert, are not considered meals (Figure 1.3 on next page) A meal contains a main course and side dishes, typically a meat, vegetable, and starch. In the western African nation of Cameroon, a meal is a snack unless *cassava* (manioc) paste is served. In many Asian cultures a meal is not considered a meal unless rice is included, no matter how much other food is consumed.

The elements that define a meal must also be served in their proper order. In the United States, appetizers come before soup or salad, followed by the entree, and then by dessert; in France the salad is served after the entree. All foods are served simultaneously in Vietnam so that each person may combine flavors and textures according to taste. Further, the foods served should be appropriate for the meal or situation. Although some cultures do not differentiate among foods that can be served at different meals, eggs and bacon are considered

A one-pot dish is considered a meal if it contains all the elements of a full meal: For example, American casserole dishes often feature meat, vegetables, and starch, such as shepherd's pie (ground beef, green beans, and tomato sauce topped with mashed potatoes) or tuna casserole (tuna, peas, and noodles).

FIGURE 1.3
Each culture defines which foods are needed to constitute a meal.

Source: Blondie. Reprinted by permission of King Features Syndicate.

The market for Coca-Cola as a breakfast beverage is estimated to be more than $200 million annually.

The sprig of parsley added to a plate of food may have originated as a way to safeguard the meal from evil.

breakfast foods in the United States, while cheese and olives are popular in the Middle East for the morning meal. Soup is commonly served at breakfast in Southeast Asia; in the United States, soup is a lunch or dinner food, and, in parts of Europe, fruit soup is sometimes served as dessert. Cake and ice cream are appropriate for a child's birthday party in the United States; wine and cheese are not.

Other aspects of the meal message include who prepares the meal and what culturally specific preparation rules are used. In the United States, catsup goes with french fries; in Great Britain, vinegar is sprinkled on *chips* (fried potatoes). Orthodox Jews consume meat only if it has been slaughtered by an approved butcher in an approved manner and has been prepared in a particular way (see Chapter 2 for more information on Judaism). Who eats the meal is also important. A meal is frequently used to define the boundaries of interpersonal relationships. Americans are comfortable inviting friends for dinner, but they usually invite acquaintances for only drinks and hors d'oeuvres. For a family dinner, people may include only some of the elements that constitute a meal, but serving a meal to guests requires that all elements be included in their proper order.

Beyond the individual meal is the cycle in which meals occur. These include the everyday routine, such as how many meals are usually eaten and when. In much of Europe a large main meal is traditionally consumed at noontime, for example, while in most of the United States today the main meal is eaten in the evening. In poor societies only one meal per day may be eaten, whereas in wealthy cultures three or four meals are standard. In most cultures the meal cycle also includes feasting or fasting, and often both.

Special dishes that include costly ingredients or are time consuming to prepare are characteristic of feasting in many cultures. (© Robert Brenner/PhotoEdit.)

Feasting celebrates special events. Religious holidays such as Christmas and Passover; secular holidays such as Thanksgiving and the Vietnamese New Year's Day, known as *Tet;* and even personal events such as births, marriages, and deaths are observed with appropriate foods. In many cultures, feasting means simply more of the foods consumed daily and is considered a time of plenty when even the poor have enough to eat. Special dishes that include costly ingredients or are time consuming to prepare also are characteristic of feasting. The elements of a feast rarely differ from those of an everyday meal. There may be more of an everyday food or several main courses with additional side dishes and a selection of desserts, but the meal structure does not change. For example, Thanksgiving typically includes turkey and often another entree, such as ham or lasagna (meat); several vegetables; bread or rolls, potatoes, sweet potatoes, and stuffing (starch); as well as pumpkin, mincemeat, and pecan pies, or other dessert selections. Appetizers, soups, and salads may also be included.

Fasting may be partial, the elimination of just some items from the diet, such as the traditional Roman Catholic omission of meat on Fridays or a Hindu personal fast day, when only foods cooked in milk are eaten. Complete fasts are less common. During the holy month of *Ramadan,* Muslims are prohibited from taking food or drink from sunrise to sunset, but they may eat in the evening. *Yom Kippur,* the day of atonement observed by Jews, is a total fast from sunset to sunset (see Chapter 2, for more details).

Therapeutic Use of Foods

No examination of culturally based food habits would be complete without mentioning the ways food is used to maintain health and prevent illness. There is broad intercultural agreement that a good diet is essential to well-being, but beliefs about which specific foods constitute a health-promoting diet vary. Three "square" meals each day make up a good diet for many majority Americans. Asians may seek harmony through the proper proportion of yin and yang foods. Middle Easterners may be concerned with sufficient quantity at a meal, and some Asian Indians follow a diet that promotes purity of the body and soul.

General dietary guidelines usually emphasize the concept of balance. In some cultures the proper amount of certain foods is dictated not only by an individual's health status, but also according to age, personality characteristics, the time of year, or spiritual need. In regions where hunger persists, sufficiency of food is important. In areas of plenty, moderation becomes an issue. Further, nearly all cultures classify certain foods as necessary to strength, vigor, and mental acuity.

In the United States, current recommendations include a foundation of complex carbohydrates in the form of whole grains, vegetables, and fruits, supplemented by smaller amounts of protein foods such as meats, legumes, and dairy products, with limited intakes of fats and sugar. A survey of American dietary habits found that vegetables and fruits were the items selected most often by respondents as the foods needed to achieve a healthy diet (American Dietetic Association, 1993). The Chinese system of yin-yang encourages a balance of those foods classified as *yin* (items that are typically raw, soothing, cooked at low temperatures, white or light green in color) with those classified as *yang* (mostly high-calorie foods, cooked in high heat, spicy, red-orange-yellow in color), avoiding extremes in both. Some staple foods, such as boiled rice, are believed to be perfectly balanced and are therefore neutral (Anderson, 1987). Although which foods are considered yin or yang varies regionally in China, the concept of keeping the body in harmony through diet remains the same. The proportion of yin and yang foods in the diet is usually adjusted seasonally to compensate for external changes in temperature and for physiological conditions such as age and gender (see Chapter 7 on Asians for more information).

Aspects of the yin-yang diet theory are found in many other Asian nations, and a similar system of balance focused on the hot-cold classification of foods is practiced in the Middle East, parts of Latin America, the Philippines, and India. Hot-cold concepts developed out of ancient Greek humoral medicine that identified four characteristics in the natural world (air—cold, earth—dry, fire—hot, water—moist) associated with four body humors: hot and moist (blood), cold and

In ancient China, nutritionists were ranked highest among health professionals.

The neutral category of foods is usually expanded by those Asians who prefer western medicine and believe that traditional health systems are unsophisticated (Anderson, 1987).

The humoral qualities of dry and moist are found in the traditional Italian meal, which features a wet (*minestra*) or a dry (*asciutta*) course before the entree.

moist (phlegm), hot and dry (yellow/green bile), and cold and dry (black bile). Applied to daily food habits, this system usually focuses on only the hot and cold aspects of food (defined by characteristics such as taste, preparation method, or proximity to the sun) balanced to account for personal constitution and the weather. In Lebanon, it is believed that the body must have time to adjust to a hot food before a cold item can be eaten. In Mexico the categorization of hot and cold foods is related to a congruous relationship with the natural world. Asian Indians associate a hot-cold balanced diet with spirituality.

Quantity of food is frequently associated with health. African Americans, for example, traditionally eat heavy meals, reserving light foods for ill and recuperating family members. In the Middle East, ample food is necessary for good health, and a poor appetite is sometimes regarded as an illness in itself. As discussed previously, being overweight indicates well-being in many cultures.

Beyond a balanced and adequate diet, the therapeutic use of foods includes specific items identified with improved strength or vigor. In the United States, milk builds strong bones, carrots improve eyesight, and candy provides quick energy. Navajos consider milk to be a "weak" food, but meat and blue cornmeal are "strong" foods. Asians call strengthening items *pu* or *bo* foods, including protein-rich soups with pork liver or oxtail in China and bone marrow or dog meat soup in Korea. Puerto Ricans drink eggnog or malt-type beverages to improve vitality.

The *sympathetic quality* of a food, meaning a characteristic that looks like a human body part or organ, accounts for many health food beliefs. American weightlifters eat meat to build muscle; Asian Indians eat walnuts to increase brain power; Italians drink red wine to improve blood; and Vietnamese eat gelatinized tiger bones to become strong. Throughout Asia and parts of the United States, ginseng, which is a root that resembles a human figure, is believed to increase stamina.

Other foods are believed to prevent certain illnesses. Americans, for instance, are urged to eat cabbage family (cruciferous) vegetables to reduce their risk of some cancers. Oatmeal, and fish, which is high in omega-3 fatty acids, have both been promoted as preventing heart disease.

Some cultures believe that locally grown foods prepared at home are healthiest, and, in the United States, organic foods (those produced without the use of chemical additives or pesticides) have increased in popularity. Vegetarianism, macrobiotics, customized diets that account for an individual's food sensitivities or allergies, and diets very low in fat are some of the many other ways in which health is promoted by some people through food habits.

Just as a good diet promotes health, poor diet is often considered the cause of illness. For instance, studies suggest that acculturation of traditional food habits to those of the majority American diet may increase the risk of hypertension and heart disease (Henry & Cassel,

Chicken soup, a traditional tonic among eastern European Jews, has become a well-accepted health-promoting food throughout the United States.

Ritualistic cannibalism, especially the consumption of the heart or liver of a brave or worthy enemy, is an extreme example of the sympathetic qualities of food.

Many juice bars, coffee bars, and even traditional alcoholic beverage bars are now offering "smart" drinks, usually protein and vitamin cocktails (with or without alcohol) that purportedly improve mental abilities.

Macrobiotics is a Japanese diet based on brown rice, miso soup, and vegetables that was promoted in Europe in the 1920s. Serious nutritional deficiencies have been identified in infants and toddlers on this restricted diet (Dagnelie & van Stavern, 1994).

In his popular books and lectures, Dr. Dean Ornish has recommended the use of a very low-fat diet (less than 10% of calories) to reverse the buildup of cholesterol-rich plaque in the arteries and to reduce the risk of heart disease.

The Chinese say *gan zhu nu*—the liver is the host of anger. The heart is associated with anxiety, the spleen with melancholia, and the kidney with declining vitality (Ots, 1990).

Anorexia nervosa is identified by an intense fear of fat, a refusal to maintain body weight (resulting in a weight 15% or more below that recommended), and the absence of three consecutive menstrual cycles in women of menstruating age. A 1985 survey reported that 9 percent of girls 13–18 years old believe they have symptoms of anorexia (Banks, 1992).

1969; Marmot & Syme, 1976; Dressler et al.,1987); obesity (McGarvey, 1991); non–insulin-dependent diabetes (Ekoe, 1988; Swinburn et al., 1991); and cancer (Whittemore et al., 1990).

Diet-related folk illnesses, which are conditions recognized in specific cultures, are common. The disorders of *high blood* and *low blood* in African Americans are an example (see Chapter 5 on Africans for more details). Imbalance in the digestive system causes different symptoms in different cultures. It results in numbness of the extremities (*si zhi ma mu*) in some Chinese; nausea and the feeling of a wad of food stuck in the stomach (*empacho*) in some Mexicans; and paralysis in some Puerto Ricans (*pasmo*). The eating disorder anorexia nervosa is described by many researchers as a culture-bound syndrome in the United States and other westernized nations, associated with issues such as body image, femininity and control, and, in some cases, religious asceticism (Swartz, 1987; Banks, 1992).

Applications

What is the impact of diverse cultural food habits on the American diet? To understand how religious and ethnic cuisines have influenced what is eaten throughout the nation, it is important to become familiar with the demographic trends shaping food habits in the United States.

Pluralism in the U.S. Population

Beginning in the 1970s, the United States has moved steadily toward a *cultural plurality,* where no single ethnic group is a majority. Pluralities already exist in 186 U.S. counties according to the 1990 U.S. census data, including those with the cities of New York and Los Angeles. Nationwide, demographers estimate that non-Hispanic whites will become less than 50 percent of the total population by the year 2050.

This change can be seen in the dramatic differences in ethnic group growth between 1980 and 1990 (see Figure 1.4). Although the total population increased by about 10 percent, many ethnic groups, such as Asian Indians, Chinese, Koreans, and Vietnamese, more than doubled their populations; Aleuts, Filipinos, Guamanians, Mexicans, and Samoans experienced growth rates five times the national average.

As of 1997, there are more Latino youths than African American children in the United States, even though blacks still outnumber Latinos over all.

Notably, many American ethnic populations have an average age significantly lower than that of the total population. In 1993, U.S. census figures indicated that the non-Hispanic white population of adults and children totaled 73 percent, while the number of non-Hispanic white youth under 5 years of age was only 64 percent. Predicted demographic changes are often seen first among children and young adults, disproportionately affecting the services and products targeted at youth.

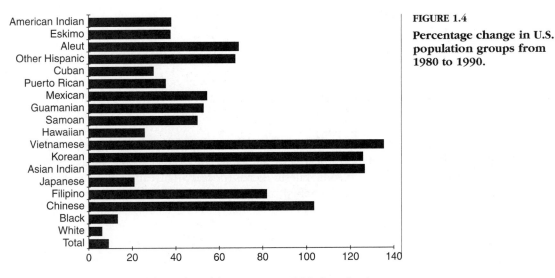

FIGURE 1.4

Percentage change in U.S. population groups from 1980 to 1990.

Note: The category Other Hispanic includes Brazilians, Chileans, Costa Ricans, El Salvadorans, Jamaicans, Nicaraguans, etc.

The Who, What, Where, When, and Why of Food Habits

Changing U.S. demographics are the reason the study of culturally based food habits is essential in all facets of food production and consumption. Decisions about which foods are grown or imported, what new items are developed, how foods are marketed, even what menu items are available at public institutions and restaurants are often dependent on the preferences of a targeted population. Learning about religious and ethnic food habits leads to understanding who is eating what, where, when, and why.

Ethnic populations in the United States are growing not only in numbers, but also in purchasing power. While total buying power has increased about 41 percent since 1990, the buying power of blacks has increased by over 54 percent and that of Latinos by nearly 66 percent (Apfel, 1998). Asians, who are the fastest growing American ethnic market, represent some of the wealthiest immigrant groups (although it is important to note that other Asian groups are among the poorest minorities in the United States).

The specific food habits of each ethnic group are useful factors not only in determining what foods to market, where, and when, but also in understanding the cross-over potential of certain products. For example, tropical fruit baby foods were developed for appeal in the Latino market, but have since proved popular with many other ethnic groups (Mogelonsky, 1995). Kosher foods are produced for the Jewish market, yet it is estimated that nearly 75 percent of sales are to consumers other than Jews, mostly other religious groups (particularly Muslims and Seventh-Day Adventists) and health-conscious patrons concerned about quality control and product purity. In

Data from the Bureau of Labor Statistics' Consumer Expenditure Study show African Americans tend to spend more per capita on pork, chicken, fish, rice, flour, sugar, and salt than do whites and others (including Asians and Native Americans); Hispanics spend more per capita on beef, lamb, organ meats, fats/oils, milk, tropical fruits, and tomatoes than do non-Hispanics. Asians and other ethnic groups are not tracked separately in the survey.

The combined buying power of African Americans, Latinos, and Asians in the United States is estimated at more than $500 billion annually.

Since 1990, U.S. sales of salsa have been greater than those of catsup.

Diversity in Canada

The Canadian census is conducted differently than the U.S. count. Canadians in 1996 were asked to list their ethnicity in an open-ended question, and multiple responses listing one or more ethnicities were accepted. This has provided a broader picture of ancestry, particularly as single responses and multiple responses were reported separately. For example, of the 1.1 million Aboriginals (including Native American Indians, Métis—people of mixed Aboriginal and non-Aboriginal heritage—, and Inuit), 477,630 listed this ethnicity as a single response and 624,330 listed it as part of a multiple response.

A separate question inquired if the census respondent was a member of a *visible minority,* defined by the Employment Equity Act as "persons, other than Aboriginal peoples, who are non-Caucasian in race or non-white in color." The act specifically lists Chinese, South Asians (i.e., Asian Indians, Pakistanis, Sri Lankans), blacks, Arabs and West Asians, Filipinos, Latin Americans, Japanese, Koreans, and Pacific Islanders.

Immigration growth (14.5%) in Canada has dramatically exceeded overall population growth (4%) in recent years. Immigrants, as of 1996, represent over 17 percent of the total Canadian population, the largest share in over 50 years. Of greater importance, immigration patterns have shifted during the past three decades. In 1961, 90 percent of immigrants came from Europe; by 1991, only 19 percent were of European background. Most recent immigrants are visible minorities, with over 57 percent from Asia.

Nearly all (93%) recent immigrants to Canada have settled in urban areas. Seven out of ten live in three metropolitan areas: Toronto, Vancouver, and Montreal. Toronto is most popular, with over 42 percent of Canada's total visible minority population, although only 15 percent of the overall national population live in the city. Almost half of all Canadian South Asians and blacks, and 40 percent of Canadian Chinese, Koreans, and Filipinos have made Toronto home. Vancouver has 18 percent of the visible minority population, 90 percent of whom are Asian. The largest concentration of Japanese Canadians lives in Vancouver. Montreal also has sizeable visible minority communities, including the largest Arab and West Asian population in the country. Over 21 percent of blacks, 22 percent of Southeast Asians, and 26 percent of Latin Americans live in the city. Other urban areas with disproportionately large recent immigrant populations include Calgary, Edmonton, and Ottawa-Hull. While Winnipeg and Halifax have lower visible minority populations than the nation as a whole, Winnipeg hosts a notable Filipino community, and significant numbers of blacks and Arabs live in Halifax.

There is some concern that as nationwide food companies recognize the potential of the ethnic foods market and acquire smaller, traditional food firms, ethnic flavors will be lost as products are homogenized for American palates.

addition to traditionally butchered meats, kosher certification has been given to specially formulated products, including pizza, luncheon meats, doughnuts, taco shells, and breakfast cereals (see Chapter 2 for more information on religious food practices).

Equally important is knowing which foods are *not* likely to appeal to a variety of cultural groups due to religious interdictions or traditional ethnic inclinations. Blood products are an example. Although blood sausages, puddings, and stews are common in much of Europe, Africa, Latin America, the Philippines, and other regions, most Americans are notoriously squeamish about such foods. More specifically, Jews are prohibited from eating any item with blood in it.

The study of culturally based food habits is especially useful in the foodservice and hospitality industry. Institutional and restaurant foodservice must meet the needs of a rapidly changing clientele. In particular, changing youth demographics are affecting school cafeterias and fast-food businesses. Over all, the eating-away-from-home market will grow to over 30 percent non-white by 2005 (Apfel, 1998).

Foodservice operations are responding to increasing religious and ethnic diversity in numerous ways. In institutional settings, providing culturally appropriate menu items is becoming more common. For example, school foodservice has found success in offering round-the-world theme meals, ethnic specials and appetizers, international holiday dishes, and the creations of guest chefs from the community (Fitzgerald, 1998). One study of hospital foodservice showed that 78 percent offered rice or tortillas on request. Religious preferences, including kosher meals for Jews, non-pork alternatives for Muslims, and vegetarian entrees for Hindus, were also accommodated. Although the percentage of ethnic dishes offered was low compared to the percentage of hospital days experienced by ethnic groups, in many cases, families are allowed to bring in preferred foods (Wong et al., 1995).

Consumer demand for "new and bold" flavors is prompting many restaurants to offer ethnic dishes, according to one survey. Ninety percent of commercial foodservice managers say they offer both typical American dishes and ethnic-style items, primarily Italian (50%), Mexican/Latino/Tex Mex (29%), or Asian (14%) dishes (Land O'Lakes FoodWire, 1997). National Restaurant Association surveys have found that one-third of entrees on menus are adaptations of ethnic dishes and that three out of every five menus feature at least one ethnic entree (Monsen, 1992; National Restaurant Association, 1998). Ethnic restaurants are also gaining in popularity. During the 1980s the restaurant business gained 10 percent, while the growth of Italian, Mexican, and Asian restaurants increased by 26 percent, 43 percent, and 54 percent respectively (Zelinsky, 1987). Ethnic diversity did not necessarily correlate with the number of ethnic restaurants in an area, however, nor did the concentration of a specific ethnic group. For instance, Thai and Ethiopian restaurants are particularly popular with restaurant patrons as a whole. At the time of the research, Chinese, Italian, and Mexican cuisines dominated the ethnic restaurant market.

Changing American demographics offer challenges other than menu selection in foodservice. Waiting tables is one of the fastest growing job opportunities in the United States, and it is expected that ethnic group participation in all foodservice work will increase in coming years. African Americans, Latinos, and Asians are already disproportionately represented in restaurant and hospitality employment

Blood drinking has had a reputation for promoting good health in many cultures. During the 1800s, British women made trips to the slaughterhouses once a week to drink a cup of the fresh red liquid to ward off tuberculosis (Livingston & Livingston, 1993).

Over two million students (K–12) in the United States are considered of limited proficiency in English: The primary native languages spoken are Spanish, Vietnamese, Hmong, Cantonese, Cambodian, Korean, Laotian, Navajo, and Tagalog (Gryder, 1998).

Hispanics frequent restaurants more often than any other ethnic group in the United States: 53 percent of Hispanic adults eat out daily, compared to 43 percent of adults nationally.

Many of the most popular items on a typical school foodservice menu are ethnic-style items, including pizza, burritos, and spaghetti.

The United States is considered the most religiously diverse nation in the world, with over 200 distinct denominations. During the past two decades the fastest growing religions have been Buddhism, Hinduism, and Islam; among Christians the largest increases have been seen in the Pentecostal, Mormon, and Jehovah's Witnesses communities.

A nationwide survey showed that 74 percent of Americans consider themselves somewhat or extremely "adventurous" when it comes to eating ethnic foods (Land O'Lakes Food-Wire, 1997). Other data show that one-half of all Americans would like to eat ethnic meals more often (Monsen, 1992).

Only 17 percent of restaurant foodservice operators surveyed said that they provide ethnic dishes because their customers "seek flavors from their home countries." Fifteen percent of operators report they offer ethnic foods because they "wish to share cuisine and the tradition of their own culture " (Land O'Lakes FoodWire, 1997).

(Apfel, 1998; Miller et al., 1998). Although one survey found that the ethnicity of cafeteria workers reflects the general U.S. population, managers were 85 percent white (American School Foodservice Association, 1998). Communication problems, high employee turnover rates, and even food safety issues may develop in a pluralistic workforce. With culturally sensitive management, institutional and restaurant foodservice can save money, boost productivity, resolve conflicts, and recruit and retain high-quality employees (Ward, 1998) (see Chapter 12 for more information on intercultural communication).

The American Melting Pot

The term *melting pot* has been used to describe cultural pluralism in the United States. It suggests not just separate ethnic and religious groups living in the same country, but a physical and spiritual blending of all cultures through exposure to a diversity of values, beliefs,

Asian tofu is the main ingredient in this vegetarian adaptation of shepard's pie, a traditional British entrée popular in the United States. (Luigart-Stayner/Corbis)

and practices. Cultural foods are a part of this mix. Although many Americans of every ethnic background enjoy hamburgers and french fries, American cuisine goes far beyond meat and potatoes. Just as it is impossible to describe "the American diet," it cannot be said that members of American ethnic groups eat only their traditional foods. Exotic combinations of ingredients and preparation techniques result in new American dishes, such as tofu lasagna, tuna croissant sandwiches, and chili-topped spaghetti. It is this unique blending of the traditional and the new that makes the study of American foods and food habits so exciting and challenging.

In 1995, Americqns consumed 14 million hamburgers each day.

One example of a multicultural creation is the California roll, the addition of avocado in traditional Japanese crab sushi. It is called American sushi in Japan.

SELF-EVALUATION OF FOOD HABITS

Demographics

Did your family immigrate to the United States? If yes, how many generations ago?

What is your ethnic background?

What is your religious affiliation?

What is your socioeconomic status (lower-, middle-, upper-class, or other)?

Ingredients/Common Foods

List food(s) that you eat *every* day.

List one food that you eat once a week; once a month.

How often (daily, weekly, occasionally, never, or other) do you eat foods traditionally consumed by your ethnic group?

Are there some foods you eat or avoid eating for religious reasons?

List two foods you consider inedible.

List two foods you consider edible by animals, but that you don't eat.

List two foods edible by persons of your group, but that you won't eat (because of preference or belief).

List two foods you consider to be high-status items.

Are there certain foods you would like to eat more often if cost wasn't a factor?

List food(s) commonly eaten in your region of the country.

List food(s) you consider to be eaten primarily by women, men, children or infants, and seniors.

Meal Composition/Cycle

How many meals do you eat each day?

What elements (bread, rice, meat, vegetables, or other) are needed to make a meal for you?

Is the meal served in "courses"? If yes, what are they? What is the order of service?

How often do you snack each day? What types of foods do you consider a snack?

What are the major holidays you and your family celebrate each year?

What special foods are served for these holidays?

Do you ever fast? If yes, when? What, if any, foods are avoided and/or consumed?

Rules

What, if any, utensils do you use when you eat?

At a family meal, who would be present?

Is someone at the family meal served first? If yes, who and why?

List three rules (i.e., don't eat with your mouth open) that you follow when you eat a meal.

Do these rules change if you eat informally? If yes, how?

Attitudes

Were you aware of your own food habit norms before you completed this evaluation?

List two personal biases you discovered through this evaluation.

Are there any food habits that you find morally or ethically repugnant?

What is your opinion about people who do not share your food habit norms?

Application

How do your food habits differ from your family norms? those of friends? those of people you work with? those of clients? In what significant ways do they differ?

How can you personally avoid ethnocentric judgments regarding food habits?

Are you willing to try new foods?

2

Food and Religion

The function of religion is to explain the inexplicable, thus providing humans with a sense of control over a chaotic world. Food, because it sustains life, is an important part of religious symbols, rites, and customs, those acts of daily life that are intended to bring about an orderly relationship with the spiritual or supernatural realm.

In the western world, Judaism, Christianity, and Islam are the most prevalent religions, whereas Hinduism and Buddhism are common in the East. The western religions, originating in the Middle East, are equated with the worship of a single God and the belief that that God is omnipotent and omniscient. It is for God to command and for humankind to obey. This life is a time of testing and a preparation for life everlasting, when humans will be held accountable to God for their actions on Earth.

The eastern religions Hinduism and Buddhism developed in India. Unlike the western religions, they do not teach that God is the lord and maker of the universe who demands that humankind be righteous. Rather, the principal goal of the Indian religions is deliverance or liberation of the human soul, which is immortal, from the bondage of the body. Moreover, nearly all Indian religions teach that liberation, given the right disposition and training, can be experienced in the present life.

This chapter discusses the beliefs and food practices of the world's major religions. Other religions of importance to specific cultures are introduced in the following chapters on each ethnic group.

Nearly 148 million Americans claim membership in a religion; of those, the majority belong to a western faith: Approximately 60 percent are Protestant Christians, 26 percent are Roman Catholics, 4 percent are Jewish, 4 percent are Muslims, and 2 percent are Eastern Orthodox. Estimates often differ in each faith due to variations in how membership is defined.

In the 1991 Canadian census, nearly half of all people in the nation were identified as Roman Catholics, and another 36 percent were listed as Protestant, many of whom belong to the United Church or the Anglican Church. It is estimated that there are 387,000 followers of the Eastern Orthodox Church (1.5% of the population); 318,100 adherents of Judaism; 253,300 Muslims; 163,400 Hindus; 157,000 Buddhists; and 147,000 Sikhs.

WESTERN RELIGIONS

Judaism

The Jewish religion, estimated to be 4,000 years old, started when Abraham received God's earliest covenant with the Jews. Judaism was originally a nation as well as a religion. However, after the destruction of its capital, Jerusalem, and its main sanctuary, the Temple of Solomon, in 70 CE by the Romans, it had no homeland until the birth of Israel in 1948.

During the Diaspora (the dispersion of Jews outside the homeland of Israel), Jews scattered and settled all over the ancient world. Two sects of Judaism eventually developed: the *Ashkenazi,* who prospered in Germany, northern France, and the eastern European countries; and the *Sephardim,* originally from Spain, who now inhabit most southern European and Middle Eastern countries. *Hasidic* Jews are observant Ashkenazi Jews who believe salvation is to be found in joyous communion with God as well as in the Bible. Hasidic men are evident in larger U.S. cities by their dress, which includes long black coats and black or fur-trimmed hats (worn on Saturdays and holidays only), and by their long beards with side curls.

The cornerstone of the Jewish religion is the Hebrew Bible, particularly the first five books of the Bible, the Pentateuch, also known as the books of Moses, or the *Torah.* It consists of Genesis, Exodus, Leviticus, Numbers, and Deuteronomy. The Torah chronicles the beginnings of Judaism and contains the basic laws that express the will of God to the Jews. The Torah not only sets down the Ten Commandments, but also describes the right way to prepare food, give to charity, and conduct one's life in all ways. The interpretation of the Torah and commentary on it are found in the *Talmud.*

The basic tenet of Judaism is that there is only one God, and His will must be obeyed. Jews do not believe in original sin (that humans are born sinful), but rather that all people can choose to act in a right or wrong way. Sin is attributed to human weakness. Humans can achieve, unaided, their own redemption by asking for God's absolution (if they have sinned against God) or by asking forgiveness of the person they sinned against. The existence of the hereafter is recognized, but the main concern in Judaism is with this life and adherence to the laws of the Torah. Many Jews belong to or attend a *synagogue* (temple), which is led by a *rabbi,* who is a scholar, teacher, and spiritual leader. In the United States, congregations are usually classified as Orthodox, Conservative, or Reform, although American Jews represent a spectrum of beliefs and practices. The main division among the three groups is their position on the Jewish laws. Orthodox Jews believe that all Jewish laws, as the direct commandments of God, must be observed in all details. Reform Jews do not believe that the laws are permanently binding, but that the moral law is valid. They believe that the laws are still being interpreted and that some laws may be irrelevant or out of date, and they observe only certain religious practices. Conservative Jews hold the middle ground between Orthodox and Reform beliefs.

Immigration to the United States

In the early nineteenth century, Jews, primarily from Germany, sought economic opportunities in the New World. By 1860 there were approximately 280,000 Jews living in the United States. Peak Jewish immigration occurred around the turn of the century (1880–1920); vast numbers of Jews moved from eastern Europe because of poverty and *pogroms* (organized massacres practiced by the Russians against the Jews before World War II).

During the Great Depression, Jews continued to immigrate into the United States, primarily to escape from Nazi Germany. Their numbers were few, however, because of restrictions in the immigration quota system. Today Jews continue to come to the United States, especially from Russia. Some come from Israel as well. The Jewish population in the United States is approximately 6 million; more than one-half of these Jews live in the northeastern region of the nation. Large populations are found in New York, Chicago, and Los Angeles. Most Jews in the United States are Ashkenazi: 10 percent identify themselves as Orthodox, 34 percent as Conservative, 29 percent as Reform, and the rest are not affiliated with a specific congregation.

Kashrut, the Jewish Dietary Laws

Some people in the United States believe that Jewish food consists of dill pickles, bagels and lox (smoked salmon), and chicken soup. In actuality, the foods Jews eat reflect the region where their families originated. Because most Jews in the United States are Ashkenazi, their diet includes the foods of Germany and eastern Europe. Sephardic Jews tend to eat foods similar to those of southern Europe and the Middle Eastern countries, while Jews from India prefer curries and other Asian foods.

All Orthodox and some Conservative Jews follow the dietary laws, *kashrut,* that were set down in the Torah and explained in the Talmud. *Kosher* or *kasher* means "fit" and is a popular term for Jewish dietary laws and permitted food items. *Glatt kosher* means that the strictest kosher standards are used in obtaining and preparing the food.

Kashrut is one of the pillars of Jewish religious life and is concerned with the fitness of food. Many health-related explanations have been postulated about the origins of the Jewish dietary restrictions;

Lender's Bagels, founded in 1927 by Polish immigrant Harry Lender, was the first company to popularize bagels outside New York City, including the creation of green bagels for St. Patrick's Day.

however, it is spiritual health, not physical health or any other factor, that is the sole reason for their observance. Jews who "keep kosher" are expressing their sense of obligation to God, to their fellow Jews, and to themselves.

The dietary laws governing the use of animal foods can be classified into the following categories:

1. *Which animals are permitted for food and which are not:* Any mammal that has a completely cloven foot and also chews the cud may be eaten, and its milk may be drunk. Examples of permitted, or clean, animals are all cattle, deer, goats, oxen, and sheep. Unclean animals include swine, carnivorous animals, and rabbits. Clean birds must have a crop, gizzard, and an extra talon, as do chickens, ducks, geese, and turkeys. Their eggs are also considered clean. All birds of prey, and their eggs, are unclean and cannot be eaten. Among fish, everything that has fins and scales is permitted; everything else is unclean. Examples of unclean fish are catfish, eels, rays, sharks, and all shellfish. All reptiles, amphibians, and invertebrates are also unclean.

2. *Method of slaughtering animals:* The meat of permitted animals can be eaten only if the life of the animal is taken by a special process known as *shehitah.* If an animal dies a natural death or is killed by any other method, it may not be eaten. The *shohet* (person who kills the animal) must be trained and licensed to perform the killing, which is done by slitting the neck with a sharp knife, cutting the jugular vein and trachea at the same time. This method, which is quick and painless, also causes most of the blood to be drained from the carcass.

3. *Examination of the slaughtered animal:* After the animal is slaughtered, it is examined by the shohet for any blemishes in the meat or the organs that would render the animal *trefah,* meaning unfit for consumption. Disease in any part of the animal makes the whole animal unfit to eat.

4. *The parts of a permitted animal that are forbidden:* Two parts of the animal body are prohibited. Blood from any animal is strictly forbidden; even an egg with a small bloodspot in the yolk must be discarded. *Heleb* (fat that is not intermingled with the flesh, forms a separate solid layer that may be encrusted with skin or membrane, and can easily be peeled off) is also proscribed. The prohibition against heleb only applies to four-footed animals.

5. *The preparation of the meat:* For meat to be kosher, the heleb, blood, blood vessels, and sciatic nerve must be removed. Much of this work is now done by the Jewish butcher, although some Jewish homemakers still choose to remove the blood. This is known as *koshering,* or *kashering,* the meat. It is accomplished by soaking the meat (within 72 hours after slaughter) in water and then covering it with kosher salt. After the blood has been drawn out,

Most gelatin is obtained from processed pig tissues. Kosher, gelatin-like products are available.

Orthodox rabbis consider swordfish a prohibited food; Conservative authorities list it as kosher. Swordfish are born with scales but lose them as they mature (Greenberg, 1989).

Kosher cheese must be made with rennet obtained from a calf that was killed according to the Jewish laws of slaughtering.

"Whoever it be that eateth any blood, that soul shall be cut off from his people." Leviticus 7:27

The prohibition of the sciatic nerve is based on the biblical story of Jacob's nighttime fight with a mysterious being who touched him on the thigh, causing him to limp. Because the nerve is difficult to remove, the entire hindquarter of the animal is usually avoided.

the meat is rinsed several times with water. The liver cannot be made kosher in the ordinary way because it contains too much blood. Instead, its surface must be cut across or pierced several times, then it must be rinsed in water, and finally it must be broiled or grilled on an open flame until it turns a greyish white color.

6. *The law of meat and milk:* Meat (*fleischig*) and dairy (*milchig*) products may not be eaten together. It is generally accepted that after eating meat a person must wait 6 hours before eating any dairy products. Only 1 hour is necessary if dairy products are consumed first. Many Jews are lactose intolerant and do not drink milk. However, other dairy items such as cheese, sour cream, and yogurt are often included in the diet. Separate sets of dishes, pots, and utensils for preparing and eating meat and dairy products are usually maintained. Often there are separate linens and washing implements. Eggs, fruits, vegetables, and grains are *pareve,* neither meat nor dairy, and can be eaten with both.

7. *Products of forbidden animals:* The only exception to the rule that products of unclean animals are also unclean is honey. Although bees are not fit for consumption, honey is kosher because it is believed that it does not contain any parts from the insect.

8. *Examination for insects and worms:* Because small insects and worms can hide on fruits, vegetables, and grains, these foods must be carefully examined before being eaten.

A processed food product (including therapeutic dietary formulas) is considered kosher only if a reliable rabbinical authority's name or insignia appears on the package. The most common insignia is a "K," permitted by the U.S. Food and Drug Administration (FDA), indicating rabbinical supervision by the processing company. Other registered symbols include those found in Figure 2.1 (Greenberg, 1989).

Because it is not known how much salt remains on the meat after rinsing, Orthodox Jews with hypertension are often advised to restrict their meat consumption.

Olives are considered dairy foods, prohibited with meat, if they are prepared using lactic acid.

Tevilah is the ritual purification of metal or glass pots, dishes, and utensils through immersion in the running water of a river or ocean. China and ceramic items are exempt.

Religious Holidays

The Sabbath

The Jewish Sabbath, the day of rest, is observed from shortly before sundown on Friday until after nightfall on Saturday. Traditionally the Sabbath is a day devoted to prayer and rest, and no work is allowed. All cooked meals must be prepared before sundown on Friday, because no fires can be kindled on the Sabbath. *Challah,* a braided bread, is commonly served with the Friday night meal. In most Ashkenazi homes the meal would traditionally contain fish or chicken or *cholent,* a bean and potato dish that can be prepared Friday afternoon and left simmering until the evening meal on Saturday. *Kugel,* a pudding, often made with noodles, is a typical side dish.

Two breads, or one bread with a smaller one braided on top, are usually served on the Sabbath, symbolic of the double portion of *manna* (nourishment) provided by God on Fridays to help sustain the Israelites when they wandered in the desert for 40 years after their exodus from Egypt.

FIGURE 2.1

Examples of kosher food symbols.

 The Union of Orthodox Jewish Congregations
New York, New York

 O.K. (Organized Kashrut) Laboratories
Brooklyn, New York

 Kosher Supervision Service
Teaneck, New Jersey

 Asian-American Kashrus Services
San Rafael, California

 The Heart "K" Kehila Kosher
Los Angeles, California

 Chicago Rabbinical Council
Chicago, Illinois

 Orthodox Vaad of Philadelphia
Philadelphia, Pennsylvania

 Vaad Hakahrus of Dallas, Inc.
Dallas, Texas

Vaad Harabonim of Greater Detroit and Merkaz
Southfield, Michigan

 Orthodox Rabbinical Council of South Florida
(Vaad Harabonim De Darom Florida)
Miami Beach, Florida

 Vaad Horabonim of Massachusetts
Boston, Massachusetts

 Vaad Hakashrus of the Orthodox Jewish
Council of Baltimore
Baltimore, Maryland

 Atlanta Kashruth Commission
Atlanta, Georgia

 Vaad Hakashrus of Denver
Denver, Colorado

 Vaad Harabonim of Greater Seattle
Seattle, Washington

 Kashruth Council Orthodox Division
Toronto Jewish Congress
Willowdale, Ontario, Canada

Montreal Vaad Hair
Montreal, Canada

 Vancouver Kashruth
British Columbia, Canada

In poor Ashkenazi homes, *gefilte* (filled) fish became popular on the Sabbath. Similar to the concept of meatloaf, it is made by extending the fish through pulverizing it with eggs, bread, onion, sugar, salt, and pepper, then stewing the balls or patties with more onions.

Rosh Hashanah

The Jewish religious year begins with the New Year, or Rosh Hashanah, which means "head of the year." Rosh Hashanah is also the beginning of a 10-day period of penitence that ends with the Day of Atonement, *Yom Kippur.* Rosh Hashanah occurs in September or October; as with all Jewish holidays, the actual date varies from year to year because the Jewish calendar is based on lunar months counted according to biblical custom and does not coincide with the secular calendar.

For this holiday the challah is baked in a round shape that symbolizes life without end and a year of uninterrupted health and happiness. Apples are dipped in honey, and a special prayer is said for a sweet and pleasant year. No sour or bitter foods are served on this holiday and special sweets and delicacies, such as honey cakes, are usually prepared.

Yom Kippur, the Day of Atonement

Yom Kippur falls 10 days after Rosh Hashanah and is the holiest day of the year. On this day, every Jew atones for sins committed against God and resolves to improve and once again follow all the Jewish laws.

Yom Kippur is a complete fast day (no food or water; medications are allowed) from sunset to sunset. Everyone fasts, except boys under 13 years old, girls under 12 years old, persons who are very ill, and women in childbirth. The meal before Yom Kippur is usually bland to prevent thirst during the fast. The meal that breaks the fast is typically light, including dairy foods or fish, fruit, and vegetables.

Sukkot, Feast of Tabernacles

Sukkot is a festival of thanksgiving. It occurs in September or October and lasts 1 week. On the last day, *Simchat Torah,* the reading of the Torah (a portion is read every day of the year), is completed for the year and started again. This festival is very joyous, and there is much singing and dancing. Orthodox families build a *sukkah* (hut) in their yards and hang fruit and flowers from the rafters, which are built far enough apart so that the sky and stars are visible. Meals are eaten in the sukkah during Sukkot.

Hanukkah, the Festival of Lights

Hanukkah is celebrated for 8 days, usually during the month of December, to commemorate the recapture of the Temple in Jerusalem in 169 CE. Families celebrate Hanukkah by lighting one extra candle on the *menorah* (candelabra) each night, so that on the last night all eight candles are lit. Traditionally potato pancakes, called *latkes,* are eaten during Hanukkah. Other foods cooked in oil, such as doughnuts, are sometimes eaten as well.

Purim

Purim, a joyous celebration that takes place in February or March, commemorates the rescue of the Persian Jews from the villainous Haman by Queen Esther. One traditional Purim recipe is for cookies filled with fruit preserves or poppy seeds called *hamantaschen* (named after Haman's pocket, but made in the triangular shape of his hat).

It is considered a mitzvah ("good deed") to eat an abundant meal on Purim in honor of the deliverance.

Passover

Passover, called *Pesach* in Hebrew, is the 8-day festival of spring and of freedom. It occurs in March or April and celebrates the anniversary of the Jewish exodus from Egypt. The Passover *seder,* a ceremony carried out at home, includes readings from the seder book, the *Haggadah,* recounting the story of the exodus, of the Jews' redemption

It is customary to invite strangers to share the Passover meal.

Ashkenazi Jews traditionally avoided pepper during Passover because it was sometimes mixed with bread crumbs or flour by spice traders.

In some Sephardic homes, matzah is layered with vegetables and cheese or meat for the Passover meal.

The Torah prohibits the drinking of wine made by non-Jews because it might have been produced for the worship of idols. Some Orthodox Jews extend the prohibition to any grape product, such as grape juice or grape jelly.

Double-yolked eggs were once believed by some Jews to cure infertility in women.

from slavery, and of the God-given right of all humankind to life and liberty. A festive meal is a part of the seder; the menu usually includes chicken soup, matzo balls, and meat or chicken.

When Moses led the Jews out of Egypt, they left in such haste that there was no time for their bread to rise. Today *matzah,* a white flour cracker, is the descendant of the unleavened bread or "bread of affliction." During the 8 days of Passover, no food that is subject to a leavening process or that has come in contact with leavened foods can be eaten. The foods that are forbidden are wheat, barley, rye, and oats. Wheat flour can be eaten only in the form of matzah or matzah meal, which is used to make *matzo* balls. In addition, beans, peas, lentils, maize, millet, and mustard are also avoided. No leavening agents, malt liquors, or beers can be used.

Observant Jewish families have two sets (as milk and meat cannot be mixed at any time) of special dishes, utensils, and pots that are used only for Passover. The entire house, especially the kitchen, must be cleaned and any foods subject to leavening removed before Passover. It is customary for Orthodox Jews to sell their leavened products and flours to a non-Jew before Passover. It is very important that all processed foods, including wine, be prepared for Passover use and be marked "Kosher for Passover."

The seder table is set with the best silverware and china and must include candles, kosher wine, the Haggadah, three pieces of *matzot* (the plural of matzah) covered separately in the folds of a napkin or special Passover cover, and a seder plate. The following items go on the seder plate:

1. *Z'roah.* Z'roah is a roasted shank bone, symbolic of the ancient paschal lamb in Egypt, which was eaten roasted.
2. *Beitzah.* Beitzah is a roasted egg, representing the required offering brought to the Temple at festivals. Although the egg itself was not sacrificed, it is used in the seder as a symbol of mourning. In this case, it is for the loss of the Temple in Jerusalem.
3. *Marror.* Marror are bitter herbs, usually horseradish (although not an herb), symbolic of the Jews' bitter suffering under slavery. The marror is usually eaten between two small pieces of matzot.
4. *Haroset.* Haroset is a mixture of chopped apple, nuts, cinnamon, and wine. Its appearance is a reminder of the mortar used by the Jews to build the palaces and pyramids of Egypt during centuries of slavery. The haroset is also eaten on a small piece of matzo.
5. *Karpas.* A green vegetable, such as lettuce or parsley, is placed to the left of the haroset, symbolic of the meager diet of the Jews in bondage. It is dipped into salt water in remembrance of the tears shed during this time. It also symbolizes springtime, the season of Passover.
6. A special cup, usually beautifully decorated, is set on the seder table for Elijah, the prophet who strove to restore purity of divine

Typical seder meal.
(© Michael Newman/
PhotoEdit.)

worship and labored for social justice. (Elijah is also believed to be a messenger of God, whose task it will be to announce the coming of the Messiah and the consequent peace and divine kingdom of righteousness on Earth.)

Shavout, Season of the Giving of the Torah

The 2-day festival of Shavout occurs 7 weeks after the second day of Passover and commemorates the revelation of the Torah to Moses on Mt. Sinai. Traditional Ashkenazi foods associated with the holiday include *blintzes* (pancakes rolled with meat or cheese filling, topped with sour cream), *kreplach* (triangular or heart-shaped dough filled with meat or cheese then boiled, similar to Italian ravioli), and *knishes* (dough filled with a potato, meat, cheese, or fruit mixture, then baked).

Cottage cheese is associated with Shavout because the Israelites were late in returning home after receiving the Ten Commandments and the milk had curdled. Many dishes served during the holiday contain cheese fillings.

Fast Days

There are several Jewish fast days in addition to Yom Kippur (see Table 2.1). On Yom Kippur and on *Tisha b'Av,* the fast lasts from sunset to sunset and no food or water can be consumed. All other fast days are observed from sunrise to sunset. Most Jews usually fast on Yom Kippur, but other fast days are observed only by Orthodox Jews. All fasts can be broken if it is dangerous to a person's health; those who are pregnant or nursing are exempt from fasting.

TABLE 2.1
Jewish Fast Days

Fast Day	Time of Year	Purpose
Tzom Gedaliah	Day after Rosh Hashanah	In memory of Gedaliah, who ruled after the first Temple was destroyed
Yom Kippur	10 days after Rosh Hashanah	Day of Atonement
Tenth of Tevet	December	Commemorate an assortment of national calamities listed in the Talmud
Seventeenth of Tamuz	July	
Ta'anit Ester	Eve of Purim	In grateful memory of Queen Esther, who fasted when seeking divine guidance
Ta'anit Bechorim	Eve of Passover	Gratitude to God for having spared the first-born of Israel. Usually only the first-born son fasts.
Tisha b'Av	August	Commemorates the destruction of the Temple in Jerusalem

Additional information about Jewish dietary laws and customs associated with Jewish holidays can usually be obtained from the rabbi at a local synagogue. The Union of Orthodox Jewish Congregations of America also publishes a directory of kosher products.

Christianity

Throughout the world, more people follow Christianity than any other single religion. The three dominant Christian branches are Roman Catholicism, Eastern Orthodox Christianity, and Protestantism. Christianity is founded on recorded events surrounding the life of Christ, believed to be the Son of God and the Messiah, that are chronicled in the New Testament of the Bible. The central convictions of the Christian faith are found in the Apostles' and the Nicene Creed. The creed explains that people are saved through God's grace and Christ's life, death, and resurrection.

For most Christians the sacraments mark the key stages of worship and sustain the individual worshiper. A sacrament is an outward act derived from something Christ did or said, through which an individual receives God's grace. The sacraments observed and the way they are observed vary among Christian groups. The seven sacraments of Roman Catholicism, for example, are baptism (entering Christ's church), confirmation (the soul receiving the Holy Ghost), communion (partaking of the sacred presence by sharing bread and wine), marriage, unction (sick and dying are reassured of salvation), reconciliation (penance and confession), and ordination of the clergy.

The commemoration of the Last Supper is called *Corpus Christi,* when Jesus instructed his disciples that bread was his body and wine his blood. In Spain and many Latin American countries, Corpus Christi is celebrated by parading the bread (called the *Host*) through streets covered with flowers.

Roman Catholicism

The largest number of persons adhering to one Christian faith in the United States are Roman Catholics (approximately 57 million people in 1990). The head of the worldwide church is the Pope, considered infallible when defining faith and morals. The seven sacraments are conferred on the faithful.

Although some Roman Catholics immigrated to the United States during the colonial period, substantial numbers came from Germany, Poland, Italy, and Ireland in the 1800s and from Mexico and the Caribbean in the twentieth century. There are small groups of French Catholics in New England (primarily in Maine) and in Louisiana. In addition, most Filipinos and some Vietnamese people living in the United States are also Catholics.

Feast Days

Most Americans are familiar with Christmas (the birth of Christ) and Easter (the resurrection of Christ after the crucifixion). Other holidays that are observed by more devout Catholics are the Annunciation (March 25th), Palm Sunday (the Sunday before Easter), Ascension (40 days after Easter), and Pentecost (Trinity) Sunday (50 days after Easter).

Holiday fare depends on the family's country of origin. For example, the French traditionally serve *bûche de Noël* (a rich cake in the shape of a Yule log) on Christmas for dessert, while the Italians may serve *panettone,* a fruited sweet bread (see individual chapters on each ethnic group for specific foods associated with holidays).

Fast Days

Before 1966, abstinence from meat was observed on every Friday that did not fall on a holy day of obligation. In the United States the 6 days of obligation are New Year's Day (January 1st), Ascension Thursday (40 days after Easter), Assumption (August 15th), All Saints' Day (November 1st), Immaculate Conception (December 8th), and Christmas (December 25th). In addition, fasting and abstinence were observed on Ash Wednesday (the first day of Lent) and Good Friday (the Friday before Easter). Abstinence forbids the use of meat, but not of eggs, dairy products, or condiments made of animal fat. Fasting permits only one full meal per day. It does not prohibit the taking of some food in the morning and evening; however, local custom as to the quantity and quality of this supplementary nourishment varies. Only Catholics older than the age of 14 and younger than the age of 60 are required to observe the dietary laws. In 1966 the U.S. Catholic Conference abolished most dietary restrictions, although Catholics are still required to abstain from eating meat on the Fridays of Lent in remembrance of the sacrificial death of Christ and to fast and abstain on Ash Wednesday and Good Friday. Some older or more devout Catholics still observe the previous rules of fasting and abstinence. Catholics are also required to avoid liquids (except water) and food 1 hour before receiving communion.

St. Agnes Day, celebrated on January 21st in Great Britain, honors the patron saint of girls. On the eve of the day, British girls traditionally baked a cake and walked upstairs backward saying a prayer to Agnes and making a wish for the man of their dreams.

The patron saint of cows and the dairy trade, St. Brigid, is honored in Ireland on February 1st.

St. Valentine's Day traditions may date back to *Lupercalia,* a Roman festival held in mid-February at which a young man would draw the name of a young woman out of a box to be his sweetheart for a day.

Lent is the 40 days before Easter; the word originally meant "spring."

The last day before Lent is a traditional festival of exuberant feasting and drinking in many regions where Lenten fasting is observed. In France and in Louisiana, it is known as *Mardi Gras;* in Britain, *Shrove Tuesday;* in Germany, *Fastnacht;* and *Carnival* throughout the Caribbean and in Brazil.

Italian American Catholics often serve *panettone,* a sweet bread with dried fruits, on feast days, especially Christmas. (Courtesy of Grossich and Bond, Inc.)

In the Eastern Orthodox religion the leavened communion bread called *Phosphoron* is prepared by the women of the church.

Eastern Orthodox Christianity

The Eastern Orthodox Church is as old as the Roman Catholic branch of Christianity, although not as prevalent in the United States. In the year 300 CE, there were two centers of Christianity, one in Rome and the other in Constantinople (now Istanbul, Turkey). Differences arose over theological interpretations of the Bible and the governing of the church, and in 1054 the fellowship between the Latin and Byzantine churches was finally broken. Some of the differences between the two churches concerned the interpretation of the Trinity (the Father, the Son, and the Holy Ghost), the use of unleavened bread for the communion, the celibacy of the clergy, and the position of the Pope. In the Eastern Orthodox Church, leavened bread is used for communion, the clergy are allowed to marry before entering the priesthood, and the authority of the Pope is not recognized.

The Orthodox Church consists of fourteen self-governing churches, five of which—Constantinople, Alexandria (the Egyptian Coptic Church), Antioch, Jerusalem, and Cyprus—date back to the time of the Byzantine Empire. Six other churches represent the nations where the majority of people are Orthodox (Russia, Rumania, Serbia, Bulgaria, Greece, and the former Soviet state of Georgia). Three other churches exist independently in countries where only a minority profess the religion. The beliefs of the churches are similar; only the language of the service differs.

The first Eastern Orthodox church in America was started by Russians on the West Coast in the late 1700s. It is estimated that more than 3 million persons in the United States are members of the Eastern Orthodox religion, with the largest following (2 million) being Greek. Most Eastern Orthodox churches in the United States recognize the patriarch of Constantinople as their spiritual leader.

Feast Days

All the feast days are listed in Table 2.2. Easter is the most important holiday in the Eastern Orthodox religion and is celebrated on the first Sunday after the full moon after March 21st, but not before the Jewish Passover. Lent is preceded by a pre-Lenten period lasting 10 weeks before Easter or 3 weeks before Lent. On the third Sunday before Lent (Meat Fare Sunday), all the meat in the house is eaten. On the Sunday before Lent (Cheese Fare Sunday), all the cheese, eggs, and butter in the house are eaten. On the next day, Clean Monday, the Lenten fast begins. Fish is allowed on Palm Sunday and on the Annunciation Day

The Ethiopian church is an Orthodox denomination that is similar to the Egyptian Coptic Church. On *Buhe*, they celebrate the transfiguration of Christ on Mount Tabor; groups of children go from house to house singing and are rewarded with special loaves of bread.

Koljivo, boiled whole wheat kernels mixed with nuts, dried fruit, and sugar, must be offered before the church altar 3, 9, and 40 days after the death of a family member. After the koljivo is blessed by the priest, it is distributed to the friends of the deceased. The boiled wheat represents everlasting life and the fruit represents sweetness and plenty.

TABLE 2.2
Eastern Orthodox Feast Days

Feast Day	Date*
Christmas	Dec. 25, Jan. 7
Theophany	Jan. 6, Jan. 19
Presentation of Our Lord into the Temple	Feb. 2, Feb. 15
Annunciation	Mar. 25, Apr. 7
Easter	See text for date
Ascension	40 days after Easter
Pentecost (Trinity) Sunday	50 days after Easter
Transfiguration	Aug. 6, Aug. 19
Dormition of the Holy Theotokos	Aug. 15, Aug. 28
Nativity of the Holy Theotokos	Sept. 8, Sept. 21
Presentation of the Holy Theotokos	Nov. 21, Dec. 4

*Date depends on whether the Julian or Gregorian calendar is followed.

The red Easter egg symbolizes the tomb of Christ (the egg) and is a sign of mourning (the red color). The breaking of the eggs on Easter represents the opening of the tomb and belief in the resurrection.

In Greece the three great saints of the Orthodox Church, St. Basil, St. Gregory, and St. John Chrysotom, are honored on January 30th, the Holiday of the Three Hierarchs.

of the Virgin Mary. The Lenten fast is traditionally broken after the midnight services on Easter Sunday. Easter eggs in the Eastern Orthodox religion range from the highly ornate (eastern Europe and Russia) to the solid red ones used by the Greeks.

Fast Days

In the Eastern Orthodox religion there are numerous fast days (see Table 2.3). Further, those receiving Holy Communion on Sunday abstain from food and drink before the service. Fasting is considered an opportunity to prove that the soul can rule the body. On fast days no meat or animal products (milk, eggs, butter, and cheese) are consumed. Fish is also avoided, but shellfish is allowed. Older or more devout Greek Orthodox followers do not use olive oil on fast days, but will eat olives.

TABLE 2.3
Eastern Orthodox Fast Days and Periods

Fast Days

Every Wednesday and Friday except during fast-free weeks:
    Week following Christmas till Eve of Theophany (12 days after Christmas)
    Bright Week, week following Easter
    Trinity Week, week following Trinity Sunday
Eve of Theophany (Jan. 6 or 18)
Beheading of John the Baptist (Aug. 29 or Sept. 27)
The Elevation of the Holy Cross (Sept. 14 or 27)

Fast Periods

Nativity Fast (Advent): Nov. 15 or 28 to Dec. 24 or Jan. 6
Great Lent and Holy Week: 7 weeks before Easter
Fast of the Apostles: May 23 or June 5 to June 16 or 29
Fast of the Dormition of the Holy Theotokos (Aug. 1 or 14 to Aug. 15 or 28)

Dates depend on whether the Julian or Gregorian calendar is followed.

Protestantism

The sixteenth-century religious movement known as the Reformation established the Protestant churches by questioning the practices of the Roman Catholic Church and eventually breaking away from its teachings. The man primarily responsible for the Reformation was Martin Luther, a German Augustinian monk who taught theology. He started the movement when, in 1517, he nailed a document containing ninety-five protests against certain Catholic practices on the door of the castle church in Wittenberg. He later broadened his position. A decade later, several countries and German principalities organized the Protestant Lutheran Church based on Martin Luther's teachings.

Luther placed great emphasis on the individual's direct responsibility to God. He believed that every person can reach God through direct prayer without the intercession of a priest or saint; thus every believer is, in effect, a minister. Although everyone is prone to sin and is inherently wicked, a person can be saved by faith in Christ, who by His death on the Cross atoned for the sins of all people. Consequently, to Luther, faith was all-important and good works alone could not negate evil deeds. Luther's theology removed the priest's mystical function, encouraging everyone to read the Bible and interpret the Scriptures.

The beliefs taught by Martin Luther established the foundation of most Protestant faiths. Other reformers who followed Luther are associated with specific denominations. In the mid-sixteenth century, John Calvin developed the ideas that led to the formation of the Presbyterian, Congregationalist, and Baptist churches; John Wesley founded the Methodist movement in the eighteenth century. Other denominations in the United States include Episcopalians (related to the English Anglican Church started under King Henry VIII); Seventh-Day Adventists; Jehovah's Witnesses; Disciples of Christ; Church of Jesus Christ of Latter Day Saints (Mormons); Church of Christ, Scientist (Christian Scientists); and Friends (Quakers).

Christmas and Easter are the primary holidays celebrated in the Protestant tradition. Although the role of food is important in these holidays, the choice of items served is determined by family ethnicity and preference rather than religious practice. Fasting is also uncommon in most Protestant denominations. Some churches or individuals may use occasional fasting, however, to facilitate prayer and worship. Only a few of the Protestant denominations, such as the Mormons and the Seventh-Day Adventists, have dietary practices integral to their faith.

Mormons

The Church of Jesus Christ of Latter Day Saints is a purely American institution that emerged in the early 1800s. Its founder, Joseph Smith, Jr., had a vision of the Angel Moroni, who told him of golden plates hidden in a hill and the means by which to decipher them. The resulting *Book of Mormon* was published in 1829, and in 1830 a new religious faith was born.

The Book of Mormon details the story of two bands of Israelites who settled in America and from whom certain Native Americans are descended. Christ visited them after His resurrection, and thus they preserved Christianity in its pure form. The tribes did not survive, but the last member, Moroni, hid the nation's sacred writings, compiled by his father, Mormon.

Welch's Grape Juice was developed by Dr. Thomas Welch, dentist, Methodist, and ardent prohibitionist, in 1869 as an alternative to communion wine.

When seven millers got together in 1891 to market oatmeal, they chose the name Quaker Oats even though none were members of the Friends, because that religious group was generally regarded as pure and wholesome.

The Mormons believe that God reveals Himself and His will through His apostles and prophets. The Mormon Church is organized along biblical lines. Members of the priesthood are graded upward in six degrees (deacons, teachers, priests, elders, seventies, and high priests). From the priesthood are chosen, by the church at large, a council of twelve apostles, which constitutes a group of ruling elders; from these, by seniority, a church president rules with life tenure. There is no paid clergy. Sunday services are held by groups of Mormons, and selected church members give the sermon.

To escape local persecution, Brigham Young led the people of the Mormon Church to Utah in 1847. Today Utah is more than 80 percent Mormon and many western states have significant numbers of church members. The main branch of the church is headquartered in Salt Lake City, but a smaller branch, the Reorganized Church of Jesus Christ of Latter Day Saints, is centered in Independence, Missouri. All Mormons believe that Independence will be the capital of the world when Christ returns.

Joseph Smith, through a revelation, prescribed the Mormon laws of health, dealing particularly with dietary matters. They prohibit the use of tobacco, strong drink, and hot drinks. Strong drink is defined as alcoholic beverages; hot drinks means tea and coffee. Many Mormons do not use any product that contains caffeine. Followers are advised to eat meat sparingly, and to base their diets on grains, especially wheat. In addition, all Mormons are required to store a year's supply of food and clothing for each person in the family. Many also fast 1 day per month (donating the money that would have been spent on food to the poor).

Seventh-Day Adventists

In the early 1800s, many people believed that the Second Coming of Christ was imminent. In the United States, William Miller predicted that Christ would return in 1843 or 1844. When both years passed and the prediction did not materialize, many of his followers became disillusioned. However, one group continued to believe that the prediction was not wrong, but that the date was actually the beginning of the world's end preceding the coming of Christ. They became known as the Seventh-Day Adventists and were officially organized in 1863.

The spiritual guide for the new church was Ellen G. Harmon, who later became Mrs. James White. Her inspirations were the result of more than 2,000 prophetic visions and dreams she reportedly had during her life. Mrs. White claimed to be not a prophet, but a conduit that relayed God's desires and admonitions to humankind.

Today, there are more than half a million Seventh-Day Adventists in the United States and more than 1 million worldwide. Besides the main belief in Christ's advent, or second coming, the Seventh-Day Adventists practice the principles of Protestantism. They believe that the advent will be preceded by a monstrous war, pestilence, and plague, resulting in the destruction of Satan and all wicked people; the earth will be purified by holocaust. Although the hour of Christ's return is not known, they believe that dedication to His work will hasten it.

The church adheres strictly to the teachings of the Bible. The Sabbath is observed from sundown on Friday to sundown on Saturday and is wholly dedicated to the Lord. Food must be prepared on Friday and dishes washed on Sunday. Church members dress simply, avoid ostentation, and wear only functional jewelry. The church's headquarters are in Tacoma Park, Maryland, near Washington, DC, where they were moved after a series of fires ravaged the previous center in Battle Creek, Michigan. Each congregation is led by a pastor (a teacher more than a minister), and all the churches are under the leadership of the president of the general conference of Seventh-Day Adventists.

Adventists follow Apostle Paul's teaching that the human body is the temple of the Holy Spirit. Many of Mrs. White's writings concern health and diet and have been compiled into such books as *The Ministry of Healing, Counsels on Diet and Foods,* and *Counsels on Health.*

Adventists believe that sickness is a result of the violation of the laws of health. One can preserve health by eating the right kinds of foods in moderation and by getting enough rest and exercise. Overeating is discouraged. Vegetarianism is widely practiced because the Bible states that the diet in Eden did not include flesh foods. Most Adventists are lacto-ovo-vegetarians (eating milk products and eggs, but not meat). Some do consume meat, although they avoid pork and shellfish. Mrs. White advocated the use of nuts and beans instead of meat, substituting vegetable oil for animal fat, and using whole grains in breads. Like the Mormons, the Adventists do not consume tea, coffee, or alcohol and do not use tobacco products. Water is considered the best liquid and should be consumed only before and after the meal, not during the meal. Meals are not highly seasoned, and condiments such as mustard and pepper are avoided. Eating between meals is discouraged so that food can be properly digested. Mrs. White recommended that 5 or 6 hours elapse between meals.

Loma Linda Foods began as a bakery in 1906 providing whole wheat bread and cookies to the patients and staff of Loma Linda University Medical Center in southern California.

The American breakfast cereal industry is the result of the dietary and health practices of the Seventh-Day Adventists. In 1886, Dr. John Kellogg became director of the Adventists' sanitarium in Battle Creek, Michigan, and in his efforts to find a tasty substitute for meat, he invented corn flakes.

Islam

Islam is the second largest religious group in the world. Although not widely practiced in the United States, Islam is the dominant religion in the Middle East, northern Africa, Pakistan, Indonesia, and Malaysia. Large numbers of people also follow the religion in parts of sub-Saharan Africa, India, Russia, and Southeast Asia.

Islam, which means "submission" (to the will of God), is not only a religion but also a way of life. One who adheres to Islam is called a Muslim, "he who submits." Islam's founder, Mohammed, was neither a savior nor a messiah, but rather a prophet through whom God delivered His messages. He was born in 570 CE in Mecca, Saudi Arabia, a city located along the spice trade route. Early in Mohammed's life he acquired a respect for Jewish and Christian monotheism. Later the archangel Gabriel appeared to him in many visions. These revelations continued for a decade or more, and the archangel told Mohammed that he was a prophet of Allah, the one true God.

Mohammed's teachings met with hostility in Mecca, and in 622 he fled to Yathrib. The year of the flight (*hegira*) is the first year in the Muslim calendar. At Yathrib, later named Medina, Mohammed became a religious and political leader. Eight years after fleeing Mecca, he returned triumphant and declared Mecca a holy place to Allah.

The most sacred writings of Islam are found in the *Koran* (sometimes spelled *Quran* or *Qur'an*), believed to contain the words spoken by Allah through Mohammed. It includes many legends and traditions that parallel those of the Old and New Testaments, as well as Arabian folk tales. The Koran also contains the basic laws of Islam, and its analysis and interpretation by religious scholars have provided the guidelines by which Muslims lead their daily lives.

The Muslims believe that the one true God, Allah, is basically the God of Judaism and Christianity, but that His word was incompletely expressed in the Old and New Testaments and was only fulfilled in the Koran. Similarly, they believe that Mohammed was the last prophet, superseding Christ, who is considered a prophet and not the Son of God. The primary doctrines of Islam are monotheism and the concept of the last judgment, the day of final resurrection when all will be deemed worthy of either the delights of heaven or the terrors of hell.

Mohammed did not institute an organized priesthood or sacraments but instead advocated the following ritualistic observances, known as the Five Pillars of Islam:

1. *Faith,* shown by the proclamation of the unity of God, and belief in that unity, as expressed in the creed, "There is no God but Allah; Mohammed is the Messenger of Allah."

2. *Prayer,* performed five times daily (at dawn, noon, midafternoon, sunset, and nightfall), facing Mecca, wherever one may be; and on Fridays, the day of public prayer, in the *mosque* (a building used for public worship). On Fridays, sermons are delivered in the mosque after the noon prayer.

3. *Almsgiving, zakat,* as an offering to the poor and an act of piety. In some Islamic countries, Muslims are expected to give 2.5 percent of their net savings or assets in money or goods. The money is used to help the poor or to support the religious organization in countries where Islam is not the dominant religion. In addition, zakat is given to the needy on certain feast and fast days (see the next section on dietary practices for more details).

If one is unable to attend a mosque, the prayers are said on a prayer rug facing Mecca.

4. *Fasting,* to fulfill a religious obligation, to earn the pleasure of Allah, to wipe out previous sins, and to appreciate the hunger of the poor and the needy.
5. *Pilgrimage to Mecca, hadj,* once in a lifetime if means are available. No non-Muslim can enter Mecca. Pilgrims must wear seamless white garments; go without head covering or shoes; practice sexual continence; abstain from shaving or having their hair cut; and avoid harming any living thing, animal or vegetable.

There are no priests in Islam; every Muslim can communicate directly with God, so a mediator is not needed. The successors of the prophet Mohammed and the leaders of the Islamic community were the *caliphes* (or *kalifah*). No caliphes exist today. A *mufti,* like a lawyer, gives legal advice based on the sacred laws of the Koran. An *imam* is the person appointed to lead prayer in the mosque and deliver the Friday sermon.

The following prominent sects in Islam have their origin in conflicting theories on the office of caliph (*caliphate*): (1) The *Sunni,* who form the largest number of Muslims and hold that the caliphate is an elected office that must be occupied by a member of the tribe of Koreish, the tribe of Mohammed. (2) The *Shi'ites,* the second largest group, who believe that the caliphate was a God-given office held rightfully by Ali, Mohammed's son-in-law, and his descendants. The Shi'ites are found primarily in Iran, Iraq, Yemen, and India. (3) The *Khawarij,* who believe that the office of caliph is open to any believer whom the faithful consider fit for it. Followers of this sect are found primarily in eastern Arabia and North Africa. (4) The *Sufis,* ascetic mystics who seek a close union with God now, rather than in the hereafter. Only 3 percent of present-day Muslims are Sufis.

It is estimated that nearly 6 million Muslims live in the United States; many came from the Middle East. In addition, some African Americans believe Allah is the one true God; they follow the Koran and traditional Muslim rituals in their temple services. The movement was originally known as the Nation of Islam and its adherents identified as Black Muslims. A split in the Nation of Islam resulted in one faction of Black Muslims becoming an orthodox Islamic religion called the World Community of Al-Islam in the West. It is accepted as a branch of Islam. The other Black Muslim faction has continued as the Nation of Islam under the leadership of Louis Farrakhan.

The *Kaaba,* in Mecca, is the holiest shrine of Islam and contains the Black Stone given to Abraham and Ishmael by the Archangel Gabriel. During the hadj, each pilgrim touches the stone and circles the shrine.

No one claiming title to the office of caliphate has been recognized by all Muslim sects since its abolition by the Turkish government in 1924 following the fall of the Ottoman Empire. The role of the caliphate in modern Islam is uncertain.

Halal, Islamic Dietary Laws

In Islam, eating is considered to be a matter of worship. Muslims are expected to eat for survival and good health; self-indulgence is not permitted. Muslims are advised not to eat more than two-thirds of their capacity, and sharing food is recommended. Food is never to be

Islamic laws consider eating to be a matter of worship, and Muslims are encouraged to share meals. (J. Boisberranger/Viesti Associates.)

"Eat of the good things. We have provided for your sustenance, but commit no excess therein." Koran 20:81

thrown away, wasted, or treated with contempt. The hands and mouth are washed before and after meals. If eating utensils are not used, only the right hand is used for eating, as the left hand is considered unclean.

Permitted or lawful foods are called *halal*. Unless specifically prohibited, all food is edible. Unlawful or prohibited (*haram*) foods prescribed in the Koran include:

1. All swine, four-footed animals that catch their prey with their mouths, and birds of prey that seize their prey with their talons.

2. Improperly slaughtered animals. An animal must be killed in a manner similar to that described in the Jewish laws, by slitting the front of the throat; cutting the jugular vein, carotid artery, and windpipe; and allowing the blood to drain completely. In addition, the person who kills the animal must repeat at the instant of slaughter, "In the name of God, God is great." Fish and seafood are exempt from this requirement.

   Some Muslims believe that a Jew or a Christian can slaughter an animal to be consumed by Muslims as long as it is done properly. Others will eat only kosher meat, while some abstain from meat unless they know it is properly slaughtered by a Muslim or can arrange to kill the animal themselves. Meat of animals slaughtered by people other than Muslims, Jews, or Christians is prohibited. Meat is also prohibited if it came from an animal that was slaughtered when any name besides God's was mentioned.

3. Alcoholic beverages and intoxicating drugs, unless medically necessary. The drinking of stimulants, such as coffee and tea, is discouraged, as is smoking; however, these prohibitions are practiced only by the most devout Muslims.

A Muslim can eat or drink prohibited food under certain conditions, such as when the food is taken by mistake, is forced by others, or there is fear of dying by hunger or disease. When in doubt regarding whether a food is halal or haram, a Muslim is encouraged to avoid the item. Foods that are in compliance with Islamic dietary laws are sometimes marked with symbols that are registered with the Islamic Food and Nutrition Council of America (IFNCA) (Figure 2.2), signifying the food is fit for consumption by Muslims anywhere in the world (Hussaini, 1993).

Feast Days

The following are the feast days in the Islamic religion:

1. *Eid al-Fitr,* the Feast of Fast Breaking—the end of Ramadan is celebrated by a feast and the giving of alms.
2. *Eid al-Azha,* the Festival of Sacrifice—the commemoration of Abraham's willingness to sacrifice his son, Ishmael, for God. It is customary to sacrifice a sheep and distribute its meat to friends, relatives, and the needy.
3. *Shab-i-Barat,* the night in the middle of *Shaban*—originally a fast day, this is now a feast day, often marked with fireworks. It is believed that God determines the actions of every person for the next year on this night.
4. *Nau-Roz,* New Year's Day—primarily celebrated by the Iranians, it is the first day after the sun crosses the vernal equinox.
5. *Maulud n'Nabi*—the birthday of Mohammed.

Feasting also occurs at birth, after the consummation of marriage, at *Bismillah* (when a child first starts reading the Koranic alphabet), after circumcision of boys, at the harvest, and at death.

Fast Days

On fast days, Muslims abstain from food, drink, smoking, and coitus from dawn to sunset. Food can be eaten before the sun comes up and again after it sets. Muslims are required to fast during *Ramadan,* the ninth month of the Islamic calendar. It is believed that during Ramadan, "the gates of Heaven are open, the gates of Hell closed, and the devil put in chains." At sunset the fast is usually broken by taking a liquid, typically water, along with an odd number of dates.

Iranians celebrate the new year with a display of seven items beginning with the letter "s," denoting life, rebirth, happiness, prosperity, joy, beauty, and health. These are vinegar (*serke*), apple (*seeb*), dried fruit or olives (*sanjed*), sumac seasoning (*sumagh*), sweet wheat pudding (*samanu*), garlic (*seer*), or hyacinth (*sonbul*), and sprouted seeds (*sabzi*), respectively.

The month of Ramadan can fall during any part of the year. The Muslim calendar is lunar but does not have a leap month; thus the months occur at different times each year.

FIGURE 2.2

Examples of halal food symbols.

Women who wish to undertake voluntary fasts must seek permission from their husbands.

All Muslims past the age of puberty (15 years old) are required to fast during Ramadan. A number of groups are exempt from fasting, but most must make up the days before the next Ramadan. They include sick individuals with a recoverable illness; people who are traveling; women during pregnancy, lactation, or menstruation; elders who are physically unable to fast; insane people; and those engaged in hard labor. During Ramadan, it is customary to invite guests to break the fast and dine in the evening; special foods are eaten, especially sweets. Food is often given to neighbors, relatives, and needy individuals or families.

Muslims are also encouraged to fast 6 days during *Shawwal,* the month following Ramadan; the tenth day of the month of *Muhurram;* and the ninth day of *Zul Hijjah,* but not during the pilgrimage to Mecca. A Muslim may fast voluntarily, preferably on Mondays and Thursdays. Muslims are not allowed to fast on 2 festival days, *Eid al-Fitr* and *Eid al-Azha* (see the previous section for more information) or on the days of sacrificial slaughter (*Tashriq*—the twelfth, thirteenth, and fourteenth days of *Dhu-al-Hijjah*). It is also undesirable for Muslims to fast excessively (because Allah provides food and drink to consume) or to fast on Fridays.

EASTERN RELIGIONS

Hinduism

Some Hindu worshipers break coconuts on the temple grounds to symbolize the spiritual experience: The hard shell is a metaphor for the human ego, and once it is cracked open, the soft, sweet meat representing the inner self is open to becoming one with the Supreme Being (Dresser, 1996).

Hinduism is considered to be the world's oldest religion, and, like Judaism, it is the basis of other religions such as Buddhism. Although Hinduism was once popular throughout much of Asia, most Hindus now live in India, its birthplace.

The common Hindu scriptures are the *Vedas,* the *Epics,* and the *Bhagavata Purana.* The Vedas form the supreme authority for Hinduism. There are four Vedas: the *Rigveda,* the *Samaveda,* the *Yajurveda,* and the *Aatharvaveda.* Each consists of four parts.

The goal of Hinduism is not to make humans perfect beings or life a heaven on earth but to make humans one with the Universal Spirit or Supreme Being. When this state is achieved, there is no cause and effect, no time and space, no good and evil; all dualities are merged into oneness. This goal cannot be reached by being a good person, but it can be obtained by transforming human consciousness or liberation, *moksha,* into a new realm of divine consciousness that sees individual parts of the universe as deriving their true significance from the central unity of spirit. The transformation of human consciousness into divine consciousness is not achieved in one lifetime, and Hindus believe that the present life is only one in a series of lives, or reincarnations. Hindus believe in the law of rebirth, which postulates that every person passes through a series of lives before obtaining liberation; the law of *karma;* and that one's present life is the result of what one thought or did in one's past life. In each new incarnation an individual's soul moves up or down the spiritual ladder; the goal for all souls is liberation.

There is one supreme being, Brahmin, and all the various gods worshiped by men are partial manifestations of him. Hindus choose the form of the supreme being that satisfies their spirit and make it an object of love and adoration. This aspect of worship makes Hinduism very tolerant of other gods and their followers; many different religions have been absorbed into Hinduism.

The three most important functions of the supreme being are the creation, protection, and destruction of the world, and these functions have become personified as three great gods—Brahma, Vishnu, and Siva (the Hindu triad or trinity). The supreme being as Vishnu is the protector of the world. Vishnu is also an *avatara,* meaning he can take on human forms whenever the world is threatened by evil. Rama and Krishna are regarded as two such embodiments and are also objects of worship.

Hindus believe that the world passes through repeating cycles; the most common version of the creation is connected to the life of Vishnu. From Vishnu's navel grows a lotus, and from its unfolding petals is born the god Brahma who creates the world. Vishnu governs the world until he sleeps; then Siva destroys it and the world is absorbed into Vishnu's body to be created once again.

The principles of Hinduism are purity, self-control, detachment, truth, and nonviolence. Purity is both a ceremonial goal and a moral ideal. All rituals for purification and the elaborate rules regarding food and drink are meant to lead to purity of mind and spirit. Self-control governs both the flesh and the mind. Hinduism does not teach its followers to suppress the flesh completely, but to regulate its appetites and cravings. The highest aspect of self-control is detachment. Complete liberation from this world and union with the divine are not possible if one clings to the good or evil of this existence. Pursuit of truth is indispensable to the progress of man, and truth is always

According to legend, Vishnu rested on a 1,000-headed cobra between the creation and destruction of the world. During the festivities of *Naga Panchami,* snakes are venerated at Hindu temples, and milk is offered to cobras to prevent snakebite.

Gandhi's birthday is commemorated in India on October 3rd with devotional songs and the spinning of cotton thread in honor of his support for textile workers.

associated with nonviolence, *ahimsa*. These principles are considered to be the highest virtues. India's greatest exponent of this ideal was Mahatma Gandhi, who taught that nonviolence must be practiced not only by individuals, but also by communities and nations.

One common belief of Hinduism is that the world evolved in successive stages, beginning with matter and going on through life, consciousness, and intelligence to spiritual bliss or perfection. Spirit first appears as life in plants, then as consciousness in animals, intelligence in humans, and finally bliss in the supreme spirit. A good person is closer to the supreme spirit than a bad person is, and a person is closer than an animal. Truth, beauty, love, and righteousness are of higher importance than intellectual values (e.g., clarity, cogency, subtlety, skill) or biological values (e.g., health, strength, vitality). Material values (e.g., riches, possessions, pleasure) are valued least.

The organization of society grows from the principle of spiritual progression. The Hindu lawgivers tried to construct an ideal society in which people are ranked by their spiritual progress and culture, not according to their wealth or power. The social system reflects this ideal, which is represented by four estates, or castes, associated originally with certain occupations. The four castes are the *Brahmins* (teachers and priests), the *Kshatriyas* (soldiers), the *Vaisyas* (merchants and farmers), and the *Sundras* (laborers). Existing outside social recognition are the untouchables (e.g., butchers, leather workers), a group of persons who do not fall into the other four categories; this designation was outlawed by the Indian government in 1950.

The four castes are represented as forming parts of the Creator's body, respectively his mouth, arms, thighs, and feet. The untouchables were created from darkness that Brahma discarded in the process of creation. The castes also conform to the law of spiritual progression, in that the most spiritual caste occupies the top and the least spiritual the bottom. The Hindus believe that nature has three fundamental qualities: purity, energy, and inertia. Those in whom purity predominates form the first caste, energy the second caste, and inertia the third and fourth caste. Each caste should perform its own duties, follow its hereditary occupation, and cooperate with the others for the common welfare. People's good actions in this life earn them promotion to a higher caste in the next life.

There are thousands of subdivisions of the four main castes. The subcastes often reflect a trade or profession, but some scholars contend that the latter was imposed on the former. In reality, the subcaste is very important to daily life, while what major caste one belongs to makes little difference to non-Brahmins (see Chapter 10 for more information).

The ideal life of a Hindu is divided into four successive stages, called *asramas*. The first stage is that of the student and is devoted entirely to study and discipline. The *guru* becomes an individual's spiritual parent. After this period of preparation the student should settle down and serve his or her marriage, community, and country. When this active period of citizenship is over, he or she should retire to a quiet place in the country and meditate on the higher aspects of the spirit (become a recluse). The recluse then becomes a *sannyasin,* one who has renounced all earthly possessions and ties. This stage is the crown of human life. The goals of life are *dharma* (righteousness), *artha* (worldly prosperity), *kama* (enjoyment), and *moksha* (liberation). The ultimate aim of life is liberation, but, on their way to this final goal, people must satisfy the animal wants of the bodies, as well as the economic and other demands of their families and communities. However, all should be done within the moral law of dharma.

Common practices in Hinduism include rituals and forms of mental discipline. All Hindus are advised to choose a deity on whose form, features, and qualities they can concentrate their mind and whose image they can worship every day with flowers and incense. The deity is only a means of realizing the supreme being by means of ritualistic worship. Externally the deity is worshiped as a king or honored guest. Internal worship consists of prayer and meditation. Mental discipline is indicated by the word *yoga.* Along with mental discipline, yoga has come to mean a method of restraining the functions of the mind and their physiologic consequences.

Hindus can be divided into three broad sects according to their view of the supreme being. They are the *Vaishnava,* the *Saiva,* and the *Sakta,* who maintain the supremacy of Vishnu, Siva, and the Sakti (the female and active aspects of Siva), respectively. Different sects are popular in different regions of India. Many Hindus do not worship one God exclusively. Vishnu may be worshiped in one of his full (Krishna or Rama) or partial embodiments. In addition there are hundreds of lesser deities, much like saints. One is Siva's son, the elephant-headed Ganesh, who is believed to bring good luck and remove obstacles.

There may be as many as 950,000 Hindus in the United States, although it is not known for certain how many Hindus live here, because the religion is not centered around a temple nor are its affairs conducted by priests. It is assumed that a significant percentage of the Asian Indian population in America is Hindu. A small percentage of non-Indian Americans have become followers of the Hindu religion. The International Society for Krishna Consciousness, founded in 1966 by devotees of a sixteenth-century Bengali ascetic, has the largest number of converts.

Yoga means yoke, as in yoking together or union.

Ganesh got his elephant head when he angered his father, Siva, who cut off his human head. When his mother pleaded with Siva to replace his head, Siva used the head of a nearby elephant. Hindus honor Ganesh through offerings of the foods he favored.

Hindu Dietary Practices

In general, Hindus avoid foods that are believed to hamper the development of the body or mental abilities. Bad food habits will prevent

Students who are studying the Vedas and other celibates are usually vegetarians and may restrict irritating or exciting foods, such as honey.

Hindus are encouraged to practice moderation—they are advised not to eat too early, not to eat too late, and not to eat too much.

Water is the beverage of choice at meals. Standing water is easily defiled if it is touched by a member of a lower caste; flowing water is so pure that even an untouchable standing in it does not pollute it.

The Hindu calendar is lunar; thus its religious holidays do not always fall on the same day on the western calendar. Every 3 to 5 years the Hindu calendar adds a thirteenth leap month (a very auspicious period) to reconcile the months with the seasons.

Each Hindu month is divided into the light half when the moon is waxing and the dark half when the moon is waning.

one from reaching mental purity and communion with God. Dietary restrictions and attitudes vary among the castes.

The Laws of Manu state that "no sin is attached to eating flesh or drinking wine, or gratifying the sexual urge, for these are the natural propensities of men; but abstinence from these bears greater fruits." Many Hindus are vegetarians. They adhere to the concept of ahimsa, avoiding the infliction of pain on an animal by not eating meat. Although the consumption of meat is allowed, the cow is considered sacred and is not to be killed or eaten. If meat is eaten, pork as well as beef is usually avoided. Fish that have ugly forms, and the heads of snakes, snails, crabs, fowl, cranes, ducks, camels, and boars are forbidden. No fish or meat should be eaten until it has been sanctified by the repetition of mantras offering it to the gods. Pious Hindus may also abstain from drinking alcohol. Garlic, turnips, onions, mushrooms, and red-colored foods such as tomatoes and red lentils may be avoided.

Intertwined in Hindu food customs is the concept of purity and pollution. Complex rules regarding food and drink are meant to lead to purity of mind and spirit. Pollution is the opposite of purity and should be avoided or ameliorated. To remain pure is to remain free from pollution; to become pure is to remove pollution.

Certain substances are considered both pure in themselves and purifying in their application. These include the products of the living cow, such as milk products, dung, and urine, and water from sources of special sanctity, such as the Ganges River. They also include materials commonly employed in rituals, such as turmeric and sandalwood paste. All body products (feces, urine, saliva, menstrual flow, and afterbirth) are polluting. Use of water is the most common method of purification, because water easily absorbs pollution and carries it away.

Feast Days

The Hindu calendar has eighteen major festivals every year. Additional important feast days are those of marriages, births, and deaths. Each region of India has its own special festivals; it has been said that there is a celebration going on somewhere in India every day of the year. All members of the community eat generously on festive occasions, and these may be the only days that very poor people eat adequately. Feasting is a way of sharing food among the population, because the wealthy are responsible for helping the poor celebrate the holidays.

One of the gayest and most colorful of the Hindu festivals is *Holi,* the spring equinox and the celebration of one of Krishna's triumphs. According to legend, Krishna had an evil uncle who sent an ogress named Holika to burn down Krishna's house. Instead, Krishna

The numerous religious holidays and secular events celebrated in India include feasting, which serves to distribute food throughout the community. (United Nations/J. Isaac.)

escaped and Holika burned in the blaze. It is traditional for Indians to throw colored water or powder at passersby during this holiday.

The 10-day celebration of *Dusshera* in late September or early October commemorates the victory of Prince Rama (one of Vishnu's embodiments) over the army of the demon Ravana and is a grateful tribute to the goddess Durga, who aided Rama. The first 9 days are spent in worshiping the deity, and the tenth day is spent celebrating Rama's victory.

Divali, celebrated throughout India in November, marks the darkest night of the year, when souls return to earth and must be shown the way by the lights in the houses. For many, Divali is also the beginning of the new year, when everyone should buy new clothes, settle old debts and quarrels, and wish everyone else good fortune.

Prince Rama was aided by Hanuman, a monkey hero; thus monkeys are revered throughout India despite the serious crop damage they cause.

In southern India the rice harvest is celebrated in the festival called *Pongal*—new rice is cooked in milk and when it begins to bubble, the family shouts, "pongal!" ("It boils!").

Fast Days

In India, fasting practices vary according to one's caste, family, age, sex, and degree of orthodoxy. A devoutly religious person may fast more often and more strictly than one who is less religious. Fasting may mean eating no food at all or abstaining from only specific foods or meals. It is rare for an individual to go without any food at all, because there are numerous fast days in Hinduism. The fast days in the Hindu calendar include the first day of the new and full moon of each lunar month; the tenth and eleventh days of each month; the feast of *Sivaratri;* the ninth day of the lunar month *Cheitra;* the eighth day of *Sravana;* days of eclipses, equinoxes, solstices, and conjunction of planets; the anniversary of the death of one's father or mother; and Sundays.

Buddhism

Siddhartha Gautama, who later became known as Buddha (the Enlightened One), founded this eastern religion in India in the sixth century BCE. Buddhism flourished in India until 500 CE, when it declined and gradually became absorbed into Hinduism. Meanwhile, it had spread throughout southeastern and central Asia. Buddhism remains a vital religion in many Asian countries, where it has been adapted to local needs and traditions.

Buddhism was a protestant revolt against orthodox Hinduism, but it accepted certain Hindu concepts, such as the idea that all living beings go through countless cycles of death and rebirth, the doctrine of karma, spiritual liberation from the flesh, and that the path to wisdom includes taming the appetites and passions of the body. Buddha disagreed with the Hindus about the methods by which these objectives were to be achieved. He advocated the "Middle Way" between asceticism and self-indulgence, stating that both extremes in life should be avoided. He also disagreed with the Hindus on caste distinctions, believing that all persons were equal in spiritual potential.

The basic teachings of Buddha are found in the *Four Noble Truths* and the *Noble Eightfold Path.* The Four Noble Truths are

1. *The Noble Truth of Suffering:* Suffering is part of living. Persons suffer when they experience birth, old age, sickness, and death. They also suffer when they fail to obtain what they want.
2. *The Noble Truth of the Cause of Suffering:* Suffering is caused by a person's craving for life, which causes rebirth.
3. *The Noble Truth of the Cessation of Suffering:* A person no longer suffers if all cravings are relinquished.
4. *The Noble Truth to the Path That Leads to the Cessation of Suffering:* This is the Eightfold Path. By following this path (right view, right thought, right speech, right action, right livelihood, right effort, right mindfulness, and right concentration), craving is extinguished and deliverance from suffering ensues.

The third and fourth phases of the Eightfold Path (Figure 2.3), right speech and right action, have been extended into a practical code of conduct that is known as the Five Precepts. These are (1) to abstain from the taking of life, (2) to abstain from the taking of what

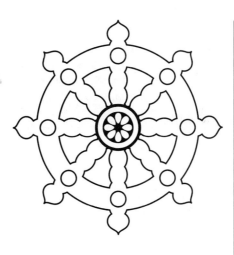

FIGURE 2.3

The Buddhist Wheel of Law—the spokes represent the Eightfold Path.

is not given, (3) to abstain from all illegal sexual pleasures, (4) to abstain from lying, and (5) to abstain from consumption of intoxicants because they tend to cloud the mind.

The person who perfects Buddha's teachings achieves *nirvana,* a state of calm insight, passionlessness, and wisdom. In addition, the person is no longer subject to rebirth into the sorrows of existence. Because the ideal practice of Buddhism is impractical in the turmoil of daily life, Buddhism has encouraged a monastic lifestyle. The ideal Buddhists are monks, following a life of simplicity and spending considerable time in meditation. They own no personal property and obtain food by begging. They are usually vegetarians and are permitted to eat only before noon. The monk confers a favor or merit (good karma) on those who give him food.

There are numerous sects in Buddhism and two great schools of doctrine: *Theravada* (also known as *Hinayana*) Buddhism, which is followed in India and Southeast Asia; and *Mahayana* Buddhism, which is followed in China, Japan, Korea, Tibet, and Mongolia. Theravada Buddhism is primarily a spiritual philosophy and system of ethics. It places little or no emphasis on deities, teaching that the goal of the faithful is to achieve nirvana. In Mahayana, a later form of Buddhism, Buddha is eternal and cosmic, appearing variously in many worlds to make known his truth, called *dharma.* This has resulted in a pantheon of Buddhas who are sometimes deified and, for some sects, a hierarchy of demons. Some sects promise the worshiper a real paradise, rather than the perfected spiritual state of nirvana.

The number of Buddists in the United States may be as high as 2 million; the majority are immigrants from Japan, China, and Southeast Asia and their descendants. There is also a small number of non-Asians who have more recently converted to Buddhism. *Zen* Buddhism, a Chinese sect that spread to Japan around the year 1200, has gained followers in the West.

At some Buddhist temples a vegetarian lunch is offered after the service. The congregation eats after the monks have finished their meal.

In both Theravada and Mahayana temples, worshipers may offer food at the altar, such as apples, bananas, grapes, oranges, pineapples, candy, rice, dried mushrooms, and oil.

A Zen Buddhist monastery, Tassajara, located in central California, is famous for its vegetarian restaurant and popular cookbook.

Zen macrobiotics is not associated with Zen Buddhism. It is a Japanese diet created in the twentieth century and popularized in Europe as a way to achieve health and spiritual enlightenment.

Dietary Practices

Buddhist dietary restrictions vary considerably depending on the sect and country. Buddhist doctrine forbids the taking of life; therefore many followers are lacto-ovo-vegetarians (eating dairy products and eggs, but no meat), some eat fish, and others abstain only from beef. Others believe that if they were not personally responsible for killing the animal, it is permissible to eat its flesh.

Feasts and Fasts

Buddhist festivals vary according to region. From July to October, Buddhist monks are directed to remain in retreat and meditate, coinciding with the rainy season and the sprouting of rice in the fields. The first day of retreat is a time for worshipers to bring gifts of food and articles of clothing to the monks; the retreat ends with *pravarana,* the end of the rainy season, when worshipers once again offer gifts to the monks, invite them to a meal, and organize processions. Mahayana Buddhists commemorate the birth of Buddha, his enlightenment, and his death on 3 separate days (which vary according to the regional calendar); Theravada Buddhists honor the Buddha on a single holiday called *Vesak,* celebrated during April or May. Buddhist monks may fast twice a month, on the days of the new and full moon. They also do not eat any solid food after noon.

Some Buddhists celebrate *Magha Puja,* the Four Miracles Assembly, in February or March when Buddha appointed the first Buddhist brotherhood of monks at a coincidental meeting of 1,250 disciples at a shrine.

Buddhist monks in Tibet carve sculptures in butter (as high as 15 feet) and parade them during an evening in March, lit by lanterns, for *Chogna Choeba,* the Butter Lamp Festival. Afterward they are dismantled and thrown in the river, symbolic of the impermanence of life.

3

Native Americans

The designation "Native American" includes the greatest number of ethnic groups of any minority population in the United States. Each of the approximately 400 American Indian and Alaska Native nations has its own distinct cultural heritage.

There are nearly 2 million self-declared Native Americans in the United States, just under 1 percent of the total population. The vast majority of Native Americans today live west of the Mississippi River. Roughly half live in rural areas, either on government reservations or on nearby farms. Native American ethnic identity varies tremendously, from tenacious maintenance of heritage to total adoption of the majority culture.

Traditional Native American foods have made significant contributions to today's American diet. Corn, squash, beans, cranberries, and maple syrup are just a few of the items Native Americans introduced to European settlers. Historians question whether the original British colonists would have survived their first years in America without the supplies they obtained and cooking methods they learned from the Native Americans. The diet of Native Americans has changed dramatically from its origins, yet recent renewed interest in Native American culture has prevented the complete disappearance of many traditional foods and food habits. This chapter reviews both the past and present diet of Native American ethnic groups.

Cultural Perspective

History of Native Americans

Settlement Patterns

It is hypothesized that the Native Americans came to North America approximately 20,000 to 50,000 years ago across the Bering Strait, which links Asia to Alaska, although some evidence suggests that earlier migrations may have occurred. Archaeological research provides little insight into the settlement patterns and diversification of Native American culture in the years before European contact in the 1600s. Further, the Native American languages were entirely verbal, so written historical records are nonexistent. There are, consequently, enormous gaps in what is known of early Native American societies.

In contrast, the observations of the Native Americans by white settlers have been well documented. They identified three major centers of Native American culture during the seventeenth century. In the Southeast the sophisticated social organization of the Cherokees, Chickasaws, Choctaws, Creeks, and Seminoles led the Europeans to call them the "Five Civilized Tribes." The Iroquois, in what is now New York State, ruled a democratic confederacy of five nations. Religion and the arts flourished in Pueblo communities adjacent to the Rio Grande and Little Colorado rivers in the Southwest.

During the early nineteenth century the Cherokee had a written language, a bilingual newspaper, a school system, a court system, and a Cherokee Nation constitution. They were a prosperous tribe; many owned black slaves.

Traditional Native American foods: Some typical foods in traditional Native American diets include beans, berries, corn, fish, *jerky,* maple syrup, squash, and tomatoes. (Photo by Laurie Macfee.)

The introduction of horses, firearms, and metal knives changed the lifestyles of many nations, especially those that used the new tools to exploit the resources of the Great Plains. This initial interaction between white settlers and Plains Indians resulted in the development of the stereotype of the buffalo-hunting horseman with feathered headdress who came to represent all Native American ethnic groups in the white imagination.

European diseases and the massacre of whole nations reduced the number of both Native American individuals and ethnic groups. In addition, many Native Americans were forced to migrate west to accommodate white expansion. It is estimated that the hardships of involuntary relocation and the deaths caused by illness and assault caused the extinction of nearly one-quarter of all Native American ethnic groups.

Native American lands dwindled as white settlers moved westward. By the late nineteenth century the majority of Native Americans lived on lands held in trust for them by the U.S. government called federal reservations. Still others resided in state reservation communities. Although they were not required by law to live on reservations, there were few other viable Native American communities.

The Bureau of Indian Affairs (BIA) took over the administration of the reservations near the turn of the twentieth century. They established a program of cultural assimilation designed to bring the Native American residents into mainstream American society. Before the 1930s, Native American children were sent to off-reservation boarding schools where white values were encouraged. Later, public reservation schools attempted similar indoctrination. The BIA program usually failed to force Native Americans to accept white values, however. The Native Americans changed their dress, occupation, and social structure, but they did not fully assimilate. In many cases their religious beliefs, crafts, music, and dance were strengthened to support their ethnic identity.

Current Demographics

Many Native Americans left the reservations for the employment opportunities available during World War II (Figure 3.1). Some joined the armed services, where they became fluent in English and the ways of the majority society. Others took war-related industry jobs. In the 1950s and 1960s the BIA Employment Assistance Program was a major factor in the continuing outmigration of Native Americans from the reservations to the cities. By 1980 just more than one-half of all Native Americans resided in urban areas and towns outside of reservations. The cities with the largest Native American populations are (in descending order) Los Angeles, the San Francisco Bay Area, Tulsa, Minneapolis–St. Paul, Oklahoma City, Chicago, and Phoenix. The remainder of the Native American population resides in rural areas,

The largest Native American populations are the Cherokee (369,000) and the Navajo (225,000).

including reservations. Many first-generation urban Native Americans maintain close ties with the reservation of their ethnic group and travel often between the city and tribal land. Members of the second generation living in urban regions are more likely to think of the city as their permanent home.

Efforts to increase prosperity on reservations include utilization of natural resources and establishment of gambling operations, which are legal on tribal lands.

Socioeconomic Status

The socioeconomic status of Native Americans declined drastically with the forced migrations of the nineteenth century. Even those Native American nations that were agriculturally self-sufficient suf-

FIGURE 3.1

Native American nations in the United States.

Source: Adapted from Taylor, T. W. 1972. *The States and Their Indian Citizens.* In Thernstrom et al. [Eds.], *The Harvard Encyclopedia of American Ethnic Groups.* Harvard University Press. Copyright 1980. Reprinted with permission by the President and Fellows of Harvard College.

fered when relocated to regions with poor growing conditions. Further, there were few native occupations that were valued in the job market outside the reservations. BIA education efforts were generally unsuccessful, and most Native Americans did not begin to find employment until World War II and the development of the BIA Employment Assistance Program. More recently the Indian Self-Determination and Education Act of 1975 was enacted to promote Native American participation in government and education.

Economic improvement has been slow. Although unemployment rates among Native Americans dropped slightly in the 1980s (unemployment rates are two to three times the national average), poverty levels have increased. Nearly one-third (32%) of Native American families fell below the poverty level in the 1990 U.S. census. Congressional amendments to the Older Americans Act in 1987 found that 61 percent of Native American elders older than the age of 60 also live in poverty. Rates of formal education have been improving, yet 43 percent of all adult Native Americans have not finished high school or obtained an equivalency diploma.

Native American Organizations

Few Native American neighborhoods develop in urban areas. Native Americans who settle in the cities usually arrive as individuals or small family groups and typically do not live near others of their nation. Sometimes longtime city residents exhibit a sense of superiority over recent arrivals from the reservations. In general, the difficulties of adjusting to urban white society stimulate many young Native Americans to identify not only with Native Americans of other nations but also with people from other ethnic groups. Activists for Native American rights often come from the cities and are not always supported by Native Americans who live on tribal lands. Native American organizations have done much to maintain Indian identity. Most areas with large Native American populations have their own clubs and service associations. Organizations to promote ethnic identity have been founded by the Navajo, Pueblos, Tlingit, Haida, and Pomo. Other groups serve the social needs of the pan-Native American community, such as athletic clubs and dance groups. The United South and Eastern Tribes works to strengthen Native American unity; the All Indian Pueblo Council advocates on behalf of Pueblo tribes. The National American Indian Council was founded in 1982 to represent the needs of urban Native Americans.

Worldview

Harmony best describes the Native American approach to life. Each individual strives to maintain a balance between spiritual, social, and physical needs in a holistic approach. Only what is necessary for life is taken from the natural environment; it is believed that the earth should be cared for and treated with respect. Generosity is esteemed and competitiveness is discouraged, yet individual rights are also highly regarded. Personal autonomy is protected through the principle of noninterference. Among the Navajo, for example, an individual would never presume to speak for another, even a close family member. For most Native Americans, time is conceptualized as being without beginning or end, and the culture is present-oriented, meaning that the needs of the moment are emphasized over the possible rewards of the future.

Religion

Traditional Native American religions vary from an uncomplicated belief in the power of a self-declared evangelist to elaborate theological systems with organized hierarchies of priests. Yet they all share one characteristic—the religion permeates all aspects of life. Rather than a separate set of beliefs practiced at certain times in specific settings, religion is an integral part of the Native American holistic worldview. Religious concepts influence both the physical and emotional well-being of the individual.

Many Native American nations have rejected all attempts at Christian conversion, especially in the Southwest. The Navajo, Arizona Hopi, Rio Grande Pueblos, Potawatomi, and the Sioux have retained most of their native religious values and rituals. Other religions unique to Native Americans emerged after European contact, such as the Drum Dance cult and the Medicine Bundle religions, which combine spiritual elements from several different ethnic groups. In addition, religions that mix Christianity with traditional beliefs have been popular since the late nineteenth century; the Native American Church has been especially successful. Other groups claim Christian fellowship but continue to practice native religions as well. Finally, many Native Americans now adhere to Roman Catholicism or some form of Protestantism, especially in urban areas, where churches have been established to serve all Native American congregations.

Family

The primary social unit of Native Americans is the extended family. Children are valued highly and there is great respect for elders. All blood kin of all generations are considered equal; there is no differentiation between close and distant relatives. Aunts and uncles are often considered to be like grandparents, and cousins are viewed as brothers or sisters. Even other tribal members are sometimes accepted as close kin. In many Native American societies an individual without relatives is considered poor. Many Native American

The primary social unit of Native Americans is the extended family, which includes all close and distant kin. (© Lionel Delevingne/Stock, Boston.)

nations are matrilineal, meaning that lineage is inherited from the mother. Even in such systems the men are the family providers and heads of the household; women are typically in charge of domestic matters. Native American children are expected to assist their parents in running the home.

Communication

Most Native Americans appreciate a quiet, unhurried conversational style. Many are comfortable with long periods of silence while they compose their thoughts and responses. Privacy is important, and some Native Americans may consider questions about their personal life to be very intrusive.

Nonverbal communication among some Native Americans is very sophisticated. It has been reported that some children are not taught to speak until other senses are developed (Wilson, 1983). A smile and a handshake are customary greetings, but an overly vigorous handshake may be interpreted as a sign of aggressiveness. Direct eye contact may be considered rude, and many Native Americans avert their eyes while listening to show respect to the speaker.

Traditional Food Habits

The traditional food habits of Native Americans were influenced primarily by geography and climate. Each Native American nation adopted a way of life that allowed it to maximize indigenous resources. Many were agriculturally based societies, others were predominantly hunters and gatherers, and some survived mainly on fish. Most of each day was spent procuring food.

Ingredients and Common Foods

Indigenous Foods

Archaeological records and early descriptions of America by European settlers indicate that Native Americans on the East Coast enjoyed an abundance of food. Fruits, including blueberries, cranberries, currants, grapes, persimmons, plums, and strawberries, as well as vegetables, such as beans, corn, and pumpkins, were mentioned by the New England colonists. They also describe rivers so full of life that fish could be caught with frying pans, sturgeon so large they were called "Albany beef," and lobster so plentiful that they would pile up along the shoreline after a storm. Game included deer, moose, partridge, pigeon, rabbit, raccoon, squirrel, and turkey. Maple syrup was

The tradition of the Pacific Northwest *potlatch* reflects the abundance of the region. Commonly held for important events such as marriage or birth of a son, these ostentatious feasts with excessive amounts of food were followed by gift giving of items such as blankets, canoes, edible oils, furs, jewelry, and wood carvings. The potlatch established the wealth and socioeconomic status of the host. The nations of this region were the only Native American groups to develop a class system based on possession of material goods. Anthropologists suggest that the potlatch was also a method of food distribution among nations from different areas.

used to sweeten foods. Farther south, Native Americans cultivated groundnuts (*Apios Americana,* also known as "Indian potatoes") and tomatoes, and collected wild Jerusalem artichokes (a starchy tuber related to the sunflower). Native Americans of the Pacific Northwest collected enough food, such as salmon and fruit, during the summer to support them for the remainder of the year. Peoples of the plains hunted buffalo and those of the northeastern woodlands gathered wild rice; nations of the Southwest cultivated chile peppers and squash amidst their corn. (See Table 3.1 for a listing of foods native to the Americas.)

Native Americans not only introduced whites to indigenous foods, but they shared their methods of cultivation and food preparation as well. Legend has it that the Pilgrims nearly starved despite the plentiful food supply because they were unfamiliar with the local foods. One version of the tale is that Squanto, the sole surviving member of the Pautuxets (the other members had succumbed to smallpox following contact with earlier European explorers), saved the Pilgrims, who were mostly merchants, by teaching them to grow corn. He

TABLE 3.1
Indigenous Foods of the Americas*

Fruits	Berries (blackberries, blueberries, cranberries, gooseberries, huckleberries, loganberries, raspberries, strawberries), cactus fruit (*tuna*), cherimoya, cherries (acerola cherries, chokecherries, ground-cherries), grapes (e.g., Concord), guava, mamey, papaya, passion fruit (*granadilla*), pawpaw, persimmon (American), pineapple, plums (American, beach), soursop (*guanabana*), zapote (*sapodilla*)
Vegetables	Avocado (alligator pear), bell peppers (sweet peppers, pimento), cactus (*nopales, nopalitos*), chayote (*christophine, chocho, huisquil, mirliton,* vegetable pear), pumpkins, squash, tomatillo, tomatoes
Tubers/roots	Arrowroot, cassava (*yuca, manioc, tapioca*), groundnut, Indian bread-root, Jerusalem artichoke, jicama, malanga (*yautia*), potatoes, sweet potatoes
Grains/cereals	Amaranth, corn (maize), quinoa, wild rice
Nuts/seeds	Brazil nuts, cashews, hickory nuts, pecans, pumpkin seeds (*pepitas*), sunflower seeds, walnuts (black)
Legumes	Beans (green beans, most dried beans), peanuts
Poultry	Turkey
Seasonings/flavorings	Allspice, chiles (e.g., hot and sweet chiles), chocolate (cocoa), maple syrup, sassafras (filé powder), spicebush, vanilla

*Foods native to North, Central, or South America. Some items not indigenous to the United States (e.g., pineapple, potatoes) were popularized only after acceptance in Europe and introduction by European settlers. Other foods (e.g., avocado, jicama, tomatillo) have become more common in the United States with the growing Latino population.

showed them the Native American method of planting corn kernels in mounds with a fish head for fertilizer and using the corn stalks as supports for beans. In Virginia, Native Americans are attributed with providing the Cavaliers, also from England, with enough food to ensure their survival.

Foods Introduced from Europe

Foods introduced by the Europeans, especially the French Jesuits in the North and the Spanish in the South, were well accepted by Native Americans. Apples, apricots, carrots, lentils, peaches, purslane, and turnips were some of the more successful new foods. Settler William Penn noted that he found peaches in every large Native American farm he encountered, barely 100 years after they were introduced to the Iroquois. The Europeans also brought rye and wheat. However, few Native American nations replaced corn with these new grains.

Livestock made a much greater impact on Native American life than did the new fruits and vegetables. Cattle, hogs, and sheep reduced the Native Americans' dependence on game meats. The Creeks and Cherokees of the Southeast fed their cattle on corn and fattened their suckling pigs and young lambs on apples and nuts. The Powhatans of Virginia fed their hogs peanuts, then cured the meat over hickory smoke. Lamb and mutton became staples in the Navajo diet after the introduction of sheep by the Spanish. In addition, the Europeans brought horses and firearms, which made hunting easier, and metal knives and iron pots, which simplified food preparation. They also introduced the Native Americans to distilled spirits.

Staples

The great diversity of Native American cultures has resulted in a broad variety of cuisines. The cooking of one region was as different from that of another as French food is from German food today. Native American cooking featured local ingredients and often reflected the need to preserve foods for future shortages. The only staple foods common to many, though not all, Native American nations were beans, corn, and squash. The Cultural Food Groups list is found in Table 3.2.

Regional Variations

Native American fare has been divided by regions into five major types: northeastern, southern, plains, southwestern, and Pacific Northwest/Alaska Native. Although each area encompasses many different Native American nations, they share similarities in foods and food habits.

Although the wild turkey was found in the Plymouth area, it may not have been eaten at the first Thanksgiving. Goose was the preferred holiday bird during colonial times.

Carrots escaped vegetable gardens in many areas, reverting to the uncultivated flowering form known as Queen Anne's lace.

Corn is the largest crop grown in the United States today. It is the American staple grain, although most corn is used for sweeteners or animal feed, and is ultimately consumed in the form of soft drinks, meat, and poultry. Some estimates suggest that up to 30 percent of food eaten in the United States derives from corn.

TABLE 3.2
Cultural Food Groups: Native American

Group	Comments
PROTEIN FOODS	
Milk/milk products	High incidence of lactose intolerance among Native Americans with a high percentage of Native American heritage
Meats/poultry/fish/ eggs/legumes	Meat highly valued, considered healthful Meats mostly grilled or stewed, preserved through drying and smoking Beans an important protein source
CEREALS/GRAINS	Corn primary grain; wild rice available in some areas
FRUITS/VEGETABLES	Indigenous plants major source of calories in diet of some Native American nations Fruits and vegetables either gathered or cultivated; fruit a popular snack food
ADDITIONAL FOODS	
Seasonings	
Nuts/seeds	Nuts and seeds often an important food source, acorns sometimes a staple
Beverages	
Fats/oils	
Sweeteners	

TABLE 3.2
Cultural Food Groups: Native American—continued

Common Foods	Postcontact Adaptation
No common milk products in traditional diets	Powdered milk and evaporated milk are typical commodity products; usually added to coffee, cereal, and traditional baked goods; ice cream popular with some groups
	Some reports of frequent milk consumption
Meat: bear, buffalo (including jerky, pemmican), deer, elk, moose, oppossum, otter, porcupine, rabbit, raccoon, squirrel	Beef well accepted; lamb and pork also popular
Poultry and Small Birds: duck, goose, grouse, lark, pheasant, quail, seagull, wild turkey	Canned and cured meats (bacon, luncheon meat) may be common if income is limited
	Game rarely eaten
Fish, Seafood, and Marine Mammals: abalone, bass, catfish, clams, cod, crab, eel, flounder, frogs, halibut, herring, lobster, mussels, olechan, oysters, perch, red snapper, salmon, seal, shad, shrimp, smelts, sole, sturgeon, trout, turtle, walrus, whale	Meats remain a favorite food
Eggs: bird, fish	Chicken eggs commonly eaten
Legumes: many varieties of the common bean (kidney, navy, pinto, etc.), *tepary* beans	
Cornmeal breads (baked; steamed), hominy, gruels, corn tortillas, *piki,* toasted corn; wild rice	Wheat has widely replaced corn; store-bought or commodity breads and sugared cereals common
	Cakes, cookies, pastries popular
Fruits: blackberries, blueberries, buffalo berries, cactus fruit (*tuna*), chokeberries, cherries, crab apples, cranberries, currants, elderberries, grapes, groundcherries, huckleberries, persimmons, plums, raspberries, salal, salmonberries, strawberries (beach and wild), thimbleberries, wild rhubarb	Apples common after European introduction
	Apples, bananas, oranges, peaches, pineapple well accepted; canned fruits popular
	Wild berries still gathered in rural areas
Vegetables: camass root, cacti (*nopales*), chiles, fiddleheads, groundnuts, Indian breadroot, Jerusalem artichokes, lichen, moss, mushrooms, nettles, onions, potatoes, pumpkin, squash, squash blossoms, sweet potatoes, tomatoes, wild greens (cattail, clover, cow parsnip, creases, dandelion, ferns, milkweed, pigweed, pokeweed, saxifrage, sunflower leaves, watercress, winter cress), wild turnips, *yuca* (cassava)	Some traditional vegetables eaten when available
	Green peas, string beans, instant potatoes common commodity items
	Intake of vegetables low; variety limited
	Potato chips and corn chips often popular as snacks
Chiles, garlic, hickory nut cream, onions, peppermint, sage, salt, sassafras, seaweed, spearmint, and other indigenous herbs and spices	
Acorn meal, black walnuts, buckeyes, chestnuts, hazelnuts, hickory nuts, mesquite tree beans, pecans, peanuts, *piñon* nuts (pine nuts), pumpkin seeds, squash seeds, sunflower seeds, seeds of wild grasses	
Teas of buffalo berries, mint, peyote, rose hip, sassafras, spicebush, sumac berries, *yerba buena;* honey and water	Coffee, tea, soft drinks common beverages
	Alcoholism prevalent
Fats rendered from buffalo, caribou, moose, and other land mammals; seal and whale fat	Butter, lard, margarine, vegetable oils have replaced rendered fats in most regions; seal and whale fat still consumed by Inuits and Aleuts
Maple syrup, other tree saps, honey	Sugar primary sweetener; candy, cookies, jams, and jellies popular

One Native American tale about the discovery of maple syrup is that a woman who was cooking a pot of moose stew was too busy to go to the creek for water, so she filled the pot with "water" dripping from a nearby tree. As it cooked, she found that the meat was in a delicious, thick, sweet syrup instead of gravy.

Maple syrup is produced from the sap of the maple tree found in New England and eastern Canada. It takes 40 gallons of sap (the entire year's production from one mature tree) to make 1 gallon of syrup. Maple sugar is made by condensing the syrup further until it solidifies.

Northeastern The northeastern region of the United States was heavily wooded, with numerous freshwater lakes and a long Atlantic coastline. It provided the local Native Americans, including the Iroquois and Powhatan, with abundant indigenous fruits, vegetables, fish, and game. Most nations also cultivated crops such as beans, corn, and squash. Many of the foods that are associated with the cooking of New England have their origins in northeastern Native American recipes. The clambake was created when the Narragansett and the Penobscot steamed their clams in beach pits lined with hot rocks and seaweed. Dried beans were simmered for days with maple syrup (the precursor of Boston baked beans). The dish that today is called succotash comes from a stew common in the diet of most Native Americans; it combined corn, beans, and fish or game. In the Northeast, it was usually flavored with maple syrup. Clam chowder, codfish balls, brown bread, corn pudding, pumpkin pie, and the dessert known as Indian pudding are all variations of northeastern Native American recipes.

In addition to clams, the Native Americans of the region ate lobster, oysters, mussels, eels, and many kinds of salt- and freshwater fish. Game, such as deer and rabbit, was eaten when available. Wild ducks, geese, and turkeys were roasted with stuffings featuring crab apples,

Modern Indian corn compared to Indian corn circa 500 CE. (From LaFarge, 1956, with permission from Crown Publishers, Inc.)

grapes, cranberries, or local mushrooms. Corn was the staple food. It was prepared in many ways, such as roasting the young ears; cooking the kernels or meal in soups, gruels, and breads; steaming it in puddings; or preparing it as popcorn. Pumpkins and squash were baked almost daily, and beans were added to soups and stews. Local green leafy vegetables were served fresh. Sweets included cherries stewed with maple syrup, cranberry pudding, crab apple sauce, and hazelnut cakes.

Southern   The great variety of foods found in the northeastern region of the United States was matched in the plentiful fauna and lush flora of the South. Oysters, shrimp, and blue crabs washed up on the warm Atlantic beaches during tropical storms. The woodlands and swamplands teemed with fish, fowl, and game, including bear, deer, raccoon, and turtle, as well as ample fresh fruit, vegetables, and nuts. The Native Americans of this region, such as the Cherokee, Creek, and Seminole, were accomplished farmers, growing crops of beans, corn, and squash.

Many of the flavors typical of modern southern cooking come from traditional Native American foods. Hominy (dried corn kernels with the hulls removed) and grits (made of coarsely ground hominy) were introduced to the settlers by the Native Americans. The chicken dish known as Brunswick stew is an adaptation of a southern Native American recipe for squirrel. The Native Americans also made sophisticated use of native plants for seasoning, and they thickened their soups and stews with sassafras. The staple foods of corn, beans, and squash were supplemented with the indigenous woodland fruits and vegetables. Blackberries, gooseberries, huckleberries, raspberries, strawberries, crab apples, grapes, groundcherries, Jerusalem artichokes, green leafy vegetables, persimmons (pounded into a paste for puddings and cakes), and plums were some of the numerous edible native plants. The Native Americans of the South also used beechnuts, hazelnuts, hickory nuts, pecans, and black walnuts in their cooking. The thick, creamlike oil extracted from hickory nuts was used to flavor corn puddings and gruels. Honey was the sweetener used most frequently, and it was mixed with water for a cooling drink. Teas were made from mint, sassafras, or spicebush (*Lindera benzoin*), and during the summer "lemonade" was made from citrus-flavored sumac berries.

Plains   The Native Americans who lived in the area that is now the American Midwest were mostly nomadic hunters, following the great herds of bison across the flat plains for sustenance. The land was rugged and generally unsuitable for agriculture. Those nations that settled along the fertile Mississippi and Missouri river valleys, however, developed farm-based societies supported by crops of beans, corn, and squash.

When Africans were first brought as slaves to America, they were often housed at the periphery of farms. There was initially a great deal of interaction between blacks and local Native Americans, who taught them how to hunt the native game without guns and to use the indigenous plants. Some of the Native American cooking techniques were later introduced into white southern cuisine by African American cooks.

Dried, ground sassafras was called *filé* (meaning "thread") powder by the French settlers of the South due to the stringy consistency it gave to soups and stews when boiled. Filé powder, which often includes ground thyme in addition to sassafras, is still used in southern cooking today.

The Sioux word for Jerusalem artichokes is *topeka,* also the name of the capital of Kansas.

Bison meat was the staple food for most plains nations such as the Arapaho, Cheyenne, Crow, Dakota, and Pawnee. The more tender cuts were roasted or broiled, while the tougher ribs, joints, and other bones with marrow were prepared in stews and soups. Pieces of meat, water, and sometimes vegetables would be placed in a hole in the ground lined with cleaned buffalo skin. The stew would then be "stone-boiled": Rocks that had been heated in the fire would be added to the broth until the mixture was thoroughly cooked. All parts of the bison were eaten, including the liver and kidneys (which were consumed raw immediately after the animal was slaughtered), udder, tongue, and hump. Extra meat was preserved by cutting it into very thin strips and then dehydrating it in the sun or over the fire. This tough, dried meat would keep for several years and was known as *jerked* buffalo or *jerky*. The jerky would be pulverized and mixed with water or corn gruel, or, in emergencies, eaten dry. Most often it was shredded and mixed with buffalo fat and berries, then formed into cakes called *pemmican*.

The term "jerked" or "jerky" is believed to have come from the Spanish word for meat dried in the sun, *charqui*.

When bison were unavailable, the plains nations would hunt deer, rabbit, and game birds. Fresh green leafy vegetables were consumed in season and root vegetables, such as wild onions, were eaten throughout the year. Wild rice was collected in the northern parts of the Midwest, where it was served with bison or venison and used as a stuffing for grouse, partridge, and duck. Blackberries, cherries, crab apples, grapes, persimmons, and plums were available in some areas, but the most popular fruit was the scarlet buffalo berry (*Shepherdia canadensis*), so called because it was so often served in sauces for bison meat or dried for pemmican.

Wild rice may have provided 25 percent of the total diet of the Ojibwa Indians.

Southwestern Some of the oldest Native American settlements in North America were located along the river valleys of the arid Southwest. Despite the semidesert conditions, many Native Americans such as the Hopi, Pima, Pueblo, and Zuni lived in *pueblo* (Spanish for "town" or "village") communities and were mostly farmers, cultivating beans, chiles, corn, and squash. Others, including the Apache and Navajo, were originally roving hunters and gatherers. After the Spanish introduced livestock, some of these nomadic groups began to raise sheep. Mutton has since become associated as a traditional staple food of the region.

Until the arrival of livestock, the diet of the region was predominantly plant-based, providing a nourishing diet when supplemented with small game such as rabbit and turkey. Corn was the primary food and at least five different colors of corn were cultivated. Each color symbolized one of the cardinal points for the Zuni, and each had its own use in cooking. White corn (East) was ground into a fine meal and was used in gruels and breads. Yellow corn (North) was roasted and eaten in kernel form or off the ear. The rarer red (South), blue (West), and black (the nadir) corn was used more for special dishes, such as the lacy, flat Hopi bread made from blue cornmeal known as *piki*. Multicolored corn represented the zenith. The Hopi also attached importance to the color of corn and cultivated twenty different varieties. In many areas, corn was prepared in ways similar to those of the northern Mexican Native Americans—*tortillas* (flat, griddle-fried cornmeal bread), *pozole* (hominy), and the *tamale*-like *chukuviki* (stuffed cornmeal dough packets). Juniper ash was often added to cornmeal dishes for flavoring (Christensen et al., 1998).

Beans were the second most important crop of the southwestern region. Many varieties were grown, including the domesticated indigenous *tepary* beans and pinto beans from Mexico. Both squash and pumpkins were commonly consumed, and squash blossoms were fried or added to soups and salads. Squash and pumpkin seeds were also used to flavor dishes and chiles were used as vegetables and to season stews. Muskmelons were also grown after they were introduced by the Spanish.

When crops were insufficient, the southwestern Native Americans relied on wild plants and to add variety Tender amaranth greens were eaten in summer. *Piñon* seeds (also called pine nuts) flavored stews and soups. Both the fruit (*tunas*) and the pads (*nopales*) of the prickly pear cactus were eaten, as were the pulp and fruit of other succulents, such as yucca (the starchy fruit known today as "Navajo bananas"). The beans of the mesquite tree were a staple in some desert regions; they were ground into a flour and used in gruels, breads, and sunbaked cakes.

Northwest Coast/Alaska Natives   This culinary region incorporates a diverse geographic area. The climate of the Pacific Northwest coast is temperate. The luxuriantly forested hills and mountain slopes abound with edible plants and game, and the sea supplies fish, shellfish, and marine mammals. Farther north, in Alaska and Canada, the growing season shortens to only a few summer months and temperatures in the winter regularly plunge to $-50°F$. Two-thirds of Alaska is affected by permafrost, and the vast stretches of tundra are inhospitable to humans.

The Native American ethnic groups that inhabit this region include Indians as well as Inuits (Eskimos) and Aleuts, known as Alaska Natives. Native American nations such as the Tlingit and Kwakiutl inhabit the northwest coastal area and some interior Alaskan regions. The Aleuts live on the 1,000-mile-long chain of volcanic islands that arch into the Pacific from Alaska called the Aleutians. The Inuits live in the northern and western areas of Alaska, as well as in Canada, Greenland, and Siberia.

The Native Americans of the Northwest Coast had no need for agriculture. Food was plentiful, and salmon was their staple. The fish were caught annually in the summer as they swam upstream to spawn. They were roasted over the fire when fresh, and the eggs,

It was up to the Hopi woman to propose marriage to a man. She did this by preparing a blue cornmeal cake called a *piki* and placing it on her intended's doorstep. If the piki was taken into the house, her proposal was accepted.

The word *Eskimo* comes from the Algonquin word *eskimantik,* meaning "eater of raw flesh." *Inuit,* meaning "the people," is the name preferred by the nation.

Inuit women preparing a dead seal for butchering. (Corbis/Bettmann.)

Adult salmon, which are normally ocean-dwelling fish, swim up rivers to spawn and then die. The Native Americans of the Pacific Northwest believed that salmon were immortal. It was thought that the salmon came yearly to the rivers to feed the people, then returned to the oceans, where they were reborn. The Native Americans would ceremoniously return the fish skeletons to the river so that this rebirth could occur.

In some areas, birch sap was collected and concentrated into a syrup. An Alaskan association revived the recipe in 1990 and is now marketing birch syrup commercially.

known today as red caviar, were a favorite treat when dried in the sun into chewy strips. Extra fish were smoked to preserve them for the winter. In addition, cod, clams, crabs, halibut, herring, shrimp, sole, smelt, sturgeon, and trout were consumed. Ocean mammals such as otter, seal, and whale were also hunted. Bear, deer, elk, and mountain goats were eaten, as were numerous wild fowl and game birds.

Despite the abundant fish and game, wild plants made up more than half the diet of the Northwest Coast Native Americans. More than 100 varieties of indigenous fruits, vegetables, and even lichen were consumed, including acorns, blackberries, blueberries, camass roots (*Camassia quamash*), chokecherries (*Prunus virginiana*), desert parsley, leafy green vegetables, hazelnuts, huckleberries, mint, raspberries, salal (*Gaultheria shallon*), and strawberries. Roots were roasted or baked, and fresh greens were popular.

In contrast to the plenty of the Northwest Coast, the diet of many Alaska Natives was often marginal. The Inuits and Aleuts were usually seminomadic, traveling as necessary to fish and hunt. Fish and sea mammals such as seal, walrus, and whale were the staple foods. Arctic hare, caribou, ducks, geese, mountain goats, moose, musk oxen (hunted to extinction in Alaska by the 1870s), polar bear, and mountain sheep were consumed when available. Some items were boiled, but many were eaten raw due to the lack of wood or other fuel. The fat of animals was especially valued as food. *Muktuk* (also called *muntak* or *onattak* is still a commonly consumed item, consisting of chunks of meat with the layer of fat and skin attached. Muktuk is typically frozen before use. Walrus or whale muktuk can also be preserved by rolling it in herbs (with no salt) and fermenting it in a pit for several months, to make a treat known as *kopalchen*. *Akutok,* a favored dish, was a mixture of seal oil, berries, and caribou fat. Even the stomachs of certain game were examined for edible undigested foods, such as lichen in elk and clams in walruses. Wild plants were limited to mosses, lichen, and a few blueberries and cranberries.

Other Native American Cuisines Many traditional Native American diets do not fit conveniently within the five major regional cuisines. Among them was the fare of the population found in what is now Nevada and parts of California, called "Digger Indians" by the first whites to encounter them because they subsisted mostly on dug-up roots, such as Indian breadroot, supplemented by small game and insects. In central California, numerous nations, such as the Miwok and Pomo, had an acorn-based diet. In the rugged northern mountains and plains lived nations such as the Blackfeet, Crow, Shoshone, and Sioux, who were nomadic hunters of game. Although many may have hunted bison at one time, they were limited to the local bear, deer, moose, rabbits, wildfowl, and freshwater fish when the expansion of other Native Americans and whites into the Midwest pushed them northward and westward. Wild plants added variety to their diet.

Meal Composition and Cycle

Daily Patterns

Traditional meal patterns varied according to ethnic group and locality. In the Northeast, one large, hearty meal was consumed before noon, and snacks were available throughout the day. Two meals per day were more common in the Southwest. The women would rise before dawn to prepare breakfast, eaten at sunrise. The afternoon was spent cooking the evening meal, which was eaten before sunset. Two meals per day were also the pattern among the Native Americans of the Pacific Northwest.

In regions with limited resources, meals were often monotonous. The two daily meals of the southwestern Native Americans, for example, regularly consisted of cornmeal gruel or bread and boiled dehydrated vegetables. No distinction was made between morning or evening menus. Other dishes such as game, fresh vegetables, or fruit were included when seasonally available. The single meal of the northeastern Native Americans often included roasted game; the Northwest Coast Native Americans frequently included some form of salmon twice a day in addition to the many local edible greens and roots.

In 1995 the Makahs of northwest Washington petitioned the International Whaling Commission for the right to resume the hunting of grey whales (with a limit of five per year). It is widely thought that other Native American coastal groups also will seek approval.

Acorns contain tannic acid, a bitter-tasting substance that is toxic in large quantities. To make the acorns edible, Native American women would first crack and remove the hard hull, then grind the meat into a meal, add water to make a dough, and then leach the tannic acid from the dough by repeatedly pouring hot water through it. Acorns were sometimes leached at sandy-bottomed streams as well.

Baking bread in a southwestern outdoor oven. (Corbis/Bettmann.)

Food was simply prepared. It was roasted over the fire or in the ashes, or cooked in soups or stews. The northeastern and Northwest Coast Native Americans steamed seafood in pits; southwestern Native Americans baked cornmeal bread in adobe ovens called *hornos*. (After the introduction of hogs, flat breads were commonly fried in lard.) Seasonal items were preserved by drying them in the sun or smoking them over a fire; for meat, fish, and oysters, special wood was often used to impart a distinctive flavor. Other foods were ground into a meal or pounded into a paste. In Alaska, meats, greens, and berries were preserved in "fermented" (aged) blubber. All nations liked sweets, but they were limited to fruits and dishes flavored with maple syrup, honey, or other indigenous sweeteners.

Special Occasions

Many Native American religious ceremonies were accompanied by feasts. Among the northeastern Iroquois, seasonal celebrations were held for the maple, planting, strawberry, green corn, harvest, and New Year's festivals. The southern nations held an elaborate Green Corn Festival in thanks for a plentiful summer harvest. No one was allowed to eat any of the new corn until the ceremony was complete. Each home was thoroughly cleaned, the fires were extinguished, and all old pieces of pottery and clothing were replaced with newly made items. The adult men bathed and purged with an emetic. When everything and everyone was thoroughly clean in body and spirit, a central fire was traditionally lit by rubbing two sticks together and each hearth fire was relit with its flames. The feasting on new corn then began. Amnesty was granted for all offenses except murder, and the festival signified the beginning of a new year for marriages, divorces, and periods of mourning.

Role of Food in Native American Culture

Many Native American nations, especially in the inland regions, experienced frequent food shortages. Food is valued as sacred and, in the holistic worldview shared by most Native American ethnic groups, food is also considered a gift of the natural realm. In some nations, elaborate ceremonies accompanied cultivation of crops, and prayers were offered for a successful hunt.

The men in many nations were traditionally responsible for hunting or the care of livestock. The job of food gathering, preparation, and storage usually belonged to the women; they also made the cooking utensils, such as watertight baskets or clay pots. In predominantly horticultural societies, both men and women were frequently involved in cultivation of the crops. Among the nations of the Northeast the men ate first, followed by women and children. In the Southwest, men prepared the game they caught and served it to the women.

Sharing food is an important aspect of most Native American societies. Food is usually offered to guests, and extra food is often given to members of the extended family. In some nations of the Southwest, meals are prepared and eaten communally. Each woman makes a large amount of one dish and shares it with the other families, who in turn share what they have prepared. Many Native Americans find the idea of "selling" food inconceivable; it is suggested that this is one reason that there are few restaurants featuring Native American specialties.

Among the nations of the Southwest, food is considered a valuable gift from a woman to a man or from a woman to another woman. A present of firewood, clothing, or game is considered more appropriate from a man to a woman.

Therapeutic Uses of Food

The role of food in spiritual and physical health is still important for many Native Americans, and many food plants provide medicine in some form. Corn is of significance in some healing ceremonies.

Cornmeal may be sprinkled around the bed of a patient to protect him or her against further illness. Corn pollen may be used to ease heart palpitations, and fine cornmeal is rubbed on children's rashes. Navajo women drink blue cornmeal gruel to promote the production of milk after childbirth, and Pueblo women use a mixture of water and corn ear smut (ustilaginales, a kind of fungus) to relieve diarrhea and to cure irregular menstruation. A similar drink was given to Zuni women to speed childbirth and to prevent postpartum hemorrhaging. Corn silk tea was used as a diuretic and was prescribed for bladder infections.

Numerous other indigenous plants are used by Native Americans for medicinal purposes. For example, *agave* leaves (from a succulent common in the Southwest) are chewed as a general tonic, and the juice is applied to fresh wounds. Pumpkin pastes soothe burns. Chile peppers are used in compresses for arthritis and applied directly to warts. Infusions are used for many remedies, such as wild strawberries for diarrhea and mint tea to ease colic, indigestion, and nausea. Traditionally, maple sugar lozenges were used for sore throats.

Often the concept of "like cures like" (*sympathetic* healing) is used in selecting medicinal plants: The white fluid from dandelion stems is given to nursing mothers to increase milk, bloodroot is used to stop bleeding because its juice is red, and sinous wormroot is given for intestinal parasites (worms) or twisting convulsions. Bitter purges and emetics are also administered because they are distasteful and repugnant to any evil spirits that might cause illness (Vogel, 1981).

Food restrictions are still common during illness. Depending on the nation, many Native Americans believe that cabbage, eggs, fish, meat, milk, onions, or organ meats should be eliminated from a patient's diet. Conversely, some foods may be considered important to maintain strength during sickness, such as meat among the Seminole in Florida (Joos, 1980) and both meat and blue cornmeal among the Navajo (Schilling & Brannon, 1986). Some foods are prohibited after childbirth, such as cod, halibut, huckleberries, and spring salmon for Nootka women of the Northwest Coast.

Many plants were found by the Native Americans to have psychotherapeutic properties. They were used to relax and sedate patients, to stupefy enemies, and to induce hypnotic trances during religious ceremonies. The opiates in the roots of California poppies dulled the pain of toothache, for example. Lobelia was smoked as an antispasmodic for asthma and bronchitis. In the Southwest, knobs from the peyote cactus were used to produce hallucinations, sometimes in combination with other intoxicants. Jimsonweed (*Datura stramonium*) was used to keep boys in a semiconscious state for 20 days so that they could forget their childhood during Algonquin puberty rites (Emboden, 1976).

The Winnebago nation held feasts at the onset of any epidemic in an effort to halt the spread of illness.

Bloodroot *(Sanguinaria canadensis)* contains strong alkaloids that work as a nervous system depressant.

An Iroquois Thanksgiving prayer illustrates the relationship between food and health: "We return thanks for all herbs, which furnish medicines for the cure of our diseases. We return thanks to the corn, and to her sisters, the beans and squash, which give us life. We return thanks to the bushes and trees, which provide us with fruit."

Some Native Americans steeped willow bark as a tea for use as a pain killer. It is high in salicyclic acid, the active ingredient in aspirin.

Contemporary Food Habits

Native American ethnic identity is changing. Traditional beliefs and values are often in direct conflict with those of the majority society, and Native Americans' self-concept has undergone tremendous changes in the process of acculturation. A 1978 study described three transitional adaptations of members of the Ojibwa (also called Chippewa), identified by three different lifestyles; these may serve as a model for the adaptations made by members of other Native American groups (Primeaux & Henderson, 1981). The first stage of adaptation is traditional in which parents and grandparents speak the *Ojibwa* language at home, practice the *Midewiwin* religion, and participate in Native American cultural activities such as feasts and pow-wows. The second stage is more acculturated. English is the primary language, although some Ojibwa also is spoken. Catholicism is the preferred religion, and the family is involved in activities of the majority society. In the third Ojibwa lifestyle, the pan-traditional stage, the family speaks either English or Ojibwa exclusively; practices a religion that is a combination of Native American and Christian beliefs, such as the Native American Church; and is actively involved in activities from both traditional Native American and white societies.

Adaptation of Food Habits

Food habits reflect changes in Native American ethnic identity. Many Native Americans eat a diet that includes few traditional foods. Others are consciously attempting to revive the foods and dishes of their ancestors.

Ingredients and Common Foods

When Native Americans were uprooted from their lands and their known food supplies, many immediately became dependent on the foods provided to the reservations. One study evaluating the diets of Havasupai Indians living on a reservation in Arizona found that 58 percent of the subjects ate only foods purchased or acquired on the reservation during the 24-hour recall period (Vaughn et al., 1997). Commodity foods currently include items such as canned and chopped meats, poultry, fruit juices, peanut butter, eggs, evaporated and powdered milk, dried beans, instant potatoes, peas, and string beans. Researchers report that many of these foods such as kidney beans, noodles, and peanut butter are discarded by the Navajo; powdered milk may also be rejected because it is considered a "weak" food suitable only for infants or the elderly (Kunitz & Levy, 1981).

Native American food is becoming trendy, especially the fare of the Southwest. In 1984 the late James Beard, considered the father of American gastronomy, wrote a glowing article praising the delicious dishes served at a New York celebration of Native American cuisine.

A study that examined Dogrib food habits in acculturating communities in Canada found that new food items are added to traditional diets rather than substituted for traditional foods, resulting in an increase in total calorie intake compared to less acculturated communities (Szarthmay et al., 1987).

Other sources of food include gardening (reportedly practiced by between 43 and 91% of rural Native Americans), fishing, hunting, gathering indigenous plants, and raising livestock. One study of California Miwok, for instance, reports that 67 percent of respondents recall that their grandparents harvested wild greens, nuts, berries, and mushrooms, and that 47 percent of respondents continue to supplement their diet this way (Ikeda et al., 1993). Among Baffin Inuit, traditional foods (e.g., sea and land mammals, fish) make up about one-third of energy intake. Men were found to eat more traditional items than women (Kuhnlein, 1995).

Over the years, traditional foods and methods of preparation were lost and substitutions were made. For example, beef is a commonly accepted substitute for game among many Native American ethnic groups. Traditional foods compose less than 25 percent of the daily diet among the Hopi. Older Hopi women lament the fact that younger Hopi are no longer learning how to cook these dishes (Kuhnlein et al., 1979). In a study of Cherokee women (Terry & Bass, 1984) the consumption of traditional foods was found to be directly related to the amount of Native American inheritance of the woman in charge of the food supply in the home. Corn and corn products such as hominy were among the most popular traditional foods; game meat, hickory nuts, raspberries, and winter squash were the least commonly served. Among Cherokee teenagers, traditional items such as fry bread, bean bread (corn bread with pinto beans), and chestnut bread (made from chestnuts and cornmeal) were well accepted. Although more than 80 percent of the adolescents were familiar with typical Cherokee dishes, including native greens and game meat (bear, deer, groundhog, rabbit, raccoon, squirrel, and wild boar), these foods were rarely eaten (Storey et al., 1986). Pima consume traditional items, such as tepary beans and cactus stew, mostly at community get-togethers (Smith et al., 1996). California Miwok list mostly southwestern items such as beans, rice, and tortillas as those they most associate with Native American foods and recall numerous items eaten by their grandparents but not consumed now, such as squirrels, rabbit, deer, acorn mush, and certain insects. Access to wild game is limited due to hunting restrictions.

Navajo women eat traditional foods infrequently, with the exception of fry bread, mutton, and tortillas. Blue cornmeal mush (with ash), hominy, and sumac berry pudding are a few of the native dishes consumed occasionally (Wolfe & Sanjur, 1988). Dakota women of all ages take pride in traditional foods but prepare them only when it is convenient or for special occasions. Uncooked meat is consumed in some nations; it has been noted that some Native Americans do not care about the temperature of foods (Bass & Wakefield, 1974).

Fry bread, a flat bread made from wheat flour and typically cooked in lard, has been prepared in the Southwest for about 100 years. Although made from ingredients introduced by the Europeans, it is frequently identified as a traditional food.

Meal Composition and Cycle

Little has been reported regarding current Native American meal patterns. It is assumed that three meals per day has become the norm, especially in families without income constraints, though irregular meals have been described among Alaska Natives (Halderson, 1993).

One study of Dakotas noted that there was little variety in daily menus (Bass & Wakefield, 1974). Cereal with milk; fried potatoes; fried eggs, chopped meat, milk, and bread with butter; oatmeal or cornmeal mush; or just bread with butter was eaten for breakfast. Coffee was the most popular beverage. Lunch was the main meal, consisting of bologna sandwiches with potato chips and a carbonated beverage or just fried potatoes. Fried potatoes and chopped meat were eaten for dinner. Similar foods were found to be eaten by Navajo women; fry bread or tortillas, potatoes, eggs, sugar, and coffee were most frequently consumed. Fried foods were preferred for breakfast, and lunch and dinner consisted of one boiled meal and one fried or roasted meal. Pima in Arizona prefer eggs, bacon or sausage, and fried potatoes for breakfast, while Southwest specialties, such as tacos, tamales, and chili con carne, are common at other meals.

Snacking is common in some Native American groups, including fruit, soft drinks, potato or corn chips, crackers, cookies or cake, candy, and ice cream (Halderson, 1993; Ikeda et al., 1993). Eating at fast-food restaurants is popular among the Navajo (Wolfe & Sanjur, 1988) but is infrequent among the Pima (Smith et al., 1996).

A Native American hotel chef, George Crum, is attributed with the invention of potato chips in 1853. Today Americans consume an average of 17 pounds of potato chips per person each year.

Special Occasions

Numerous traditional celebrations are maintained by Native American tribal groups (Kavasch, 1995). Among the largest is the 5-day Navajo Nation Fair held each Labor Day weekend; the Pawnee Veteran's Day Dance and Gathering where ground meat with pecans and corn with yellow squash are served; the Miccosukee Arts Festival and the Seminole Fair in Miami, where alligator meat is featured; the Iroquois Midwinter Festival held in January to mark the new year; the Upper Mattaponi Spring Festival in Virginia over Memorial Day Weekend; the 3-day Creek Nation Festival and Rodeo; the Yukon International Storytelling Festival at which wild game such as caribou and musk ox are available; and the Apache Sunrise Ceremony which features gathered foods such as amaranth leaves and the pulp and fruit from the saguaro and prickly pear cacti. More local festivities are also common. Pueblo Feast Days are observed in honor of the Catholic patron saint of each village with a soup of posole (hominy) and beef or pork ribs. Northwest Coast potlatches are common in the spring, featuring herring roe, fish or venison stews, euchalon, salmon, and other traditional foods. In addition, there are all-Indian festivals which draw attendees

The adoption of the new Cherokee Nation constitution (following their forced dislocation) is commemorated on September 6th. The event honors reunification of all Cherokees and is celebrated over the Labor Day weekend with a State of the Nation address, parade, arts and crafts, and games.

from throughout the country, such as O'Odham Tash Indian Days in Casa Grande Arizona, the Red Earth Festival in Oklahoma City, and the Gallup Intertribal Indian Ceremonial in New Mexico. Native Americans may also eat traditional foods on special occasions such as birthdays, but for holidays of the majority culture, other foods are considered appropriate. For example, turkey with all the trimmings is served by Dakotas for Thanksgiving and Christmas (Bass & Wakefield, 1974).

4

Europeans

The majority of Americans share a common European ancestry. Even within this population, however, there are numerous ethnic and religious groups. The culturally diverse southern, northern, central, and eastern Europeans are represented in the United States in significant numbers. Today much of American cuisine reflects the traditional foods and food habits of these early settlers; European immigrants started arriving in what is now the United States in the sixteenth century and are still coming. Each group has brought a unique cuisine that, mixed with indigenous ingredients, blended with other European regional cuisines, and influenced by the cooking of Africans, Asians, and Latinos, has created what is now considered the typical American diet. This chapter discusses the traditional cuisines of northern, southern, and central Europe and Russia, as well as Scandinavia, and examines their contributions to American foods and food habits. Before discussing individual regions in Europe, a brief history of Europe following the end of the Roman Empire to the fifteenth century is presented.

EARLY EUROPEAN HISTORY

After the fall of Rome in 476, warring tribes fought for control of the empire. By the mid-sixth century the former Western Empire of Rome was almost completely occupied by barbarian tribes. The Jutes,

The decline of the Roman Empire is believed due in part to the spice trade. The Roman demand for cinnamon, ginger, pepper, and other seasonings led to a trade imbalance that weakened the entire economy.

Angles, and Saxons settled in Britain; the Franks and Burgundians inhabited France; and the Ostrogoths invaded Italy. Eastern Europe, in turn, was threatened by the Germans and Huns, as well as by Arabs and Persians. The Celts had dominated western and central Europe before the Roman conquest. In the fifth century they converted to Christianity, as did many other barbarian tribes. However, by then the Celtic foothold in Europe was confined to Ireland, Wales, and Scotland. In the late eighth century, pagan Scandinavians, known as Vikings, attacked western Europe. They eventually settled in Britain, northern France (Normandy), and parts of eastern Europe. The Scandinavians converted to Christianity by the tenth century.

The years between the fifth and fifteenth centuries are known as the Middle Ages, or the medieval period, the time between the ancient and modern periods. During this time, local feudalism ordered the social and governmental hierarchy. By the eleventh century, trade developed and towns emerged, while politically monarchies started to assert centralized authority over individual nobles.

The Crusades, military and religious pilgrimages to the Holy Lands that took place during the eleventh and twelfth centuries, were one factor that stimulated trade and exchange of ideas between Europe and the then more civilized East. Beginning in Italy during the fourteenth century, the Renaissance, which means "rebirth," spread to other European countries. During this period, Europe was in transition, moving away from a religious worldview to a more secular, materialistic outlook. Art, music, literature, science, medicine, and technology flourished by enlarging, modifying, and questioning the knowledge handed down from the Middle Ages and antiquity. Roman Catholicism was also undergoing change; during this period the Reformation led to the establishment of the Protestant movement in Christianity (see Chapter 2).

By the fifteenth century the Spanish, French, and English monarchies dominated western Europe, and the Holy Roman Empire of the Germanies ruled central Europe. In southeastern Europe, the Ottoman Turks were well established in the Balkans and were threatening Italy and central Europe. European states expanded their influence worldwide through overseas empires. One result of this imperialism was the establishment of colonies in North America by the British, French, and Spanish.

The nation-states in western Europe were continually threatened by other states that attempted to absorb or control them. Endangered states often joined together to fight off the threat and maintain the status quo. Throughout European history, boundaries have been in flux. Current national boundaries reflect agreements reached following the last war in Europe, World War II; the collapse of the Soviet Union in 1991; and recent ethnic independence movements. (See Figure 4.1.)

FIGURE 4.1
Europe.

NORTHERN EUROPEANS

Great Britain includes the countries of England, Scotland, Wales, and Northern Ireland. Ireland is now a sovereign country. Although quite northern, the climate is temperate due to the warming influence of the Gulf Stream, and the lowlands are arable.

Just across the English Channel is France, regarded for centuries as the center of western culture politically, as well as in the arts and sciences. Its capital, Paris, is one of the world's most beautiful and famed cities. France contains some of the best farmland in Europe, and three-fifths of its land is under cultivation. It is especially well known for premium wine production.

In 1607, people from Great Britain began immigrating to what has become the United States. They brought with them British trade practices and the English language, literature, law, and religion. By the time the United States gained independence from Britain, the British and their descendants constituted one-half of the American population. They produced a culture that remains unmistakably British-flavored, even today. The French came to the United States later, and in smaller numbers, yet have made significant regional contributions. The traditional foods of northern Europe and their influence on American cuisine are examined in this next section.

Cultural Perspective

History of Northern Europe

Great Britain and Ireland

The ethnic origins of the British are Celtic, Roman, Anglo-Saxon, and Norman. The Angles and Saxons were Germanic tribes that arrived in the British Isles starting in the third century. The Normans invaded and conquered England in the eleventh century and their leader, William of Normandy (northern France), then ruled as William I. William's reign was succeeded by that of the Plantagenets, another French family, whose heirs included Richard the Lionhearted and his brother, John. English rulers continued to press their claims to lands in France, which led to the Hundred Years War in the fourteenth century.

In the mid-fifteenth century, rival claims to the English throne triggered the War of the Roses and led to the establishment of the Tudor reign in 1485. Under the Tudor King Henry VIII, Protestantism was established in England as a result of his split with the Roman Catholic church over his divorce from his first wife and his subsequent marriage to Anne Boleyn. The Tudors continued on the throne through the reign of Elizabeth I, who was succeeded in 1603 by James I, the first Stuart monarch. James was also king of Scotland.

Civil war and revolution due to religious and class divisions rocked England in the seventeenth century. Conflict between Catholicism and the Protestant Church of England resulted in the Glorious Revolution of 1689. George I, a German prince, assumed the

Traditional foods of northern Europe. Some typical foods in the northern European diet include apples, bacon, beef, cheese, cream, French bread, oatmeal, salt cod, and tripe. (Photo by Laurie Macfee.)

throne in 1714, and his descendants have ruled Great Britain ever since.

Scotland, a Protestant country, joined into a successful union with England in 1707. This unification is symbolized by the Scottish cross of St. Andrew and the English cross of St. George on one flag, the Union Jack.

In contrast to the Scots, the Irish, who supported the Catholic cause, have had a bitter existence under English rule. English presence in Ireland had been sporadic for several centuries, but the Irish Rebellion of 1643, in which thousands of Protestants were massacred, led England to retaliate by murdering thousands of Irish Catholics. The resulting war led to a British victory, followed by the imposition of penal laws, which forbade Irish Catholics from voting or being elected to public office, practicing law, studying or teaching at a university, sending their children abroad for education, or practicing their religion. In addition, Irish Catholics could not lease land for longer than 31 years, and the land they inherited had to be distributed among all the descendants. The English attempted to secure their rule in Ireland by encouraging lowland Scots, considered to be loyal Protestants, to migrate to northern Ireland, primarily in County Ulster. Ulster rapidly industrialized and became an important textile center.

The Liberty Bell in Philadelphia cracked when it was rung to celebrate the repeal of the Irish penal laws.

The oppressive penal laws were eventually repealed in 1829, but repeated crop failure and rising rent for land kept the Irish poor. The majority of Ireland gained independence from England in 1921 and is now governed by a parliamentary democracy. Northern Ireland is still under English control and there is ongoing conflict between resident Irish Catholics and Protestants, and between both groups and the British army. The Northern Ireland Peace Accord of 1998 provides for a democratically elected assembly to govern the Northern Ireland province.

During the eighteenth and nineteenth centuries, Britain became a great colonial and maritime power abroad. Even though the American colonies were lost in the Revolutionary War, this loss was balanced by the gain of India. The twentieth century brought a decline in Britain's power; most of its colonies achieved independence, which contributed to the slow erosion of its economic base. Today Great Britain is governed by a democratic constitutional monarchy.

France

France emerged from the Middle Ages as the leading nation-state in Europe. French power and influence expanded under Cardinal Richelieu, minister to Louis XIII (1610–1643). The reign of Louis XIV was the golden era in the history of the French monarchy. The French Revolution (1789) destroyed the monarchy, and the First Republic was established in 1792.

Napoleon, crowned emperor in 1804, dominated European politics for the next decade. He battled, acquired territory, and lost it again repeatedly. After his defeat in 1815 by the combined forces of England, Russia, Austria, Sweden, and Prussia, a short restoration of the French monarchy was followed by the Second Republic (1848–1852) and then the Second Empire (1852–1870) under the nephew of the first Napoleon. His defeat by Prussia in 1870 led to the establishment of the Third Republic.

During the nineteenth century, France competed with Great Britain in establishing a colonial empire. Since the seventeenth century the French had been exploring vast areas of America, and by the eighteenth century they had established a territory extending from the Gulf of Mexico to Canada, known as the Louisiana Territory. The United States purchased this land from France in 1803. Most of France's colonies obtained independence by the twentieth century.

Although the nation was a victor in World War I, France suffered great human and economic loss. In World War II, France was unprepared for Germany's air and armored attacks. The country fell in 1940 and was occupied by German forces until liberated by the Allies in 1944. The Fifth Republic was established in 1962, and today France is governed by a constitutional democracy that features a strong presidency.

History of Northern Europeans in the United States

Immigration Patterns

Great Britain The British who immigrated in the seventeenth century settled primarily in New England, Virginia, and Maryland. While many originally came to avoid religious persecution, such as the Puritans in New England and the Catholics in Maryland, most later immigrants earned their passage to America by signing on as indentured servants.

By the eighteenth century, British immigration had slowed. After independence, British immigration to the United States further declined due to American hostility and disapproval by the British government. However, reported arrivals of British in the nineteenth century increased substantially. Early in the century most immigrants were families from rural areas of southern and western England. In the latter half of the century the majority of immigrants were from large English towns; many were seasonal unskilled workers who repeatedly returned to Britain.

It is said that there have been Scots in America as long as there have been Europeans on the continent. More than 100 towns and cities in the United States bear Scottish names, and it has been estimated that 1.5 million Scots immigrated to America. Although the majority of Scots came during the eighteenth and nineteenth centuries, 400,000 immigrated between 1921 and 1931, when Scotland suffered a severe economic depression. The Scottish settled over most of the United States and were often professionals or skilled laborers.

Although British immigration did not decline in the early twentieth century, the United States was no longer the country of first choice for those leaving Great Britain. During the Great Depression in the 1930s, more British people returned to Britain than came to America. After World War II an increase in immigration was attributable to British war brides returning to the United States with their American husbands. Since the 1970s, British immigration has been constant at about 10,000 to 20,000 persons per year.

Ireland The first Irish people to immigrate in substantial numbers to the United States were the descendants of Scottish Presbyterians who settled in Northern Ireland in the seventeenth century. Large-scale immigration began in the eighteenth century, and by 1775 there were an estimated 250,000 Scotch Irish living in the American colonies. Most of the immigration was the result of an economic depression brought on by a textile slump in Ireland.

Initially the Scotch Irish settled in Pennsylvania. Before long the direction of Scotch Irish immigration was westward to the frontier, first up the Delaware River and then beyond the Susquehanna into the rich farmlands of the Cumberland Valley. The Scotch Irish played

St. Patrick's Day in Savannah. (© Robert Brenner/PhotoEdit.)

an important role in the settlement of the trans-Allegheny region and eventually clustered around the site of Pittsburgh and in other areas of southwestern Pennsylvania. They also settled in the frontier regions of western Maryland, the Shenandoah valley of Virginia, and the backcountry of Georgia.

Irish Catholics started to arrive in the United States by 1820, and their immigration reached an apex between 1840 and 1860, when approximately 2 million people arrived. The impetus to leave Ireland was not only religious persecution but also repeated crop failures. The potato blight that destroyed their principal crop in 1845 resulted in death by starvation of 1 million Irish people.

The Irish Catholics were the first great ethnic minority in American cities, and their early history set the pattern for later minority immigrant groups. They settled in the northeastern cities and were at the bottom of the socioeconomic ladder. While the Scotch Irish, who were often of relatively high economic standing and Protestant, found it fairly easy to move into mainstream American society, the Irish Catholics were often stereotyped as drunkards, brawlers, and incompetents. The Irish achieved success with painful slowness. For many, their first entry into the American mainstream came by way of city politics.

France Immigration directly from France has been the smallest, yet most constant, of that from any European country, but the return rate has been high. Most of the estimated 1 million persons who have immigrated to the United States from France have been middle class, skilled, and have come for economic opportunity. A smaller number came because of religious persecution. More than 12,000 Huguenots, French Protestants, settled in the American colonies in the eighteenth century. They were considered to be excellent skilled workers.

Generally, French people who settled in the United States were eager to assimilate and able to do so because they were economically successful. Few pockets of French culture remain in the United States, with the exception of southern Louisiana, originally a French holding, and northern New England. However, the Frenchness of these areas is probably due more to the influence of French Canadian immigration than to direct French immigration.

French Canadians are the descendants of explorers and settlers who came from France, primarily Normandy and Brittany, during the seventeenth century. They established New France in what is today known as Canada. When the English gained control of Canada, many French Canadians moved to the United States; in some instances they were deported from Canada. Most settled in northern New England, especially Maine, and their descendants are known as Franco-Americans. Others from Acadia (Nova Scotia, New Brunswick, Prince Edward Island, and part of Maine) relocated, often not by choice, to central and southern Louisiana; their descendants are known as *Cajuns*.

Current Demographics and Socioeconomic Status

British and Irish The British assimilated into American mainstream society easily. Distinct groups from specific regions of Great Britain can still be found, however. For example, Cornish immigrants of the nineteenth century were often miners, and their descendants are still living in certain old mining regions, such as Grass Valley, California; Butte City, Montana; and the areas around Lake Superior. The Welsh who immigrated in the nineteenth century were miners and millworkers. They settled in the mid-Atlantic and midwestern states, especially Ohio and Pennsylvania; many were Baptist, Calvinist, or Methodist. Remnants of Welsh communities in the United States still celebrate St. David's Day (the feast day of the patron saint of Wales) and the annual festival of the National Gymanfa Ganu Association (an assembly that sings Welsh hymns or folk songs). Forty-three million Americans listed English or British ancestry in the 1990 U.S. census.

Close to 5 million Irish Catholics have immigrated to the United States, and today there are approximately 38 million Americans (about 15% of the total population) who claim to be of Irish descent. Although they started out on a lower economic rung than other older immigrant groups, they are now scattered throughout the occupational structure. In the 1950s the Irish were overrepresented as clergymen, fire fighters, and police officers. Today there are disproportionately more in law, medicine, and the sciences. Numerous Irish

The Welsh honor the patron saint of Wales, St. David, by wearing a leek stalk on their lapel. St. David identified his followers by placing a leek in the brim of their caps.

people have also excelled in the literary arts and in sports, especially boxing and baseball. Although Irish Catholics have to some extent assimilated into mainstream American society, they still remain an identifiable ethnic group.

The Scotch Irish are widely dispersed and are not easily identifiable. It has been estimated that one in every thirty Americans (some 8 million people) is of Scotch Irish descent.

French It is believed that more than 2 million people of French Canadian descent live in the United States. In Louisiana, more than 800,000 are of Acadian ancestry. The Cajuns settled in rural and inaccessible areas of southern Louisiana, the bayous, and along the Mississippi River. Primarily farmers, fishermen, and herders, they were self-sufficient and kept to themselves. Today they are still rural, but their occupations reflect local economic conditions.

The French Canadians who settled in the New England states were less likely to be farmers; instead, they worked in factories that processed textiles, lumber, and bricks. Since 1950 there has been an increase in the percentage of Franco-Americans holding white-collar jobs, but they still lag behind other ethnic groups economically. Compared to the French who immigrated directly from France and assimilated rapidly into American culture, the descendants of French Canadians have clung to their heritage, including language, customs, and religious affiliation.

Cultural Organizations

British The oldest British cultural organization is St. George's Society of New York, founded in 1770. Membership is open to citizens of Great Britain, their descendants, and other citizens of the British Commonwealth. It provides aid to needy British immigrants residing in the New York area. The North American Conference on British Studies promotes British history and culture. The British Social and Athletic Club encourages British social and recreational activities, such as cricket and soccer. It has branches worldwide.

Irish Once the Irish Catholics had settled into the urban Northeast, the predominant organizations that contributed to and often dominated life were the Catholic church, politics, and the labor unions.

One of the earliest and most spectacular successes of Irish Americans was in politics, especially in the Democratic party. The Irish controlled the political machinery in many large cities for decades. Their achievements have been attributed to their previous experience in Ireland when they campaigned against the English and to a loyal political body that would vote in a bloc. An Irish politician's supporters could depend on him for help in times of trouble. Lastly, the Irish are said to excel at public speaking, and this has aided their political ascent. Although the influence of the Irish has declined, the majority of Americans of Irish Catholic descent remain politically liberal.

The Irish, concerned over low wages and poor working conditions, often helped establish workers' unions. By 1900, Irish Americans held the presidencies of more than half of the 110 unions in the American Federation of Labor (AFL). The Irish still remain important as members and officers in U.S. labor unions.

Today the largest Irish cultural organization is the Ancient Order of Hibernians in America, with more than 200,000 members.

French In both Louisiana and New England, ethnic revival in the 1970s brought increased awareness of Cajuns and Franco-Americans. The French language is receiving greater emphasis in public schools in Louisiana and New England. There is a renewed interest in Cajun food, music, humor, and celebrations; Franco-American festivals have been revived. Several organizations are dedicated to the preservation of Cajun and Franco-American tradition, such as the Federation of French American Women and the National Association of Franco-Americans.

Religion

British Nearly all early British immigrants to America were Protestant. Although many came to escape persecution by the Church of England, others maintained this faith and established congregations throughout the American colonies. The Church of England in the United States became the Episcopal church during the late eighteenth century.

New England Puritans and English Quakers were among the first in the United States to promote free public education.

British ethnicity was often expressed through religious affiliation, particularly with the Episcopal, Methodist, Baptist, and Quaker faiths. Many immigrants established distinctively English congregations, but, within a generation, most became indistinguishable from other American churches. Today Americans of British descent participate in most U.S. faiths.

Irish Religion is a cornerstone of Irish Catholic society, and in the United States, it is centered around the parish. Over time the Catholic church in America came to be dominated by the Irish, often to the resentment of other Catholic immigrants. The church spared no effort to aid its members; it established schools, hospitals, and orphanages across the United States. The church helped to bridge the cultural gap for many Irish immigrants through advice, job placement, savings clubs, and temperance societies. Today religion plays a less important role in Irish Catholic life, although the role of the Irish in the church is still significant.

French   Among French Americans the Catholic church provided the nucleus of the community, gave it stability, and helped preserve the language and traditions of the people. The church today still plays a central role.

Family

British   The immigrant English family formed the model for the typical American family. It included a father, a mother, and their children. This family group would sometimes reside near other relatives, but more often would establish solitary households. The father was in charge of the public and business aspects of the family, while the mother controlled the domestic and social responsibilities. Traditionally the oldest children in the home were well educated and were sent to private schools, if affordable. Such an education was considered an investment in the future, and children were expected to continue the family businss and to maintain the family's social position.

Due to the similarities between the British family and the emerging American family, new immigrants from England assimilated quickly. It was very common for British immigrants to marry non-English spouses.

Irish   Many of the characteristics of the Irish family in the nineteenth century persisted into the twentieth century. Irish Catholics tended to marry at a late age, have large families, and divorce rarely. Today, however, most first- and second-generation Irish Catholics are likely to marry outside their group and, with increasing frequency, outside Catholicism. Traditionally the father was the breadwinner in the Irish Catholic family, but the mother's position was a strong one. Daughters were often as well educated as sons. The Irish people's relatively egalitarian attitudes toward sex roles may be responsible for the high concentration of Irish American women in professional jobs and white-collar work.

French   Until the twentieth century, Cajuns lived in rural areas in extended family households with as many as ten or twelve children per couple. The whole family worked as a unit, and decisions that affected the group were made jointly by all the adults. Until 1945, many Cajuns were illiterate and spoke only Cajun French. The use of Cajun French was prohibited by the public schools in 1921; as a result, many younger Cajuns today do not speak or understand French. The average family size today is smaller and there is more marriage outside the community, but Cajuns still retain strong ties to their families.

The Franco-Americans in New England are similar to the Cajuns in that they maintained French traditions; this was not due to isolation, however, but rather to their continued contact with French relatives in Quebec. They had little desire to acculturate. During the 1930s the bond to Canada weakened because of new laws restricting reentry into the United States and the Great Depression, which diminished new French Canadian immigration. Today the descendants of the French Canadians speak French infrequently and often marry outsiders. Family ties are still strong, but, as with the Cajuns, family size has decreased. Franco-American women have traditionally had higher status and more authority than their counterparts in France.

Communication

In general the British, Irish, and French are more formal than Americans; politeness is expected, and speaking in complete sentences is appreciated. Asking about what a person does for a living and discussing topics such as religion and politics should be avoided. Many British and Irish are typically reserved (even stoic in the face of difficulties), whereas the French tend to be expressive. A light handshake is an appropriate greeting. Eye contact is direct for all northern Europeans. People from the south of France prefer to sit closely together when conversing, and they touch frequently. The British and Irish are monochronistic and the French are polychronistic, undertaking several activities simultaneously. Most Americans of British, Irish, or French descent are fully acculturated.

Traditional Food Habits

The influence of France on the food habits of Great Britain and Ireland and vice versa has led to many similarities in the cuisines of these countries, although the ingredients of southern French cooking differ in that they are more like those of Mediterranean countries. The influence of these northern European cuisines on American foods and food habits has been extensive.

Ingredients and Common Foods

Staples and Regional Variations

Great Britain and Ireland   Animal products are of key importance in Great Britain and Ireland. Some form of meat or fish is present at most meals, in addition to eggs, milk, and cheese. In Britain and Ireland, lamb is a commonly eaten meat, as is roast beef, which is often made for Sunday dinner with *Yorkshire pudding* (a popover cooked in meat drippings). Pork is often served as sausages (*bangers*) and bacon. Various game birds also are eaten. The Cultural Food Groups list (Table 4.1) includes a more complete detailing of ingredients.

The Irish and British diet also contains a variety of seafood. A well-known fast-food item is *fish and chips*. The fish is battered and deep-fried, served with fried potatoes, and seasoned with salt and malt vinegar. Fish is often preserved and served as an appetizer or at breakfast. Examples are smoked Scottish salmon and *kippers,* salted and smoked fish.

Dairy products and eggs also play an important role in the diet of the British and Irish. Eggs are traditionally served for breakfast, and cheese is the key ingredient in the traditional *ploughman's lunch* served in pubs. It consists of a piece of cheddar cheese, bread, pickled onions, and a pint of beer. Other cheeses produced in England are the slightly salty, nutty Cheshire and Stilton, a blue cheese. Devonshire is known for its rich cream products, such as double cream (which has twice as much butter fat as ordinary cream) and clotted cream, a slightly fermented, thickened cream. It is often spread on *scones,* biscuits made with baking powder.

Although not the main focus of the meal, breads are not over-looked. In Ireland, soda bread, a bread made with baking soda instead of yeast, was traditionally prepared every day to accompany the meal. Wheat flour is commonly used for baking, and oatmeal is eaten as a porridge for breakfast in Scotland or used in making bread and biscuits throughout Britain and Ireland. Biscuits, or "biskcake," in England can refer to bread, cake, cookies, crackers, or what are known in America as biscuits. Scottish shortbread is an example of a sweet, buttery biscuit.

Fruits and vegetables are limited to those that grow best in cool climates. Potatoes, brought to Ireland from the New World in the seventeenth century, are the mainstay of the Irish diet and are found in British fare as well. Potatoes are found in stews or pies, such as *stobhach Gaelach,* an Irish stew of lamb's neck, and *shepherd's* or *cottage pie,* a meat pie made of leftover ground meat and onions and topped with mashed potatoes. Mashed potatoes are often just referred to as "mash," as in "bangers and mash" (sausages and mashed potatoes). Some side dishes made of potatoes are *boxty,* a type of potato pancake; *bubble and squeak,* a dish made of leftover cabbage and potatoes, chopped and fried together; and *colcannon,* mashed and seasoned boiled white vegetables with onions or leeks.

The most common beverages consumed by adults in Ireland and England are tea, beer, and whiskey. Tea, which has become synonymous with a meal or break in the afternoon, was introduced to England in 1662 by the wife of Charles II. Drunk with most meals and as a refreshment, strong black tea is preferred, served with milk and sugar. Frequently consumed alcoholic beverages include beer and whiskey. The British and the Irish do not drink the bottom-fermented style of beer common in the United States. Instead, in Ireland a

A *pub*, or public house, is a bar that serves beer, wine, hard liquor, and light meals. The British pub is often the place where friends and family meet to socialize.

Oatcakes, called *bannocks*, were traditionally eaten to celebrate the pagan Celtic holiday of Beltane on May 1st. One section was burnt or covered with ash; the unlucky person who received the marked portion was sacrificed (in more recent times the victim would leap through a small bonfire three times instead).

Colcannon was customarily served for the harvest dinner and on Halloween in Ireland. For Halloween, coins were wrapped and buried in the dish so the children could find them as they ate.

favorite is *stout,* a dark, rich, heavy beer that can provide substantial calories to the diet; in Britain the pubs usually serve "bitters," a rich amber-colored beer, strongly flavored with hops. Both beers are served at cellar temperature and are naturally carbonated.

Whiskey is made in both Ireland and Scotland, but the Irish are usually credited with its invention and name. In Ireland it is distilled from mashed, fermented barley. Scotch, or Scotch whisky (spelled without the "e"), is distilled from a blend of malted whiskey (where the barley germinated before fermentation) and unmalted whiskey. Scotch is traditionally a much stronger, smokier-tasting beverage than Irish whiskey. Other alcoholic drinks popular in Britain are gin, port (a brandy-fortified wine made in Portugal), and sherry (also a fortified wine, from Spain). A less common beverage but still popular in some regions is *mead,* a type of honey wine made from the fermentation of honey and water. The Welsh prefer a stronger, highly spiced variety, called *metheglyn.*

France   The cooking of France has traditionally been divided into classic French cuisine (*haute* or *grande* cuisine) and provincial or regional cooking. Classic French cooking is elegant and formal, mostly prepared in restaurants using the best ingredients from throughout the country. Provincial cuisine is simpler fare made at home featuring fresh local ingredients.

The ancestors of most French Americans are from two of France's northern provinces, Brittany and Normandy. Brittany, known as *Bretagne,* is located in the northwest; its shores are washed by the English Channel and the Bay of Biscay. Seafood, simply prepared, is common, and delicate Belon oysters are shipped throughout France. It is said that mutton and vegetables from the region have a naturally salty taste because of the salt spray. Apples are the prevalent fruit, and cider is widely exported.

Located along the English Channel and east of Brittany is Normandy, also known for its seafood and apples. *Calvados,* an apple brandy, is thought to be the mother of applejack, an alcoholic apple drink used to clear the palate during meals in Louisiana. Another alcoholic drink produced in the region is *Bénédictine,* named after the Roman Catholic monks who still make it at the monastery in Fecamp. Normandy is also renowned for its rich dairy products; its butter is considered one of the best in France. *Camembert,* a semisoft cheese with a mild flavor, and *Pont-l'Évêque,* a hearty aromatic cheese, are produced in the area. Dishes from Normandy are often prepared with rich cream sauces. *Crêpes,* very thin, unleavened pancakes, originated in this region; they are typically served topped with sweet or savory sauces or rolled with meat, poultry, fish or seafood, cheese, or fruit fillings.

Champagne, bordered by the English Channel and Belgium, has a cuisine influenced by the Germanic cultures. Beer is popular, as are sausages, such as *andouille* and *andouillette,* large and small

The Guinness Book of World Records was originally published by the family who makes Guinness stout to help settle pub arguments.

The term "honeymoon" originated with the European custom of newlyweds drinking mead for the first lunar month following their wedding.

Fresh cream is called *fleurette* and is often added to sauces or whipped for dessert. Also popular is *crème fraîche,* cream that is fermented until it is thickened and slightly tangy.

TABLE 4.1
Cultural Food Groups: Northern European

Group	Comments
PROTEIN FOODS	
Milk/milk products	The English and Irish drink milk as a beverage; the French may not.
Meat/poultry/fish/eggs/legumes	Meat, poultry, or fish is usually the centerpiece of the meal.
	Meats are generally roasted or broiled in Great Britain; also prepared as stews or in pies.
	Smoked, salted, or dried fish is popular in England.
CEREALS/GRAINS	Wheat bread usually accompanies the meal.
	In Britain and Ireland, oatmeal or porridge is common for breakfast.
FRUITS/VEGETABLES	Potatoes are frequently eaten in Ireland.
	Arrowroot starch is used as thickener and tapioca (from cassava tubers) is eaten.
ADDITIONAL FOODS	
Seasonings	
Nuts/seeds	
Beverages	
Fats/oils	
Sweeteners	

TABLE 4.1
Cultural Food Groups: Northern European—continued

Common Foods	Adaptations in the United States
Cheese (cow, sheep, and goat milk), cream, milk, sour cream, yogurt	The Irish consume more animal protein.
Meat: Beef (roasts; variety cuts such as brains, kidneys, liver, sweetbreads, tongue, and tripe), horse-meat, lamb, oxtail, pork, rabbit, snails, veal, venison	
Poultry and small birds: chicken, duck, goose, partridge, pheasant, pigeon, quail, thrush, turkey	
Fish and shellfish: anchovies, bass, clams, cod, crab, crawfish, haddock, herring, lobster, mackerel, mullet, mussels, oysters, perch, pike, pompano, salmon, sardines, scallops, shad, shrimp, skate, sole, sturgeon, trout, whiting	
Eggs: poultry and fish	
Legumes: kidney beans, lentils, lima beans, split peas	
Barley, hops, oats, rice, rye, wheat	Corn and corn products are consumed more.
Fruits: apples, apricots, cherries, currants, gooseberries, grapes (many varieties), lemons, melons, oranges, peaches, pears, plums, prunes, raisins, raspberries, rhubarb, strawberries	Native and transplanted fruits and vegetables, such as bananas, blueberries, okra, and squash, were added to the diet.
Vegetables: artichokes, asparagus, beets, brussels sprouts, cabbage, carrots, cauliflower, celery, celery root, cucumbers, eggplant, fennel, green beans, green peppers, lettuce (many varieties), leeks, mushrooms (including chanterelles, cèpes), olives, onions, parsnips, peas, potatoes, radishes, salsify, scallions, sorrel, spinach, tomatoes, turnips, truffles, watercress	
Angelica (licorice-flavored plant), bay leaf, capers, chiles, chives, chocolate, chutney, cinnamon, cloves, coffee, cognac, fennel seeds, garlic, ginger, horseradish, juniper berries, mace, malt vinegar, marjoram, mint, mustard, nutmeg, oregano, paprika, parsley, pepper (black, white, green, and pink), rosemary, saffron, sage, shallots, sweet basil, Tabasco sauce (and other hot sauces), tarragon, thyme, vanilla, Worcestershire sauce	Cajun and Creole cooking are highly spiced. Stews are thickened with *filé* powder (sassafras).
Nuts: almonds (sweet and bitter), chestnuts, filberts (hazelnuts), pecans, walnuts (including black)	
Seeds: sesame	
Beer (ale, stout, bitters), black and herbal tea (mint, anise, chamomile, etc.), cider, coffee, gin, hot chocolate, liqueurs, port, sherry, whiskey, wine (red, white, champagne, and fruit/vegetable)	
Butter, goose fat, lard, margarine, olive oil, vegetable oil, salt pork	
Honey, sugar	
	Molasses and maple syrup are used as sweeteners.
	Irish Americans use more sugar than members of other groups.

Tea time in Great Britain has become an afternoon meal, with small sandwiches, scones (on the second rack of the silver tray), and an assortment of cookies and pastries. (Courtesy of Grossich and Partners.)

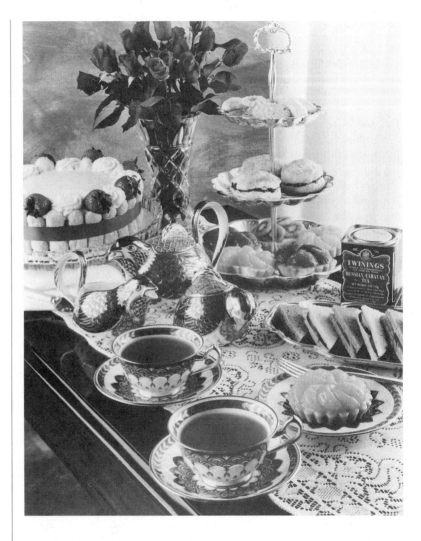

In the seventeenth century the method for producing sparkling wine was discovered by the monk Dom Perignon, who reputedly shouted when he first sipped the beverage, "I think I am drinking stars!" Today the champagne bearing his name is considered one of the finest in the world.

intestinal casings stuffed with pork or lamb stomach. *Charcuterie,* cold meat dishes such as sausages, *pâtés,* and *terrines,* which often are sold in specialty stores, are especially good from this region. Throughout the world, Champagne is probably best known for its naturally carbonated wines. Only sparkling wines produced in this region can be legally called *champagne* in France.

The province that borders Germany, Alsace-Lorraine, has been alternately ruled by France and Germany. One of its principal cities is Strasbourg. Many German foods are favored in the region, such as goose, sausages, and sauerkraut. Goose fat is often used for cooking, and one of the specialties of the area is *pâté de fois gras,* pâté made from the enlarged livers of force-fed geese. Another famous dish is *quiche Lorraine,* pie pastry baked with a filling of cream, beaten eggs, and bacon. Alsace-Lorraine is a wine-producing area; its wines are similar to the German Rhine wines but are usually not as sweet. Distilled liquors produced in the region are *kirsch,* a cherry brandy, and the brandy *eau de vie de framboise,* made from raspberries.

Located south of Normandy and Brittany in the west-central part of France is Touraine, the province that includes the fertile Loire valley. Along the river one can see the beautiful chateaux or palaces built by the French nobility. Known as the "garden of France," Touraine produces some of the finest fruits and vegetables in the country. A dry white wine produced in the area is *Vouvray.* In the north-central region is the area surrounding the city of Paris called the *Ile-de-France,* the home of classic French cuisine. Some of the finest beef and veal, as well as a variety of fruits and vegetables, are produced in this fertile region. *Brie,* semisoft and mild-flavored, is the best-known cheese of the area. Dishes of the Ile-de-France include *lobster à l'américaine,* lobster prepared with tomatoes, shallots, herbs, white wine, and brandy; *potage St. Germain,* pea soup; and *filet de bœuf béarnaise,* filet of beef with a béarnaise sauce.

Located southeast of Paris is Burgundy, one of the foremost wine-producing regions of France. Burgundy's robust dishes start to take on the flavor of southern France; they contain garlic and are often prepared with olive oil. Dijon, a principal city, is also the name of the mustards of the region prepared with white wine and herbs. Dishes of the area are *escargot,* snails (raised on grape vines) cooked in a garlic butter and served in the shell; *coq au vin,* rooster or chicken cooked in wine; and *bœuf bourguignon,* a hearty red wine beef stew. In Burgundy the red wines are primarily made from the pinot noir grape and the white wines from the chardonnay grape. The great wines of the area are usually named after the villages in which they are produced; for example, Gevrey-Chambertin, Vosne-Romanée, and Volnay. *Cassis,* a black currant liquor, is also produced in the region, and brandy from Cognac is a specialty. To the east, along the border with Switzerland, is the mountainous Franche-Comte region, known for its exceptionally tender and flavorful Bresse chicken.

The other major wine-producing region of France is Bordeaux, which is also the name of its principal city. Famous for its hearty dishes, the term *à la bordelaise* can mean (1) prepared in a seasoned sauce containing red or white wine, marrow, tomatoes, butter, and shallots; (2) use of *mirepoix,* a finely minced mixture of carrots, onions, and celery seasoned with bay leaves and thyme; (3) accompanied by *cèpes,* large fleshy mushrooms; or (4) accompanied by an artichoke and potato garnish.

A red Bordeaux wine is full-bodied and made primarily from the cabernet sauvignon grape. (In Great Britain, Bordeaux is called

Pâté is a spread of finely ground, cooked, seasoned meats. A *terrine* is commonly made with leftover meats cut into small pieces, mixed with spices and a jelling substance, then baked in a loaf pan.

Home of French mustard, Dijon, France.

Tomatoes were introduced to Europe in 1523 from the New World. Reaction was mixed; some people thought they were poisonous, while others believed they brought luck. Tomato-like pin cushions developed from the latter superstition.

claret.) Among the wines produced are St. Julien, Margaux, Graves, St. Emilion, Pomerol, and Sauternes, a sweet white dessert wine.

In the south of France is Languedoc, famous for *cassoulet,* a complex dish containing duck or goose, pork or mutton, sausage, and white beans, among other ingredients. Provence, located on the Mediterranean Sea, is a favorite vacation spot because of its warm Riviera beaches. Provence is also known for the large old port city of Marseilles, its perfumes from the city of Grasse, and the international film festival in Cannes.

The cooking of Provence is similar to that of Italy and Spain. Staple ingredients are tomatoes, garlic, and olive oil; *à la Provençal* means that a dish contains these three items. Other common food items are seafood from the Mediterranean, eggplant, and zucchini. Popular dishes from the region are *bouillabaisse,* the famed fish stew made with tomatoes, garlic, olive oil, and several types of seafood, seasoned with saffron, and usually served with *rouille,* a hot red pepper sauce; *ratatouille,* tomatoes, eggplant, and zucchini cooked in olive oil; *salade Niçoise,* a salad originating in Nice, containing tuna, tomatoes, olives, lettuce, other raw vegetables, and sometimes hard-boiled eggs; and *pan bagna,* a French bread sandwich slathered with olive oil and containing a variety of ingredients, such as anchovies, tomatoes, green peppers, onions, olives, hard-boiled eggs, and capers. One unique specialty item in the region associated with haute cuisine is black truffles. This costly, pungent underground fungus flavors or garnishes many classic French dishes.

Cooking Styles

Although the ingredients of the countries on the opposite sides of the English Channel are not substantially different, their cooking styles vary greatly. France's cuisine is admired and imitated around the world, while Britain and Ireland's cuisine is often described as being simple and hearty.

Great Britain and Ireland Both the British and the Irish take pride in the naturalness of their fare and their ability to cook foods so that the flavors are enhanced rather than obscured. Meat is usually roasted or broiled, depending on the cut, and lightly seasoned with herbs and spices. Strong-flavored condiments like *Worcestershire sauce* (flavored with anchovies, vinegar, soy, garlic, and assorted spices) on roast beef or mint jelly on lamb are often served. *Chutneys,* highly spiced fruit or vegetable pickles originally from India, are also popular. Leftover meat is finely chopped, then served in a stew, pie, or pudding.

While most Americans think of pies and puddings as being sweet desserts, in Britain and Ireland this is not necessarily the case. A pie is a baked pastry consisting of a mixture of meats, game, fish, and vegetables, or fruit, covered with or enclosed in a crust. A *Cornish pasty* is a small, pillow-shaped pie filled with meat, onions, and potatoes, and sometimes fruit (a handy all-in-one meal of meat, side vegetable, and dessert) that miners took down in the mines to eat for lunch or dinner. Another well-known British dish is steak and kidney pie.

Pudding is a steamed, boiled, or baked dish that may be based on anything from custards and fruits to meat and vegetables. An example of a sweet pudding is *plum pudding,* which is served traditionally at Christmas. It is a steamed dish of suet, dried and candied fruit, and other ingredients. *Trifle* is a layered dessert made from custard, pound cake, raspberry jam, whipped cream, sherry, and almonds.

France Classic French cuisine implies a carefully planned meal that balances the texture, color, and flavor of the dishes. The soul of French cooking is its sauces, often painstakingly prepared from stocks that are simmered for hours to bring out the flavor. A white stock is made from fish, chicken, or veal, and a brown stock is made from beef or veal.

Sauces are subtly flavored with natural ingredients, such as vegetables, wine, and herbs. They must never overwhelm the food, but rather complement it. The five basic sauces are *espagnole* (or brown sauce), made with brown stock, mirepoix, and *roux* (thickening agent made from flour cooked in butter or fat drippings)*; velouté,* made with white stock, roux, onions, and spices; *béchamel* (or cream sauce), made with white stock, milk, and roux; tomato, made with white stock, tomatoes, onions, carrots, garlic, and roux; and, *hollandaise,* which combines egg yolks and drawn butter (béarnaise is

Mincemeat pies, which are traditionally served at Christmas and Thanksgiving in some parts of the United States, were originally prepared with seasoned, ground meats, suet, and fruit, but today they are usually made with only dried and candied fruit, nuts, and spices.

It is said that the devil refused to visit Cornwall because the wives of Cornish miners had a reputation for putting anything in a pasty (Lockwood & Lockwood, 1991).

In Elizabethan England, prunes (dried plums) were offered free to brothel guests because of their reputation as an aphrodisiac.

similar, flavored with tarragon). Examples of classic cold sauces are mayonnaise and *vinaigrette,* a mixture of vinegar and oil.

Some common rules in preparing French dishes are (1) never mix sweet and sour flavors in the same dish; (2) never serve sweet sauces over fish; (3) do not under- or overcook food; (4) with the exception of salad and fruit, do not serve uncooked food; (5) always use the freshest, best-tasting ingredients; and (6) wine is an integral part of the meal and must complement the food.

French breads and pastries are particularly noteworthy. Breads are typically made with white flour, shaped into long loaves (e.g., thin *baguettes*), rounds, braids, or rings, then baked in a wood-fired oven. Sweeter breads, such as eggy *brioche* or buttery, flaky *croissants,* are between breads and pastries. Specialty doughs, such as cream puff pastry, multilayered puff pastry, and the classic sponge cake *génoise,* are used to create the numerous desserts of France, such as cakes, *petits fours* (small, bite-size pastries), and tarts. Chocolate, fresh fruits, and pastry cream thickened with egg yolks enrich these pastries.

Meal Composition and Cycle

Daily Pattern

Great Britain and Ireland In Britain, four meals are traditionally served each day—breakfast, lunch, tea, and an evening meal (dinner). In the nineteenth and early twentieth centuries, breakfast was a very substantial meal, consisting of oatmeal; bacon, ham, or sausage; eggs (prepared several ways); bread, fried in bacon grease; toast with jam or marmalade; grilled tomatoes or mushrooms; and possibly smoked fish or deviled kidneys. All this was washed down with tea. In Scotland, oatmeal is usually eaten for breakfast, while in England today, packaged breakfast cereals are often eaten during the week and the more extensive breakfast is reserved for weekends and special occasions.

Lunch was originally a hearty meal and still is on Sunday, but during the week it is squeezed in between work hours. It may include a meat pie, fish and chips, or a light meal at the pub with a pint of bitters. Both Sunday lunch and the weekday dinner are much like an American dinner. They consist of meat or fish, vegetable, and starch. The starch is often potatoes or rice, and bread also accompanies the meal. Dessert (often called pudding) follows the main course.

In the late afternoon in Britain and Ireland, most people take a break and have a pot of tea and a light snack. In some areas a "high tea" is served. This can be a substantial meal that includes potted meat, fish, shrimp, ham salad, salmon cakes, fruits, and a selection of cakes and pastries. Children often eat their dinner at tea time.

The French do not usually use bread plates, but place their portion directly on the table.

The first eating chocolate was introduced by the British in 1847. Europeans now consume 20–25 pounds of chocolate per person each year—twice the amount eaten by U.S. citizens.

Deviled describes a dish prepared with a spicy hot sauce or seasoning.

Potted is an English term for fish, meat, poultry, or game pounded with lard or butter into a coarse or smooth pâté, then preserved in jars or pots.

France   The French eat only three meals a day—breakfast, lunch, and dinner. There is very little snacking between meals. Breakfast, in contrast to the British meal, is very light, consisting of a *croissant* or French bread with butter and jam, and strong coffee with hot milk or hot chocolate. The French breakfast is what is known in the United States as a "continental breakfast." Lunch is traditionally the largest meal of the day and, in many regions of France, businesses close at midday for 2 hours so that people can return home to eat. The meal usually starts with an appetizer (*hors d'oeuvre*) such as pâté. The main course is a meat, fish, or egg dish accompanied by a vegetable and bread. If salad is eaten, it is served after the main course. Dessert at home is usually cheese and fruit. In a restaurant, ice cream (more like a fruit sherbet or sorbet), cakes, custards, and pastries are served in addition to fruit and cheese. Wine is served with the meal and coffee after the meal.

Special Occasions

Christmas and Easter are the most important Christian holidays celebrated in England, Ireland, and France. Ireland and France are predominantly Catholic countries and tend to observe all the holy days of obligation and patron saints' days. France commemorates the beginning of the French Revolution on July 14th, Bastille Day.

Great Britain and Ireland   The British celebrate Christmas by serving hot punch or mulled wine; roast goose, turkey, or ham; plum pudding and mince pies; and, afterward, port with nuts and dried fruit. The plum pudding is traditionally splashed with brandy, then flamed before serving. Boxing Day, the day after Christmas, is when friends and relatives visit one another.

Foods served at Easter include hot cross buns and *Shrewsbury simnel.* In ancient times the cross on the buns is believed to have symbolized both sun and fire; the four quarters represented the seasons. Today the cross represents Christ and the resurrection. Shrewsbury simnel is a rich spice cake topped with twelve decorative balls of marzipan originally representative of the astrological signs. It is also served on Mother's Day.

Another holiday celebrated throughout Great Britain is New Year's Day on January 1st. The Scottish traditionally eat *haggis* on New Year's Eve. It is a sheep's stomach stuffed with a pudding made of sheep's innards and oatmeal. After it is served, the diners drench their portions with Scotch whisky before eating.

St. Patrick's Day began as a religious commemoration for the patron saint of Ireland. The Irish American custom of eating a corned beef and cabbage meal on March 17th is now as popular in Ireland as it is in America.

The Associated Press reported in 1995 that the number of small neighborhood cafés in France, known as *bistros,* was declining. Nearly 500,000 existed in 1900; only 50,000 are open today. The popularity of fast foods and less time to socialize are some of the reasons responsible for the lifestyle changes.

In Britain a piece of mincemeat pie is eaten at midnight on New Year's Eve while making a wish for the upcoming year.

Traditionally a sprig of holly is placed on top of the Christmas pudding; the leaves represent Christ's crown of thorns, the red berries His blood.

When the Christmas pudding is prepared, it is a British superstition for each family member to take a turn stirring it clockwise (the direction the sun was in ancient times assumed to rotate around the earth). To stir counterclockwise is to ask for trouble.

In 1992, U.S. customs officials prevented a shipment of *haggis* from entering the country claiming it unfit for human consumption.

"Corn" originally meant "a grain." Before the invention of refrigeration, meats were often preserved in a brine made with grains of salt in a process called "corning."

France   In France the main Christmas meal is served after mass on the night of December 24th. Two traditional dishes are a black or white "pudding" (blood or pork sausage) and a goose or turkey with chestnuts. In Provence the Christmas Eve meal is meatless, usually cod, but the highlight is that it is followed by thirteen desserts.

On Shrove Tuesday (*Mardi Gras*) the French feast on pancakes, fritters, waffles, and various biscuits and cakes. During Lent, no eggs, fat, or meat are eaten. Dishes served during Lent often contain cod or herring. Cod is also the traditional dish served on Good Friday; in some regions, lentils are eaten to "wash away one's sins." Easter marks the return of the normal diet, and eggs are often served hard-boiled (also colored), in omelets, or in breads and pastries. French toast (*croûtes dorée*) is a traditional Easter dish. Also common are pies filled with minced meats.

Therapeutic Uses of Food

Most northern Europeans share a belief that a "good" diet is essential to maintaining health. Traditional home remedies for minor illness include chicken soup, tea with honey or lemon or whiskey, hot milk, or hot whiskey with cloves in it. Practices less common today are taking sulfur with molasses as a laxative, and regular use of cod liver oil.

The French Canadians who settled in Louisiana brought numerous traditional therapeutics to the region. In addition, the Native Americans were admired for their knowledge of indigenous plants and cures. Today Americans of French descent, including Cajuns and urban dwellers of all socioeconomic groups, often use home remedies. Teas made from magnolia leaves, elderberry flowers, sassafras, or citronella are just a few of the infusions commonly prescribed for colds. Sore throats are treated by gargling herbal teas or hot water with dissolved honey, salt, and baking soda. Nausea is abated with an infusion of flies or chicken gizzards, sassafras tea is used to cleanse the blood, and garlic is ingested for worms.

Contemporary Food Habits in the United States

Adaptations of Food Habits

Ingredients and Common Foods

British and Irish   Many American dishes have their origins in Great Britain. The Puritans, adapting Native American fare, made a pudding with cornmeal, milk, molasses, and spices. Today this is called *Indian pudding*. Pumpkin pie is just a custard pie to which the native American squash, pumpkin, is added. *Sally Lunn,* a sweet hot bread

Some Cajuns believe that milk and fish should not be consumed together at the same meal.

Cornish pasties are still popular in parts of the country where immigrants from Cornwall came to work in the mines, such as the Upper Peninsula in Michigan, where May 24th was declared Pasty Day in 1968.

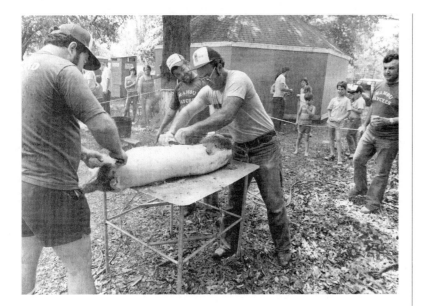

La Boucherie: French-speaking Cajuns in Louisiana maintain the hog-butchering traditions of their past. Before the days of refrigeration, everyone in the community helped to prepare the meat and lard. Participants went home with fresh pork cuts and spicy sausages called *boudin*. La boucherie continues today at many Cajun festivals. (Courtesy of the Louisiana Office of Tourism.)

made in Virginia, is said to have been sold on the streets of Bath, England, by a young lass who gave it her name. Others claim that the name is a corruption of the French *sol et lune,* a sun and moon cake. *Syllabub,* a milk and wine punch drunk in the American South at Christmastime, is also an English recipe.

French French cooking has had less influence on everyday American cooking (except for french fries), but there are probably few cities that don't have a French restaurant (which may or may not be owned by a French immigrant). French Americans adapted their cuisine and meal patterns to the available ingredients and other ethnic cooking styles. The best example of this is found in Louisiana, where *Creole* and *Cajun* cooking developed. Creole cooking is to Cajun cooking what French grande cuisine is to provincial cooking. Some dishes may sound typically French, such as the fish stew *bouillabaisse,* but it is made with fish from the Gulf of Mexico, not from the Mediterranean. Even the coffee is slightly different, as it is flavored with the bitter chicory root.

Ingredients for Cajun cooking reflect the environment of Louisiana: "Bayou Cajun" foods are from lake and swamp areas, while

Crawfish are also known as crayfish (especially in New Orleans), crawdads, crawdaddy crab (in the Great Lakes area), clawfish, and mudbugs, among others. They are small crustaceans that look like miniature lobsters, found in the fresh waters of Louisiana, Lake Michigan, California, and the Pacific Northwest.

Gumbo is the African Bantu word for okra.

Louis Armstrong, the famous jazz trumpeter from New Orleans, always signed his letters, "Red beans and ricefully yours."

"prairie Cajun" dishes are found in inland areas. Fish and shellfish abound, notably crawfish, crabs, oysters, pompano, redfish, and shrimp, to name just a few. Shellfish is commonly eaten raw on the half shell (oysters) or boiled in a spicy mixture. *Gumbo* and *jambalaya* are often made with seafood. Gumbo is a thick, spicy soup made with a variety of seafood, meat, and vegetables. It is thickened with either okra or filé powder and then ladled over rice. Jambalaya, also a highly seasoned stew made with a combination of seafood, meats, and vegetables, was brought to New Orleans by the Spanish. Originally made only with ham (*jambon*), it was later modified. The base for these stews and gravies is roux; however, the Cajun roux is unique in that the flour and fat (usually vegetable oil) are cooked very slowly until the mixture turns brown and has a nutlike aroma and taste.

Other key ingredients in Cajun cooking are rice (which has been grown in Louisiana since the early 1700s), red beans, tomatoes, chayote squash, eggplant, spicy hot sauce, and a variety of pork products. One of the better-known hot sauces, *Tabasco,* is produced in the bayous of southern Louisiana from fermented chile peppers, vinegar, and spices. A deep-fried rice fritter, *calas,* is the Louisiana version of a doughnut. Other rice dishes are *red beans and rice* and *dirty rice.* Dirty rice derives its name from the fact that its ingredients, bits of chicken gizzards and liver, give the rice a brown appearance. Cajun *boudin* sausages are a specialty. *Boudin blanc* is made with pork and rice; *boudin rouge* has pork blood added to it. *Cochon de lait,* a suckling pig roasted over a wood fire, is prepared at Cajun festivals in central Louisiana. *Fricot* is a popular soup made with potatoes and sausage or shredded meat. Cracklings, known as *gratons,* are fried, bite-size bits of pork skin (often with meat attached) that are popular in some regions.

Pecan *pralines* are a famous New Orleans candy. Pecans are native to Louisiana; pralines are large flat patties made from brown sugar, water or cream, and butter. Another confection eaten often with coffee are *beignets,* round or square puffed French doughnuts dusted with powdered sugar. French toast, or *pain perdu,* is another French specialty that was transported to New Orleans and is now familiar to most Americans.

The cuisine of French Americans in New England tends to be traditionally French, but it is influenced by common New England foods and food habits. Franco-Americans use more herbs and spices than other New Englanders and take time to prepare the best-tasting food. Traditional French dishes are pork pâté, called *creton* by the Franco-Americans, and the traditional yule log cake (*bûche de Noël*) served at Christmas. Franco-American cuisine offers numerous soups and stews. One of the most elaborate of the stews, which is also called a pie, is *cipate,* known as *cipaille, si-pallie, six-pates,* and "sea pie" in some areas. A typical recipe calls for chicken, pork, veal, and beef plus four or five kinds of vegetables layered in a heavy kettle, covered with pie crust. It is slowly cooked after chicken stock has been added through vents in the crust.

Maple syrup is commonly used. One unique breakfast dish is eggs poached in the syrup. Maple syrup is also served over bread dumplings or just plain bread. Franco-Americans appreciate wine and distilled spirits. One unusual combination of both is *caribou,* a mixture of "white whiskey" (a distilled, colorless liquor) and red wine, which is drunk on festive occasions. (See also Chapter 11, "Regional Americans.")

Meal Composition and Cycle

British and Irish   American food habits have been greatly influenced by British and Irish immigrants. Meal patterns and composition are very similar to those in Great Britain. Americans eat a hearty breakfast that often includes ham or bacon and eggs. The heart of the evening meal is usually meat, accompanied by a vegetable and a starch. Bread is served with most meals.

Festive meals also reflect the British and Irish influence. A traditional Christmas dinner includes roast turkey or ham, stuffing, and mashed vegetables. For dessert a pie is customary, often mincemeat. Two holidays that Americans think of as being typically American, Thanksgiving and Halloween, are actually of British and Irish origin. Thanksgiving combined the tradition of an old British harvest festival with the Pilgrims' celebration of surviving in their new environment. In Great Britain and Ireland, Halloween, or *All Hallow's Eve,* is believed to have originated in ancient times. Ghosts and witches were thought likely to wander abroad on Halloween night.

French   Americans of French descent have adopted the American meal cycle with the main meal in the evening. In Louisiana, the best-known celebration is Mardi Gras, culminating on Shrove Tuesday, just before the beginning of Lent. In New Orleans there are parades, masquerading, and general revelry; the festival reaches its climax at a grand ball before midnight. After this day and night of rich eating and grand merriment the 40 days of fasting and penitence of Lent begin. In the Cajun countryside, Mardi Gras is celebrated with "run": Men on horseback ride from farmhouse to farmhouse collecting chickens and sausages to add to a community gumbo. Participants enjoy beer, boudin, and *faire le maque* ("make like a monkey" or clown around) at each stop. During the rest of the year, Cajuns sponsor many local festivals, such as the crawfish, rice, and yam festivals.

Franco-Americans, like their French ancestors, serve meat pies on religious holidays. The special pie for Easter has sliced hard-boiled eggs laid down on the bottom crust, then a layer of cooked meat topped with well-seasoned pork and beef meatballs. For Christmas, *tourtière,* a pie made with simmered seasoned pork, is eaten cold after midnight Mass.

SOUTHERN EUROPEANS

Southern European countries lie along the Mediterranean Sea and include Italy, southern France, Spain, and Portugal. Italy, shaped like a boot, sticks out into the Mediterranean and includes the island of Sicily, which lies off the boot toe. Italy is separated from the rest of Europe by the Alps, which form its northern border. Spain, located to the west of France (the Pyrenees Mountains form a natural border between the two countries), occupies the majority of the Iberian Peninsula. Portugal sits on the western end of the peninsula, but also includes the Azore and Madeira islands located in the Atlantic Ocean. Most of southern Europe enjoys a warm Mediterranean climate except in the cooler mountainous regions.

Immigration to the United States from southern Europe has been considerable, primarily from the poorer regions of southern Italy. Many Americans, even those of non-European descent, enjoy Italian cuisine in some form. The foods of Spain and Portugal are similar to those of Italy and France because of both the Greek and Roman influence in the region and the shared climate, but their preparations differ.

The following section reviews the traditional diets of Italy, Spain, and Portugal. The influence of these cuisines on American fare is also discussed.

Cultural Perspective

History of Southern Europe

At the peak of its empire, Rome occupied and ruled most of Europe, including southern France (Gaul) and the Iberian Peninsula. Before the Romans, however, Phoenicians and Greeks had settled all along the Mediterranean coast. Muslims from North Africa invaded Spain, Portugal, and southern Italy in the eighth century and dominated much of the region for more than 500 years. They introduced Iberia to their eastern civilization, including their advances in agriculture, art and architecture, and technology. Palermo, the capital of Sicily, became a center of learning during this period.

Rome gave the Carthaginian name of Hispania to what is known as Spain today, because of its abundance of rabbits, *sphan.*

The word *salary* comes from the Latin word for salt, because Roman soldiers were paid with rations of the mineral.

Traditional foods of southern Europe. Some foods typical of the traditional southern European diet include almonds, artichokes, basil, cheese, eggplant, garlic, chickpeas, olive oil, olives, onions, pasta, *prosciutto,* salt cod, sweet bread, and tomatoes. (Photo by Laurie Macfee.)

Italy

Italy was politically divided from the fall of the Roman Empire until 1870. Parts of northern Italy had been ruled by a variety of European countries, including France and Austria, or existed as independent city-states. Southern Italy and Sicily were ruled at various times by the Muslims, the Normans, and the Spanish. The Catholic church also exerted control over parts of Italy, especially near Rome. Vatican City is still a separate sovereignty.

Today Italy is a prosperous industrialized nation. Its present form of government, a constitutional democracy, was established after the defeat of the fascist dictatorship that ruled during World War II.

Spain and Portugal

The Christians eventually drove the Muslims out of Spain, and the country was unified under the rule of Ferdinand and Isabella in 1492, the same year Columbus discovered the New World. Portugal, also a Christian country, had successfully ousted the Muslims many years before the Spanish eviction. Both Portugal and Spain became sea powers, and the effects of their colonization of new lands are still evident today, especially in Latin America. In 1497, Portuguese explorer Vasco da Gama successfully navigated an ocean route to the East via the Cape of Good Hope.

In Piedmont, the northern Italian state that borders France, the dish *chicken Marengo* was supposedly created for Napoleon after his defeat of the Austrians. Legend has it his cooks invented the dish from locally available ingredients, including chicken, eggs, crawfish, tomatoes, and garlic. Napoleon liked it so much he ordered it to be served after every battle.

The Spanish word *olé,* used to express excitement and approval, is thought to be from the Arabic word for God, *Allah.*

Spain became a major European power in the sixteenth century but declined in strength after its navy, the Armada, was defeated by the English in 1588. It eventually lost its colonies in the Americas and its influence in other European countries, notably Italy and the Low Countries. In the twentieth century, Spain's government alternated between dictatorship and democracy. Today it has a parliamentary democracy and a monarchy; it is one of the poorer nations in Europe.

Portugal's power also steadily declined, and by 1820 it had lost most of its major colonies. Portugal was ruled by a dictator from 1928 to 1968. In 1974, revolution resulted in the establishment of a democratic government.

History of Southern Europeans in the United States

Immigration Patterns

The majority of immigrants from southern Europe were Italians, who swelled the population of U.S. cities on the eastern seaboard during the late nineteenth and early twentieth centuries. Next in number were the Portuguese, primarily from the Azore Islands. Smaller numbers of Spanish immigrants have been documented.

The market for processed spaghetti sauce in the United States is more than $500 million annually.

Italians According to immigration records, more than 5 million Italians have settled in the United States. The majority came from the poorer southern Italian provinces and from Sicily between 1880 and 1920. Although earlier immigrants from northern Italy settled on the west coast of the United States during the gold rush, most of the later immigrants settled in the large industrial cities on the east coast. Several cities still boast Italian neighborhoods such as the North End in Boston and North Beach in San Francisco.

Many Italians came to America for economic reasons; more than one-half of the immigrants, mostly men, returned to their homeland after accumulating money. Peasants in their native land, Italians in the United States often became laborers in skilled or semiskilled professions, especially the building trades and the clothing industry. Immigration from Italy fell sharply after World War I, yet more than 500,000 Italians have immigrated since World War II.

Spaniards More than one-quarter of a million people from Spain have immigrated to the United States since 1820. However, the majority of the Spanish-speaking population in the United States comes from American acquisition of Spanish territories and the immigration of people from Latin American countries (see Chapter 6 for more detail).

Half of the Spanish immigrants to the United States came in the late nineteenth and early twentieth centuries, probably because of depressed economic conditions in Spain. In 1939, after the fall of the second Spanish republic, a small number of refugees immigrated for political reasons. Many of the early Spanish immigrants were from the Basque region, located in northeastern Spain on the border with France (there are also French Basques). They came to the United States in the nineteenth century, settling first in California, then spreading north and east throughout the West. The Basques are thought to be one of the oldest surviving ethnic groups in Europe; they lived in their homeland before the invasion of the Indo-Europeans around 2000 BCE. Their language, *Euskera,* is not known to be related to any other living language.

Portuguese   Beginning in the early nineteenth century, two waves of Portuguese immigrants arrived in the United States. Early immigrants were primarily from the Azore Islands, and they often located in the whaling ports of New England and Hawaii. The gold rush attracted a large number of Portuguese to the San Francisco Bay area. Many of these immigrants came for economic opportunity.

After World War II a small number of Portuguese from Macao, a Portuguese settlement on the coast of China near Hong Kong, settled in California. They are well educated and many hold professional jobs. A much more significant number of Portuguese, more than 150,000, entered the United States after 1958, again mostly from the Azore Islands, following a series of volcanic eruptions that devastated the region. It has been estimated that the Portuguese currently have one of the higher rates of new arrivals among European groups.

Current Demographics and Socioeconomic Status

Italians   Today there are approximately 14 million Americans of Italian descent, most of whom live in or around major cities. Economically, Italian Americans shared in the general prosperity after World War II, and today most are employed in white-collar jobs or as skilled laborers.

Four generations of Italians living in the United States have been identified. The elderly living in urban Italian neighborhoods are one group, those who are middle age and living in either urban or suburban settings are the second generation, the well-educated younger Italian Americans living in mostly suburban areas are the third generation, and fourth are the very recent immigrants from Italy (Harwood, 1981).

Spaniards   More than 500,000 citizens identified themselves as Spaniards in the 1990 U.S. census; another 93,000 claimed to be Spanish Americans. Unlike the Spaniards, who settled in cities such as New York and later Tampa, Florida, the Basques settled mostly in the rural regions of California, Nevada, Idaho, Montana, Wyoming, Colorado, New Mexico, and Arizona and became ranchers. Some Basque immigrants, however, were drawn to the mining jobs of West Virginia and the rubber and steel plants of Ohio, Illinois, Michigan, and Pennsylvania. There are between 50,000 and 100,000 Basque Americans living

Among the Basques, it is said that the devil once came to the region to learn their language, *Euskera,* so that he could entrap the inhabitants. He gave up after 7 years when he was only able to master two words: *bai* and *ez* ("yes" and "no").

Boise, Idaho, is considered the Basque capital of the United States.

in the United States. Today most Basque descendants are involved in some aspect of animal husbandry or small business; few have entered other professions. Newer Basque communities now exist in Connecticut and Florida because *jai alai* (a Basque sport) facilities were established there.

Portuguese In 1993, over 1,150,000 Americans were of Portuguese descent. Initially the Portuguese Americans on the West Coast were farmers and ranchers, but eventually their descendants moved into professional and skilled labor occupations. On the East Coast the descendants of the Portuguese who settled in the whaling ports now make up a significant part of the fishing industry.

Cultural Organizations

Italian One institution that aided the adjustment of early Italian immigrants was the mutual benefit society, which provided a form of health and life insurance during times of crisis. Many of these societies have since merged or disbanded; the largest one existing today is known as the Order of the Sons of Italy in America.

Spanish The Basque Americans were slow to form ethnic associations. In 1972, most of the Basque social clubs in the West joined together to form the North American Basque Organization, Inc., to foster regional interaction. A resurgence in Basque pride is evident in the National Basque Festival, celebrated annually on the Fourth of July in Nevada since 1964. However, one older and unique Basque institution is the Basque hotel. Throughout the West, these hotels served as mailing addresses for Basque herdsmen and boardinghouses for their families, as well as providing an ethnic haven. To outsiders, they were known for their hearty cuisine and friendly family atmosphere.

Portuguese Portuguese cultural organizations, such as social clubs, folklore groups, mutual aid societies, credit unions, Portuguese language newspapers, and radio programs, are closely associated with the Catholic church. Most important are the fraternal benefit societies, the largest ones being the Portuguese Union of the State of California (UPEC) and the Portuguese Continental Union of the United States of America, located in San Leandro, California, and Boston, respectively.

Worldview

Religion

Italians In Italy the Roman Catholic church was a part of everyday life. Immigrants to America, however, found the church to be more remote and puritanical, as well as staffed by the Irish. The church responded by establishing national parishes (parishes geared toward one ethnic group with a priest from that group), which helped immigrants adjust to America. Some religious festivals, part of daily spiritual life in Italy, were transferred to America and are still celebrated today, such as the Feast of San Gennaro in New York's Little Italy.

Spanish   Most Spaniards are Roman Catholic. The Jesuit Order was founded in Basque country and has significantly influenced Basque devotion. Basque Americans are very involved in their parishes, and there is the expectation that religion is part of daily life and sacrifice.

Portuguese   The Roman Catholic church also helped ease the Portuguese into the mainstream of American life. Local churches and special parishes often sponsor traditional religious *festas* that include Portuguese foods, dances, and colorful costumes.

Family

Italians   The social structure of rural villages in southern Italy was based on the family, whose interests and needs molded each individual's attitudes toward the state, church, and school. The family was self-reliant and distrusted outsiders. Each member was expected to uphold the family honor and fulfill familial responsibilities. The father was head of the household; he maintained his authority with strict discipline. The mother, although subordinate, controlled the day-to-day activities in the home and was often responsible for the family budget.

Once in America, the children broke free of parental control due to economic necessity. Although sons had always been allowed some independence, daughters soon gained their freedom as well, because they were expected to work outside the home like their brothers. Education eventually also changed the family. Early immigrants repeatedly denied their children schooling, sending them to work instead. However, by 1920, education was considered an important stepping stone for Italian Americans.

Spanish   In the traditional Spanish family the father spent much of his time working and socializing outside the home, while the mother devoted her life to her children. Typically one daughter would choose not to marry and would care for her parents as they aged. In the United States, Spanish American families are usually limited to immediate members, although the obligation to parents remains stronger than for most Americans. An elder may live part of the year with one child, then part of the year with another child. Independent living and retirement homes are also common.

The Basque family was customarily extended. Basques in Spain are prohibited from marrying non-Basques, but in the United States many Basques marry other nationalities. Basques accept all members who marry into their family.

Spanish women hold unique status among southern Europeans. Class distinctions are more important than gender when it comes to educational and professional attainment. The Basque women are historically recognized for their equality. Since ancient times their duties have been as valued as those of men, and jobs are often not gender-specific.

Portuguese   Like the Italians, the Portuguese have close family solidarity and have had some success in maintaining the traditional family structure. Grown sons and daughters often live close to their parents and family members try to care for the sick at home. Men strongly dominate the family and, as a result, some Portuguese women marry outside the group.

Communication

Conversational style of southern Europeans is animated, warm, and expressive. Feelings are more important than objective facts in a discussion. Women may be modest and resist discussing personal topics until another person is well known, and certain topics, such as religion, politics, and off-color jokes, are often avoided. Shaking hands with everyone in the room in greeting and leaving is appropriate; some men include pats on the back, and women may quickly embrace or kiss on the cheeks. Eye contact among elders tends to be frequent and quick, whereas younger people may prefer steady eye contact. Touching is very common, especially between members of the same sex.

Traditional Food Habits

Spaghetti comes from the Italian word for string, *spago*.

A *tortilla* in Spain is an egg omelet, not the cornmeal flatbread eaten by the Mexicans. It is believed that the Spanish called the Mexican bread by that name because of its similar shape.

Although the foods of the southern European countries are similar, as detailed in the Cultural Food Groups list (Table 4.2), there are notable differences in preparation and presentation. Many Americans think of Italian cooking as consisting of pizza and spaghetti. In reality, these dishes are only a small part of the regional cuisine of southern Italy, the ancestral homeland of most Italian Americans. Spanish food is mistakenly equated with the hot and spicy cuisine of Mexico. Although Mexico was a colony of Spain, foods and food habits of the two countries differ substantially. Portugal and Spain have very similar cuisines, but most of the Portuguese immigrants to the United States are from the Azore Islands and the island of Madeira. Their diet was less varied than that of the mainland Portuguese.

Ingredients and Common Foods

Foreign Influence

The Phoenicians and Greeks, who settled along the Mediterranean coast in ancient times, are believed to have brought the olive tree and chickpeas (garbanzo beans) to the region. In addition, fish stew, known as *bouillabaisse* in France and *zuppa di pesce alla marinara* in Italy, may be of Greek origin. The Muslims brought lemons, oranges, sugar cane, rice, and a variety of sweetmeats and spices. *Marzipan,* a sweetened almond paste used extensively in Italian desserts, and rice flavored with saffron, as in the northern Italian dish *risotto alla Milanese,* are both believed to have Muslim origins. In Spain the Muslim influence is seen in saffron-colored rice and the use of ground nuts to thicken sauces, and in candies and desserts.

It was the food of the New World colonies, however, that shaped much of Italian, Spanish, and Portuguese cuisine. Chocolate, vanilla, tomatoes, pimentos, pineapple, white and sweet potatoes, maize (corn), many varieties of squash, and turkey were brought back from the Americas. The tomato is of particular importance to the character of southern European cooking. Asian ingredients have had a significant impact in the fare of Portugal and, to a lesser degree, the dishes of Spain and Italy. From India and the Far East came coconuts, bananas, mangoes, sweet oranges, and numerous spices, such as pepper, nutmeg, cinnamon, and cloves.

Rice was brought to Italy by the Muslims; the Italians eat more rice than any other Europeans. Thomas Jefferson supposedly smuggled rice out of Italy to the United States, where his first attempts to cultivate it were unsuccessful.

Staples

Italy   Although the cooking style and ingredients vary from region to region in Italy, some general statements can be made about the differences between the foods of northern and southern Italy. Pasta is a common dish throughout Italy, but in the north it is usually made with eggs and in the shape of flat ribbons. In the agriculturally poorer south the pasta is made without eggs, generally in a tubular form, such as macaroni. In the north, pasta (e.g., *ravioli*) is commonly stuffed with cheese or bits of meat, then topped with a cream sauce, while in the south it is usually served unfilled, with a tomato sauce. Other differences are that northern fare uses more butter, dairy products, rice, and meat than the south, which is notable for the use of olive oil, little meat, and more beans and vegetables, such as artichokes, eggplants, bell peppers, and tomatoes. Seasonings common to all of Italy are garlic, parsley, and basil.

Roman soldiers are credited with sowing garlic throughout their conquered lands.

There are reputedly more than 300 different varieties of olives.

Spain   The rugged terrain in Spain is suitable for raising small animals and crops, such as grapes and olives. In fact, Spain is the largest producer of olives in the world.

Entrees usually feature eggs, lamb, pork, poultry, or dried and salted fish, especially cod, called *bacalao*. Sausages, such as the

TABLE 4.2
Cultural Food Groups: Southern European

Group	Comments
PROTEIN FOODS	
Milk/milk products	Most adults do not drink milk but do eat cheese. Dairy products are often used in desserts. Many adults suffer from lactose intolerance.
Meat/poultry/fish/eggs/legumes	Dried salt cod eaten frequently. Small fish, such as sardines, eaten whole, provide substantial dietary calcium.
CEREALS/GRAINS	Bread, pasta, or grain products usually accompany the meal.
FRUITS/VEGETABLES	Fruit is often eaten as dessert. Fresh fruits and vegetables are preferred.
ADDITIONAL FOODS	
Seasonings	
Nuts/seeds	
Beverages	
Fats/oils	
Sweeteners	

TABLE 4.2
Cultural Food Groups: Southern European—continued

Common Foods	Adaptations in the United States
Cheese (cow, sheep, buffalo, goat), milk	It is assumed that second- and third-generation southern Europeans drink more milk into their adulthood than their ancestors did.
Meat: beef, goat, lamb, pork, veal (and most varietal cuts) *Poultry:* chicken, duck, goose, pigeon, turkey, woodcock *Fish:* anchovies, bream, cod, haddock, halibut, herring, mullet, salmon, sardines, trout, tuna, turbot, whiting, octopus, squid *Shellfish:* barnacles, clams, conch, crab, lobster, mussels, scallops, shrimp *Eggs:* chicken *Legumes:* broad beans, chickpeas, fava and kidney beans, lentils, white beans	More meat and less fish is eaten than in Europe.
Cornmeal, rice, wheat (bread, farina, a variety of pastas)	
Fruits: apples, apricots, bananas, cherries, citron, dates, figs, grapefruit, grapes, lemons, medlars, peaches, pears, pineapples, plums (prunes), pomegranates, quinces, oranges, raisins, Seville oranges, tangerines *Vegetables: arugala,* artichokes, asparagus, broccoli, cabbage, cardoon, cauliflower, celery, chicory, cucumber, eggplant, endive, escarole, fava beans, fennel, green beans, lettuce, lima beans, kale, kohlrabi, mushrooms, mustard greens, olives, parsnips, peas, peppers (green and red), pimentoes, potatoes, *radicchio,* swiss chard, tomatoes, turnips, zucchini	First- and second-generation southern Europeans generally eat only fresh fruit and vegetables. Fruit and vegetable consumption tends to reflect general American food habits by the third generation.
Basil, bay leaf, black pepper, capers, cayenne pepper, chocolate, chervil, cinnamon, cloves, coriander, cumin, dill, fennel, garlic, leeks, lemon juice, marjoram, mint, mustard, nutmeg, onion, oregano, parsley (Italian and curley leaf), rosemary, saffron, sage, tarragon, thyme, vinegar Almonds, hazelnuts, *pignolis* (pine nuts), walnuts, lupine seeds Coffee, chocolate, liqueurs, port, Madeira, sherry, flavored sodas (e.g., *orzata*), tea, wine	
Butter, lard, olive oil, vegetable oil	There is decreased use of olive oil.
Honey, sugar	

Pastas, such as spaghetti and rotini, are traditionally topped with tomato-based sauces in southern Italy. Filled pastas, such as ravioli, are more common in northern Italy. (Corbis/Michelle Garrett.)

The name *gazpacho* may have come from the vinegar-and-water drink called *posca,* reportedly offered to Christ on the Cross.

paprika- and garlic-flavored *chorizo*, are common, and seafood is popular in coastal regions. Meats are often combined with vegetables in savory stews. Each region has its own recipe for *paella,* which typically includes saffron-spiced rice topped with chicken, mussels, shrimp, sausage, tomatoes, and peas. *Cocido,* a stew of chickpeas, vegetables (e.g., cabbage, carrots, potatoes), and meats (e.g., beef, chicken, pork, meatballs, sausages), also varies from area to area, but is always served in three courses. The strained broth with added noodles is eaten first, followed by a plate of the boiled vegetables, and concluded with a plate of cooked meats. Crusty bread is served with the meal.

Garlic and tomatoes flavor many Spanish dishes, for example, *gazpacho,* a refreshing pureed vegetable soup that is usually served cold, and *zarzuela* (meaning "operetta"), a fresh seafood stew. Olive oil is also a common ingredient used in almost all cooking, even deep-frying pastries, such as the ridged, cylindrical doughnuts known as *churros.* Sauces accompany many dishes. *Alioli* is made from garlic pulverized with olive oil, salt, and a little lemon juice. It is served with grilled or boiled meats and fish. Another popular sauce, called *romescu,* is sometimes mixed with alioli to taste by each diner at the table. It combines pureed almonds, garlic, paprika, and tomatoes with vinegar and olive oil. Spain's best-known dessert is *flan,* a sweet milk and egg custard topped with caramel.

Wine usually accompanies the meal. *Sangria,* made with red wine and fresh fruit juices, is served chilled in the summer. Spain is probably most famous in the United States for its sherries.

Portugal   In addition to the ingredients listed for Spanish cooking, the Portuguese in the Azore and Madeira islands use cornmeal. It is often mixed with water and baked on flat hearth stones. *Açorda d'azedo,* a dish eaten for breakfast, combines onions, garlic, vinegar, lard, saffron, and cornbread, all boiled in enough water to moisten the bread. Broad beans and *tremocos,* or lupine seeds, are popular. Fish dominates the diet of the Portuguese; they are said to prepare *bacalhau* (dried salt cod) in 125 different ways. Sardines are often grilled or cooked in a tomato and vegetable sauce. *Chouriço,* similar to the Spanish pork sausage, chorizo, and *linguiça,* a pork and garlic sausage, are often eaten at breakfast. Other typical dishes are *cacoila,* a stew made from pig hearts and liver, then served with beans or potatoes; *isca de figado,* beef liver seasoned with vinegar, pepper, and garlic, then fried in olive oil or lard; and *assada no espeto,* meat roasted on a spit. A common soup is *caldo verde,* or green broth, made from kale or cabbage and potatoes. Portuguese sweet breads, *pan doce,* and doughnuts, *malassadas,* are also quite popular.

Regional Variations

Italy   Some of the regional specialities in the northern area around Milan are *risotto,* a creamy rice dish cooked in butter and chicken stock, flavored with Parmesan cheese and saffron; *polenta,* cornmeal mush (thought to have been made originally from semolina wheat), often served with cheese or sauce; and *panettone,* a type of fruitcake. The cheeses of the region include *Gorgonzola,* a tangy, blue-veined cheese made from sheep's milk, and *Bel paese,* a soft, mild-flavored cheese. The area is also known for its apperitifs, such as bittersweet *Vermouth.*

Venice, located on the east coast and known for its romantic canals (although the city actually consists of 120 mud islands), has a cuisine centered around seafood. Its best-known dish is *scampi,* made from large shrimp seasoned with oil, garlic, parsley, and lemon juice. Inland is Verona, famous for its delicate white wines, such as *Soave.* Turin, the capital of the western province of Piedmont, is known for its *grissini,* the slender breadsticks popular throughout Italy, and *bagna cauda* (meaning "hot bath"), a dip for raw vegetables consisting of anchovies and garlic blended to a paste with olive oil or butter. Located on the northwest coast of Italy, Genoa is known for its *burrida,* a fish stew containing octopus and squid, and *pesto,* an herb,

Olive oil is labeled according to method of processing and the percent of acidity, from *extra virgin* to *virgin* (or "pure") olive oil. In the United States, only the oils derived from the first press of the olives can be called virgin; a blend of refined and virgin olive oils developed to reduce acidity must be labeled "pure."

Linguiça comes from the Portuguese word meaning tongue, a reference to the shape of the sausage.

Italian folklore has it that basil can only develop its full flavor if the gardener curses daily at it.

The city of Bologna is nicknamed *la grossa* (the "fat") and is proud of it.

Catherine de' Medici's son, Henry III, is said to have introduced the fork to the French court, after he observed it being used in Venice. Although originally from Constantinople, the three-pronged fork was created in Italy for eating pasta.

cheese, and nut paste (usually made with basil), which has become popular in the United States.

Moving southward, the city of Bologna is the center of a rich gastronomic region. Pasta specialties of the area include *lasagne verdi al forno,* spinach-flavored lasagna noodles baked in a *ragú* (meat sauce) and white sauce, flavored with Parmesan cheese; and *tortellini,* egg pasta stuffed with bits of meat, cheese, and eggs, served in soup or a rich cream sauce. It is traditionally served on Christmas Eve. A similar stuffed pasta is *cappelleti,* named for its shape, a "little hat." Other specialities are *mortadella,* a pork sausage (similar to American bologna); *prosciutto,* a raw, smoked ham served thinly sliced, often as an appetizer with melon or fresh figs; and *Parmesan* cheese, a sharply flavored cow's milk cheese with a finely grained texture.

Florence, the capital of Tuscany, has a long history of culinary expertise. In 1533, Catherine de' Medici (the Medici family ruled Florence) married into the royal family of France. She is often credited with introducing Italian fare, at the time the most sophisticated cuisine in Europe, to France. Florence is renowned for its green spinach noodles that are served with butter and grated Parmesan cheese. The term *alla Fiorentina* refers to a dish garnished with or containing finely chopped spinach. Tuscany is also famous for its full-bodied red wine, *Chianti,* and its use of chestnuts, which are featured in a cake eaten at Lent called *castagnaccio alla Fiorentina.*

Rome, the capital of Italy, has its own regional cooking and is probably best known for *fettucine Alfredo,* long, flat egg noodles mixed with butter, cream, and grated cheese. Another dish is *saltimbocca,* meaning "jumps in the mouth"—thin slices of veal rolled with ham and cooked in butter and Marsala wine. *Gnocchi,* which are dumplings, are eaten throughout Italy, but in Rome they are made out of semolina and baked in the oven. Fried artichokes are popular at Easter time, as is roast baby lamb or kid. *Pecorino romano* is the hard sheep's milk cheese of Rome, similar to Parmesan but with a sharper flavor.

The capital of Campania in southern Italy is Naples, considered the culinary capital of the south. Pasta is the staple food and a favorite way of serving it is simply with olive oil and garlic, or mixed with beans, as *pasta e fagiole.* Pizza is native to Naples and is said to date back to the sixteenth century. Another form of pizza is *calzone,* which is pizza dough folded over a filling of cheese, ham, or salami, then baked or fried. The area's best-known cheeses are *Mozzarella,* an elastic, white cheese originally made from buffalo milk; *Provolone,* a firm smoked cheese; and *Ricotta,* a soft, white, unsalted cheese made from sheep's milk and often used in desserts.

Sicily and other regions of southern Italy use kid and lamb as their principal meat. Along the coast, fresh fish, such as tuna and sardines, are used extensively; *baccalo,* dried salt cod, is often served on fast days. The North African influence shows up in Sicily in the use of *couscous,* called *cuscus* in Italy, which is commonly served with fish stews. Southern Italy's cuisine is probably best known for its desserts. Many examples can be found in Italian American bakeries and espresso bars: *cannoli,* crisp, deep-fried tubular pastry shells filled with sweetened ricotta cheese, shaved bittersweet chocolate, and citron; *cassata,* a cake composed of sponge cake layers with a ricotta filling and a chocolate- or almond-flavored sugar frosting; *gelato,* fruit or nut (e.g., black currant or pistachio) ice cream; and *granita,* intensely flavored ices. *Spumoni* is chocolate and vanilla ice cream with a layer of rum-flavored whipped cream containing nuts and fruits. Another popular sweet is *zeppole,* a deep-fried doughnut covered with powdered sugar. The sweet dessert wine *Marsala* is also a specialty in the region.

Spain Most Spanish dishes prepared in the United States reflect the cooking of Spain's southern region, with its seafood, abundant fruits and vegetables, and Muslim influence. Central Spain has a more limited diet; roast suckling pig and baby roast lamb are specialties. In the Basque provinces, lamb is the primary meat and charcoal-grilled lamb is a specialty. Other favored Basque dishes are *bacalao al pil-pil* (dried salt cod cooked in olive oil and garlic), *bacalao a la vizcaina,* (dried salt cod cooked in a sauce of onions, garlic, pimento, and tomatoes), and *angulas* (tiny eel spawn cooked with olive oil, garlic, and red peppers).

Meal Composition and Cycle

Daily Patterns

Italy A traditional Italian breakfast tends to be light, including coffee with milk (*caffe latte*), tea, or a chocolate drink, accompanied by bread and jam. Lunch is the main meal of the day and may be followed by a nap. It usually starts with *antipasto,* an appetizer course, such as ham, sausages, pickled vegetables, and olives. Next is *minestra* (wet course), usually soup or *asciutta* (dry course) of pasta, risotto, or gnocchi. The main course is fish, meat, or poultry served with a starchy or green vegetable, followed by a salad. Dessert often consists of fruit and cheese; pastries and ice creams are served on special occasions. Dinner is served at about 7:30 PM and is a lighter version of lunch. Wine usually accompanies lunch and dinner. Coffee or *espresso* is enjoyed after dinner, either at home or in a coffeehouse. Marsala may be drunk after dinner, and is often used in the preparation of desserts. One such sweet, now prepared all over Europe, is *zabaglione,* a wine custard.

Spain By American standards, the Spanish appear to eat all the time. The traditional pattern, four meals plus several snacks, is spread

The art of making ice cream is believed to have been invented by the Chinese, who brought it to India; from there it spread to the Persians and Arabs. The Muslims brought it to Italy, and it was a Sicilian, Francisco Procopio, who introduced ice cream to Paris in the 1660s. The British discovered it soon after, and later brought ice cream to America.

Bread may be served during the meal in Italy with olive oil and a strong, aged, red wine vinegar known as balsamic vinegar. Each person mixes the oil and vinegar as desired, then dips the bread.

Espresso, which means "made expressly for you," is made from finely ground dark roast coffee through which water is forced by steam pressure. *Cappuccino* is espresso topped with frothy, steamed milk.

Zabaglione was supposedly created to increase male vigor by a Franciscan monk who tired of hearing the confessional complaints from women about their tired husbands.

It was the Spanish in the 1600s who first added sugar to the bitter chocolate beverage native to Mexico. Its popularity spread quickly through Europe, even though certain clerics tried to ban it due to its association with the "heathen" Aztecs.

The word *tapas* means "lid," and the first tapas were pieces of bread used to cover wine glasses to keep out flies. Tapas are differentiated from appetizers in Spain in that they are strictly finger foods, such as olives, almonds, stuffed mushrooms, shrimp, sausage bits, and so on.

across the day. A light breakfast (*desayuno*) of coffee or chocolate, bread, or churros is eaten about 8:00 AM, followed by a midmorning breakfast around 11:00 AM of grilled sausages, fried squid, bread with tomato, or an omelet. A light snack, *tapa*, is consumed around 1:00 PM as a prelude to a three-course lunch (*comida*) at around 2:00 PM, consisting of soup or salad, fish or meat, and dessert, which is often followed by fruit and cheese. Many businesses close for several hours in the afternoon to accommodate lunch and a nap. Tea and pastries (*merienda*) are eaten between 5:00 and 6:00 PM and more tapas are enjoyed at 8:00 or 9:00 PM. Finally supper, including three light courses such as soup or omelets and fruit, is consumed between 10:00 PM and midnight. Tapas are usually served in bars and cafés and are accompanied by sherry or wine; the variety of tapas is tremendous and it is not unusual for more than twenty kinds to be offered on a menu. The evening meal may be skipped if a substantial number of tapas are eaten at night. The main meal of the day is lunch, which is generally eaten at home and consists of three hefty courses.

Portugal Portuguese meal patterns are similar to those of Spain, although the evening meal is usually eaten earlier. As in Spain, red wine usually accompanies the meal. Portugal is famous for its sweet, rich wines—Port and Madeira; the latter is often drunk with dessert.

Special Occasions

Italy Italy celebrates few national holidays, probably because of its divided history. Most *festas* are local and honor a patron saint. Other significant religious holidays are usually observed by families at home, although some cities, such as Venice, have a public pre-Lenten carnival. In some areas of the United States, where southern Italians predominate, St. Joseph, the patron saint of Sicily, is honored during Lent. Breads in the shape of a cross blessed by the parish priest, pasta with sardines, and other meatless dishes are featured.

Among Italian Americans it is traditional to serve seven seafood dishes on Christmas Eve. During the Easter holidays, Italian American bakeries sell an Easter bread that has hard-boiled eggs still in their shells braided into it. Special desserts may accompany the holiday meal, such as *panettone, amaretti* (almond macaroons), and *torrone* (nougats) at Christmastime and *cassata* at Easter. Colored, sugar-coated Jordan almonds, which the Italians call *confetti*, meaning "little candies," are served at weddings.

Spain The most elaborate of Spanish festivals is Holy Week, the week between Palm Sunday and Easter. It is a time of Catholic processions; confections and liqueurs such as coffee, chocolate, and *anisette* (licorice-flavored) are served. Holiday sweets include *tortas de aceite,* cakes made with olive oil, sesame seeds, and anise; *cortados rellenos de cidra,* small rectangular tarts filled with pureed sweetened squash; *torteras,* large round cakes made with cinnamon and squash and decorated with powdered sugar; and *yemas de San Leandro,* a sweet made by pouring egg yolks through tiny holes into boiling syrup. It is often served with marzipan.

Special dishes are also prepared for Christmas and Easter. The Basques eat roasted chestnuts and *pastel de Navidad,* individual walnut and raisin pies, at Christmas; an orange-flavored doughnut, called *causerras,* is featured on Easter. At New Year's, it is customary for the Spanish (and the Portuguese) to eat twelve grapes or raisins at the twelve strokes of midnight. It is believed to bring luck for each month of the coming year.

Portugal   Christmas Eve typically features two meals in Portugal: dinner and a post–midnight Mass buffet in the early hours of Christmas morning. Dinner often includes a casserole of bacalhua and potatoes, as well as meringue cookies known as *suspiros* ("sighs"). The buffet offers mostly finger foods, such as fried cod puffs and sausages.

In America, the Holy Ghost (Spirit) Festival is the most popular and colorful social and religious event in the Portuguese community. Although the origins of the event are obscure, it is believed to date back to Isabel (Elizabeth) of Aragon, wife of Portugal's poet king, Dom Diniz (1326). One story is that the festival derives its character from the belief that Isabel was particularly devoted to the Holy Ghost and that she wanted to give an example of charity in the annual distribution of food to the poor. In the United States the festival is usually scheduled for a week after Easter and before the end of July and is held at the local church or Hall of the Holy Ghost (also called an I.D.E.S. Hall). The main event of the festival takes place on the last day, Sunday, with a procession to the church and the crowning of a queen after the service. The donated food, which was originally distributed to needy persons on Sunday afternoon but is now often served at a free community banquet, is blessed by the priest. The most traditional foods at the feast are a Holy Ghost soup of meat, bread, and potatoes, and a sweet bread called *massa sovoda.* The bread is sometimes shaped like little doves, called *pombas.*

Also celebrated in the United States is the Feast of the Most Blessed Sacrament, which was started in New Bedford, Massachusetts by four Madeirans in gratitude for their salvation from a shipwreck en route to the United States in 1915. Other festivities are associated with the Madeiran cult of Our Lady of the Mount (a shrine on the island of Madeira).

Although the Spanish are fond of chocolate, it is used mostly as a beverage and is rarely added to pastries or confections.

The Holy Ghost Festival is not widely celebrated in Portugal. It was most likely brought to the United States by immigrants from the Azores.

Both balsamic vinegar and olive oil are believed to be health-promoting foods in Italy.

Some Italians believe that wine mixed with milk in the stomach causes too much acid, so milk is avoided at meals and consumed mostly with snacks.

Some diet books advocate a traditional Mediterranean diet to promote weight loss and lessen the risk of heart disease.

Therapeutic Uses of Food

Many Italians, particularly older immigrants, categorize foods as being "heavy" or "light," "wet" or "dry," and "acid" or "nonacid" (Ragucci, 1981). Heavy foods, such as fried items and red meats, are considered difficult to digest; light foods, including gelatin, custards, and soups, are believed to be easy to digest and appropriate for people who are ill. Wet and dry refer to how foods are prepared (with or without ample broth or fluid) as well as to their inherent qualities. For example, leafy greens like escarole, spinach, and cabbage are considered wet. A wet meal is served once a week by some Italian Americans to "cleanse out the system." Wet meals, especially soups, are considered necessary when a person is sick, because illness is associated with dryness in the body. Citrus fruits, raw tomatoes, and peaches are thought to be acidic foods that may cause skin ailments and are avoided if such conditions exist.

Other Italian beliefs about foods are that liver, red wine, and leafy vegetables are good for the blood, and that too many dairy products make the urine "hard" (kidney stones).

Contemporary Food Habits in the United States

Adaptations of Food Habits

It is generally assumed that second- and third-generation Americans of southern European descent have adopted the majority American diet and meal patterns, preserving some traditional dishes for special occasions. These assimilated Americans consume more milk and meat but less fish, fresh produce, and legumes than their ancestors. Olive oil is still used often, although not exclusively; pasta remains popular with Italians.

CENTRAL EUROPEANS AND RUSSIANS

Central Europe stretches from the North and Baltic Seas, south to the Alps, and east to the Baltic States. It includes the nations of Germany, Austria, Hungary, the Czech Republic, Slovakia, and Poland, as well as

Traditional foods of central Europe and Russia. Some foods typical of the traditional diet of central Europe and Russia include beets, cabbage, ham, herring, *kasha,* potatoes, rye bread, sausages, and sour cream. (Photo by Laurie Macfee.)

Switzerland and Liechtenstein. Most of the countries share common borders; Austria, Hungary, the Czech Republic, and Slovakia are situated south of Germany and Poland. Switzerland, a small, isolated nation, is surrounded by Germany, Austria, France, Italy, and Liechtenstein. The climate of central Europe is harsher and colder than that of southern Europe, but much of the land is fertile. Russia and its former territories, including the Commonwealth of Independent States (CIS) and the Baltic States, extend east to the border with China and the Pacific Ocean. Its vast geography includes the Arctic and parts of the Middle East. Except in the southern republics, the harsh winters of Russia affect agricultural capacity.

The large number of immigrants from central Europe made significant contributions to the literature, music, and cuisine of the United States. Many central European foods have become standard fare. What would a baseball game be without hot dogs and beer, or a picnic without potato salad? Croissants, originally from Budapest, are now a common item at fast-food restaurants. This next section explores the traditional foods and food habits of central Europe and Russia, and their impact on the American diet.

"Eastern Europe" is the term sometimes used to define the region that is also called European Russia (the western half of the country; east of the Ural mountains is known as Siberia or Asian Russia). Before the breakup of the USSR, "Eastern Europe" was sometimes used to describe those countries under Soviet control (e.g., Czechoslovakia, Hungary, East Germany, etc.).

According to legend, *croissants* were first created by the bakers of Budapest, who expressed their joy regarding their city's victory over the Turks in 1683 with a roll in the shape of the Islamic crescent. Crescent-shaped rolls symbolizing the moon were made as early as the eighth century in Europe, however.

Cultural Perspective

History of Central Europe and Russia

Germany and the Austrian Empire

Although Germany's influence in the twentieth century and its role in two world wars suggest that it has been a major force in Europe for centuries, it was not until the nineteenth century that Germany became a unified country.

Until the dissolution of the Holy Roman Empire in 1806, Germany was a patchwork of numerous small principalities and free cities stretching from the Netherlands and France to Poland and the former Czechoslovakia, many of which were prosperous and exerted economic influence throughout Europe. The most powerful state to emerge in the seventeenth and eighteenth centuries was Prussia (eastern Germany), and in 1866, it triumphed militarily over its rival, Austria, resulting in the establishing of a united German nation.

The current boundaries of Austria date only from 1918, and during the past ten centuries the term "Austria" has designated a variety of geographic and political configurations. Although it is a landlocked country of mostly mountainous terrain, Austria is located at the crossroads of Europe and has often been a center of power. The Hapsburg family came to power in the thirteenth century, and from the fifteenth until the nineteenth century the Holy Roman emperors were chosen from this dynasty. The land controlled by the Hapsburgs was considerable, including parts of modern-day Germany, Poland, Italy, Slovenia, Bosnia, Croatia, and Russia, as well as most of Hungary, the Czech Republic, Slovakia, and Rumania. The Austro-Prussian War of 1866 resulted in the Hungarians gaining control of their internal affairs, but they remained united with Austria in the Austro-Hungarian Empire.

In the early twentieth century, nationalistic movements grew within the empire and led to the onset of World War I, eventually causing the empire to crumble. In 1918, Poland, Czechoslovakia, and Hungary each proclaimed their independence.

Germany, after World War I, became a democratic republic. However, the economic crisis of the postwar years, high unemployment, and inflation resulted in the rise of the National Socialist (Nazi) party. Adolf Hitler became chancellor of Germany in 1933. This turn of events led to World War II. In the early years of the war, Germany had great success; it conquered Czechoslovakia, Poland, Denmark, Norway, Belgium, the Netherlands, Luxembourg, France, the Balkan States, and Greece. Hitler attempted to eliminate all persons he considered undesirable, such as Jews, dissidents, Gypsies, and homosexuals. It has been estimated that more than 10 million persons died in concentration camps and by other means. More than 6 million of those killed were Jews.

It was the 1914 assassination of Archduke Ferdinand, heir to the Austrian crown, in Sarajevo (in the former Yugoslavia) that precipitated World War I between the countries of the Three Emperors' League (Austria, Hungary, and Germany) and the Triple Entente (France, England, and Russia).

Switzerland, due to its isolated location, developed without external interference. Founded in 1291, it is known for its political tradition of armed neutrality, which kept it out of both WWI and WWII.

In May 1945, one month after Hitler committed suicide, Germany agreed to an unconditional surrender to the Allies (the Soviet Union, Great Britain, Free France, and the United States). As a result of the war, the Allies, at the Yalta Conference, divided Germany into two countries: the German Federal Republic (West) and the German Democratic Republic (East).

Following World War II, West Germany and Austria became independent democracies, and East Germany, Hungary, and Czechoslovakia were communist countries under control of the Soviet Union. Hungary, in 1956, and Czechoslovakia, in 1968, revolted against their communist regimes; both rebellions were put down by the Soviet Union. Communism collapsed in Czechoslovakia in 1988. Efforts to maintain a unified country failed, and in 1993, two nations were created—the Czech Republic and Slovakia. Hungary succeeded in becoming an independent democracy in 1989.

In 1990 the Soviet Union released its hold on East Germany, resulting in the dramatic dismantling of the Berlin Wall dividing east from west. The nation of East Germany was dissolved and absorbed as a state within the unified German Federal Republic.

Poland

Since the seventeenth century, Poland's borders have varied considerably. Poland's golden age, in the sixteenth century, was a period when its empire reached from the Baltic Sea to the Black Sea, and the arts and sciences flourished. By the end of the seventeenth century, Poland was increasingly influenced by its powerful neighbors, Russia, Prussia, and Austria. By 1795, Poland had almost disappeared from the European map because of Russian expansion. Poland was declared an independent state in 1918 after World War I. In 1939, Germany invaded Poland; after World War II, Poland was again declared independent, although it was under Soviet influence. Today it is a democracy struggling with the transition to a free market economy.

Russia

The early history of Russia is marked by repeated invasions: the German Goths in the third century, the Asian Huns in the fourth century, and the Turkish Avars in the sixth century. By the ninth century, Slavs had settled in parts of western Russia but were under Turkish control. The first Russian dynasty was founded by the Varangians, who were Scandinavian traders and warriors. They united the Slavs and freed them from the Turks. Vladimir I, a descendant of the Varangians and ruler of Russia, converted the Russians to the Eastern Orthodox Church in 998. It is said that his first choice was the Islamic religion, until he discovered that alcohol was forbidden to its followers.

The Mongols (commonly called the Tartars), under Butu Khan, invaded Russia in the thirteenth century, destroyed most of the cities, and established an empire that lasted until 1480. Ultimately the princes of Moscow ended the Tartar rule, and later, Ivan the Terrible (1533–1584) was crowned the first *czar,* or emperor.

In 1613 the Romanov dynasty began its rule, which lasted until 1917. Russia in the seventeenth century was still feudal and was not considered a member of the European community. During the reign of Peter I, known as Peter the Great (1689–1725), Russia's government and culture were altered through a program of modernization and the nation rapidly became a European power.

Napoleon began the French invasion of Russia in 1812 and took Moscow, but his army was nearly destroyed in the freezing winter. Despite other countries' attempts to obtain Russian lands during the second half of the nineteenth century, Russia was able to continue its territorial expansion and industrialization. In the beginning of the twentieth century the last czar, Nicholas II, ruled Russia. Lenin, a communist, took control of the government after the February Revolution of 1917. Civil war broke out shortly afterward and the Soviet regime won in 1920. Poland, Finland, and the Baltic countries became independent states after the civil war. Russia proclaimed itself the Union of Soviet Socialist Republics (USSR) in 1922. After World War II the Soviet Union forcibly annexed the Baltic States and exerted political control over the other countries on its eastern border.

The changing socioeconomic systems of Russia have created marketing opportunities for U.S. food firms. In 1992 the National Peanut Council gave away 50,000 pounds of peanut butter in Moscow to introduce the product.

Economic pressures weakened communist power in the Soviet Union in the 1980s, leading to the release of bordering countries in 1988 and 1989. In the following 2 years, numerous Soviet republics declared independence. The Baltic States (Estonia, Latvia, and Lithuania), as well as Armenia, Azerbaijan, Belarus, Georgia, Kazakhstan, Kyrgyzstan, Tajikistan, and Turkmenistan, have formed a loose alliance with Russia called the Commonwealth of Independent States (CIS). Internal conflict continues within some regions of Russia that also desire independence; sovereignty issues have yet to be resolved.

In 1993, Russian voters approved a new constitution modeled on that of France. It includes provisions for a democratically elected president.

History of Central Europeans and Russians in the United States

Immigration Patterns

Germans   For almost three centuries, Germans have been one of the most significant elements in the U.S. population. In the 1990 U.S. census, it was estimated that 58 million people identified themselves as being of German descent. Germans are also one of the least visible of any American ethnic group.

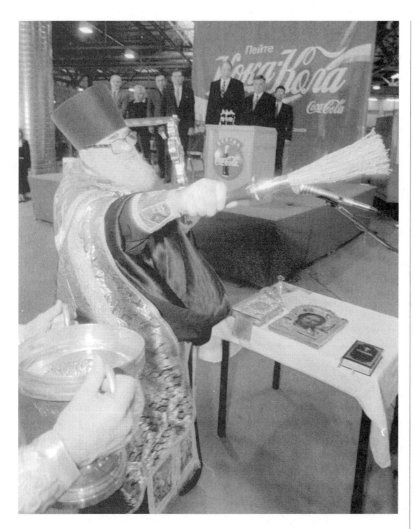

Eastern Orthodox priest blessing the Coca-Cola plant in Moscow, 1996. (AP/Wide World Photos)

The earliest German settlement in the American colonies was Germantown, Pennsylvania, founded in 1681. By 1709, large-scale immigration began, primarily from the Palatinate region of southwestern Germany. Most of the immigrants settled in Pennsylvania. The majority were farmers who steadily pushed westward searching for new lands for their expanding families. Those in Pennsylvania, Ohio, and Indiana became known as the *Pennsylvania Dutch*.

Immigration dropped off between 1775 and 1815, but an economic crisis in Europe once again prompted numerous Germans to come to the United States. It is estimated that approximately 5 million Germans immigrated to America between 1820 and 1900. Like the

The word "Dutch" is a corruption of *Deutsch,* meaning German, and has nothing to do with the Netherlands.

earlier settlers, most were farmers who arrived with their families, although by the end of the century there were increasing numbers of young, single people who were agricultural laborers and servants. Many of these settled in the Mississippi, Ohio, and Missouri River valleys, the Great Lakes area, or the Midwest. Most Germans avoided settling in the southern United States, but there are sizeable German settlements in Texas and New Orleans.

A third phase of immigration began after the turn of the twentieth century, when approximately 1.5 million Germans came to America. Many were unmarried industrial workers seeking higher pay, and others were the descendants of Germans who had settled in ethnically isolated colonies in Russia as early as the sixteenth century. Discrimination and the revolution of 1917 led to their departure. Most of these third-phase immigrants joined growing numbers of second- and third-generation Germans living in urban areas. Cities with considerable German populations included Cleveland, New York, Toledo, Detroit, Chicago, Milwaukee, and St. Louis. Russian Germans, however, tended to settle in rural areas; many settled in Colorado.

During the 1930s, many of the German immigrants were Jewish refugees. After World War II, displaced persons of German descent and East German refugees made up the sizeable German immigrant group who settled in the United States.

Poles   Although the Poles have arrived in the United States continuously since 1608, the largest wave of immigration occurred between 1860 and 1914, mostly for economic reasons. The early phase was dominated by Poles (approximately 500,000) from German-ruled areas of Poland (Pomerania and Poznan) or by Poles who worked in western Germany. German Poles often became part of the German or Czech communities or established farming settlements in the Southwest and Midwest.

The number of Polish immigrants from Germany began to decline after 1890, but the slack was taken up by the arrival of more than 2 million Poles from areas under Russian and Austrian rule. The German Poles left their homeland to become permanent settlers, but the Russian and Austrian Poles came as temporary workers. Although 30 percent returned to Poland, many eventually moved back to the United States permanently. The Austrian and Russian Poles tended to settle in the rapidly developing cities of the middle Atlantic and midwestern states, especially Chicago, Buffalo, and Cleveland.

Polish emigration after World War I was usually not for economic reasons. Most (more than 250,000) left because of political dissatisfaction: government instability and dictatorship in the 1920s and 1930s, the German invasion and occupation from 1939 to 1945, and the pro-Soviet communist government after 1945. Many settled in urban areas in which there were substantial existing Polish populations. More recently, small numbers of younger Poles have taken advantage of the freedom resulting from post-communist rule to come to the United States.

Other Central Europeans   Nearly 4 million Austrians, Hungarians, Czechs, Slovaks, and Swiss have come to the United States, primarily during the late nineteenth and early twentieth centuries, for economic and political reasons.

Austrian immigration patterns are not entirely known because Austrians and Hungarians were classified as a single group in U.S. statistics until 1910. It is believed that more than 2 million Austrians came to the United States in the decade following 1900, searching for economic opportunities. Most were unskilled and many were fathers who left families in Austria with the hopes of making their fortune. Many Austrians never found the advancement they were seeking, and approximately 35 percent returned home. A second, smaller wave of immigration occurred in the 1930s, when 29,000 well-educated, urban Austrian Jews fled Hitler's arrival.

The first group of Hungarians to arrive in the United States were several thousand political refugees following the Revolution of 1848. Most were men—well-educated, wealthy, and often titled. Later Hungarian immigrants who immigrated at the turn of the century were often poor, young, single men who found job opportunities in the expanding industrial workplace. Many worked in the coal mines of eastern Ohio, West Virginia, northern Illinois, and Indiana. Cities that developed large Hungarian populations were primarily located in the Northeast and Midwest. More than 50,000 additional Hungarians entered the United States as refugees after World War II and the 1956 uprising against the communist government. They first settled in the industrial towns populated by earlier Hungarian immigrants, but many, mostly professionals, soon moved to other cities that offered better jobs.

Czech immigrants initially tended to be farmers or skilled agricultural workers who settled in the states of Nebraska, Wisconsin, Texas, Iowa, and Minnesota, often near the Germans. Later Czech immigrants were skilled laborers; they settled in the urban areas of New York, Cleveland, and especially Chicago.

The majority of the Slovak immigrants were young male agricultural workers who arrived before World War II. Those who decided to remain in America later sent for their wives and families. The majority settled in the industrial Northeast and Midwest; they labored in coal mines, steel mills, and oil refineries.

Immigrants from Switzerland came to the United States for economic opportunities. The majority arrived prior to World War I, seeking jobs as artisans or professionals in the urban areas of New York, Philadelphia, Chicago, Cincinnati, St. Louis, San Francisco, and Los Angeles.

Both the Czechs and the Slovaks are descendants of Slavic tribes.

Swiss immigrants of the early nineteenth century were often Mennonites, who established religious communities in Ohio, Pennsylvania, and Virginia.

The Gypsies are an insular ethnic group found throughout the world. When they first arrived in Europe in the 1300s from India, they were mistaken for Egyptians. Their name derives from this error.

Another group without national boundaries found throughout central Europe (as well as in northern and southern Europe) are the Gypsies. Gypsy immigrants to the United States are not counted in U.S. census figures. Estimates are that there are between 200,000 and 1,000,000 Gypsies in America, from a variety of Gypsy groups, and speaking different dialects. Although they originate from numerous European countries, it is believed that the majority living in the United States came from central and eastern Europe.

Russians   Russian immigrants originally came to Alaska and the West Coast, rather than to the eastern states. Most of their settlements were forts or outposts, used to protect their fur trade and to shelter missionaries. When Russia sold Alaska to the United States in 1867, half of the settlers returned home and many of the others moved to California. Subsequent immigration was primarily to the East Coast, although some Russians (Molokans, followers of a religion that had rejected the Russian Eastern Orthodox Church) immigrated to the West Coast in the early twentieth century.

Russians, mainly impoverished peasants seeking a better life, began to arrive in large numbers during the 1880s. A second wave of immigrants came after the 1917 revolution, when more than 2 million people fled the country; 30,000 settled in the United States. After World War II, only small numbers of Soviet refugees, primarily Jews, were allowed to emigrate. Following the breakup of the Soviet Union, nearly 200,000 Russians settled in the United States between 1990 and 1993.

The settlement patterns of Russians are similar to those of other immigrants from central Europe. For the later wave of immigrants the port of entry was New York City. Many remained in New York, and others settled in nearby industrial areas that offered employment in the mines and factories.

Current Demographics and Socioeconomic Status

Germans   Germans differ little from the national norms demographically, although they are slightly higher in economic achievement and are generally conservative in attitudinal ratings. Only the Pennsylvania Dutch, and the rural-dwelling Germans from Russia who settled in the Midwest and in a few concentrated communities in Texas, retain some aspects of their cultural heritage.

Nearly one in every four Americans is of German descent, the largest ethnic group in the United States.

The high degree of German acculturation is attributed to their large numbers, their occupations, and the time of their arrival in the United States. Further, entry of the United States into World War I created a storm of anti-German feeling in America. German-composed music was banned, German-named foods were renamed, and German books were burned. As a result, German Americans rapidly assimilated, abandoning the customs still common in other ethnic groups, such as ethnic associations and use of their oral and written language.

Poles Polish Americans form one of the largest ethnic groups in the United States today. In 1990, it was estimated that there were more than 9.5 million Americans of Polish descent; many still live in the urban areas of the Northeast and upper Midwest where their ancestors originally settled. Economically the third-generation Polish American has moved modestly upward, but the majority of Polish Americans still live just below or solidly at middle-class level. Forty-five percent of the males have white-collar jobs, and 40 percent of working Polish women are semiskilled or unskilled laborers. Poles have been active in the formation and leadership of U.S. labor unions. More recent immigrants usually possess higher occupational skills and educational backgrounds than earlier immigrants.

Other Central Europeans There is continued confusion over Austrian ethnicity dating back to changing national boundaries and names. It is believed that although only 950,000 Americans identify themselves as being of Austrian descent in the 1990 U.S. census, as many as 4 million U.S. citizens may actually be of Austrian ancestry. Though early immigrants settled mostly in the Northeast, the largest populations of Austrian Americans are now found in New York, California, and Florida. At the turn of the century, Austrians were involved in clothing and tailoring, mining, and the food industry, including bakeries, meatpacking operations, and restaurants. Today Austrians are found in a diverse range of occupations.

In the 1990 U.S. census, it was estimated that there were more than 1.5 million Hungarian Americans in the United States. Most settled originally in the Northeast, but younger generations have migrated to California and Texas, while many Hungarian retirees have moved to Florida. Economically the Hungarians differ little from other central European immigrants. Most live in urban areas and work mostly in white-collar occupations. First- and second-generation Hungarian Americans encouraged their children to become engineers, a science that was respected by the Hungarian aristocracy at the turn of the century.

More than 1,296,000 Americans of Czech descent were identified in the 1990 U.S. census. As of 1970, most Czechs lived in cities or rural nonfarm areas; statistics show that 450,000 of them grew up in homes where Czech was spoken. Cities and states with large Czech populations are California, Chicago, Iowa, Minnesota, Nebraska, New York City, Texas, and Wisconsin. Occupationally, only a small number of Czech Americans are still farmers; a majority now hold sales, machinist, or white-collar jobs. Many Czechs have been successful in industry, founding businesses in the production of cigars, beer, and watches.

There are nearly 2 million Americans of Slovak descent, according to the 1990 U.S. census. The first two generations of Slovaks grew up in tightly knit communities anchored by work, church, family, and social activities. The third and fourth generations have sought higher education, work in white-collar jobs, and live in the suburbs; the 1990 U.S. census revealed only 26 percent of Slovaks hold jobs in areas such as manufacturing and construction. As of 1989 the median family income was $40,000, far above the national median. Less than 4 percent of Slovaks live in poverty. Cultural ties are still strong among the later generations of Slovaks.

More than 600,000 citizens declared Swiss ancestry in the 1990 U.S. census. Most Swiss were multilingual and often multicultural when they arrived, assimilating quickly into American culture. The few Swiss who come to the United States today work mostly in the U.S. branches of Swiss companies.

Gypsies retain their reputation for roving after arrival in the United States; their exact numbers are unknown and they are a very mobile population, often living in trailer parks. Many renovate apartments and houses to accommodate large social gatherings, then pass the homes on to other Gypsy Americans when they move. It is estimated that approximately half live in rural areas, and half live in urban regions. The cities with the largest concentrations of Gypsies are Los Angeles, San Francisco, New York, Chicago, Boston, Atlanta, Dallas, Houston, Seattle, and Portland. Traditionally tinkers and traders, Gypsies have entered the car dealership profession in large numbers. They also are a strong presence in the mystical arts, including fortune-telling.

Russians In 1990 there were approximately 3 million Russian Americans living in the United States. They have mostly moved out of the inner-city settlements to the suburbs. Approximately 181,000 Russian Jews immigrated to the United States between 1971 and 1991. Most of these recent émigrés have settled in urban areas, including New York, Chicago, Los Angeles, and San Francisco. Immigrants who have arrived since 1920 have come from relatively high educational and professional backgrounds.

Since World War II the relations between the Russian American community and American society at large have largely been dependent on the political climate between the United States and Russia. During the 1950s, anti-Soviet and anti-communist sentiments in the United States caused many Russian Americans to assume a low profile that hastened their acculturation.

Cultural Organizations

Germans Although few Germans belong to ethnic organizations due to extensive acculturation, the National Committee for Amish Religious Freedom was formed to provide legal counsel to the Amish

Seventy-three percent of the population in Switzerland speaks German Swiss, 20 percent speaks French Swiss, and 5 percent speaks Italian Swiss; in addition, most Swiss speak one or two other languages.

Policy in the former Soviet Union required aging parents to leave if their children wished to emigrate. One result is that Russian immigrants are one of the oldest populations in the United States: 20 percent are older than 65 years.

(a Pennsylvania Dutch sect), who for religious reasons are reluctant to defend themselves.

Poles Polish societies, such as the Polish National Alliance and the Polish Roman Catholic Union (both based in Chicago), were originally set up to aid the newly arrived immigrants. These organizations remain a vital part of Polish American life, supporting cultural preservation and educational projects in the community. The largest association is the Polish American Congress, which promotes an improved quality of life for Polish Americans.

Other Central Europeans Austrians have founded numerous local fraternal or cultural associations, while the Hungarians have created two national groups that serve as umbrella organizations lobbying on behalf of Hungarian causes—the American Hungarian Federation is the oldest (established in 1906) and the National Federation of Hungarian Americans is the largest.

Many Czechs formed fraternal organizations, often to provide health and life insurance. The Czechoslovak Society, with more than 200 lodges, is the oldest existing Czech fraternal benefit society still operating. Children's gymnastic societies, called *sokols* ("falcon"), are also popular. The American Sokol Educational and Physical Cultural Organization (ASEPCO) has seventy branches and 9,000 members who participate in gymnastic classes, cultural activities, summer camps, and ethnic festivals.

Leisure activities among the first two generations of Slovaks revolved around community associations. Many belonged to fraternal lodges that organized dances, plays, and sporting competitions. Lodge membership has dropped off among members of the third and fourth generations. The Slovak League of America is active in promoting Slovak culture.

Russians The Tolstoy Foundation, founded in New York by the daughter of famous Russian author Leo Tolstoy, serves the needs of recent immigrants. It maintains a cultural center and a home for senior citizens. The Congress of Russian Americans, Inc., is a national organization devoted to the promotion of Russian heritage and the protection of immigrant rights.

Worldview

Religion

Germans The majority of German immigrants were Lutheran; a minority were Jewish or Roman Catholic. Today the Pennsylvania Dutch and the rural Germans from Russia faithfully maintain their religious heritage. Both groups are primarily Protestant, mostly Lutheran

The Amish and Mennonites are referred to as the "Plain People." The more liberal and worldly members of the Lutheran and Reformed Churches are called the "Gay Dutch," "Fancy Dutch," or "Church People."

The Amish live by the acronym JOY—Jesus first, Others in between, and Yourself last.

or Mennonite. Mennonites are a religious group derived from the Anabaptist movement, which advocated baptism and church membership for adult believers only. They are noted for their simple lifestyle and rejection of oaths, public office, and military service. The Amish, a strict sect of the Mennonites, follow the Bible literally. They till the soil and shun worldly vanities such as electricity and automobiles. Their life centers on *Gelassenheit*, meaning submission to a higher authority through reserved and humble behavior, placing the needs of others before the needs of the individual.

Poles Most Polish immigrants were devout Catholics; they quickly established parish churches in the United States. The Catholic church is still a vital part of the Polish American community, although Polish Americans have been found to marry outside the church more than other Catholics.

Other Central Europeans Austrians are mostly Roman Catholic and have been actively involved in promoting Catholicism in America. In 1829 the *Leopoldine Stiftung* was founded in Austria to collect money throughout Europe to introduce religion to the U.S. frontier, resulting in more than 400 Catholic churches established in the East, the Midwest, and in what was known as "Indian" country. There are also small numbers of Austrian Jews. The majority of Hungarians are Catholic, although in the United States, nearly 25 percent are Protestant.

In Europe, most Czechs were Roman Catholics, but one-half to two-thirds of nineteenth-century Czech immigrants from rural areas left the church and were considered "free thinkers" who believed in a strong separation of church and state. Subsequent generations now belong to a variety of faiths.

Religion is still an important factor in the lives of Slovaks. Most are Roman Catholics who attend services regularly. First- and second-generation Slovaks usually send their children to parochial schools supported by the ethnic parish.

Traditional spirituality for the Gypsies is derived from Asian Indian religions, such as Hinduism and Zoroastrianism (see Chapter 2 regarding Eastern religions and Chapter 10 for more information on Asian Indian faiths), but many Gypsy Americans are Christians. Gypsies are often members of fundamentalist congregations, and some churches have specifically combined Gypsy spiritual concepts with Christian practices.

Russians Except for the Soviet Jews, the primary organization of the Russian American community today is the Russian Orthodox Church. Religion has always played a central role in the Russian community, and the Orthodox church has tried to preserve the culture. However, the largest branch of the Eastern church, officially known as the Orthodox Church in America (formerly the Russian Orthodox

Church Outside Russia), now includes people from other central European countries and the Russian traditions have been de-emphasized.

Family

Germans The traditional German family was based on an agricultural system that valued large families in which every member worked in the fields to support the household. Even when German immigrants moved to urban areas, family members were expected to help out in the family business. It is assumed that most German families today have adopted the smaller American nuclear configuration. The exception may be among the Pennsylvania Dutch, particularly the Amish, who continue to have large families of seven to ten children. It is not unusual for an Amish person to know as many as seventy-five first cousins or for a grandparent to have thirty-five grandchildren (Kraybill, 1995).

Poles Traditionally the Polish American family was patriarchal and the father exerted strong control over the children, especially the daughters. The mother took care of the home, and if the children worked, it was near the home or the father's workplace. Since the 1920s the overwhelming majority of Polish American families have been solely supported by the father's income; wives and children have rarely worked.

Other Central Europeans Tight nuclear families typify traditional Austrian households. Although the father is in charge of family finances, it is the mother who rules home life. Assimilation in the United States has led to a deterioration of the nuclear family, including an increased divorce rate. Traditional Czech and Hungarian families were male-dominated and included many relatives. In the United States, participation in church activities, fraternal societies, and political organizations often served to replace the extended family for both men and women. The role of women has become less circumscribed; children are typically encouraged to pursue higher education and professional careers. Family ties are strong among the Slovaks. Parents are respected; they are frequently visited and cared for in their old age. Weddings are still a major event, although they are not celebrated for several days as they once were.

Gypsies traditionally maintain extended families, although in the United States more nuclear families have been established. The father is in charge of all public matters, but, at home, women often make most of the family income and manage money matters. Women also retain some power through their ability to communicate with the supernatural world.

Russians Traditionally Russians lived in very large family groups with women legally dependent on their husbands. This structure changed, however, with the education and employment opportunities offered to women during the communist rule of the Soviet Union. Most women worked, and families became smaller. Even when employed full-time, however, women remained responsible for all household chores.

In the United States, Russian family structure has shrunk even further. Russian couples have significantly fewer children than the national average for American families. Education is emphasized, especially if it can be obtained at a Russian-language school. Many first-generation immigrants attempted to maintain ethnic identity by restricting their children to spouses from their immediate group, but marriage to non-Russians is now the norm.

Communication

Good manners and formality are expected in German conversations. Education is respected, and use of titles is important. Honesty and directness are appreciated. Germans are monochronistic and prefer to deal with one topic at a time. Direct eye contact is a sign of attentiveness and trust. A handshake is used in greeting, but there is little other touching between acquaintances.

Poles tend to speak more quietly than Americans and feel uncomfortable with loud behavior. Discussions about politics are avoided. Direct eye contact and a handshake of greeting and when leaving are appropriate.

Russians expect formality between acquaintances, and first names are saved for close friends and relatives. Russians may initially respond to any question that requires an affirmative or negative answer with a "no." Direct eye contact is the norm. A quick three kisses on the cheeks or a handshake is used in greeting. Touching becomes more prominent with familiarity. Russians may consider it impolite to sit with the legs splayed or with an ankle resting on the knee.

Gypsies are often very adaptive and may use many forms of communication, depending on the situation. Gypsies prefer minimal contact with non-Gypsies.

Many Americans of central European or Russian descent are highly acculturated.

Traditional Food Habits

Ingredients and Common Foods

Staples and Regional Variations

The regional variations in central European and Russian cuisine are minor. Ingredients in traditional dishes were dictated by what could be grown in the cold, often damp climate.

Legend has it that it was the Mongols who showed the central Europeans how to broil meat, make yogurt and other fermented dairy products, and preserve cabbage in brine.

Common ingredients are potatoes, beans, cabbage and members of the cabbage family, beets, eggs, dairy products, pork, beef, fish and seafood from the Baltic Sea, freshwater fish from local lakes and rivers, apples, rye, wheat, and barley (see Table 4.3 for the Cultural Food Groups). Foods were often dried, pickled, or fermented for preservation—for example, cucumber pickles, sour cream, and sauerkraut.

Bread is a staple item and there are more than 100 different varieties. Because the climate makes wheat harder to grow, bread is often made with rye and other grains; thus it is darker in color than bread made from wheat flour. Another common breadlike food in the region is dumplings (called *knedliky* in Czech, *Knödel* in German, and *kletski* in Russian), which can be made with flour or potatoes and with or without yeast. Stuffed dumplings, filled with meat, liver, bacon, potatoes, or fruit, are called *pierogi* (Polish), *pelmeni* (Russian), or *varenyky* (Ukranian). Dumplings are usually boiled in water. Related to the dumpling is stuffed pastry dough, which is baked or fried. It is customarily filled with meat or cabbage. Small individual pastries are called *pirozhki* in Russian, and a large oval pie is known as a *pirog* (also called as *kulebi*).

Next to bread, meat is probably the most important element of the diet. Pork is the most popular. *Schnitzel* is a meat cutlet, often lightly breaded and then fried. Ham is served fresh or cured; Poland is famous for its smoked ham, and in Germany, *Westphalian* ham is lightly smoked, cured, and cut into paper-thin slices. Beef is also common. In Germany, *Sauerbraten,* a marinated beef roast, is the national dish. Poultry is well liked. Germans often eat roast goose, stuffed with onions, apples, and herbs, on holidays. In Russia, chicken is stewed on special occasions. A famous Russian dish is *chicken Kiev,* breaded, fried chicken breasts filled with herbed butter.

In the past, meat was often scarce and expensive; thus many traditional recipes stretched it as far as possible. Dishes common throughout the region are ground meat that has been seasoned, mixed with a binder such as bread crumbs, milk, or eggs, formed into patties, then fried. In Germany, ground beef (and sometimes pork or veal) is served raw on toast as *steak Tartar.* Ground meat is also used to stuff vegetables (such as stuffed cabbage) or pastry, or is cooked as meatballs. Cut-up meat is often served in soups, stews, or one-pot dishes. In Germany a slowly simmered one-pot dish of meat, vegetables, potatoes, or dumplings is called *Eintopf.* Hungary is known for its *gulyás,* a paprika-spiced stew known as goulash in the United States. Sweet Hungarian paprika is ground, dried, red chile peppers to which sugar has been added. As chiles are a New World food, it is thought the Hungarians used black pepper to season their food before the discovery of the Americas.

Ground meats are also made into sausages. In Germany there are four basic types of sausage (*Wurst*). *Rohwurst,* similar to American-style

In Germanic regions the shape of bread is thought to be derived from pagan offerings to the gods; the bread substituted for animals in ritual sacrifices. Pretzels may once have been the ancient symbol for the solar cycle.

Pumpernickel is a very dark rye bread. Its German name derives from its supposed gas-producing qualities: *Pump,* meaning a small hollow sound, and *Nickel,* a dwarf.

Spätzle are tiny dumplings common in southern Germany. They are made by forcing the dough through a large spoon with small holes into boiling water. They are usually served as a side dish.

Game meats are traditional favorites throughout central Europe. In Germany the *wildfleisch* season is observed in winter, when venison, rabbit, and wild boar are featured at restaurants and markets.

A *frankfurter* means a sausage from the German city of Frankfurt. There are differing opinions as to how the frankfurter was introduced to America, but it soon became a favorite at baseball games. The cartoonist T. A. Dorgan drew a sausage with a tail, legs, and a head so that it looked like a dachshund, leading to the nickname "hot dog."

TABLE 4.3
Cultural Food Groups: Central European and Russian

Group	Comments
PROTEIN FOODS	
Milk/milk products	Dairy items, fresh or fermented, are frequently consumed.
	Whipped cream is popular.
Meat/poultry/fish/eggs/legumes	Meats are often extended by grinding and stewing.
	Russians tend to eat their meat very well done.
CEREALS/GRAINS	Bread or rolls are commonly served at all meals. Dumplings and *kasha* are also common.
	Numerous cakes, cookies, and pastries are popular.
	Rye flour is commonly used.
FRUITS/VEGETABLES	Potatoes are used extensively, as are all the cold-weather vegetables.
	Cabbage is fermented to make sauerkraut.
	Fruits and vegetables are often preserved by canning, drying, or pickling.
	Fruit is often added to meat dishes.
ADDITIONAL FOODS	
Seasonings	Central Europeans tend to season their dishes with sour-tasting flavors, such as sour cream and vinegar.
Nuts/seeds	Poppy seeds are often used in pastries; caraway seeds flavor cabbage and bread.
Beverages	Central Europeans drink coffee; Russians drink tea.
	Many varieties of beer are produced.
	Hungarians and Austrians tend to drink more wine than other central European people.
Fats/oils	

liverwurst, is cured and smoked by the butcher and can be eaten as is. *Bruhwurst* (the frankfurter is one type) is smoked and scalded by the butcher; it may be eaten as is or heated by simmering. *Knock-wurst,* which is like a cold cut, may be smoked and is fully cooked by the butcher. *Bratwurst,* such as breakfast sausage links, is sold raw by the butcher and must be pan-fried or grilled before eating.

TABLE 4.3
Cultural Food Groups: Central European and Russian—continued

Common Foods	Adaptations in the United States
Milk (cow, sheep) fresh and fermented (buttermilk, sour cream, yogurt), cheese, cream	Milk products still frequently consumed.
Meat: beef, boar, hare, lamb, pork (bacon, ham, pig's feet, head cheese), sausage, variety meats, veal, venison	Consumption of meat and poultry increased; use of variety meats decreased.
Fish: carp, flounder, frog, haddock, halibut, herring, mackerel, perch, pike, salmon, sardines, shad, shark, smelts, sturgeon, trout	Sausages often eaten.
Shellfish: crab, crawfish, eel, lobster, oysters, scallops, shrimp, turtle	
Poultry and small birds: chicken, cornish hen, duck, goose, grouse, partridge, pheasant, quail, squab, turkey	
Eggs: hens, fish (caviar)	
Legumes: kidney beans, lentils, navy beans, split peas (green and yellow)	
Barley, buckwheat (*kasha*), corn, millet, oats, potato starch, rice, rye, wheat	More white bread, less rye and pumpernickel bread is eaten.
Fruits: apples, apricots, blackberries, blueberries, sour cherries, sweet cherries, cranberries, currants, dates, gooseberries, grapefruit, grapes, lemons, lingonberries, melons, oranges, peaches, pears, plums, prunes, quinces, raisins, raspberries, rhubarb, strawberries	
Vegetables: asparagus, beets, broccoli, brussels sprouts, cabbage (red and green), carrots, cauliflower, celery, celery root, chard, cucumbers, eggplant, endive, green beans, kohlrabi, leeks, lettuce, mushrooms (domestic and wild), olives, onions, parsnips, peas, green peppers, potatoes, radishes, sorrel, spinach, tomatoes, turnips	
Allspice, anise, basil, bay leaves, borage, capers, caraway, cardamom, chervil, chives, cinnamon, cloves, curry powder, dill, garlic, ginger, horseradish, juniper, lemon, lovage, mace, marjoram, mint, mustard, paprika, parsley, pepper (black and white), poppy seeds, rosemary, rose water, saffron, sage, savory (summer and winter), tarragon, thyme, vanilla, vinegar, woodruff	Saffron is a popular spice in Pennsylvania Dutch fare.
Nuts: almonds (sweet and bitter), chestnuts, filberts, pecans, walnuts	
Seeds: poppy seeds, sunflower seeds	
Beer, hot chocolate, coffee, syrups and juices, fruit brandies, herbal teas, milk, tea, vodka, wine	
Butter, bacon, chicken fat, flaxseed oil, goose fat, lard, olive oil, salt pork, suet, vegetable oil	
Honey, sugar (white and brown), molasses	

The Polish are famous for *kielbasa,* a garlic-flavored pork sausage. In Austria, some sausages are called *wieners.* Two popular sausages with both the Czechs and Slovaks are *jaternice,* made from pork, and *jelita,* a blood sausage, which can be boiled or fried.

Fresh- and saltwater fish and seafood are often eaten smoked or cured. In Germany, herring is commonly pickled and eaten as a snack

With the collapse of state control over the countries of the former Soviet Union, caviar production is now unregulated. Quality control has disappeared, and overharvesting threatens to destroy the sturgeon population.

The national dish of Switzerland is cheese fondue (chunks of bread dipped into melted cheese). The Swiss are known for their zesty cheeses, with holes, such as *Emmenthal* (the original Swiss cheese) and *Gruyère*.

The dense chocolate cake known as *Sachertorte* was the subject of a 7-year court battle in Vienna over who had the right to claim the original recipe—the Hotel Sacher or Demel's, a famous bakery. The Hotel Sacher won.

The French Swiss introduced viticulture to the U.S. Midwest and the Italian Swiss introduced it to parts of California. Italian Swiss Colony Winery, founded in 1881, is one successful example.

Malzbier is a German beer (1% alcohol) that is considered appropriate for young children and nursing mothers.

or at the main meal. Eel is also popular. In Russia, smoked salmon and sturgeon are considered delicacies, as is *caviar,* which is fish roe. Caviar is classified according to its quality and source. *Beluga,* the choicest caviar, is taken from the largest sturgeon and has the largest eggs; its color varies from black to gray. *Sevruga* and *osetrova,* taken from smaller sturgeon, have smaller eggs and are sometimes a darker color. The finest caviar is sieved by hand to remove membranes and is lightly salted. Less choice roes are more heavily salted and pressed into bricks.

Dairy products are eaten daily. Cheeses may be served at any meal, from the fresh, sweet varieties to the strongly flavored aged types like Limburger. Fresh milk is drunk; butter is the preferred cooking fat. Buttermilk, sour cream, and fresh cream are also common ingredients in sauces, soups, stews, and baked products. In Austria and Germany, whipped cream is part of the daily diet, served with coffee or pastries.

In much of central Europe sweets are enjoyed daily. They are eaten at coffeehouses in the morning or afternoon, or bought at the local bakery and served as dessert. There are numerous types, such as cheesecakes, coffee cakes, doughnuts, and nut- or fruit-filled individual pastries. Austria is reputed to be the home of apple strudel, made from paper-thin sheets of dough rolled around cinnamon-spiced apple pieces. Germany is known for *Schwarzwälder Kirschtorte* (Black Forest cake), a rich chocolate cake layered with cherries, whipped cream, and *Kirsch* (cherry liqueur). *Dobosch torte,* a multilayered sponge cake with chocolate filling and caramel topping, is a favorite in Hungary.

In central Europe the common hot beverage is coffee. In Russia, strong tea, diluted with hot water from a *samovar,* is drunk instead of coffee. A samovar is a brass urn, which may be very ornate, heated by charcoal inserted in a vertical tube running through the center.

Although southwestern Germany, Austria, and Hungary produce excellent white wine, the most popular alcoholic drink in the region is beer. The Czechs are known for *pilsner* beer, which is bitter tasting but light in color and body. German beers can be sweet, bitter, weak, or strong, and are typically bottom-fermented (meaning the yeast sinks during brewing). *Lager,* a bottom-fermented beer that is aged for about 6 weeks, is the most common type. *Bock* beer is the strongest flavored, traditionally made once a year when the brewing tanks are cleaned. *Märzenbier,* a strong beer midway between a pilsner and a bock beer, is served at Oktoberfest (see section on "Special Occasions") in Munich.

Vodka, which is commonly drunk in Poland and Russia, is a distilled spirit made from potatoes. It is served ice cold and is often flavored with seasonings, such as lemon or black pepper. In Poland, one vodka, *goldwasser,* contains flakes of pure gold.

Meal Composition and Cycle

Daily Patterns

Central Europe   In the past, people of this region would eat five or six large meals a day, if they could afford it. The poor, and usually the people who worked the land, had fewer meals, which were often meatless. Today modern work schedules have affected the meal pattern, resulting in three meals with snacks each day.

In Germany and the countries of central Europe the first meal of the day is breakfast, which consists of bread served with butter and jam. Sometimes it is accompanied by soft-boiled eggs, cheese, and ham. At midmorning, many people have their second breakfast, which may include coffee and pastries, bread and fruit, or a small sandwich. Lunch is the main meal of the day. Traditionally people ate lunch at home, but today they are more likely to go to a cafeteria or restaurant. A proper lunch begins with soup, followed by a fish course, then one or two meat dishes served with vegetables, and perhaps stewed fruit. Dessert is the final course and is usually served with whipped cream. A quicker and lighter lunch may consist of only a stew or a one-pot meal.

A coffee break is taken at midafternoon, if time permits. It typically includes coffee and cake or cookies. The evening meal tends to be light, usually salads and an assortment of pickled or smoked fish, cheese, ham, and sausages eaten with a selection of breads. Guests are usually not invited for dinner but may come for dessert and wine later in the evening.

Gypsies customarily eat two meals each day, first thing in the morning and in the late afternoon. Meals are typically social occasions, featuring the dishes common in their adopted homeland; stews, fried foods, and unleavened breads are especially popular.

Russia   In Czarist times the aristocracy ate four complete meals per day; dinner was the largest. The majority of the population never ate as lavishly or as often. One part of the traditional Czarist evening meal, *zakuski* (meaning "small bites"), is still part of dinner in Russia today. The meal starts with zakuski, an array of appetizers, which may range from two simple dishes, such as cucumbers in sour cream and pickled herring, to an entire table spread with countless hors d'oeuvres. An assortment of zakuski usually includes a variety of small open-faced sandwiches topped with cold, smoked fish; anchovies or sardines; cold tongue and pickles; and ham, sausages, or salami. Caviar, the most elegant of zakuski, is served with an accompanying plate of chopped hard-boiled eggs and finely minced onions. Other zakuski include marinated or pickled vegetables, hot meat dishes, and eggs served a variety of ways.

The meal that peasants ate after a long day's work is still the basis of a typical dinner in present-day Russia. The staples are bread; soup

In Germany, cutting potatoes, pancakes, or dumplings with a knife is an insult to the cook or host because it suggests that these items are tough.

Sharing food is essential to Gypsy culture. The harshest punishment that can be imposed on an individual is to be banned from communal meals.

Gypsies avoid eating food with their left hands.

Buckwheat (groats) is a grain native to central Asia.

The tradition of the Christmas tree comes from Germany. Traditionally the tree was decorated with cookies (such as *Lebkuchen* and *Pfeffernüsse*) and candy ornaments. (© Miro Vintoniv/Stock, Boston.)

Hazelnuts are also called filberts because they ripen at the end of summer near St. Philibert's Day (August 22nd).

Marzipan, a paste of ground almonds and sugar, is commonly used in desserts and candies throughout central Europe.

In the Polish Easter meal the dairy products, meats, and pastries symbolize the fertility and renewal of springtime, while the horseradish is to remember the bitterness and disappointments in life.

made from beets (*borscht*), cabbage (*shchi*), or fish (*ukha*); and *kasha* (cooked grain, usually buckwheat). Beer brewed from bread, called *kvas,* usually accompanies the meal.

Special Occasions

The majority of central European holidays have a religious significance, although some traditions date back to pre-Christian times. The two major holidays in the region are Christmas and Easter. Many of the American symbols and activities associated with these holidays, such as the Christmas tree and the Easter egg hunt, were brought to the United States by central European immigrants.

Germany   Germany is a land of popular festivals: Nearly all are accompanied by food and drink. Probably the best-known celebration is Munich's Oktoberfest, which lasts for 16 days from late September through early October. Founded in 1810 to commemorate the marriage of Prince Ludwig of Bavaria, it is now an annual festival with polka bands and prodigious sausage-eating and beer-drinking.

Advent and Christmas are the holiest seasons in German-speaking countries. The Christmas tree, a remnant of pagan winter solstice rites, is lit on Christmas Eve when the presents, brought not by Santa Claus but by the Christ Child, are opened. The Christmas tree is not taken down until Epiphany, January 6th. A large festive dinner is served on Christmas Day, and it is customary for families to visit one another. Foods served during the Christmas season include carp on Christmas Eve and roast hare or goose accompanied by apples and nuts on Christmas Day. Brightly colored marzipan candies in the shape of fruits and animals are traditional Christmas sweets. Other desserts prepared during the season are spice cakes and cookies (*Pfeffernüsse* and *Lebkuchen*), fruit cakes (*Stollen*), cakes in the shape of a Christmas tree (*Baumkuchen*), and gingerbread houses.

On Easter Sunday the Easter bunny hides colored eggs in the house and garden for the children to find. Ham and pureed peas are typically served for Easter dinner. Candy Easter eggs and rabbits are also part of the festivities.

Poland   Christmas and Easter are the two most important holidays in Poland, a predominantly Catholic country. On Easter the festive table may feature a roast suckling pig, hams, coils of sausages, and roast veal. Always included are painted hard-boiled eggs, grated horseradish, and a Paschal lamb sculptured from butter or white sugar. Before the feasting begins, one of the eggs is shelled, divided, and reverently eaten. The crowning glory of the meal is the *babka*, a rich yeast cake. All the foods are blessed by the priest before being served.

On Christmas Eve, traditionally a fast day, the meal consists of soup, fish, noodle dishes, and pastries. One popular soup, *barszcz Wigilijny,* a cousin to Russian borscht, is made with mushrooms as well as beets. Carp is usually the fish served on Christmas Eve. A rich Christmas cake, *makowiec,* is shaped like a jelly roll and filled with black poppy seeds, honey, raisins, and almonds.

Jelly doughnuts, *paczki,* are eaten on New Year's Eve, while on New Year's Day, *bigos,* "hunter's stew," made with a variety of meats and vegetables (some form of cabbage is required), is washed down with plenty of vodka.

Austria, Hungary, the Czech Republic, and Slovakia At Christmastime the Czechs eat carp four different ways: breaded and fried, baked with dried prunes, cold in aspic, and in a fish soup. The Christmas Eve meal might also include pearl barley soup with mushrooms, fruits, and decorated cookies. Christmas dinner features giblet soup with noodles, roast goose with dumplings and sauerkraut, braided sweet bread (*vanocka* or *houska*), fruits and nuts, and coffee. *Kolaches,* round yeast buns filled with poppy seeds, dried fruit, or cottage cheese, are served at the Christmas meal and on most festive occasions. For Easter a baked ham or roasted kid is served with *mazanec* (vanocka dough with raisins and almonds shaped into a round loaf).

The Slovaks break the Advent fast on Christmas Eve by eating *oplatky,* small wafer-like Communion bread spread with honey. The meal may contain wild mushroom soup, cabbage and potato dumplings, stuffed cabbage (*holubjy*), and mashed potato dumplings covered with butter and cheese (*halusky*). A favorite dessert is *babalky,* pieces of bread sliced, scalded and drained, then rolled in ground poppy seeds, sugar, or honey. Mulled wine usually accompanies this meal, as do assorted poppy seed and nut pastries and a variety of fruits. For Easter the Slovaks prepare *paska,* a dessert in the form of a pyramid containing cheese, cream, butter, eggs, sugar, and candied fruits, decorated with a cross. The meal, blessed by the priest on Holy Saturday, includes ham, sausage (*klobása*), roast duck or goose, horseradish, an Easter cheese called *syrek,* and an imitation cheese ball made from eggs (*hrudka*).

In Hungary the most important religious holiday is Easter. Starting before Lent, pancakes are traditionally eaten on Shrove Tuesday; sour eggs and herring salad are served on Ash Wednesday. During Easter week, new spring vegetables are enjoyed, as well as painted Easter eggs. The Good Friday meal may include a wine-flavored soup, stuffed eggs, and baked fish. The biggest and most important meal of the year is the feast of Easter Eve, which consists of a rich chicken soup served with dumplings or noodles, followed by roasted meat (ham, pork, or lamb), then several pickled vegetables, stuffed cabbage rolls, and finally a selection of cakes and pastries served with coffee. The

Polish tradition is to invite the poor and the ill to Christmas Eve supper.

One customary Christmas Eve dish in Poland is *karp po zydowsku*, chilled slices of carp in a sweet-and-sour aspic with raisins and almonds. It is of Jewish origin, dating to when Poland was a haven for Jews in the fourteenth century.

An ancient Slavic saying is "A guest in the house is God in the house."

Vanocka, a Christmas bread popular in the Czech Republic. (Courtesy of Florida State News Bureau.)

Christmas Eve meal, which is meatless, usually features fish and potatoes. The Christmas Day meal often includes roast turkey, chicken, or goose accompanied by roast potatoes and stuffed cabbage, followed by desserts of brandied fruits or fruit compote and poppy seed and nut cakes.

In addition to Christmas and Easter the Austrians celebrate *Fasching* (a holiday also known in southern Germany). Originating as a pagan ceremony to drive out the evil spirits of winter in which a procession would parade down the main street of a town ringing cow bells, it developed into a multiday carnival associated with Lent.

Russia Before the 1917 revolution, Russians celebrated a full calendar of religious holidays. Today on fast days the observant do not eat any animal products (see Chapter 2 for the fast days in the Eastern Orthodox Church). Of all the holidays, the most important is Easter, which replaced a pre-Christian festival that marked the end of the bleak winter season.

The "Butter Festival" (*maslenitas*) precedes the 40 days of Lent. One food eaten during this period is *blini,* raised buckwheat pancakes. Blini can be served with a variety of toppings such as butter, jam, sour cream, smoked salmon, or caviar. Butter is the traditional topping because it cannot be eaten during Lent.

Traditional foods served on Easter after midnight Mass are *pascha,* similar to the Slovak paska but decorated with the letters "XB"

The term *pascha* comes from the Hebrew word for Passover, *Pesach.*

("Christ is risen"); *kulich,* a cake made from a very rich sweet yeast dough baked in a tall, cylindrical mold; and red or hand-decorated hard-boiled eggs. On Pentecost (Trinity) Sunday (50 days after Easter), kulich left over from Easter is eaten.

Twelve different dishes are served during the Christmas Eve meal. One of the traditional dishes may be *kutia,* wheat grains combined with honey, poppy seeds, and stewed dried fruit. A festive meal is served on Christmas Day. On New Year's Day, children receive gifts, and spicy ginger cakes are eaten. A pretzel-shaped sweet bread, *kren-del,* is eaten on wedding anniversaries and name days (saint's day celebrated as birthdays in the Eastern Orthodox faith).

Therapeutic Uses of Foods

A study of elderly German Americans found that they sometimes use home remedies to treat minor illnesses. Chicken soup is used for diarrhea, vomiting, or sore throat. Tea is taken for an upset stomach, and milk with honey is commonly used for a cough (Spector, 1991). Traditionally the Pennsylvania Dutch believe that cold drinks are unhealthy and that eating meat three times a day is the cornerstone of a good diet. Herbal teas are consumed for a variety of complaints (Hostetler, 1976; Yoder, 1976). Elderly Polish Americans reportedly believe that sauerkraut is good for colic, as are tea and soda water. Chamomile tea is used for cramps, tea with dried raspberries and wine for colds, cooked garlic for high blood pressure, and warm beverages (milk, tea, or lemonade) for coughs.

Gypsies have unique health beliefs, many involving food. For example, Gypsies traditionally think that fresh food is the most nourishing and that leftovers are unwholesome. Canned and frozen items may be mistrusted as not being fresh. Many Gypsies believe that non-Gypsies carry disease, and they may insist on using disposable plates and utensils anytime they must eat in a public place. Insufficient intake of "lucky" foods, such as salt, pepper, vinegar, and garlic, can predispose a person to poor health. Home remedies are common, such as tea with crushed strawberries, asafetida (called Devil's Dung), and ghost vomit (*Fuligo septica*) (Hancock, 1991; Sutherland, 1992).

Traditionally some Pennsylvania Dutch considered oysters to be an aphrodisiac and warned young women that eating them would lead to a wanton heart.

Ghost vomit (*Fuligo septica*) is a myxomycete or slime mold. The thin, yellow, creeping mass is found on rotting wood and other decaying material, where it eats bacteria.

Contemporary Food Habits in the United States

Adaptations of Food Habits

Ingredients and Common Foods

The central European and Russian diet is not significantly different from American fare. Immigrants made few changes in the types of foods they ate after they came to the United States. What did change was the quantity of certain foods. Most central European immigrants were not wealthy in their native lands, and their diets had included meager amounts of meat. After immigrating to the United States, they increased the quantity of meat they ate considerably.

The people of eastern Pennsylvania, where there is a large concentration of German Americans, still eat many traditional German dishes adapted to accommodate available ingredients. Common foods include *scrapple* (also called *ponhaus*), a pork and cornmeal sausage flavored with herbs and cooked in a loaf pan, served for breakfast with syrup; *sticky buns,* little sweet rolls thought to be descended from German cinnamon rolls known as *Schnecken; schnitz un knepp* (apples and dumplings), a one-pot dish made from boiled ham, dried apple slices, and brown sugar, topped with a dumpling dough; *boova shenkel,* beef stew with potato dumplings; *hinkel welschkarn suup,* a rich chicken soup brimming with tender kernels of corn; *apple butter,* a rich fruit spread, very much like a jam; *schmierkaes,* a German cottage cheese; *funnel cake,* a type of doughnut; *shoofly pie,* a molasses pie thought to be descended from a German crumb cake called *Streuselkuchen; fastnachts,* doughnuts, originally prepared and eaten on Shrove Tuesday to use up the fat that could not be eaten during Lent; and *sweets and sours,* sweet-and-sour relishes, such as coleslaw, crabapple jelly, pepper relish, apple butter, and bread-and-butter pickles, served with lunch and dinner. Saffron crocuses were cultivated in parts of Pennsylvania and the seasoning was used to color many dishes dark yellow, from soups to a traditional wedding cake known as *Schwenkfelder*.

Much of German cooking has been incorporated into American cuisine. Many foods still have German names, although they are so common in the United States that their source is unrecognized (e.g., sauerkraut, pretzels). Other foods contributed by the Germans are hamburgers, frankfurters, *braunschweiger* (liver sausage), *thuringer* (summer sausage), liverwurst, jelly doughnuts, and pumpernickel bread. Beer production, especially in Milwaukee, was dominated by the Germans for more than 100 years. German immigrants created a lager-style beer that is milder, lighter, and less bitter than typical German beer; it can now be described as American-style beer (see also "Regional Americans," Chapter 11).

Meal Composition and Cycle

Third- and fourth-generation central European and Russian Americans tend to consume three meals a day (with snacks), and meal composition is similar to that of a typical American meal, although more dairy products and sausages may be eaten. Some traditional foods and ingredients may not be available in areas without large central European or Russian populations.

In the 1800s, fried oysters with a glass of Schnapps was a popular Pennsylvania Dutch breakfast for men.

"Sauerkraut Yankees" was the derogatory nickname for the Pennsylvania Dutch during the Civil War.

Pennsylvania Dutch funnel cake is an unusual "doughnut" made by pouring the batter through a funnel or from a pitcher into the hot oil in a swirled pattern.

Many central European and Russian American families serve traditional foods at special occasions. Polish Americans celebrate Pulaski Day on October 11th, a national day of remembrance that features a large parade in traditional apparel down the streets of New York City. The Austrians typically observe St. Nicholas Day (December 6th), when apples and nuts are put in the stockings of well-behaved children and coal is given to the naughty ones. Hungarian Americans observe three unique holidays in the United States with a combination of patriotic and religious activities. The first is March 15th, commemorating the Revolution of 1848; the second is August 20th, St. Stephen's Day; and the attempted revolt known as the Revolution of 1956 is honored on October 23rd.

Among the Amish, many national holidays, such as the Fourth of July and Halloween, are not observed. A second day of celebration is added to Christmas, Easter, and Pentecost: The first day is reserved for sacred ceremonies; the second day for social and recreational activities. Most Amish celebrate all holidays quietly with family.

SCANDINAVIANS

The Scandinavian countries include Sweden, Norway, Denmark, Finland, and Iceland. With the exception of Denmark and the island of Iceland, they are located north of the Baltic and North seas and share

Few Icelanders have made their home in the United States; the 1990 U.S. census indicates approximately 40,000 Americans claim Icelandic descent.

Veal oscar, veal topped with a béarnaise sauce, white asparagus, and lobster or crab, is named after Swedish king Oscar II (1872–1907), a renowned gourmet.

common borders with each other and Russia. Most of the population in Scandinavia is concentrated in the warmer southern regions; the harsher northern areas extend above the Arctic Circle. Norway's weather is more temperate than that of Finland and Sweden because its long western coastline is washed in the temperate North Atlantic Drift. Denmark juts into the North Sea to the north of Germany, and its capital, Copenhagen, is directly opposite from Sweden. The majority of Scandinavian immigrants to the United States arrived in the 1800s. This next section reviews the traditional foods of Scandinavia and the Swedish, Norwegian, and Danish contributions to the American diet.

Cultural Perspective

History of the Scandinavian Countries

In the fourteenth century, Margaret of Denmark united the rule of Denmark, Sweden, and Norway (at this time Finland was under the rule of Sweden and Iceland was controlled by Norway). Norway virtually ceased to exist as a separate kingdom and was ruled by Danish governors for the following four centuries. Sweden, however, could not be controlled by Denmark, and King Gustavus I, founder of the modern Swedish state, came to rule in 1523. Sweden became the dominant Protestant (Lutheran) power of continental Europe in the seventeenth century. Norway and Finland did not become independent nations until the twentieth century—Norway in 1905 and Finland after the Russian Revolution of 1917.

All four countries have enjoyed economic prosperity and industrial development in this century. During World War II, Germany invaded Denmark and Norway, while Sweden remained neutral and Finland was aligned with the Germans. The Soviet Union invaded Finland in 1944 and eventually forced the Germans out. After the war, Finland was required to pay the Soviet Union $300 million and to cede disputed territory. Iceland became an independent nation in 1944. Today Denmark, Norway, and Sweden have constitutional monarchies, and Finland and Iceland are democratic republics.

History of Scandinavians in the United States

It is believed that the Norsemen (ancient Scandinavians), renowned seafarers and explorers, first discovered North America and colonized as far west as Minnesota in the thirteenth and fourteenth centuries. The documented presence of Scandinavians in America dates back to the seventeenth century. Jonas Bronck, a Dane, arrived in 1629 and

Danish Americans in Texas, slicing apples, 1915. (From Cynthia Thyrsen Preismeyer, Danevang, TX, copy from Institute of Texan Cultures at San Antonio.)

bought a large tract of land from the Native Americans that later became known as the Bronx in New York City.

Immigration Patterns

The majority of Scandinavians arrived in the United States in the 1800s, led by the Norwegians and the Swedes. During the nineteenth century no other country, except Ireland, contributed as large a proportion of its population to the settlement of North America as Norway. During the 1900s an additional 363,000 Norwegians, more than 1,250,000 Swedes, 363,000 Danes, and 300,000 Finns entered the United States.

The peak years of Scandinavian immigration to the United States were between 1820 and 1930. Overpopulation was the single most important reason for emigration. The population of all the Scandinavian countries had increased substantially, resulting in economies that could not absorb the unemployed and landless agrarian workers. In Sweden the problem was magnified by a severe famine in the late 1860s. For the Norwegians there was the additional lure of freedom that America offered, and the chance for emancipation from the peasant class. The Scandinavians settled in homogeneous communities.

The Norwegians and Swedes often moved to the homestead states of the Midwest, especially Illinois, Minnesota, Michigan, Iowa, and Wisconsin. One-fifth of all Swedish immigrants settled in Minnesota. Pockets of Finns and Danes also settled in this region, but they were fewer in number. Norwegians and Swedes also migrated to the coastal areas of the Northwest, working in the lumber and fishing industries.

The Scandinavians introduced the cast iron stove to the United States. Cooking was done previously in fireplaces and brick ovens.

The shipping industry attracted Norwegians to New York City, where they still live in an ethnic enclave in Brooklyn.

Although Swedes and Norwegians are often associated with the rural communities of the Midwest, by 1890, one-third of all Swedes lived in cities and many Norwegians were seeking opportunity in the urban areas. Chicago and Minneapolis still have large Scandinavian populations. The Swedes were particularly prominent in Chicago's construction industry, which was commonly referred to as a Swedish trade guild.

The Danes, in an effort to preserve their ethnicity, developed twenty-four rural communities between 1886 and 1935 in which, for a set number of years, land could be sold only to Danes. The best known of these communities are Tyler, Minnesota; Danevang, Texas; Askov, Minnesota; Dagmar, Missouri; and Solvang, California. Today most Danes live in cities, primarily on the East or West coasts. The largest concentrations of Danes are in the Los Angeles area and in Chicago.

Following World War I, U.S. immigration from Finland dropped significantly as Finns chose other countries for emigration. As the Finnish population stagnated, ethnic identity became very difficult to maintain. Second- and third-generation Finns are highly acculturated.

Current Demographics and Socioeconomic Status

According to the 1990 U.S. census, there are approximately 1.6 million Danes, 4.7 million Swedes, 3.9 million Norwegians, and 650,000 Finns and their descendants now living in the United States. Most Scandinavians assimilated rapidly into American society, rising from blue-collar to white-collar jobs within a few generations. Many Norwegians and Swedes have continued farming in the Midwest, although many Norwegian Americans are employed in management or specialty professions, and Swedish Americans have made significant contributions in writing and publishing, the arts, education, the ministry, and politics. Danes entered a variety of occupations, but they were most prominent in gardening, raising livestock, and dairy farming. Urban Danes are not associated with specific occupations. Finnish American men have been active in fields such as natural resources management, mining engineering, and geology, while women have been attracted to nursing and home economics.

Cultural Organizations

Many Scandinavian ethnic organizations grew out of the need for mutual help or cultural preservation. Although there are hundrds of such organizations at the local and regional level, the larger national ones are The Danish Brotherhood; the American Scandinavian Society; the Sons of Norway; the Swedish Council of America, which coordinates Swedish American activities; and the Finnish American League, which promotes Finnish culture in the United States. An international organization with chapters in the United States, the Norsemen's Federation, was founded in Norway to strengthen ties among Norwegians throughout the world.

Worldview

Religion

The majority of Scandinavians who immigrated to the United States were Lutheran, although each nationality had its own branch of the church. As with other immigrant groups, the church helped to ease the adjustment of recent arrivals and provided ethnic companionship. In this century, many of the Scandinavian and German Lutheran churches joined together to create the Evangelical Lutheran Church in America (ELCA).

Family

The nuclear Scandinavian family was at the center of rural life. The father controlled all family affairs (often to the dissatisfaction of the wife and children). Families were typically large; ten and twelve children were not uncommon. Kinship ties were strong. In America, families were expected to pay the way for relatives remaining in Scandinavia to come to the United States, where they would be given a room, board, and help in finding employment. The family structure was easily maintained in the early homogeneous communities and on isolated farms. The power of the father diminished as the Scandinavian Americans became more integrated in mainstream society; among the Finns it has been noted that when both parents work, they may choose to have only one child.

Communication

Scandinavians tend to be highly analytical. Emotions are controlled; superficiality and personal inquiries are avoided. Swedes and Finns are comfortable with silence during a conversation. As a rule, Danes are a little more informal than other Scandinavians or northern Europeans and may use first names. Danes and Swedes make and maintain direct eye contact, whereas Norwegians and Finns make direct eye contact intermittently. A brief, firm handshake is used in greetings. Other touching is infrequent, reserved for friends and relatives.

TABLE 4.4
Cultural Food Groups: Scandinavian

Group	Comments
PROTEIN FOODS	
Milk/milk products	Dairy products, often fermented, are used extensively.
Meat/poultry/fish/eggs/legumes	Fish is a major source of protein, often preserved by drying, pickling, fermenting, or smoking.
CEREALS/GRAINS	Wheat is used less than other grains.
	Rye is used frequently in breads.
FRUITS/VEGETABLES	Fruits with cheese are frequently served for dessert.
	Preserved fruits and pickled vegetables are common.
	Tapioca (from cassava) eaten.
ADDITIONAL FOODS	
Seasonings	
Nuts/seeds	Marzipan (sweetened almond paste) is used in many sweets.
Beverages	
Fats/oils	Butter is often used.
Sweeteners	

Traditional Food Habits

In Scandinavia they say, "Danes live to eat, Norwegians eat to live, and Swedes eat to drink."

The fare of Scandinavia is simple and hearty, featuring the abundant foods of the sea and making the best use of the limited foods produced on land. Most Scandinavian cooking and food processing

TABLE 4.4
Cultural Food Groups: Scandinavian—continued

Common Foods	Adaptations in the United States
Buttermilk, milk, cream (cow, goat, reindeer); cheese, sour cream, yogurt	
Meat: beef, goat, lamb, hare, pork (bacon, ham, sausage), reindeer, veal, venison	More meat and less fish is consumed.
Fish and shellfish: anchovies, bass, carp, cod, crab, crawfish, eel, flounder, grayling, haddock, halibut, herring, lobster, mackerel, mussels, oysters, perch, pike, plaice, roche, salmon (fresh, smoked, pickled), sardines, shrimp, sprat, trout, turbot, whitefish	
Poultry and small birds: chicken, duck, goose, grouse, partridge, pheasant, quail, turkey	
Eggs: chicken, goose, fish	
Legumes: lima beans, split peas (green and yellow)	
Barley, oats, rice, rye, wheat	More wheat used, fewer other grains.
Fruits: apples, apricots, blueberries, cherries, cloudberries, currants, lingonberries, oranges, pears, plums, prunes, raisins, raspberries, rhubarb, strawberries	A greater variety of fruits and vegetables are obtainable in the United States than in Scandinavia, but may not be eaten.
Vegetables: asparagus, beets, cabbage (red and green), carrots, cauliflower, celery, celery root, cucumber, green beans, green peppers, nettles, kohlrabi, leeks, mushrooms (many varieties), onions, parsnips, peas, potatoes, radishes, spinach, tomatoes, yellow and white turnips	
Allspice, bay leaf, capers, cardamom, chervil, cinnamon, cloves, curry powder, dill, garlic, ginger, horseradish, lemon juice, lemon and orange peel, mace, marjoram, mustard, mustard seed, nutmeg, paprika, parsley, pepper (black, cayenne, white) rose hips, saffron, salt, tarragon, thyme, vanilla, vinegar	
Almonds, chestnuts, walnuts	
Coffee, hot chocolate, milk, tea, ale, aquavit, beer, vodka, wine, liqueurs	
Butter, lard, margarine, salt pork	
Sugar (white and brown), honey, molasses	

reflect preservation methods of previous centuries. Fish was dried, smoked, or pickled, and milk was often fermented or allowed to sour before being consumed. Scandinavians still prepare a large variety of preserved foods and prefer their food salty. The basics of the Scandinavian diet are listed in the Cultural Food Groups list (Table 4.4).

Ingredients and Common Foods

Staples and Regional Variations

The Scandinavians are probably best known for their use of fish and shellfish, such as salmon, sardines, and shrimp. In Norway the fish-processing industry is believed to date back to the ninth century. Today Scandinavian dried salt cod is exported all over the world. *Lutefisk* is prepared by soaking the dried cod in a lye solution before cooking. Other fish dishes include salmon marinated in dill, called *gravlax;* smoked salmon, known as *lox;* and the many varieties of pickled herring.

The cooking of Finland mixes Swedish and Russian elements, such as *smörgåsbords, piroshkis* (meat turnovers), and *blini* (thin buckwheat pancakes). Vodka is preferred over *aquavit.*

Without fermentation the Scandinavians would not have been able to store the plentiful fresh dairy products produced in the spring and summer. Although they drink milk and cook many of their dishes with cream and butter, they also use considerable quantities of fermented dairy products, such as sour cream, cheese, and buttermilk. Popular Danish cheeses are semifirm, mellow, nutty-tasting *Tybo* (usually encased in red wax); firm and bland *Danbo;* semisoft, slightly acidic *Havarti;* rich, soft *Crèma Dania;* and Danish blue cheese.

Common fruits and vegetables are apples, potatoes, cabbage, onions, and beets. Pea soups are a winter specialty throughout Scandinavia, often served with pancakes. Several varieties of berries (particularly lingonberries) and wild mushrooms are collected from local forests.

Meat, traditionally in limited supply, was stretched by chopping it and combining it with other ingredients. Today the Scandinavians still eat many vegetables, such as onions and cabbage, stuffed with ground pork, veal, or beef. The Swedes are known for their tasty meatballs and the Danes for *fricadeller,* which are patties of ground pork and veal, breadcrumbs, and onion fried in butter.

Bread is also a staple food item and is often prepared from rye flour (white bread is called French bread in Scandinavia). The Scandinavian breads may or may not be leavened, are often hard, and vary in size and shape. To keep bread for the winter, crusty rye breads with holes punched in them are hung from the ceilings and dried. A thin round bread called *lefser,* made of potatoes cooked on an ungreased griddle, is usually eaten with butter and sugar and folded like a handkerchief.

During Advent, Danish *aebleskivers* are filled with whole almonds.

Desserts, whether they are served after a meal or at a coffee break, are rich but not overly sweet. Most are made with butter and also contain cream or sweetened cheese and the spice cardamom. *Aebleskivers* are spherical Danish pancake puffs, sometimes stuffed with fruit preserves. Another popular dessert is pancakes served with preserved berries or jam. The Scandinavians use almonds, almond paste, or *marzipan* in desserts as often as Americans use chocolate. The Danes are best known for their pastries or, as they call them, *Wienerbrød* (Vienna bread). The pastries were brought to Denmark

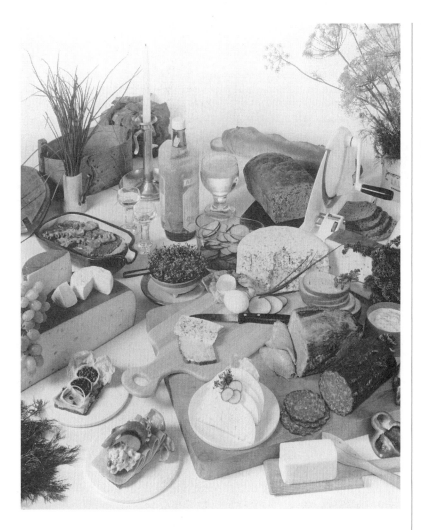

Danish *smørrebrød*: Danish Fontina and Havarti cheeses, ham, salami, and smoked salmon are a few of the toppings typical of the open-face sandwiches known in Denmark as smørrebrød. (Courtesy of Denmark Cheese Association.)

by Viennese bakers 100 years ago when the Danish bakers went on strike. When the strike was over, the Danes improved the buttery yeast dough by adding jam and other fillings.

Besides milk and other dairy drinks, common beverages are coffee, tea, beer, and *aquavit*. Aquavit, which means "water of life," is a liquor made from the distillation of potatoes or grain. It may be flavored with an herb, such as caraway, and is served ice cold in a *Y*-shaped glass. Beer is customarily consumed everyday; occasionally it is drunk with aquavit.

When Scandinavians toast, they say *skoal*, which probably derives from the word for skull. Ancient Norsemen used the empty craniums of their enemies as drinking vessels.

Øllebrød, a Danish rye bread porridge made with nonalcoholic beer, is a favorite breakfast for children.

One theory about the origin of the *smørrebrød* is that it dates back to the time before people had dishes, when rounds of bread were used for plates.

Both the Swedes and the Finns relish crawfish feasts, at which abundant amounts of the crustacean are served with melted butter and aquavit or vodka to rinse them down.

In Sweden, on the morning of December 13th, St. Lucia's Day, the eldest daughter in the home, wearing a long white dress and a crown of lingonberry greens studded with lit candles, serves her parents saffron yeast buns and coffee in bed.

The tradition of serving the two simple foods (rice and fish) for Christmas dates back at least four centuries when the Scandinavians were Catholic and Christmas was a fast, instead of a feast.

Christmas ginger cookies, *pepparkakor* in Swedish and *pebernødder* in Danish, have become a favorite in Utah. They were brought by Scandinavian Mormon converts and are known as pepper cookies.

Meal Composition and Cycle

Daily Patterns

The Scandinavians eat three meals a day, plus a coffee break midmorning, late in the afternoon, or after the evening meal. Breakfast is usually a light meal that may consist of bread or oatmeal porridge, eggs, pastries, cheese, bread, fruit, potatoes, or herring. Fruit soups may be served in the winter, topped with thick cream.

Lunch in Denmark is frequently a *smørrebrød,* which means "buttered bread," an open-faced sandwich eaten with a knife and fork. Buttered bread is topped with anything from smoked salmon to sliced boiled potatoes with bacon, small sausages, and tomato slices. Smørrebrød may also be served as a late afternoon or bedtime snack.

A buffet meal in Sweden is the *smörgåsbord* (bread and butter table), a large variety of hot and cold dishes arrayed on a table and traditionally served with aquavit. Ritual dictates the order in which foods are eaten at a smorgasbord. The Swedes start with herring, followed by other fish dishes, such as smoked salmon and fried fins. Next are the meats and salads (pâtés and cold cuts), and the final course before dessert is comprised of hot dishes, such as Swedish meatballs and mushroom omelets.

Dinner is also large, often including an appetizer, soup, entree, vegetables, and dessert. Potatoes are usually served with the evening meal. Coffee is served with the dessert course.

Special Occasions

December is the darkest month of the year in Scandinavia, and Christmas celebrations are a welcome diversion. The Christmas season lasts from Advent (4 weeks before Christmas) until January 13th, Saint Canute's Day. However, the climax of the season is on Christmas Eve, when the biggest, richest, and most lavish meal of the year is eaten.

Traditional foods eaten on Christmas Eve are rice porridge sprinkled with sugar and cinnamon; and lutefisk served with a white sauce, melted butter, green peas, boiled potatoes, and mustard. Buried in the rice porridge is one blanched almond; the person who receives it will have good fortune in the coming year. Another common food served for Christmas is pork or ham, often accompanied by sauerkraut or red cabbage. In Denmark a goose is preferred.

Dozens of cookies and cakes are prepared for the Christmas season. The cookies are often flavored with ginger and cloves; the Christmas tree may be hung with gingerbread figures. Deep-fried, brandy-flavored dough, known as *klejner, klener,* or *klenätter,* is also popular. The traditional holiday beverage is *glögg,* a hot alcoholic punch.

Midsummer's Day (June 24th) is a popular secular Scandinavian holiday. It features maypoles, bonfires, and feasting. In Sweden, fish accompanied by boiled new potatoes and wild strawberries are eaten; in Norway, *rommegrot,* a cream pudding sprinkled with cinnamon and sugar, is served; and in Finland, new potatoes with dill and smoked salmon are typical festive fare.

Contemporary Food Habits in the United States

Adaptations of Food Habits

The Scandinavians assimilated rapidly into American society, yet their diet did not change significantly. Many of their food habits are similar to the diet of the American majority, such as three large meals per day containing dairy products and animal protein. Because many Scandinavians settled in the Midwest, their consumption of fresh seafood declined, but they eat freshwater fish and prepare dishes from dried salt cod, such as lutefisk.

Scandinavian Americans still prepare traditional holiday foods such as rice porridge and lutefisk. Some Scandinavian foods, such as meatballs, Swedish butter cookies, and Danish pastries, are commonly eaten by many Americans.

Midsummer's Day is still observed by many Scandinavian Americans. In some areas of the United States, it has become *Svenskarnas* Day (Swede's Day), celebrating Swedish culture and solidarity.

St. Urho's Day (March 16th) was invented by Finnish Americans as a spoof on St. Patrick's Day. It commemorates the driving of the grasshoppers from Finland by the saint.

5

Africans

African Americans are one of the largest cultural groups in the United States, including nearly 30 million people, more than 12 percent of the total American population. The majority are blacks who came originally from West Africa, although some have immigrated from the Caribbean, Central America, and, more recently, from the famine- and strife-stricken East African nations. A small number of Americans of African heritage are white, primarily immigrants from the nation of South Africa.

Most African Americans are the only U.S. citizens whose ancestors came by force, not choice. Their long history in America has been characterized by persecution and segregation. At the same time, blacks have contributed greatly to the development of American culture. The languages, music, arts, and cuisine of Africa have mingled with European and Native American influences since the beginnings of the nation to create a unique American cultural mix.

African Americans live with this difficult dichotomy. They are in many ways a part of the majority culture, because of their early arrival, their large population, and their role in the development of the country. Much of their native African heritage has been assimilated and their cultural identity results more from their residence in the United States than from their countries of origin. Yet they are often more alienated than other ethnic groups from white American society. This chapter discusses sub-Saharan African cuisines (North African fare is more similar to that of the Middle East. See Chapter 9) and their contributions to U.S. foods and food habits. The historical influence of West African, black slave, and southern cuisines on current African American cuisine is examined.

Cultural Perspective

Africa is the second-largest continent in the world and has a population estimated in the mid-1990s at more than 670 million people. It straddles the equator, and much of its climate is tropical, yet rainfall varies tremendously. (See Figure 5.1) Rainforests, grassland savannas, high mountain forests, and temperate zones are found in the far south and along the Mediterranean. In the north the Sahara, the largest desert in the world, stretches from the Atlantic to the Red Sea, separating the Arabic northern African nations (Morocco, Algeria, Tunisia, Libya, and Egypt) from the sub-Saharan western, eastern, and southern regions.

Numerous ethnic groups have evolved in Africa, and it is estimated that between 800 and 1,700 distinct languages are spoken. Cultural identity is strong. The long history of conflict and conquest on the continent has never completely eliminated tribal affinity; most destabilization in individual nations today arises over ethnic issues.

Traditional African American foods. Some foods typical of the southern black diet include bacon, black-eyed peas, *chayote* squash, corn, greens, ham hocks, hot sauce, okra, peanuts, watermelon, and sweet potatoes. (Photo by Laurie Macfee.)

History of Africa

Knowledge of African history is fragmentary. Archaeological remains of protohuman fossils suggest that Africa is the birthplace of humankind. The prehistoric cultures were hunter-gatherer societies, evolving into horticultural villages in the west and pastoral nomadic groupings in the north and east. The earliest known sub-Saharan civilization emerged in north Ethiopia. The kingdom of *Aksum* dominated the Red Sea region in the third and fourth centuries and established trade with Greece, Rome, and Egypt. It was the model for the East African city-states that flourished until European expansion in the 1500s. (See Figure 5.1.)

The earliest West African states are thought to have developed next to trade routes established by the Egyptians. The first ruling kingdom was ancient *Ghana,* in the third century, followed by the *Mali* and *Songhai* empires. North African traders introduced the Islamic religion to West Africa, where it was widely accepted. The combined African and Muslim societies resulted in the rise of the *Gao, Hausa,* and *Kanem-Bornu* empires, which, along with the Mali, dominated West Africa between the twelfth and sixteenth centuries. Their trade economy was based on gold, slaves, and ivory, which they exchanged for cloth, tools, and weapons. A large middle class of merchants developed during this period. The rise of the *Ashanti, Dahomey,* and *Oyo* states is due to their involvement in trade.

The first European explorers to reach sub-Saharan Africa came from Portugal in the fifteenth century seeking gold and spreading Christianity. Early European settlements in the sixteenth and seventeenth centuries along the coast of West Africa and on the east coast of what is now Mozambique were trade outposts, where local Africans would barter slaves obtained from the inland areas. Contact with Europeans in the west and south, and with Arabs in the east, increased in the late 1700s. Dutch, British, and French farmers in what is now South Africa were among the first Europeans to settle in Africa. With the abolition of slavery in the mid-nineteenth century, the scramble for African natural resources began. By 1914, Belgium, Britain, France, Germany, Italy, Portugal, and Spain occupied nearly all of the continent, creating arbitrary nations and ignoring traditional ethnic and tribal boundaries. There was little united opposition, although fierce resistance by the Zulus in South Africa and by the Ethiopians slowed domination in those areas. Only Liberia, founded in 1847 by freed American slaves, remained independent.

The economic and political changes resulting from World War I, the depression of the 1930s, and World War II weakened European interest in Africa. Pressure for African representation in their own government increased and was gradually permitted by the Europeans. These African representatives formed national movements throughout the continent. Sudan became the first independent republic in

FIGURE 5.1
Sub-Saharan Africa.

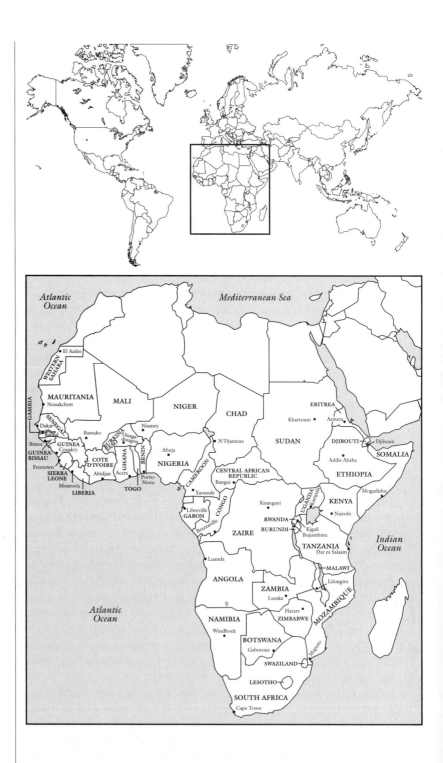

1956; Seychelles (Indian Ocean islands) was the last to become independent in 1976.

Nationhood has not translated into economic independence or political stability in most countries. The African per capita income in 1990 was less than in 1960. Interracial conflict dominated southern Africa until Rhodesia became Zimbabwe in 1979 and the laws upholding white supremacy in South Africa were repealed in 1991. Political coups and interethnic fighting have led to continuous upheaval and boundary changes. Namibia separated from Angola in 1991, and Eritrea gained independence from Ethiopia in 1993. Tribal warfare in Somalia and in Rwanda has devastated parts of East Africa in recent years.

> Not all African nations have experienced political or economic turbulence. Botswana, for example, has maintained a stable democracy since its independence in 1966 and has dramatically improved its economy through the development of mineral resources.

History of Africans in the United States

The arrival of black indentured servants taken forcefully from West Africa preceded the arrival of the Mayflower in America. In 1619, Dutch traders sold twenty West Africans to colonists in Jamestown, an early English settlement. More than 425,000 slaves were subsequently imported legally, ancestors of the majority of black Americans residing in the United States today.

Enslavement

The institution of slavery was well established before the first blacks were brought to North America. European slave traders negotiated with African slave suppliers for their human cargo; which West Africans became slaves and which sold slaves depended on intertribal conditions.

The European traders kept some records of tribal affiliation, but none of place of origin. It is believed that more than one-half the slaves in the United States came from the coastal areas of what are now Angola and Nigeria. Others came from the regions that are today Senegal, Gambia, Sierra Leone, Liberia, Togo, Ghana, Benin, Gabon, and Zaire (now The Democratic Republic of Congo). These political identities now are relatively recent, however, and the slaves identified with their tribal groups, such as *Ashanti, Bambara, Fulani, Ibo, Malinke,* or *Yoruba,* rather than with a specific country or Africa as a whole.

The tribal villages of West Africa were predominantly horticultural. Individuals viewed their existence in relation to the physical and social needs of the group. The extended family and religion were the foundations of tribal culture. It was especially difficult for individuals to be separated from their tribe because identity was so closely associated with the group. It is perhaps for this reason that enslaved individuals held on tenaciously to their African traditions. African language, ornamentation (i.e., scarification and teeth filing), and other customs were very threatening to slave owners. New

Slaves working in kitchens built outside plantation living quarters (due to fire danger) were asked to whistle as they brought food to the main house to prevent them from sampling along the way.

The word *Creole* has numerous definitions, mostly describing Africans and Europeans who moved to the U.S. South and Latin America during the colonial period. Creole Negro (typically translated to "black Creole") was the term used for Africans who developed their own American culture influenced by the British, Spanish, and French settlers in the region.

slaves, usually in small groups from eight to thirty, were often housed at the perimeter of plantations until they became acclimated. They learned English in 2 or 3 years through contact with Native Americans or white indentured servants. When they became sufficiently acculturated, they would be allowed to work in positions closer to the main plantation house.

This initial period of separation allowed slaves to maintain many cultural values despite exposure to slaves from other tribal groups, indentured servants of different ethnic groups, and the majority culture of the white owners. At the same time, frontier farming was sufficiently difficult that slave owners were quite willing to learn from the slaves' agricultural expertise; therefore intercultural communication was inevitable. Instead of becoming totally acculturated to the ways of the owners, slaves developed a black Creole, native-born culture during the early slave period, combining both white and West African influences.

After the end of slave importation in 1807 the black Creole population swelled. By law, slavery was a lifelong condition and the children of female slaves were slaves as well. Although most slaves worked on farms and on cotton, tobacco, sugar, rice, and hemp plantations, many others worked in mines and on the railroads. A large number of slaves were found in the cities, doing manual labor and service jobs. It was during this period of rapid growth in the African American population that separate racial group identities began to form in the United States.

Emancipation

The movement to free the slaves began with the American Revolution. Many of the northern states banned slavery from the beginning of independence. By the 1830s there were 300,000 "free persons of color" living in urban areas outside of the Deep South. Tension between states that supported slavery (the Confederacy) and those that opposed it (the Union) was one factor that led to the Civil War (called the War between the States in the South) in 1861.

In 1862, President Lincoln signed the Emancipation Proclamation. Union victory over the Confederacy in 1865 and the subsequent ratification of the Thirteenth Amendment gave all blacks living in the United States their freedom. Some left the South immediately, searching for relatives and a better life. However, most remained in the South because they lacked the skills needed to begin an independent life; for instance, fewer than 2 percent of former slaves were literate.

After emancipation, former slave owners continued to exploit African American labor through tenant farming and sharecropping. Under this system, black farmers were perpetually in debt to white landowners. Slowly, as competition for skilled farm labor increased, work conditions for black Americans in the South improved. Literacy rates and political representation increased. At the same time, racial persecution by white supremacists, such as members of the Ku Klux Klan, became more frequent.

At the turn of the twentieth century, depressed conditions in the South and industrial job opportunities in the northern states prompted more than 750,000 African Americans to settle in the Northeast and Midwest. Most were young men, and the majority moved to large metropolitan areas, such as New York, Boston, Detroit, Chicago, and Philadelphia. The influx of southern blacks was resented by both whites and the small numbers of middle-class blacks who had been well accepted in the northern cities. Laws that established racial segregation were enacted for the first time in the early 1900s, resulting in inner-city African American ghettos.

Because of poor economic conditions throughout the country, there was a pause in African American migration north during the Great Depression. The flow increased in the 1940s, and in the following 30 years more than 4 million African Americans left the South to settle in other regions of the country. This migration resulted in more than a change in regional demographics. It meant a change from a slow-paced rural lifestyle to a fast-paced, high-pressured, urban industrial existence.

In the 1960s the movement against the injustices of "separate but equal" laws (which permitted segregation as long as comparable facilities, such as schools, were provided for African Americans) gained momentum under the leadership of blacks such as Martin Luther King, Jr. Violent riots in city ghettos underscored the need for social reform. Civil rights activism resulted in the repeal of many overtly racist practices and passage of compensatory laws and regulations meant to reverse past discrimination, as typified by federal affirmative action requirements.

Current Demographics

Today just more than one-half of African Americans live in the U.S. South, most in suburban areas. Since 1988, more blacks have been moving to the South than to the northern states, reversing the demographic trend northward established in 1900. The remaining African American population is found predominantly in northeastern and midwestern urban areas. As of 1993, approximately 1 percent of Americans of African descent are identified as recent immigrants; nearly 100,000 from the West African nations of Nigeria, Ghana, and Senegal; 70,000 from the more eastern countries of Ethiopia and Kenya; and 44,000 from South Africa. Less than 1 percent of the black population is of Caribbean or Central American descent.

Socioeconomic Status

African Americans continue to suffer from the discriminatory practices that began with their enslavement, yet it is estimated that two-thirds are making steady economic progress and the black middle class is growing. According to 1995 census figures, high school graduation rates are equal among blacks and whites. Nevertheless, one-third suffer severe economic constraints (Bigelow, 1995). The African American unemployment rate is more than double that of whites, and average income is substantially lower than for whites. In 1996 over one-fourth (28.4%) of black families lived below the poverty line. While life expectancy rates have increased over all in the United States, they declined for male African Americans in the 1980s. Currently life expectancy is lower for black men than for any other group in the United States, primarily because of the social problems found in many African American communities, particularly access to health care.

Many African Americans believe they are not completely accepted in American society. Blacks isolated in urban ghettos frequently experience alienation. Frustration, hopelessness, and hostility often result. At the same time, discrimination has promoted ethnic identity among African Americans, due in part to a shared history of persecution. Although Americans of African descent are geographically, politically, and socioeconomically diverse, there is a strong feeling of ethnic unity, as demonstrated by the black pride movement of recent years.

On October 16, 1995, African American men gathered in Washington, DC as a demonstration of solidarity and atonement. Called the Million Man March, between 650,000 and 1,000,000 black men and their supporters participated in the event.

African American Organizations

Major African American organizations have been formed to combat racism. They include the National Association for the Advancement of Colored People (NAACP), founded in 1909; the National Urban League, created in 1911 to protect the rights of blacks in New York City, but now fighting racial discrimination nationally; the Congress of Racial Equality (CORE), which began protest activities in the 1940s; and the Southern Christian Leadership Conference, led by Martin Luther King, Jr. from its beginning in 1957 to his death in 1968. Other black American organizations active today began when African Americans who were barred from joining existing professional associations formed their own, such as the National Medical Association and the National Dental Association.

Worldview

Religion

Spirituality was integral to African tribal society, and indigenous religious affiliations were maintained by most slaves despite attempts to convert blacks to Christianity. Although the first black church, a Baptist congregation, was founded in the 1770s in South Carolina, it was only after American religious groups became involved in the anti-slavery movement that the black Creole community responded with large numbers of conversions.

Religion is as essential to African American culture today as it was to African society. For many black Americans the church represents a sanctuary from the trials of daily life. It is a place to meet with other African Americans, to share fellowship and hope. More than 75 percent of African Americans belong to a church. The largest denomination is the National Baptist Convention of the U.S.A. Others with large African American followings include the Methodist Episcopal churches and Pentecostal denominations, such as the Church of God in Christ. A small percentage of African Americans are Muslims who are members of either the World Community of Al Islam or the Nation of Islam (see Chapter 2 for more information about this religion).

Recent immigrants from Africa adhere to a variety of faiths. Approximately one-quarter of Africans today are Muslim (the fastest growing religion on the continent) and one-quarter are Christian, mostly Protestant. Many Ethiopians follow an Eastern Orthodox faith that is similar to, but separate from, the Egyptian Coptic Church. In addition, it is believed that nearly one-half of the African population participate in traditional tribal religions or combine elements of several faiths.

The Eastern Orthodox church in Ethiopia prohibits the consumption of pork, a practice that may reflect early Judaic influences in the region.

Family

The importance of the extended family to African Americans has been maintained since tribal times. It was kinship that defined the form of African societies. During the early slave period the proportion of men to women was two to one, and the family structure included many unrelated members. As the black Creole population increased, nuclear families were established but were often disrupted by the sale or loan of a parent. The extended family provided for dislocated parents and children.

In 1990, 46 percent of African American families were headed by women. More than one-half of black children are born to single mothers and nearly one-half of those to teenage girls. The family network often includes grandparents, aunts, uncles, sisters, brothers, deacons or preachers, and friends. Such extended kinship still supports and protects individuals, especially children, from the problems of a discriminatory society. The extended family has been found to be equally valued by both wealthy and poor African Americans.

Even though interracial marriages have quadrupled in the past 30 years, as of 1992, fewer than 1 percent of African Americans wed members of other races.

Communication

African American conversational style is fully engaged and very expressive. Interjections of agreement or disagreement are frequent. Words are often spoken rhythmically and passionately. Response time is very quick. A direct, but respectful, approach is appreciated. Eye contact is made while speaking, but prolonged eye contact is considered rude. African Americans may avert their eyes while listening attentively. A firm handshake and smile are the expected greeting;

hugging and kissing may also be included. Touching is common, and reluctance to touch may be interpreted as personal rejection.

Traditional Food Habits

What are traditional African American foods—foods of Africans in the seventeenth and eighteenth centuries, foods of the slaves, or foods of the black South since emancipation? African American cuisine today includes some elements from each of these diets.

Ingredients and Common Foods

Historical Influences

African American foods offer a unique glimpse into the way that a cuisine develops. Even before West Africans were brought to the United States, their food habits had changed significantly due to the introduction of New World foods such as cassava (*Manihot esculenta,* a tuber that is also called manioc), maize, chiles, peanuts, pumpkins, and tomatoes during the fifteenth and sixteenth centuries. The slaves brought a cuisine based on these new foods and native West African foods, such as watermelon, black-eyed peas, okra, sesame, and taro. Adaptations and substitutions were made based on what foods were available. Black cooks added their West African preparation methods to British, French, Spanish, and Native American techniques to produce American southern cuisine, emphasizing fried, boiled, and roasted dishes using pork, pork fat, corn, sweet potatoes, and local green leafy vegetables. The cuisines of other African regions have had little impact at this point on the typical American diet, although recent immigrants may continue to prepare and consume traditional fare.

African Fare

West African Knowledge of West African food habits before the nineteenth century is incomplete. It is mostly based on the records of North African, European, and American traders, many of whom considered the local cuisine unhealthy. Most West Africans during the slave era lived in preliterate, horticulturally based tribal groups. There was a heavy dependence on locally grown foods, although some items, such as salt and fish (usually salt-cured), could be traded at the daily markets held throughout each region.

Historically, staple foods varied in each locality. Corn, millet, and rice were used in the coastal areas and Sierra Leone. Yams were popular in Nigeria (where they were customarily boiled and pounded into a paste called *fufu*). Cassava (often roasted and ground into a

"Goober," the nickname for peanut, comes from the Angolan word for the legume, *nguba*.

Throughout Africa, women cultivate nearly all food that is consumed, while men grow export crops.

A 6-day week is used in many parts of West Africa; days are named by many tribes for the regional market that occurs on that day.

flour known as *gari*) and plantains were the dietary foundation of the more southern regions, including the Congo and Angola. The arid savanna region of West Africa bordering the Sahara desert was too dry for cultivation, so most tribes were pastoral, herding camels, sheep, goats, and cattle. In the north, these animals were eaten; in other regions, local fish and game were eaten. Chickens were also raised, although in many tribes the eggs were frequently traded, not eaten, and the chicken itself was served mostly as a special dish for guests. Chicken remains a prestigious meat in many regions today.

There were many similarities in cuisine throughout West Africa. Most foods were boiled or fried, and then small chunks were dipped in a sauce and eaten by hand. Palm oil was the predominant fat used in cooking, giving many dishes a red hue. Peanut oil, shea oil (from the nuts of the African shea tree), and occasionally coconut oil were used in some regions. The addition of tomatoes, hot chile peppers, and onions as seasoning was so common that these items were simply referred to as "the ingredients." Most dishes were preferred spicy, thick, and "sticky" (mucilaginous).

Legumes were popular throughout West Africa. Peanuts were especially valued and were eaten raw, boiled, roasted, or ground into meal, flour or paste. Cow peas (*Vigna ungulculata,* neither a standard pea nor a bean—black-eyed peas are one type of cow pea) were eaten as a substitute for meat, often combined with a staple starch such as corn, yams, or rice. *Bambara groundnuts,* similar to peanuts, were also common. Nuts and seeds were frequently used to flavor and thicken sauces. Mango seeds (called *agobono, og bono,* or *apon*), cashews, *egusi* (watermelon seeds, usually dried and ground), *kola nuts,* and sesame seeds were popular.

Many varieties of tropical and subtropical fruits and vegetables were available to West Africans, but only a few were widely eaten. *Akee apples, baobab* (both the pulp and seeds from the fruit of the baobab tree), guava, lemon, papaya (also called *pawpaw*), pineapple, and watermelon were the most common fruits. Many dishes included coconut milk. In addition to starchy staple roots and the flavoring ingredients of onions, chile peppers, and tomatoes, the most popular vegetables were eggplant, okra, pumpkin, and the leaves from plants such as cassava, sweet potato, and taro (also called *callaloo* or *cocoyam*).

West African cuisine today remains very similar to that of the past. Although fish is favored, little meat is consumed. A mostly vegetarian fare has developed based on regional staples such as beans, yams, and cassava. *Gari foto* is a popular Nigerian specialty often eaten for breakfast; it combines *gari* (cassava meal) with scrambled eggs, onions, chiles, and tomatoes. It is sometimes served with beans. Stews featuring root vegetables, okra, or peanuts and flavored with small amounts of fish, chicken, or beef are common. Curries are popular in Nigeria, often served with dozens of condiments and garnishes, such as coconut, raisins, chopped dates, peanuts, dried shrimp, and diced

---

Taboos against eating eggs still exist in some areas of Africa, including beliefs that they make childbirth difficult and that they excite children.

Okra, when sliced, releases a sticky, milky substance (made mostly of carbohydrate) that thickens liquids and produces a mucilaginous texture in soups, stews, and sauces.

Cow peas were so named by southern slave owners because they were considered animal fodder. By the turn of the twentieth century, they were well accepted as human food throughout the South.

Kola nuts are a bitter nut with twice the caffeine content of coffee beans. The original recipe for Coca-Cola, invented in 1886, included extracts from coca leaves and kola nuts.

Pods from the flowers of roselle *(Hibiscus sabdariffa)* are used to make *bissap rouge,* a sweet beverage popular in Senegal. They are also used in the popular herbal tea called *Red Zinger* (Harris, 1998).

Insects like termites (often called "white ants") and locusts are consumed in many regions of Africa.

Market scene in Ghana, West Africa. (Photo courtesy of the World Health Organization/P. Almasy.)

fruits. *Pili-pili*, a sauce of chile peppers, tomatoes, onion, garlic, and horseradish, is usually offered at the table so that each diner may spice dishes to taste.

Deep-fried fish, fried plantain chips, and balls made from steamed rice, black-eyed peas, yams, or peanuts are snack foods available at street stalls in urban areas. The favorite West African sweet is *kanya,* a peanut candy. Bananas are commonly baked and flavored with sugar, honey, or coconut for dessert. Sweetened dough balls prepared from millet or wheat flour are a specialty in many areas; in Ghana they are called *togbei* ("sheep balls") and are brightly colored with food dye before being deep-fried. They are served for special occasions such as birthdays and weddings.

Ethiopian   Mountainous plains and lowland valleys cover much of Ethiopia and the climate is mostly arid. Millet, including a variety unique to Ethiopia called *teff,* sorghum, and plantains are the staple foods produced, and coffee is the leading export crop. Other foods common to the region include barley, wheat, corn, and potatoes, as well as peanuts and other legumes. Some chicken, fish, mutton, and beef is available.

Ethiopian cuisine has been little changed by outside influences, and the restricted intake of animal products required in the Ethiopian

Ethiopians claim that coffee originated in the region of Kaffa, where it derived its name. Historically the beans were made into wine.

Eastern Orthodox religion has facilitated the development of vegetarian fare. *Wat,* meaning "stew," is the national dish of Ethiopia. It is thick, spicy, and features whole, hard-boiled eggs with lentils, chickpeas, peanuts, and root vegetables and chicken, fish, or beef. It is served with rice or the traditional Ethiopian flat bread called *injera.* Injera is prepared with a spongy, fermented dough made from teff, then cooked on a griddle in a very large circular loaf. Ethiopian foods are frequently flavored with a hot spice mixture known as *berbere,* which includes allspice, cardamom, cayenne, cinnamon, cloves, coriander, cumin, fenugreek, ginger, nutmeg, and black pepper. Honey (sometimes consumed with the bee grubs) is popular as a sweetener; it is also fermented to make *tej,* a meadlike beverage.

East African   The climate and topography of Kenya, Tanzania, and Uganda are well suited to farming and ranching. Cassava, corn, millet, sorghum, peanuts, and plantains are the foundation of the diet. Crops grown for export include coffee, tea, cashews, and cloves. Cattle are raised in the northern plateaus of Kenya; they are considered a gift of the gods (especially among the Maasai tribe) and they indicate wealth. The abundant game animals are also often sacred, although specific taboos vary from region to region. Eating fish and seafood is common along the coast.

The cuisines of East Africa are predominantly vegetarian, influenced in part by Arab, Asian Indian, and British fare. In Kenya the national dish is *ugali,* a very thick cornmeal porridge. Mashed beans, lentils, corn, plantains, and potatoes are also popular. Coconut milk, chile peppers, and curry spice blends flavor many dishes. In Uganda, peanuts are a staple food and are used in everything from stews to desserts. Plantains are the core food of Tanzania. They are used in soups (with or without beef), stews, fritters, custards, and even to make wine. Coconut milk is a frequent flavoring, as is curry powder. Throughout the region, dishes made with taro greens or other leafy vegetables and side dishes of local grains and produce, such as eggplant and papaya, round out the cuisine.

South African   South Africa has a very temperate climate favorable to many fruits and vegetables uncommon in the rest of the continent, such as cucumbers, carrots, apricots, tangerines, grapefruit, quinces, and grapes. The cuisine has been strongly influenced by the European settlers of the region, including the Dutch, British, and French. Muslim slaves imported from Malaysia and India have also had a significant impact on South African fare. Mutton, beef, pork, fish, and seafood are popular.

South African meat specialties include *sosaties,* skewered, curried mutton; *bredie,* a mutton stew that may include onions, chiles, tomatoes, potatoes, or pumpkin; *frikkadels,* braised meat patties; *bobotie,* a meatloaf flavored with curry and topped with a custard mixture

Ethiopians believe that they are God's chosen people. According to legend, God made humans from clay. When he baked the first batch, they came out burnt and black, so he tossed them into the south of Africa. The second batch was underdone, and he disposed of the pasty white figures in the north. Finally, he cooked the third batch to a perfect golden brown, and he put them in Ethiopia.

Although cattle are sacred to the Maasai, cow's milk is a staple in their diet. It is sometimes mixed with cow's blood as a pudding-like dish.

Sukuma wiki is Swahili for "stretch the week" and is a stew of leftover meats and vegetables popular in Kenya.

Zanzibar, an island just off the coast of Tanzania, was known as the Spice Island in the 1800s. It was a trade center between East and West and supplied most of the cloves used worldwide.

The Zulu do not eat fish because they believe it will turn their brave warrior hearts to water.

when baked; and *biltong,* meat strips dried and preserved over smoke. Grape-stuffed chicken or suckling pig is sometimes served for special occasions. Spicy fruit or vegetable relishes called *chutney* (for more information on Asian Indian foods see Chapter 10); *atjar,* unripe fruit or vegetables preserved in fish or vegetable oil with spices like tumeric and chile powder; and fresh grated fruit or vegetable salads flavored with lemon juice or vinegar and chiles accompany the dishes.

Sweets are very common. Dried fruits, fruit leathers called "planked" fruit, and fruit preserves or jams are popular. Many pastries are available, too, such as tarts made with raisins, sweet potatoes, coconut, or custard. Cookies are a favorite. *Koeksister* are braided crullers that are deep-fried and dipped in a cinnamon syrup, and *soetkoekies* are a spice cookie flavored with the sweet wine Madeira.

The Slave Diet

When West Africans were forcefully taken from their tribes, they were not immediately separated from their accustomed foods. Conditions on the slave ships were appalling, but most slave traders did provide a traditional diet for the tribal members on board. The basic staples of each region, plus dried salt cod (which was familiar to most West Africans), were fed to the slaves in minimal quantities. Chile peppers and the native West African *malagueta* peppercorns were used for seasoning because they were believed to prevent dysentery. It wasn't until the Africans were sold in America that significant changes in their cuisine occurred.

The diet of the field workers was largely dependent on whatever foods the slave owners provided. Salt pork and corn were the most common items. Sometimes rice (instead of corn), salted fish, and molasses were included. Greens, legumes, milk, and sweet potatoes were occasionally added. The foods provided, as well as their amount, were usually contingent on local availability and agricultural surplus. Hunger was common among the slaves. Some slave owners allowed or required their slaves to maintain garden plots or to plant needed vegetables around the periphery of the cotton or tobacco fields. Okra and cow peas from Africa were favored, as well as American cabbage, collard and mustard greens, sweet potatoes, and turnips. Herbs were collected from the surrounding woodlands, and small animals such as opossums, rabbits, raccoons, squirrels, and an occasional wild pig were trapped for supplementary meat. Children would often catch catfish and other freshwater fish.

During the hog-slaughtering season in the fall, variety pork cuts, such as *chitterlings* (intestines, pronounced *chitlins*), *maw* (stomach lining), tail, and hocks, would sometimes be given to slaves. Some slaves were encouraged to raise hogs and chickens. The eggs and the primary pork cuts were usually sold to raise cash for the purchase of

The nutritional results of the limited slave diet were seen in the many cases of pellagra, beri-beri, and "sore-mouth" caused by deficiencies in Vitamin A and many of the B vitamins. Malnourishment also left African Americans vulnerable to malaria, yellow fever, cholera, and other diseases common in the South.

A slave folktale describes the land of Diddy-Wah-Diddy, where roast hogs and chickens run about calling "Eat me!" and there are fritter ponds of oil.

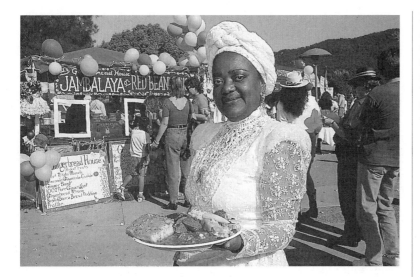

Many traditional southern foods, such as fried chicken, corn bread, spicy stews, bean dishes, and simmered greens, reflect West African influences. (© Bonnie Kamin/PhotoEdit.)

luxury foods. Chickens, a prestigious food in West Africa, continued to be reserved for special occasions.

West African cooking methods were adapted to slave conditions. Boiling and frying remained the most popular ways to prepare not only meats but also vegetables and legumes. Bean stews maintained popularity as main dishes. Corn was substituted for most West African regional staple starches and was prepared in many forms, primarily as cornmeal pudding, cornmeal breads known as *pone* or *spoon bread,* *grits* (coarsely ground cornmeal), and *hominy* (hulled, dried corn kernels with the bran and germ removed). Pork fat (lard) replaced palm oil in cooking and was used to fry or flavor everything from breads to greens. Hot pepper sauces were used instead of fresh peppers for seasoning. No substitutions were available for many of the nuts and seeds used in West African recipes, although peanuts and sesame seeds remained popular.

Food for the slave field workers had to be portable. One-dish vegetable stews were common, as were fried cakes, such as *hushpuppies* (perhaps named because they were used to quiet whining dogs), and the cornmeal cakes baked in the fire on the back of a hoe, called *hoecakes.* Meals prepared at home after a full day of labor were usually simple.

The West Africans who cooked in the homes of slave owners enjoyed a much more ample and varied diet. They popularized fried chicken and fried fish. They introduced "sticky" vegetable-based stews (thickened with okra or the herb sassafras, which when ground is called *filé* powder), such as the southern specialty *gumbo z'herbes,* nearly identical to a recipe from the Congo. Green leafy vegetables

Agricultural scientist George Washington Carver conducted numerous culinary experiments on peanuts. He is credited with the discovery of peanut butter and peanut oil, although both were in use in West Africa for centuries before his find. Today Americans eat more than 2 billion pounds of peanuts annually as butter, snacks, and candy.

It takes about 548 peanuts to produce one 12-ounce jar of peanut butter.

(simply called "greens") became a separate dish instead of being added to stews, but they were still cooked for hours and flavored with meat. Ingredients familiar to West Africans were used for pie fillings, such as nuts, beans, and squash.

Foods after Abolition of Slavery

In the years following emancipation, chickens were known as "preacher's birds" because they were commonly served to the minister when he came calling on Sunday.

The food traditions of African Americans did not change significantly after emancipation, and they differed little from those of white farmers of similar socioeconomic status. One exception was that pork variety cuts and salt pork remained the primary meats for blacks, while whites switched to beef during the post–Civil War period.

African American Southern Staples

The traditional southern African American fare that evolved from West African, slave, and post-abolition foods and food habits emphasizes texture before flavor; the West African preference for "sticky" foods continues. Pork, pork products, corn, and greens are still the foundation of the diet. The Cultural Food Groups list (Table 5.1) includes other common southern black foods. (For information about the food habits of blacks from the Caribbean, see Chapter 6 and for more information on foods of the South, see Chapter 11 on regional Americans.)

The phrase "living high on the hog" comes from the post-abolition period, meaning that a family was wealthy enough to eat the primary pork cuts, such as chops and ham.

Pork variety cuts of all types are used. Pig's feet (or knuckles) are eaten roasted or pickled; pig's ears are slowly cooked in water seasoned with herbs and vinegar and then served with gravy. Bits of pork skin (with meat or fat attached) are fried to make *cracklings.* Chitterlings also are usually fried, sometimes boiled. Sausages and head cheese (a seasoned loaf of meat from the pig's head) make use of smaller pork pieces. Barbecued pork is also common. A whole pig (or just the ribs) is slowly roasted over the fire. Each family has its own recipe for spicy sauce, and each has its opinion about whether the pork should be basted in the sauce or the sauce should be ladled over the cooked meat.

Other meats, such as poultry, are also popular. Occasionally the small game that was prevalent during the slave period, such as opossum and raccoon, is eaten. More often the meal includes local fish and shellfish, such as catfish, crab, or crawfish. Frog legs and turtle are popular in some areas. Meats, poultry, and fish are often combined in thick stews and soups, such as *gumbos* (still made sticky with okra or filé powder), that are eaten with rice. They may also be coated with cornmeal and deep-fried in lard, as in southern-fried chicken and catfish.

The vegetables most characteristic of southern African American cuisine are the many varieties of greens. Food was scarce during the

Civil War, and most southerners were forced to experiment with indigenous vegetation, in addition to cultivated greens such as chard, collard greens, kale, mustard greens, spinach, and turnip greens. Dockweed, dandelion greens, lamb's quarter, marsh marigold leaves, milkweed, pigweed, pokeweed, and purslane were added as acceptable vegetables. Traditionally the greens are cooked in water flavored with salt pork, fatback, bacon, or ham, plus hot chile peppers (or hot-pepper sauce) and lemon. As the water evaporates, the flavors intensify, resulting in a broth called *pot likker*. Both the greens and the liquid are served; hot sauce is offered for those who prefer a spicier dish.

Other common vegetables include black-eyed peas, okra, peas, and tomatoes. Onions and green peppers are frequently used for flavoring. Corn and corn products are as popular in southern black cuisine today as they were during the slave period. Corn bread and fried hominy are served sliced with butter. Wheat flour biscuits are also served with butter or, in some regions, gravy. Dumplings are sometimes added to stews and greens.

Squash is eaten as a vegetable (sometimes stuffed) and as a dessert pie sweetened with molasses. Sweet potatoes are also used both ways. Other common desserts include bread pie (bread pudding), crumb cake, chocolate or caramel cake, fruit cobblers, puddings, and shortcake, as well as sesame seed cookies and candies.

Meal Composition and Cycle

Daily Patterns

Two meals a day were typical in West Africa, one late in the morning and one in the evening. Snacking was common; in poorer tribes, snacks would replace the morning meal and only dinner would be served. Food was eaten family style or, more formally, the men would be served first, then the boys, then the girls, and last the women. Sometimes men would gather together for a meal without women. Mealtimes often were solemn; people concentrated on the attributes of the food and conversation was minimal.

The West African tradition of frequent snacking continued through the slave period and after emancipation. Meals were often irregular, perhaps due to the variable hours of agricultural labor.

The traditional southern-style meal pattern was adopted as economic conditions for both blacks and whites improved. Breakfast was typically large and leisurely, always including boiled grits and homemade biscuits. In addition, eggs, ham or bacon, and even fried sweet potatoes would be served. Coffee and tea were more common beverages than milk or juice.

Lunch, called dinner, was the main meal of the day. It was eaten at midafternoon and featured a boiled entree, such as legumes or greens with ham, or another stew-type dish. Additional vegetables or a salad

Ethiopians generally eat one meal in the early evening, snacking throughout the rest of the day.

Traditionally African Americans in the South believed that heavy meals would stay with a person; light meals were appropriate only for infants and invalids.

TABLE 5.1
Cultural Food Groups: African American (Southern United States)

Group	Comments
PROTEIN FOODS	
Milk/milk products	Dairy products uncommon in diet (incidence of lactose intolerance estimated at 60–95 percent of the population).
	Milk widely disliked in some studies; well accepted in others.
	Few cheeses or fermented dairy products eaten.
Meats/poultry/fish/eggs/legumes	Pork most popular, especially variety cuts; fish, small game, poultry also common; veal and lamb infrequently eaten.
	Bean dishes popular.
	Frying, boiling most common preparation methods; stewed dishes preferred thick and "sticky."
	Protein intake high.
CEREALS/GRAINS	Corn primary grain product; wheat flour used in many baked goods.
	Rice used in stew-type dishes.
FRUITS/VEGETABLES	Green leafy vegetables most popular, cooked with ham, salt pork, or bacon, lemon and hot sauce; broth also eaten.
	Intake of fresh fruits and vegetables low.
ADDITIONAL FOODS	
Seasonings	Dishes frequently seasoned with hot-pepper sauces.
	Onions and green pepper common flavoring ingredients.
Beverages	
Nuts/seeds	
Fats/oils	
Sweeteners	

may have been served, as well as potatoes and bread or biscuits. Dessert was mandatory and was usually a baked item, not simply fruit. In some homes a full supper of meat, vegetables, and potatoes was served in the evening. Poorer agricultural families often ate only two of these hearty meals a day.

Today few southern African Americans, or whites, continue this traditional meal pattern in full. The southern-style breakfast might be served just on weekends or holidays, for example. As in the rest of the country, a light lunch has replaced the large dinner on most days, and supper has become the main meal.

TABLE 5.1
Cultural Food Groups: African American (Southern United States)—continued

Common Foods	Regional Adaptations in the United States
Milk (consumed mostly in desserts, such as puddings and ice cream), some buttermilk; cheese	Blacks in urban areas may drink milk more often than rural blacks.
Meat: beef, pork (including *chitterlings,* ham hocks, sausages, variety cuts)	Pork remains primary protein source; prepackaged sausages and lunch meats popular.
Poultry: chicken, turkey	Small game rarely consumed.
Fish and shellfish: catfish, crab, crawfish, perch, red snapper, salmon, sardines, shrimp, tuna	Variety cuts considered to be *soul food* and eaten regardless of socioeconomic status or region.
Small game: frogs, opossum, raccoon, squirrel, turtle	Frying still popular, but more often at evening meal; boiling and baking second most common preparation methods.
Eggs: chicken	
Legumes: black-eyed peas, kidney beans, peanuts (and peanut butter), pinto beans, red beans	
Biscuits; corn (corn breads, grits, hominy); pasta; rice	Store-bought breads often replace biscuits (toasted at breakfast, used for sandwiches at lunch).
Fruits: apples, bananas, berries, peaches, watermelon	Fruits eaten according to availability and preference; intake remains low.
Vegetables: beets, broccoli, cabbage, corn, greens (chard, collard, kale, mustard, pokeweed, turnip, etc.), green peas, okra, potatoes, spinach, squash, sweet potatoes, tomatoes, yams	Green leafy vegetables (*greens*) popular in all regions; other vegetables eaten according to availability and preference; intake remains low.
Filé (sassafras powder), garlic, green peppers, hot-pepper sauce, ham hocks, salt pork or bacon (added to vegetables and stews), lemon juice, onions, salt, pepper	
Coffee, fruit drinks, fruit juice, fruit wine, soft drinks, tea	
Peanuts, pecans, sesame seeds, walnuts	
Butter, lard, meat drippings, vegetable shortening	
Honey, molasses, sugar	Cookies (and candy) are preferred snacks.

Special Occasions

Sunday dinner had become a large family meal during the slave period, and it continued to be the main meal of the week after emancipation. It was a time to eat and share favorite foods with friends and kin, a time to extend hospitality to neighbors.

Many southern African Americans still enjoy a large Sunday dinner. It is usually prepared by the mother of the house, who begins cooking in the early morning. The menu would probably include fried chicken, spareribs, chitterlings, pig's feet (or ears or tail), black-

Ethiopians in rural regions of Africa may fast every Wednesday and Friday (no food from sunrise to noon; no animal products of any type until sunset) according to their Eastern Orthodox faith.

Kwanzaa, the African American holiday celebrated from December 26th through January 1st each year, culminates with a feast featuring dishes from throughout Africa, the Caribbean, the U.S. South, and other regions where Africans now live. (© Merritt Vincent/PhotoEdit.)

eyed peas or okra, corn, corn bread, greens, potato salad, rice, sweet potato pie, and watermelon. Homemade fruit wines, such as strawberry wine, might also be offered.

Other holiday meals, especially Christmas, feature menus similar to the Sunday meal, but with added dishes and even greater amounts of food. Turkey with cornbread stuffing and baked ham are often the entrees; other vegetable dishes, such as corn pudding, sweet peas, and salads, are typical accompaniments. A profusion of baked goods, including yeast rolls, fruit cakes and cobblers, custard or cream pies, and chocolate, caramel, and coconut cake, round out the meal.

Southern black cuisine is particularly well suited to buffet meals and parties. A pan of gumbo, a pot of beans, or a side of barbecued ribs can be stretched to feed many people on festive occasions. Informal parties to celebrate a birthday, or just the fact that it's Saturday night, are still common.

The African American holiday of *Kwanzaa* has gained popularity in recent years. Created in southern California in 1966, Kwanzaa recognizes the African diaspora and celebrates the unity of all people of African heritage. It begins on December 26th and runs through New Year's Day. Each day a new candle is lit to symbolize one of seven principles: unity, self-determination, collective work and responsibility, cooperative economics, purpose, creativity, and faith. The holiday culminates with a feast featuring dishes from throughout Africa, the

"Juneteenth" celebrations, featuring traditional southern fare, are held in many African American communities to commemorate the emancipation of the slaves.

Caribbean, the U.S. South, and any other region where Africans were transported.

Role of Food in African American Society

Food was central to African village life. Human fertility, crop fertility, and spiritualism were often interlinked. Many tribes existed at subsistence level yet were generous in sharing available food among tribal members.

In the American South, food has traditionally been a catalyst for social interaction, and southern hospitality is renowned. Food is lovingly prepared for family and friends. The sharing of food is considered an important factor in the cohesiveness of African American society.

In the Dan tribe of Liberia and the Ivory Coast, special *wunkirle* spoons in a symbolically female shape are presented to the most generous woman in the village.

Therapeutic Uses of Food

Many African Americans maintain health by eating three hearty meals each day, including a hot breakfast. Numerous other beliefs about food and health are found among poor African Americans living in the rural South. Some of these dietary concepts were brought to other regions of the country during the great migrations.

The conditions known as "high blood" and "low blood" are one example. High blood (often confused with a diagnosis of high blood pressure) is thought to be caused by excess blood that migrates to one part of the body, typically the head, and is caused by eating excessive amounts of "rich" foods or foods that are red in color (beets, carrots, grape juice, red wine, and red meat, especially pork). Low blood, associated with anemia, is believed to be caused by eating too many astringent and acidic foods (vinegar, lemon juice, garlic, and pickled foods) and not enough red meat. Other blood complaints include "thin" blood that cannot nourish the body, causing a person to feel chilly; "bad" blood, due to hereditary, natural, or supernatural contamination; "unclean" blood when impurities collect over the winter months and the blood carries more heat; and "clots," when the blood thickens and settles in one area, associated with menstruation or stomach and leg cramps (Jackson, 1981).

Some African Americans believe that peppermint candies or yellowroot tea can cure diabetes. Others recommend a mixture of figs and honey to eliminate ringworm and goat's milk with cabbage juice to cure a stomach infection. In some areas, eggs and milk may be withheld from sick children to aid in their recovery.

Pica, the practice of eating nonnutritive substances such as clay, chalk, and laundry starch, is one of the most perplexing of all food habits practiced by African Americans, whites, and other ethnic

Geophagy, or clay eating, is common among the men, women, and children of Africa. It is done to alleviate hunger, to soothe the irritation of intestinal parasites, for spiritual purposes in connection with the swearing of oaths, and for medical reasons. Active trade in clay tablets and disks is found at some markets.

groups. Studies conducted between the 1950s and 1970s determined that pica is most often practiced by black women during pregnancy and the postpartum period (information on pica among other ethnic groups or age groups in the United States is limited). It is common in the South, where anywhere from 16 to 57 percent of pregnant African American women admit to pica. But pica is also found in other areas of the country where there are large populations of poor African Americans. In rural regions the substance ingested is usually clay. In urban areas, laundry starch is often the first choice, although instances of women who ate large amounts of milk of magnesia, coffee grounds, plaster, ice, and paraffin have also been reported. Many theories about the reasons for pica have been suggested—a nutritional need for minerals, hunger or nausea, a desire for special treatment, and cultural tradition are the most common hypotheses. Reasons for pica reported by rural and urban black women include a craving for clay and the belief that clay prevents birthmarks or that starch makes the skin of the baby lighter and helps the baby to slip out during delivery (Hunter, 1973; Horner et al., 1991).

Contemporary Food Habits in the United States

Most researchers have noted that the food habits of African Americans today usually reflect their current socioeconomic status, geographic location, and work schedule more than their African or southern heritage. Even in the South, many traditional foods and meal patterns have been rejected because of the pressures of a fast-paced society.

Adaptations of Food Habits

Ingredients and Common Foods

Food preferences do not vary greatly between blacks and whites in similar socioeconomic groups living in the same region of the United States. Comparisons do show that African Americans choose items such as fried chicken, barbecued ribs, corn bread, sweet potato pie, collard greens, and fruit-flavored drinks and juices as favorite foods more often than whites do. In addition, cookies or candy are preferred snack items (versus soft drinks for whites). African American households purchase cereal and bakery products, dairy products, sugar, and other sweets less often than do white households, however.

The popularity of *soul food* is notable, considering the similarities between African American and white diets. Traditional southern black cuisine was termed "soul food" in the 1960s. African Americans adopted this cuisine as a symbol of ethnic solidarity, regardless of region or social class. Today soul food serves as an emblem of identity and a recognition of black history for many African Americans.

Meal Composition and Cycle

While the common foods that African Americans eat reflect geographic location and socioeconomic status, meal composition and cycle have changed more in response to work habits than to other lifestyle considerations.

The traditional southern meal pattern of the large breakfast with fried foods, followed by the large dinner with boiled foods and a hearty supper, has given way to the pressures of industrial job schedules. One study (Jerome, 1969) showed that southern breakfast habits were maintained for only 18 months after migration to the North and then were replaced with a meal typically consisting of biscuits or toast, sausage, and coffee.

Recent research indicates that some African Americans living outside the South no longer identify certain foods, such as okra and yams, as African in origin. Many of the items known to be traditional fare are not eaten often, including pig's feet and chitterlings (the author notes that some of these foods are also associated with the poor, and respondents may be reluctant to admit eating such items). The exception was greens, which were identified most often as a traditional African American food and were also the most popular with respondents: 78 percent eat greens at least once a month (Byars, 1996).

African Americans throughout the country now eat lighter breakfasts and sandwiches at a noontime lunch. Dinner is served after work, and it has become the biggest meal of the day. Snacking throughout the day is still typical among most African Americans. In many households, meal schedules are irregular and family members eat when convenient. It is not unusual for snacks to replace a full meal.

Frying is still one of the most popular methods of preparing food. An increase in consumption of fried dinner items suggests that the customary method of making breakfast foods has been transferred to evening foods (which were traditionally boiled) when time constraints prevent a large morning meal (Jerome, 1969). Boiling and baking are second to frying in popularity (Wheeler & Haider, 1979). African Americans use convenience foods and fast foods as income permits.

Aunt Jemima Pancake Mix was named after a tune popular at turn-of-the-century minstrel shows. Uncle Ben's Converted Rice was named for a real-life African American rice farmer in Texas renowned for his quality product.

6

Latinos

Latinos are one of the largest ethnic groups in the United States, representing nearly 9 percent of the total population. If current growth trends continue, the number of Latinos in America will double within 25 years, and by early in the next century they will surpass African Americans as the largest U.S. minority. Yet they are not a single group. Latinos come from throughout Latin America, including Mexico, Puerto Rico, Cuba and other Caribbean countries; Central America; and South America. The majority share Spanish as a common language of origin.

Immigrants from Latin America bring a rich cultural history. The Olmec culture, known for its sophisticated sculpture, existed in southeastern Mexico as early as 1200 BCE. The great Aztec, Mayan, Toltec, and Inca civilizations thrived while Europe was in its dark ages. Their independent mastery of astronomy, architecture, agriculture, and art astonished later explorers.

The influence of the Spanish on Latin American history is nearly as extensive as that of the early native populations. Occupation of Mexico, the Caribbean countries, and the Central and South American nations by various European powers, as well as the importation of slave populations from Africa and Asia, has resulted in the multicultural blend seen today throughout the area.

The foods of Mexico typify this heterogeneous society. This chapter examines Mexico and the food habits of Americans of Mexican descent in depth. The foods of the Caribbean Latinos are also included, focusing on Americans of Puerto Rican and Cuban descent. The cuisines of Central America, which share many similarities with those of Mexico and the Caribbean, especially in ingredients, are outlined due to the dramatic increases in immigration from the region in the 1980s. South American fare features many of the characteristics common throughout Latin America with some differences due to historical or climatic factors. Fewer than 5 percent of all Latinos in the United States come from the fourteen different nations of South America, and little research on the food habits of immigrants from these areas has been reported. Only the traditional cooking of South America is discussed. (See Figure 6.1 for a map of Latin America.)

FIGURE 6.1

Mexico, the Caribbean Islands, Central America, and South America.

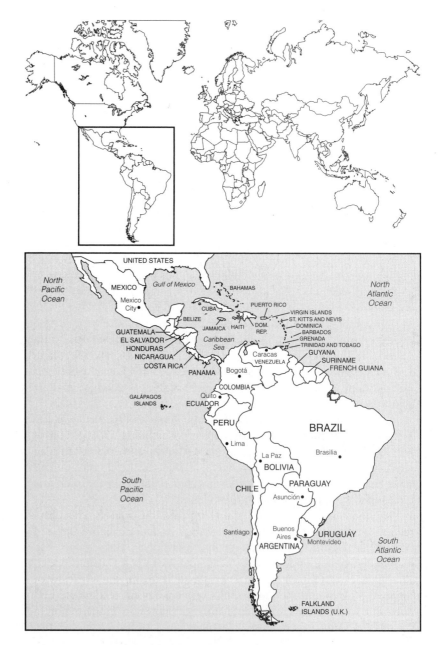

MEXICANS

Estados Unidos Mexicanos, the United Mexican States, is the northernmost Latin American country. It is more than one-fourth the size of the United States, with 756,065 square miles of territory. The varied geography includes a large central plateau surrounded by mountains except to the north. Coastal plains edge the country along the Gulf of Mexico and the Pacific. The separate Baja peninsula is found in the west and the Yucatán peninsula juts out in the southeast. Snow-capped volcanoes, such as Orizaba, Popocatépetl, Ixtacchiuatl, and El Chichón, and frequent earthquakes also affect the landscape. The climate ranges from arid desert in the northern plains to tropical lowlands in the south.

Almost two-thirds of Mexicans are *mestizos,* that is, of mixed Indian and Spanish ancestry. Thirty percent are native Indians, and about 10 percent are whites of Spanish descent. Spanish is the official language. Only 1.5 percent of Mexicans speak only an Indian language, mostly Nahuatl.

Traditional Latin American foods. Some foods typical of the traditional Latin American diet include annatto, avocado, *bacalao,* black beans, cassava *(yuca),* chile peppers, cilantro, corn tortillas, *jícama,* papaya, plantains, pinto beans, pork, *tomatillos,* and tomatoes. (Photo by Laurie Macfee.)

Cultural Perspective

History of Mexico

Current knowledge of Mexican history before Spanish contact is limited. It is believed that nomadic hunting tribes settled the area around 21,000 BCE. The *Olmec* civilization emerged about 1200 BCE in the eastern region of the country. It is not known how long the empire ruled, but by 100 BCE it had declined for unknown reasons.

The *Maya* established another early civilization in southern Mexico during the first century. At the height of their empire the Mayans occupied the Yucatán peninsula, as well as parts of what is now Guatemala and Nicaragua, establishing more than sixty cities connected by paved roads.

During this same time, approximately 900 to 1200, the *Toltecs* rose to prominence in the north. They are thought to be the ancestors of the *Tenochcas,* who later became known as the *Aztecs.* The Aztecs conquered many of the other native tribes in the region and controlled much of what is now Mexico. Their capital city of Tenochtitlan, site of present-day Mexico City, was founded in 1325. The famous emperor Montezuma II ruled from 1502 to 1520.

In 1519 the Spanish explorer Hernán Cortés arrived in Mexico. Cortés conquered the Aztecs in less than 2 years, and most of Mexico (including the Mayan Empire) was subjugated to Spanish rule by 1540 when it became the viceroyalty of New Spain. Heavy taxation and land distribution that benefited the Spanish colonists followed.

The movement toward independence grew as the Mexican-born Spanish people, called *Creoles,* became unhappy with their inferior status among Europeans. However, the original insurrections were led by Catholic priests with an Indian and mestizo following. The Creoles eventually joined in the ongoing guerilla war, and independence from Spain was achieved in 1820 under the leadership of Agustín de Itúrbide. In 1824 a federal constitution was adopted.

The territory of Texas declared independence from Mexico in 1836. In 1845 the United States annexed Texas, and a boundary dispute with Mexico led to war. The Mexican armies suffered repeated defeats, and in 1848 the United States occupied Mexico City. The ensuing Treaty of Guadalupe ceded the area that is now Texas, New Mexico, Arizona, and parts of Colorado, Nevada, and California to the United States.

A new constitution was created in 1857 to eliminate the unfair laws remaining from the colonial period. In 1862, Mexico was invaded by Britain, France, and Spain on the pretext of nonpayment of debts. After the withdrawal of Britain and Spain, Napoleon III sent the archduke of Austria, Maximilian, to be emperor of Mexico. He ruled for 3 years, but, in 1867, Maximilian was executed by liberal Mexican nationals. In 1876, Porfirio Díaz seized power in Mexico and ruled as a dictator for nearly 35 years. He was overthrown in the Mexican Revolution of 1910.

Reforms were not completed when Díaz took over. Continued pressure from peasants resulted in a new constitution in 1917. Other reforms were instituted by the Partido Nacional Revolucionario (in 1946, renamed Partido Revolucionario Institucional [PRI]) in 1934. A program of modernization was begun in 1976, but economic hardship has made progress difficult. Today Mexico is a democratic republic.

History of Mexicans in the United States

Immigration Patterns

Mexican immigration patterns have changed over the years since the Mexican-American War clearly defined the U.S.–Mexican border. Today Mexicans living in America and their descendants can be classified in the following groups: (1) *Chicanos:* those who are born in the United States (from the descendants of the wealthy Mexican landowners who controlled the area from California to Texas in the eighteenth and early nineteenth centuries to the children of the most recent arrivals), as well as those who immigrated from Mexico and became U.S. citizens; (2) *Braceros:* those who work here legally but remain Mexican citizens; and (3) undocumented residents: those who enter the country illegally.

The term *Chicano* came from the Aztec word for Mexicans, *Meshicano.*

Mexicans lived in what is now the American Southwest for hundreds of years before the United States declared its independence in 1776. Although they welcomed American settlers, they soon found themselves outnumbered and their economic and political control of the region weakened. At the end of the Mexican-American War in 1848 the 75,000 Mexicans living in the ceded territories became U.S. citizens.

Between 1900 and 1935, it is estimated that 10 percent of the Mexican population, approximately 1 million persons, emigrated north to the United States. Then, during the Great Depression, tens of thousands of undocumented aliens, plus those admitted legally under the 1917 contract labor laws, were "repatriated" and sent back to Mexico.

Approximately 1 million immigrants from South America now live in the United States, with the largest single group (379,000 in 1990) from Colombia.

After the depression the need for cheap labor increased. The Bracero program was created to meet this need. Thousands of Mexicans were offered jobs in agriculture and on the railroads. Following World War II the continued need for migrant farmworkers encouraged more than 1 million Mexicans to immigrate between 1951 and 1975. In the past 30 years, Mexicans have been the largest single group of legal immigrants to the United States.

Current Demographics

The 1990 U.S. census reported more than 13 million Chicanos and Braceros in this country, of whom nearly 5 million were born in Mexico. The census also accounted for approximately 3.5 million

In 1996, several states sued the U.S. government over inaccurate minority population counts; lower-than-actual census numbers mean reduced funding for immigrant programs. The courts ruled that the census was reasonably diligent in its count and therefore was not responsible for the faulty figures.

The most recent immigrants from Mexico have been Mexican Indians (mostly Mixtecos from Oaxaca), who are replacing mestizos in some migrant agricultural jobs. They speak neither English nor Spanish.

undocumented Mexicans living in the country, although this figure may be low due to the reluctance of undocumented residents to become involved in government procedures. Economic pressures in Mexico have increased the number of Mexican immigrants entering the United States each year. Many are attempting to escape the life-threatening poverty that affects the majority of the populace.

The majority of Chicanos live in California and Texas. Other states, such as Illinois, Arizona, and New Mexico, also host large Chicano populations. Eighty percent of the immigrants from Mexico settle in U.S. cities like Los Angeles, San Antonio, and Chicago. Other recent immigrants, legal and undocumented, settle in the urban Latino neighborhoods called *barrios*.

A continuing decline in the Mexican economy may encourage even greater emigration in the near future. More than 91,000 Mexicans entered the United States legally in 1992, the largest group from any country. However, it is the uncontrolled number of undocumented immigrants from Mexico entering the country that concerns U.S. officials. The U.S.–Mexican border is 1,931 miles long, most of it in unpopulated desert regions. More than 1.5 million Mexicans are apprehended each year as they attempt to enter the United States illegally. Some estimates suggest that twice that number may cross successfully.

Political pressures in the United States regarding taxpayer support of services for undocumented residents have led to immigration limits and social program restrictions. It is unknown how effective these changes will be long-term in preventing illegal entry into the country or how it will affect immigration patterns. What is certain is that the economic disparities between the two nations will continue to draw Mexicans to the United States.

Socioeconomic Status

Chicanos, Braceros, and undocumented aliens occupy three main socioeconomic classes. There are the migrant farmworkers, who maintain a culturally isolated community; the residents of the urban barrios, who also are segregated from much of American society; and a growing number of acculturated middle-class Chicanos.

Undocumented aliens tend to move in with family members who already reside in the United States. Usually this is in a predominantly Latino neighborhood, where they can live inconspicuously among the residents while becoming familiar with the American social and economic systems.

Despite a rapidly growing Chicano middle-to-upper class, many Americans of Mexican descent have low socioeconomic status. In 1996, nearly one in every four families fell below the poverty level. This is due in part to a disproportionate number of Chicanos employed in unskilled or semiskilled labor. Although only 3 percent of Mexican Americans are currently working in agricultural jobs, more than 50 percent are employed in manufacturing or service occupations. Approximately 16 percent hold professional or managerial positions. Just more than one-half of Chicanos graduate from high school, but this figure rises to 65 percent among second-generation Mexican Americans. As many as two-thirds of Mexican American girls do not finish high school. Nearly 5 percent of adults older than 35 have completed 4 or more years of college; more than 15 percent have less than 5 years total of education.

Cultural Organizations

Most national associations formed by Americans of Mexican descent address political and economic issues. The League of United Latin American Citizens was founded in 1928 to promote better working conditions and job training; it now has chapters throughout the country. The Mexican American Legal Defense and Education Fund protects the rights of Latinos and fights discrimination. The National Council of La Raza has almost 200 affiliates working to increase opportunities and reduce poverty for all Latinos. A group specifically interested in Hispanic women's issues is the *Comision Femenil Mexicana Nacional* (National Mexican Women's Commission).

Worldview

Chicanos, Braceros, and undocumented immigrants often live in culturally homogeneous communities. Their ethnic identity is proudly maintained; they speak Spanish and prefer Mexican music and food. The concept of *la Raza* (meaning "the people") was first promoted in the 1960s as a pride and solidarity movement for all persons of Latin American heritage.

When exposed to the mainstream American society, immigrants from Mexico can be highly adaptive. There are many Chicanos who are completely assimilated. They may speak no Spanish and consider themselves "white." Others are successfully bicultural. Cross-cultural marriages are becoming more common, especially in the northern regions of the United States.

Religion

It is estimated that between 75 and 97 percent of Americans of Mexican descent are Roman Catholics. Traditional religious ceremonies, such as baptism, communion, confirmation, marriage, and the novenas (9 days of prayer for the deceased) are important family events (see Chapter 2). Yet despite their numbers within the laity, they are underrepresented within the institutional church; as of 1992, only 5 percent of U.S. bishops were Latinos.

A strong faith in the will of God influences how immigrants from Mexico perceive their world. Many believe they have no direct control over their own fate. Nearly all Mexican Americans who are not Catholic practice Protestant faiths; evangelical churches are particularly popular in urban areas.

The Chicano Family

The most important social unit in the Chicano community is the family. In contrast to American majority society, the well-being of the family comes before the needs of the individual. The Chicano father is typically the head of the household. He is the primary decision maker and wage earner. In traditional Mexican society the wife is a homemaker. In America, this role is changing. One-half of Mexican-American women work outside the home, are responsible for household management, and are likely to be involved in family decisions. Men rarely increase involvement in chores as women increase their hours of employment. Some women find that their new roles are occasionally in conflict with their self-concept as mother and caregiver.

Children are cherished in the Chicano family, and families are usually large. Children are taught to share and to work together; sibling rivalry is minimal. When possible, an extended family is the preferred living arrangement. Grandparents are honored and are often involved in child care. Because of space limitations in the United States, however, many Chicano elders live in separate apartments. During periods of hardship, other relatives such as aunts, uncles, and godparents willingly accept the care of children. Girls were traditionally raised differently from boys and were kept at home to learn household skills; they were carefully chaperoned in public. Although such strict supervision diminished with successive generations born in the United States, family expectations may limit the educational and professional attainments of some young women.

Communication

The communication style of Mexican Americans is nonconfrontational, and a warm, personal, yet dignified approach is favored. Courtesy is expected and titles are important. A handshake is the greeting between men (but most men wait for a woman to extend her hand first); women frequently pat each other on the arm or hug. Touching is common, and pulling away may be insulting. Putting one's hands on hips or in pockets is sometimes interpreted as confrontational. Most Mexican Americans are polychronic and are comfortable doing several things at once.

Traditional Food Habits

Mexicans are very proud of their culinary heritage. It is a unique blend of native and European foods prepared with Indian (mostly

Aztec) and Spanish cooking techniques. There are even some French and Viennese influences from the Maximilian reign. The resulting cuisine is both spicy and sophisticated.

Ingredients and Common Foods

Many people associate the cooking of Mexico with chile peppers. Although chiles are used frequently, not all Mexican dishes are hot and spicy. Other New World foods such as beans, cocoa (from the Aztec word for "bitter"), corn, and tomatoes add equally important flavors to the cuisine. These indigenous ingredients were the basis of Indian fare throughout Mexico before the arrival of the Spanish.

Aztec Foods

The Aztec empire had an estimated population of 25 million people at its peak in the fifteenth century. About one-quarter of the population were an elite class of nobles who were supported by the remaining 75 percent of the Indian slave populace. The capital city of Tenochtitlan was surrounded by lakes on which were built *chinampas,* rich agricultural fields of mud scooped from the lake bottoms. It is believed that these drought-resistant fields produced enough food to feed 180,000 people annually. The monarchy stored surplus crops to protect against famine. The Aztecs were also known for their animal husbandry and game protection laws.

Documents from early Spanish expeditions recorded the enormous variety of foods enjoyed by the Aztec nobility. More than 1,000 dishes are described. Montezuma II reportedly ate up to thirty different items per meal, each kept warm on a pottery brazier. These included hot tortillas of several types; turkey pie; roast turkey, quail, and duck; fish, lobster, frog, newt, and insect dishes garnished with red, green, or yellow chiles; squash blossoms; and sauces of chiles, tomatoes, squash seeds, or green plums. *Chocolatl,* a hot unsweetened chocolate drink made from native cocoa beans, was the most popular beverage.

Corn was the staple grain. Legumes, fruits, and vegetables were plentiful; turkeys and dogs were domesticated for meat; and some small game was available. The notable deficiency of the Aztec diet was a consistent source of fat or oil.

Spanish Contributions

The Spanish arrived in Mexico with cinnamon, garlic, onions, rice, sugar cane, wheat, and, most important, hogs, which added a reliable source of domesticated protein and fat to the native diet. These additions combined with indigenous ingredients produce the classic

Another New World food is the potato, thought to have been first cultivated high in the Andes Mountains of Peru and Bolivia, where it was too cold to grow corn. Potatoes are a staple in those regions today.

The scientific name for the cocoa tree is *Theobroma,* meaning "food of the gods."

Corn is believed to have been domesticated from extinct wild varieties in southern Mexico somewhere between 8000 and 7000 BCE. It spread south into Central America and north into what is now the United States.

flavors and foods of Mexican cuisine, such as corn tortillas with pork; tomato, chile, and onion sauces or *salsas;* rice and beans; and boiled beans fried in lard, known as *frijoles refritos,* or, as they are incorrectly called in English, refried beans. The Spanish also introduced the distillation of alcohol to native Mexican fermented beverages; *tequila* and *mescal* were the result.

Staples

The cuisine of Mexico is very diverse, and many inaccessible regions have retained their native diets. Others have held onto traditional foods and food habits despite Aztec or Spanish domination. The diets of still other areas differ because of the availability of local fruits, vegetables, or meats. This variety makes it difficult to typify Mexican foods in general (Table 6.1). Nevertheless, some foods are found, in varying forms, throughout Mexico.

Tortillas are the flat bread of Mexico. Traditionally they are made by hand. Corn kernels are heated in lime solution until the skins break and separate. The treated kernels, called *nixtamal,* are then pulverized on a stone slab (*metate*). The resulting flour, *masa harina,* is combined with water to make the tortilla dough. Small balls of the dough are patted into round, flat circles, about 6 to 8 inches across. The tortillas are cooked on a griddle (often with a little lard) until soft or crisp, depending on the recipe.

Beans are ubiquitous in Mexican meals. They are served in some form at nearly every lunch and dinner and are frequently found at breakfast, too. They are often the filling in stuffed foods and are a common side dish, such as simmered *frijoles de olla* ("out of the pot") and frijoles refritos. They are popularly paired with rice as well.

One-dish meals are typical, almost always served with warm tortillas. Hearty soups or stews called *caldos* are favorite family dinner entrees. Casseroles, known as *sopas-secas,* using stale tortilla pieces, rice, or macaroni, are eaten as main dishes.

Stale tortillas can also be broken up and softened in a sauce to make *chilaquiles,* which are served as a side dish or light entree. They can also be soaked in milk overnight, then pureed to make a thick dough. This dough is used to prepare *gordos,* which are fat fried cakes, or *bolitos,* which are added to soup and are similar to dumplings.

Meats are normally prepared over high heat. They are typically grilled, as in *carne asada* (beef strips), or fried, as in *chicharrónes* (fried pork rind). Slow, moist cooking (stewing, braising, etc.) may also be used. These techniques help to tenderize the tough cuts that are generally available, as does marinating, another common preparation method. Nearly all parts of the animal are used, including the variety cuts and organs. Sausage is especially popular, such as spicy pork or beef *chorizo.*

The majority of poor Mexicans have little variety in their diet; some subsist almost entirely on corn, beans, and squash.

The snack food Fritos, based on an old Mexican recipe for fried masa harina, was invented in San Antonio, Texas.

Menudo is a tripe and hominy soup that is believed to have curative properties, particularly for hangovers. It is a popular weekend breakfast dish.

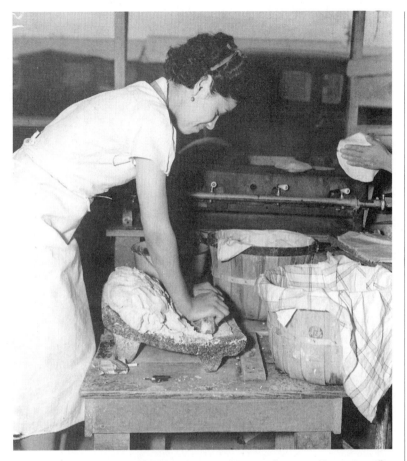

Hand-made *tortillas,* made from *masa harina* (a type of cornmeal) or wheat flour, are the staple bread of Mexico. In this photograph, taken in a tortilla factory, the lime-soaked corn kernels are pulverized on a stone *metate.* On the right a tortilla is patted into a flat circle by hand. (Courtesy of San Antonio Light Collection; copy from the Institute of Texas Cultures at San Antonio.)

Mexico is famous for its "stuffed" foods, such as *tacos, flautas, enchiladas, tamales, quesadillas,* and *burritos.* These are found throughout the country, with regional variations. Tacos are the Mexican equivalent of sandwiches. Tortillas, either soft or crisply fried, are filled with anything from just salsa to meat, vegetables, and sauce. Flautas ("flutes") are a variation on the taco, with tortillas tightly rolled around the filling, then fried until crispy. They may be served with a red or green chile sauce or guacamole. Enchiladas are tortillas softened in lard or sauce, then filled with meat, poultry, seafood,

TABLE 6.1
Cultural Food Groups: Mexican

Group	Comments
PROTEIN FOODS	
Milk/milk products	Few dairy products used (incidence of lactose intolerance estimated at two-thirds of the population). Dairy products are used more in northern Mexico than in other regions.
Meats/poultry/fish/eggs/legumes	Vegetable protein primary source for majority of rural and urban poor. Pork, goat, poultry common meats. Beef preferred in northern areas and seafood in coastal regions. Meat usually tough. Prepared by marinating, chopping, and grinding (sausages popular), or sliced thinly. Cooked by grilling, frying, stewing, or steaming. Usually mixed with vegetables and cereals.
CEREALS/GRAINS	Corn and rice products used throughout the country; wheat products more common in the north. Principal bread is *tortilla*; European-style breads and rolls also popular.
FRUITS/VEGETABLES	Vegetables usually served as part of a dish, not separately. Semitropical and tropical fruits popular in most regions (limited availability in north).
ADDITIONAL FOODS	
Seasonings	Food often heavily spiced; ninety-two varieties of chiles used. Regional sauces typical.
Nuts/seeds	Seeds often used in flavoring.
Beverages	
Fats/oils	

cheese, or egg mixtures. The tortilla rolls are then baked covered with sauce. Tamales are one of the oldest Mexican foods, dating back at least to the Aztec period. A dough made with either masa harina or leftover *pozole* (hominy) is placed in corn husks (in the north) or young leaves of avocados or bananas (in the south). The leaves are folded and then baked in hot ashes or steamed over boiling water.

TABLE 6.1
Cultural Food Groups: Mexican—continued

Common Foods	Adaptations in the United States
Milk (cow, goat), evaporated milk, hot chocolate; *atole;* unaged cheeses	Aged cheese used in place of fresh cheese; more milk (usually whole) consumed; ice cream popular.
Meats: beef, goat, pork (including *chicharrónes* and variety cuts) *Poultry:* chicken, turkey *Fish and seafood: camerones* (shrimp), *huachinango* (red snapper), other firm-fleshed fish *Eggs:* chicken *Legumes:* black beans, garbanzo beans (chickpeas), kidney beans, pinto beans	Traditional entrees remain popular. Fewer variety cuts used. Protein intake may decline in second-generation Mexican Americans. Beans eaten less frequently.
Corn (*masa harina, pozole, tortillas*); wheat (breads, rolls, *pan dulce,* pasta); rice	Wheat tortillas used more than corn tortillas; convenience breads used. Increased consumption of baked sweets, such as doughnuts, cake, and cookies. Increased consumption of sugared breakfast cereals.
Fruits: avocados, bananas, *carambola, cherimoya,* coconut, *granadilla* (passion fruit), *guanábana,* guava, lemons, limes, *mamey,* mangoes, melon, oranges, papaya, pineapple, plantains, strawberries, sugar cane, *tuna* (cactus fruit), *zapote* (fruit of the *sapodilla* tree) *Vegetables:* cactus (*nopales or nopalitos*), chiles, corn, *jícama,* onions, peas, potatoes, squashes (*chayote,* pumpkin, summer, etc.), squash blossoms, *tomatillos,* tomatoes, *yuca* (cassava)	Fruit remains popular as dessert and snack item; apples and grapes accepted after familiarization.
Anise, *achiote* (annatto), chiles, *cilantro* (coriander leaves), cinnamon, cocoa, cumin, *epazote,* garlic, mace, onions, vanilla	
Piñons (pine nuts), *pepitas* (pumpkin seeds), sesame seeds	Use of spices depends on availability.
Atole, beer, coffee (*café con lèche*), hot chocolate, soft drinks, *pulque, mescal, tequila,* whiskey, wine	Increased consumption of fruit juices, Kool-Aid, soft drinks, and beverages with caffeine; decrease in use of hard spirits.
Butter, *manteca* (lard)	Fat intake increases, including use of mayonnaise and salad dressings.

The tamale may contain plain dough, be filled with a seasoned meat or vegetable mixture, or be sweetened for a dessert. After cooking, the husk or leaf is unfolded, revealing the aromatic tamale. Quesadillas are tortillas filled with a little cheese, leftover meat, sausage, or vegetable, then folded in half and heated or crisply fried. Burritos are popular in northern Mexico. They are similar to tacos, but large, thin, wheat flour tortillas are used instead of corn tortillas. The most common filling is beans with salsa.

Vegetables are usually part of the main dish or served as a substantial garnish. Potatoes, greens, tomatoes, and onions are most common. Chile peppers are used extensively in seasonings, sauces, and even stuffed, as in *chiles rellenos* and the Independence Day dish *chiles en nogada,* garnished with the colors of the Mexican flag—white sauce, green *cilantro* (fresh coriander leaves), and red pomegranate seeds.

Sugar cane grows well in Mexico, and sweets of all kinds are popular. Dried fruits and vegetables, candied fruits and vegetables, and sugared fruit or nut pastes are eaten alone and used in more complex desserts. The Spanish make many desserts with eggs, and some of these recipes have been adopted in Mexico. *Flan,* a sweetened egg custard topped with carmelized sugar, is the most common. *Huevos reales* is another popular dessert, made with egg yolks, sugar, sherry, cinnamon, pine nuts, and raisins.

The most common beverage in Mexico is coffee, which is grown in the south. Soft drinks and fresh fruit blended with water and sugar, called *aguas naturales,* are also favored. Adults drink milk infrequently, except in sweetened, flavored beverages such as hot chocolate with cinnamon. The most popular alcoholic beverage in Mexico is beer. The Mexican wine industry is also developing rapidly, in part due to a 1982 ban on the import of foreign wine. Men drink alcoholic beverages at all occasions when they gather socially. In addition to tequila and mescal, whiskey is typically served at these times.

Regional Variations

Mexican Plains   The northern and west-central regions of Mexico consist of mostly arid plains. The Indians who originally inhabited the area were called *Chichimecs* by the Aztecs ("sons of the dog") because of their seminomadic lifestyle. It is believed that their diet consisted of corn, beans, squash, greens, cactus fruit (*tuna*), and young cactus leaves (*nopales*). They also hunted small game and ate domesticated turkeys and poultry. When the Mexican Indians mixed with the Indians of the American Southwest, they adopted piñon nuts (also called pine nuts or pignolis), pumpkin, and plums.

The Spanish introduced longhorn cattle to the northern plains, as well as wheat. Today this is the only region of Mexico where people eat substantial amounts of beef and cheese. A favorite way to prepare beef is to air-dry it in thin slices called *cecinas,* similar to American chipped beef but more assertive in flavor. Cecinas can be used in stews or soups; it can be fried or used as fillings for other foods. The most popular Mexican cheeses are unripened. There is *queso blanco,* which is similar to mozzarella, and creamy *queso fresca,* which is similar to ricotta or pot cheese. Wheat is also used in more products in the north than in the south.

Vanilla, made from the bean of a vine native to Mexico and Central America, flavors many desserts. Legend is that the goddess Xanat fell in love with a mortal Mexican youth. Distraught that she could not marry him, she became a vanilla plant to provide him happiness.

Caesar salad, romaine lettuce with a tangy dressing of lemon, vinegar, garlic, anchovy, Romano cheese, and raw egg, was invented in northern Mexico.

The sap of the maguey cactus (century plant) is credited with being a reliable substitute for fresh water in the arid countryside; it is called *aguamiel* or "honey water." Tequila is probably the best-known beverage of the region, made from the distillation of fermented aguamiel, known as *pulque*. Pulque is the sour, mildly alcoholic beverage that was drunk throughout Mexico before the arrival of the Spaniards. The Spaniards, lacking grain, tried their distillation methods on the pulque, producing *mescal*, a harsh brew. Tequila is the more refined, twice-distilled version of mescal. It is produced in the central-western state of Jalisco around the towns of Tequila and Tepatitlan from a maguey subspecies *Agave tequiliana*.

Tropical Mexico Fruits and vegetables are featured foods in the southern coastal regions of Mexico. Tomatoes, green tomato-like *tomatillos*, chayote squash, onions, *jícama* (a sweet, crispy root), sweet and starchy plantains, carambola (star fruit), *cherimoya* (custard apple), *guanábana* (soursop), *mamey* (a type of plum), pineapple, *yuca* (a tuber also called cassava or manioc), and *zapote* (the fruit of the *sapodilla* tree) are just a small sampling of the produce available in this area.

More than ninety varieties of chile peppers are found in the region, varying enormously in degree of hotness. The chemical heat of chiles comes from the alkaloid capsaicin, found mostly in the

Mayauel was the ancient goddess of pulque. She was believed to bring both intoxication and death to mortals.

A worm from the maguey plant in a bottle of mescal or tequila is a signature of authenticity.

Tropical fruit from Latin America. (Courtesy of the Florida Division of Tourism.)

Chile (with an "e") comes from the Nahuatl word *chilli*. Foods like the powders, sauces, and stews made with chiles are conventionally called *chili* (with an "i").

Avocado comes from the Nahuatl word for the fruit, *ahuactl,* meaning "testicle," which they resemble hanging from the tree.

Achiote is called annatto in the United States. It is made from the seeds of a tropical tree and used sometimes to color cheddar-style cheeses, ice creams, margarine, and some baked goods.

fleshy ribs and seeds inside the fruit. It is not known why the sting of chile-spiced foods is enjoyed. It may stimulate the appetite and digestion through irritation of the stomach lining, or it may cause the body to release pain-killing endorphins creating a comfortable, gratified feeling.

Avocados, grown in the tropical climate, vary in size from 2 to 8 inches across, in skin color from light green to black, and in flavor from bland to bitter. Their succulent, smooth flesh is added to soups, stews, and salads. They are most popular in *guacamole,* mashed avocado with onions, tomatoes, chile peppers or chili powder, and cilantro, the pungent leaf of the coriander plant. It is used as a side dish, a topping, or a filling for tortillas.

Yucatán The cuisine of the Yucatán peninsula reflects its unique history. It was isolated from the rest of the country by dense, mountainous jungles until modern times. Many of the residents are descendants of the Mayas, the early Indian dynasty of the region. Some regional favorites date from this time. For example, one popular preparation method is to steam foods, called *píbil.* Traditionally food was cooked this way in an outdoor pit, but today it is prepared more often in a covered pot. Shrimp are a local specialty; the long coastline of the Yucatán along the Gulf of Mexico provides ample seafood. Sauces made with toasted squash seeds or the bright red spice *achiote* are also common to the area.

Southern Mexico The foods of southern Mexico are similar to those of the Yucatán in that they are more tropical and more Indian influenced than the foods of other regions. They are renowned for their complex, spicy sauces that use numerous ingredients such as chiles, nuts, raisins, sesame seeds, spices, and even chocolate. These sauces come in many colors, including red, yellow, green, and black, and are called *moles,* probably from the Aztec word for sauce with chiles, *molli.* Poultry, goat, and pork are the most popular meats, although some specialties of the region are more unusual, such as *chalupines,* a cricket that is found in the corn fields.

Meal Composition and Cycle

Daily Patterns

In familes where income is not limited, the preferred meal pattern is four to five daily meals: *desayuno* (breakfast), *almuerzo* (coffee break), *comida* (lunch), *merienda* (late afternoon snack), and *cena* (dinner). Most meals are eaten at home and served family style. If there are too many people to sit at the table, each one is served individually from the stove.

Desayuno is a filling breakfast, often including tortillas, eggs, meat, beans left over from the previous night, *bolillos* (wheat rolls), *pan dulce* (sweet bread, pastry, or cake), and fresh fruit. Coffee and hot chocolate are the preferred beverages. Near 11:00 AM is almuerzo, which features pan dulce or fruit, served with *café con lèche* (coffee with milk).

Comida is traditionally the largest meal of the day, eaten about 1:00 or 2:00 PM. A complete comida includes six full courses, from soup through dessert. When possible, an afternoon rest period (*siesta*) follows this meal. Merienda is a light meal of sweet rolls, cake, or cookies eaten around 6:00 PM. Coffee, hot chocolate, or a warm drink of thin, sugared cornmeal and milk gruel, called *atole,* accompanies the sweets. A light supper, cena, follows between 8:00 and 10:00 PM. This meal may be skipped entirely or expanded into a substantial feast on holidays or other formal occasions. Recently many Mexicans have adopted the American habit of eating a light lunch and a heavy supper, eliminating merienda altogether.

Snacking is frequent in urban Mexico; munching occurs from morning to midnight. *Antojitos,* or "little whims," include foods like *tostadas* (called *chalupas* in northern Mexico), fried tortillas topped with shredded lettuce, cheese, or meat. Nearly every block offers streetside food vendors, providing everything from fresh fruits to grilled meats. In addition, many neighborhoods feature an open-air market that also offers ready-to-eat foods.

Special Occasions

In Mexico, many foods are associated with holidays. For example, the Día de los Santos Reyes (also called Día de los Reyes Magos, or Three Kings Day) on January 6th is customarily celebrated with *rosca de reyes,* a raisin-studded, ring-shaped loaf of bread. Baked inside the bread is a figurine of the infant Jesus, and the person who receives it is obligated to give a party on February 2nd.

During Lent, *capirotada* is a popular dessert. Each family has its own recipe for this holiday bread pudding. Another holiday food is bread decorated with a skull and crossbones (*pan de muerto*), eaten on All Soul's Day (November 2nd) as part of a large feast honoring the deceased. Christmas festivities, called *posadas,* frequently feature *piñatas,* brightly decorated papier-mâché animals and figures that are filled with sweets. Blindfolded children take turns swinging a large stick at the hanging piñata until it breaks and candies fly everywhere. In some regions, thin, fried, anise-spiced cookies called *buñuelos* are eaten at Christmastime. They are drenched in syrup and served in pottery bowls, which when empty are smashed on the street for good luck. On Christmas Eve a salad of fruits, nuts, and beets is served. Turkey, tamales, and *arroz con leche* (rice pudding) are special foods eaten at holidays throughout the year.

In the city of Oaxaca, artisans carve intricate nativity scenes and representations of the Virgin of Guadelupe into large (up to 2-feet long) radishes in a state-sponsored competition the night before Christmas Eve. The origins of the event are lost in history.

Role of Food in Mexican Society

In family-centered Mexican society, food-related activities facilitate interactions between family members and help delineate family roles. Meal planning is usually the responsibility of the wife. Depending on economic status, food is prepared by the wife or by servants supervised by her, because Mexican foods can be laborious to prepare. The final dishes are greatly appreciated by all who partake in the meal, and it is considered an insult not to eat everything that is served. In rural areas, food sharing is an important social activity, reflecting the Indian worldview. To reject offered food or drink is a severe breach of social conduct.

Therapeutic Uses of Food

Some Mexicans avoid cold air and drafts after eating chiles (which are classified as hot) to avoid causing an imbalance in their bodies.

Some Mexican Indians and rural poor practice a hot-cold system of diet and health. It is believed to have derived from the Arab system of humoral medicine brought to Mexico by the Spanish, combined with the native Indian worldview. Although it has parallels with other classification systems, such as the Asian practice of yin-yang (see Chapter 7 for details), the Mexican system is only applied to foods and to the prevention and treatment of illness. It does not emcompass moral or social beliefs. The Mexican hot-cold theory is based on the concept that the world's resources are limited and must remain in balance. People must stay in harmony with the environment. Hot has the connotation of strength; cold, of weakness. When the theory is applied to foods, items can be classified according to proximity to the sun, method of preparation, or how the food is thought to affect the body. Meals balanced between hot and cold foods are considered to be health-promoting. Unbalanced meals may cause illness. Thus a typical comida in a rural village would consist of rice (hot), soup (made with hot and cold ingredients), and beans (cold).

Although the hot-cold classification of foods does vary, items generally considered hot are alcohol, aromatic beverages, beef, chiles, corn husks, oils, onions, pork, radishes, and tamales. Cold foods include citrus fruits, dairy products, most fresh vegetables, goat, and tropical fruits. Some foods, such as beans, corn products, rice products, sugary foods, and wheat products, can be classified as either hot or cold depending on how they are prepared.

Mexican women sometimes eat cilantro after giving birth because it is considered a cooling food for postpartum women.

Illnesses are also believed to be hot or cold and are usually treated with a diet rich in foods of the opposite classification. Certain conditions, such as menstruation and childbirth, are considered to be hot, and some women refuse hot foods at these times, such as pork, or very cold foods that might create a sudden imbalance, including cucumbers, tomatoes, and watermelon (Kay, 1977; Maduro, 1983). Sour foods are believed to thin the blood and are avoided by menstruating women because they are thought to increase blood flow; acidic foods may also be shunned because they are said to cause menstrual cramps.

Food and herbal remedies are also used in some regions. For example, chamomile is believed to cure colic, menstrual cramps, anxiety, insomnia, and itching eyes. Garlic is chewed for yeast infections in the mouth, toothache pain, and stomach disorders; boiled peanut broth is used to cure diarrhea; boiled cornsilk is taken for kidney pain; honey and water are given to infants for colic; oregano is used for fever, dry cough, asthma, and amenorrhea; and papaya is thought to help cure digestive ailments, diabetes, asthma, tuberculosis, and intestinal parasites.

Some Mexicans believe a sprig of parsley tucked above the ear will cure a headache.

Contemporary Food Habits in the United States

The foods of Mexico have influenced cooking in the American Southwest and California. In Texas, Tex-Mex cuisine features many modified Mexican dishes, such as chili, tamale pie, and nachos. Barbecued chile-spiced meat kebobs called *anacuchos* and *capriotada* with whiskey sauce known as "drunken pudding" are other examples of Tex-Mex creativity. (See Chapter 11 on regional Americans for more information.) Chicanos, Braceros, and undocumented immigrants living in the United States may eat these and other American foods or may eat a more traditional diet, depending on length of time in the country, location, income, or other factors.

Chili con carne (beans with beef) is not a Mexican dish, although there are similar combinations of ingredients found throughout Mexico. The origins of chili are believed to be in Texas, after the Mexican-American War.

Adaptations of Food Habits

Many Mexicans in the United States eat a diet similar to that of their homeland. Recent immigrants, those who live near the U.S.–Mexican border, and migrant workers are most likely to continue traditional food habits.

Chicanos and Mexicans who are well established in the United States often become more acculturated. In one hospital, it was found that "Mexican" patients overwhelmingly preferred American foods, even when offered traditional Mexican meals (Smith, 1979). A marketing study (Wallendorf & Reilly, 1983) noted that Mexican immigrants living in the southwestern United States are more likely to eat a diet with a high intake of red meats, white bread, sugared cereals, caffeine-containing beverages, and soft drinks than their socioeconomic counterparts in Mexico or white neighbors. This suggests that, rather than adopting a diet that fell somewhere between the food

Early researchers were perplexed by the absence of the niacin deficiency disease, pellagra, in Mexicans who consumed a corn-based diet. Pellagra was common in the southern United States, where corn was also a staple. It was found that when the corn kernels were prepared for *masa harina,* the alkaline lime solution used to soften them released the niacin that was bound to a protein. The lime is also believed to add calcium to the diet.

habits of Mexico and those of the United States, the Mexican immigrants in the survey accepted the stereotypical American consumption patterns of a decade ago.

Ingredients and Common Foods

Some American foods are accepted in even the most traditional families. Doughnuts, pie, cake, cookies, ice cream, and Popsicles are popular as desserts and snacks. Sugared cereals are becoming more common at breakfast for children, and American cheeses are often used in place of unaged Mexican cheeses.

A preference for sweet or carbonated beverages usually increases in the United States. Soft drinks, Kool-Aid, and juices are popular with meals and as snacks. Beer and coffee are also consumed with meals or snacks throughout the day. Whole milk is considered a "superfood" for children, but adults, especially men, consider it to be a juvenile drink. Milk is often flavored with chocolate, eggs, and bananas in a drink called *licuado;* mixed with coffee; or mixed with cornmeal to make atole. Some adults reject milk completely, claiming that they are allergic to it (it is estimated that two-thirds of Latinos are lactose-intolerant).

More acculturated Mexican Americans buy many prepared and convenience foods. Baked goods are usually purchased, including tortillas (often wheat tortillas are chosen over corn), breads, pan dulce, and even special desserts like flan. Extra income is usually spent on meats.

Meal Composition and Cycle

Daily Patterns   Studies of low-income Latinos and Mexican migrant farmworkers indicate that, for most meals, traditional foods are preferred. These include eggs, beans or meat, and tortillas or pan dulce for breakfast; a large lunch of beans, tortillas, and meat, or a soup or stew; and a lighter dinner of tortillas, beans or meat, and rice or potatoes. As in Mexico, vegetables tend to be served as part of a soup or stew. Fruit remains a typical snack and dessert, especially familiar varieties such as bananas, oranges, mangoes, guava, pineapple, strawberries, and melon. One study determined that the largest change is in increased consumption, of both basic items and new foods, due to increased income and increased availability (Dewey et al., 1984).

Chicanos more often adopt the American meal pattern of small breakfast, small lunch, and large dinner. Although consumption of tortillas remains relatively stable, breakfast cereals have become popular with all family members and sandwiches are a common lunch item. Meats and cheese become more prevalent at meals, beans are eaten less frequently, and vegetables are served as side dishes such as salads (Romero-Gwynn et al., 1993).

Changes in preparation methods may also occur. Recent immigrants may not know how to use the baking and broiling apparatus on an oven and may continue to fry and grill foods outdoors. Newer immigrants sometimes avoid canned and frozen foods because they do not know how to prepare them.

Special Occasions The Mexican custom of saving dishes that require extensive preparation, such as tamales and enchiladas, for Sunday and holiday meals is continued in the United States. In one study (Bruhn & Pangborn, 1971), migrant workers were asked what was the main dish served at holidays. No preference was found for Easter; tamales were preferred for Christmas. Turkey with mashed potatoes was the most popular Thanksgiving entree, indicating that this American holiday was adopted along with its traditional foods.

In addition to religious holidays, two secular celebrations are significant in the Mexican American community. The first is Mexican Independence Day on September 16th, commemorating the war of liberation from Spain. Observations emphasize ethnic unity including *mariachis* and traditional clothing. Foods the color of the Mexican flag, such as white rice, green avocado, and red or green chilis are eaten. *Cinco de Mayo* (May 5th) is the second holiday, more widely recognized by all ethnic groups throughout the U.S. even though the meaning of the event (remembrance of a historic victory over France) is often forgotten amidst the parades, piñatas, and Aztec dancing that typify the day.

CARIBBEAN ISLANDERS

More than 1,000 tropical islands in the Caribbean stretch from Florida to Venezuela. They include the Bahamas, the Greater Antilles (Jamaica, Cuba, Hispaniola, and Puerto Rico), and the Lesser Antilles. The largest island is Cuba, and the smallest islands are barely more than exposed rocks. Most were claimed at one time by Spain, Britain, France, the Netherlands, Denmark, or the United States, but now include the independent nations of Antigua/Barbuda, the Bahamas, Barbados, Cuba, Dominica, Dominican Republic, Grenada, Haiti, Jamaica, St. Christopher/Nevis, St. Lucia, St. Vincent/Grenadines, and Trinidad and Tobago, as well as the U.S. territory of Puerto Rico. Many islands, such as the Virgin Islands (U.S.) and Martinique (France), are still under foreign control.

The islands are uniformly scenic. The tropical warmth and torrential rains provide the ideal climate for a lush plant cover that includes numerous indigenous fruits and vegetables. Later immigrants found the region suitable for imported crops. The Caribbean Islands share a history of domination by foreign powers and political turmoil. Native Indians, Europeans, blacks from Africa, and Asians from China and India have intermarried over the centuries to produce an extremely diverse population.

Cultural Perspective

History of the Caribbean Islands

The original inhabitants of the Caribbean Islands are believed to be the prehistoric Cibony Indians. About 1000 CE, Arawak Indians migrated to the region from South America, followed by the Carib Indians. The Arawaks were an horticulturally based society; the Caribs were hunters and warriors.

When Columbus arrived in the Bahamas in 1492, he believed that he had discovered the East Indies. When this was found to be erroneous, the area became known as the West Indies. During the century following discovery by Europeans, thousands of Spanish settlers arrived in the region searching for riches. The Arawaks were enslaved and nearly exterminated by disease and abuse. The more aggressive Caribs were driven to the remote islands and now exist in only a few small enclaves.

The great natural wealth of the West Indies, especially spices, did not go unnoticed by the other European nations. Pirates from Britain and France regularly attacked the Spanish-occupied ports. Britain, France, the Netherlands, and Denmark established colonies in the Caribbean during the seventeenth century. The Europeans also recognized the region's potential for profitable agriculture. The Spanish were the first to cultivate sugar cane, although it was the French and British who exploited the crop.

The decimated Indian population was not large enough to support the sugarcane plantations that thrived in the West Indies. Fifteen million slaves from Africa were imported to the region between 1518 to 1865 to work in the fields. Emancipation of the African slaves was granted in the Caribbean during the 1850s and 1860s. This immediately required that a new source of inexpensive labor be found. Indentured servants were brought in from Asia, mostly India, to support the plantations, particularly on islands where sugar production was a new industry. Established sugar cane–growing islands, such as Puerto Rico, had few Asian immigrants.

Colonial control of the Caribbean Islands weakened during the nineteenth century as revolutions led to independence and European interest in the region waned as plantation profits declined. Haiti established the first self-governing nation in 1804. The Dominican

Republic separated from Haiti and became an independent country soon after.

The Spanish-American War led to independence for Cuba, and Spain ceded Puerto Rico to the United States. The Virgin Islands were purchased by the United States from Denmark in 1917. Cuba, Haiti, and the Dominican Republic remained the only self-ruling Caribbean nations until the early 1960s. Each has been led by a succession of dictators. In 1959, revolutionary Fidel Castro established Cuba as a communist state. Beginning in 1962, other islands slowly gained independence, starting with Jamaica, Trinidad, and Tobago. The latest to become a nation was St. Christopher/Nevis in 1983. Puerto Rico has fluctuated between desire for independence and U.S. statehood, and now functions as a commonwealth with an autonomous government that is subject to most federal laws. Puerto Ricans are U.S. citizens, yet they cannot vote in U.S. elections, nor do they pay federal income tax.

History of Caribbean Islanders in the United States

Immigration Patterns

It is estimated that the total Latino population in the United States is more than 22 million people. Immigrants from Puerto Rico constitute approximately 12 percent of the total; those from Cuba about 5 percent. In addition, there are small groups of immigrants from other Caribbean nations, most significantly from the Dominican Republic and Haiti.

Puerto Ricans Puerto Ricans differ from most other people who come to the United States in that they are technically not immigrants. They come to the mainland as U.S. citizens and are free to travel to and from Puerto Rico without restriction. Nearly half of the population of Puerto Rico resides on the mainland of the United States, and the number of Puerto Ricans who live in New York City is more than double the number living in San Juan, the largest city in Puerto Rico.

Small numbers of political exiles from Puerto Rico arrived in America in the 1800s, but most returned home when Puerto Rico became a U.S. possession. Others arrived when unemployment increased in the depressed agricultural economy of the island during the 1920s and 1930s. It was after World War II that the largest number of Puerto Ricans moved to the mainland. Unlike other immigrants, the Puerto Rican population in the United States is in continual flux. Many Puerto Ricans live alternately between the mainland and the island, depending on economic conditions. In many years the number of Puerto Ricans leaving the mainland is greater than the number arriving.

In 1995, more than 500 Puerto Ricans renounced their U.S. citizenship, saying it was imposed against their wills and saying that they are *Boricua* (the Taino Indian word for Puerto Rican), not American. The "Boricua First" movement advocates independence for the island.

Cubans Cubans have immigrated to the United States since the early nineteenth century. In the early years the majority were those who found economic conditions disadvantageous or who were politically out of favor with the current government.

The majority of Cubans came to the United States after Fidel Castro overthrew the dictatorship of Fulgencio Batista in 1959. In the 3 years following the revolution, more than 150,000 Cubans arrived in America. Most of these were families from the upper socioeconomic group fleeing the restraints of communism. Commercial air travel between Cuba and the United States was suspended after the Cuban missile crisis in 1962. Airlifts of immigrants from 1965 to 1973 increased the total number of Cubans in the United States to nearly 700,000. Due to the political differences between the two countries, most Cubans have not been subject to the usual immigration quotas.

Immigration from Cuba slowed with the end of the airlifts. In 1980, another large group of 110,000 Cubans arrived in Florida in private boats (the Mariel boatlift) seeking asylum. Unlike earlier immigrants, these recent arrivals, called *marielitos,* were mostly poor, unskilled laborers. They were often single and black. Today a trickle of exiles continues to come to the United States. Some arrive by boat and others go through legal immigration channels from a neutral third country.

Current Demographics

Puerto Ricans Figures from the 1990 U.S. census show that almost 2 million Puerto Ricans have settled on the U.S. mainland, the majority in New York. In the 1930s, Puerto Ricans began moving into

Cuban cafeteria, Miami, Florida. (Courtesy of the Metro Dade Department of Tourism.)

East Harlem, which became known both as *El Barrio* and as "Spanish Harlem." More than 900,000 Puerto Ricans now reside in New York City, and because Puerto Ricans are a young population, they now constitute nearly one-quarter of the students in the city's public schools. Boston, Chicago, Philadelphia, Newark, Miami, San Francisco, and Los Angeles also have Puerto Rican communities.

Puerto Ricans living in Puerto Rico are not counted in the U.S. census. If all Puerto Ricans were included, they would constitute nearly one-quarter of all Latinos in the United States.

Cubans   More than 1 million Cubans were counted in the 1990 U.S. census, one-third of them noncitizens. Americans of Cuban descent prefer to live in the Miami area, which is sometimes called "Little Havana." The climate is similar to that of their homeland, and the Cuban population in the region is the largest in the United States. Efforts to resettle exiles in other areas have been only moderately successful. Many Cubans living in Los Angeles, Chicago, New York City, and Jersey City and Newark, New Jersey choose to move to Miami after gaining job skills. Those Cubans who remain in other cities are most likely to be employed in technical or professional occupations. Nearly all Cubans who live in the United States are urban dwellers.

Other Caribbean Islanders   In the 1990 U.S. census, approximately 500,000 residents from the Dominican Republic and 280,000 residents from Haiti were identified. Unofficial estimates suggest that several hundred thousand undocumented immigrants from the two nations have also settled in the United States; most live in the urban areas of New York, New Jersey, Massachusetts, and Florida, with smaller numbers in Illinois. Dominicans often immigrate to Puerto Rico first in search of employment, then come to the mainland. Haitians come directly to the United States. Many are well-educated political refugees seeking asylum.

Socioeconomic Status

Immigrants from the Caribbean vary tremendously in both economic and educational attainment. Among Latinos, Puerto Rican Americans have the highest rate of unemployment (in 1990, it was 31% of men and 59% of women) and Cuban Americans have the lowest. In 1987 the median annual income of Puerto Ricans in the mainland United States was approximately half that of the U.S. Cuban population, again the lowest and highest among Latinos, respectively. Almost 25 percent of Puerto Ricans live in poverty. Although nearly half of Cuban Americans are employed in professional, technical, managerial, sales, or administrative support positions, one-third of Cuban American families still earned less than $20,000 in 1990.

Even though large numbers of Dominican professionals have immigrated to the United States, most obtain lower-paying jobs in manufacturing and service industries. More than 22 percent of Dominican families live at the poverty level. Haitian immigrants have usually come from poor segments of their society and have entered migrant labor and service positions. It is estimated that nearly one-third of Haitians in Miami are unemployed.

Educational rates for first-generation immigrants from the Caribbean are very similar to those of other Latinos. Nearly half of all adults from Puerto Rico and Cuba did not attend high school. Differences in educational attainment appear with second-generation Americans of Caribbean descent, however. Only 27 percent of Puerto Ricans living on the mainland complete high school; 83 percent of U.S.-born Cuban Americans graduate from high school and one-quarter complete some college. Cuban Americans are more likely than any other Latino group to pay for education; nearly one-half have attended private schools. Dominicans in New York have demonstrated their commitment to education through political involvement, running for control of local school boards. Statistics of school attainment of Dominicans and Haitians in the United States are usually combined with those of other Latinos and are not generally available for individual groups.

Socioeconomic differences among Latino groups from the Caribbean are due to many factors. Puerto Ricans living on the mainland are free to travel between the United States and their homeland, and the frequent changes in residence may hamper socioeconomic improvement. Puerto Ricans have also chosen to settle primarily in New York City, where as a new ethnic minority they took over the decayed neighborhoods previously occupied by African Americans. In general, their low education levels and undeveloped job skills translate into unemployment and low-level employment. Further, it is thought that Puerto Ricans, Dominicans, and Haitians often face discrimination similar to that experienced by African Americans because many are of African heritage.

In contrast, Cubans in the United States are mostly political refugees who emigrated out of necessity, not choice. There are a disproportionate number of Cubans in the United States from the upper socioeconomic levels, and although many lost all their material goods when they emigrated, they brought upper-class values, including the importance of educational and financial success. Instead of displacing any ethnic minority in Florida, they immigrated in such numbers that they immediately became the dominant ethnic group. This is not to say that there are no well-educated, wealthy Puerto Ricans living on the mainland or no poor Cuban Americans. However, circumstances surrounding their immigration have influenced the general socioeconomic status of both groups.

Cultural Organizations

Caribbean Islander communities are often highly self-sufficient, including meeting the needs of members with little official outside contact with mainstream business or government. For example, Haitians typically form rotating credit associations, called *sangue,* to finance homes and businesses of recent immigrants and undocumented residents.

National organizations are most numerous among Puerto Ricans and Cubans. The National Puerto Rican Coalition and the National Association for Puerto Rican Civil Rights work for the economic and political well-being of Puerto Ricans; the National Conference of Puerto Rican Women promotes political, social, and economic issues advocacy; and the Association for Puerto Rican–Hispanic Culture fosters awareness of Puerto Rican values. Many Cuban groups work toward the liberation of Cuba. Others are more focused on Cuban American issues: the Cuban American Legal Defense and Education Fund fights discrimination and stereotypes; the Cuban American National Council promotes expanded social services in the Cuban community; and the National Association of Cuban American Women in the U.S.A. considers issues of importance to Cuban and Hispanic women. The Caribbean Haitian Council provides help with acculturation and advocacy for Haitians and other Caribbean Islander immigrants.

Worldview

Ethnic identity is strongly maintained in both the Puerto Rican and Cuban communities in the United States. Puerto Ricans on the mainland continue close ties with the island; Cubans believe it is important to retain their heritage because they cannot return. Spanish may be spoken exclusively in the home and used frequently to conduct business within the community.

In contrast, immigrant populations with large numbers of undocumented residents, such as Dominicans and Haitians, often try to blend into existing Latino communities or assimilate into mixed ethnic neighborhoods. It has been noted that Dominicans appear to acculturate quickly and accept many outwardly American values and aspirations.

Religion

The majority of Caribbean Islanders are Roman Catholics, although many are not faithful followers of the church. The role of the Catholic church has been less important in the Caribbean than in other regions of Latin America; it is estimated that only 63 percent of

Cuban Americans born in the United States are Catholic and that 25 percent have no religious affiliation.

There are a number of other religions in the islands, including Protestantism and Judaism, as well as some folk religions. The best known of these is *voodoo,* a unique combination of West African tribal rituals with Catholic beliefs and local customs. Saint Patrick is associated with the African snake deity Damballah, for example, and St. Christopher is identified with Bacoso, the god responsible for infectious illness. Certain rites, such as repeating the Hail Mary, making the sign of the cross, and baptism, are practiced in conjunction with ancestor worship, drums, and African dancing. Worship is family-based and there is no central leadership or organization of activities. Typically ceremonies are conducted for annual events such as Christmas and the harvest and for funerals. Voodoo originated in Haiti, although very similar Afro-Catholic cults are found on the other islands. In Cuba and Puerto Rico, they are called *santeria.* Many followers of voodoo or santeria are also members of Christian faiths and do not believe that there is any contradiction in practicing both religions simultaneously.

Family

The Puerto Rican family is based on the concept of *compadrazco,* which means co-parenting. Grandparents, aunts and uncles, cousins, and godparents are all considered part of the immediate family, responsible for the care of children (Green, 1995).

Men are the heads of households as well as being in charge of community matters. The oldest boys in the family are expected to help with supervision of younger siblings, particularly daughters. Women maintain the home. Men are expected to be aggressive; women are traditionally reserved. As in most Latino cultures, age is respected; even younger children are taught to defer to older children.

Traditional Cuban families are also patriarchal and extend to include relatives. Godparents are significant in childrearing. Children are deferential to elders and well chaperoned in public.

Caribbean Islander familes often change in the United States. Economic pressures, American values of individualism and equality, and intergenerational stress are often cited as responsible for nontraditional adaptations. Studies have shown that one-third of Dominicans, for example, live in nuclear family groupings in the United States even though only 1 percent did so in the Dominican Republic. Dominican women in the United States also have fewer children than those on the island (Buffington, 1995b). In the United States, Caribbean Islander women assume more authority in the household with their increased involvement in the workforce, and Caribbean Islander children gain greater autonomy.

Communication

Caribbean Islanders use an expressive conversational style. Respect and politeness are practiced, but it is not considered rude to interrupt a speaker. Shaking hands in greeting and in leaving is customary, and touching is very common, especially between members of the same sex, who may hug freely. Direct eye contact is expected throughout the Caribbean, with some variations: Looking away suggests disrespect or dishonesty among Cubans; Dominicans maintain eye contact depending on the situation, and men are more likely to look directly at one another than are women; Haitians may avert their eyes from authority figures.

Traditional Food Habits

Ingredients and Common Foods

Caribbean food habits are remarkably similar for an area influenced by so many other cultures. The indigenous Indians, the Spanish, French, British, Dutch, Danes, Africans, Asian Indians, and Chinese have all had an impact on the cuisine. Although each island has its specialties, the basic diet is the same throughout the region.

Indigenous Foods

Columbus likened the West Indies to paradise on earth. The islands are naturally laden with fresh fruits and vegetables that originally came from South America, including the staple *cassava* (two varieties of tuber, bitter and sweet, that are also known as *manioc* and *yuca;* tapioca is a starch product of manioc), avocados, bananas and plantains, some varieties of beans, cashew apples (fruit surrounding the cashew nut), cocoa, coconuts, guavas, *malanga* (a mild tuber), papayas, pineapple, *soursop* (a fruit with a cotton-like consistency), several types of squash (including *chayote,* called *chocho* or *christophene* in the islands), sweet potatoes, *tanier* (another type of tuber), and tomatoes. Fish and small birds are also plentiful.

As in other Latin American areas, many varieties of chile peppers grow profusely in the West Indies. The native cuisine makes frequent use of these for flavoring, especially in pepper sauces, such as *coui,* a mixture of cassava juice and hot chile peppers. Other herbs and spices include allspice and annatto.

Because of the abundance of fresh fruits and vegetables year-round, traditionally there was little need for preparation or preservation of foods. Consequently cooking techniques were underdeveloped in the native populations. Cassava was baked most

Cassava contains hydrocyanic acid, which is toxic in large amounts. The acid must be leached out and the tuber cooked before it can be eaten safely.

The American word barbecue is probably derived from *barbacoa,* the Arawak term for grilling meats.

often in a kind of bread, made from pressed, dried, grated cassava that was fried in a flat loaf. Fish and game were either covered with mud and baked in a pit or grilled over an open fire.

Foreign Influence

The Europeans who settled in the Caribbean were impressed with the abundant supply of native fruits and vegetables. Yet they longed for the accustomed tastes of home. The Spanish brought cattle, goats, hogs, and sheep to the islands, in addition to introducing rice. Plants introduced for trade by the Europeans included breadfruit, coffee, limes, mangoes, oranges, and spices such as nutmeg and mace. The African slaves brought in to work the sugarcane fields cultivated *akee* (a mild, apple-sized fruit), okra, and *taro* (also called *ado* or *dasheen;* both the roots and the leaves are eaten). The demand for Asian ingredients by later immigrants resulted in the introduction of soybean products, Asian greens, and tamarind to the Caribbean.

Staples

Legumes are eaten throughout the Caribbean; the rice and kidney beans of Puerto Rico are also found in the Dominican Republic and Jamaica. In Cuba, black beans are preferred; in Haiti, black-eyed peas are combined with the rice. The legumes in all countries are prepared similarly, flavored with lard and salt. Onions, sweet peppers, and tomatoes are added in some variations.

Examples of other foods common throughout the West Indies are found in the Cultural Food Groups list (Table 6.2). They include Indian foods like cassava bread, chili sauces, and pepper pot (a meat stew made with the boiled juice of the cassava, called *cassarep*). European-influenced items like *escabeche* (fried, marinated fish, seafood, or poultry) and *morcillas* (a type of blood sausage), as well as fried corn cakes, are popular in most Caribbean countries. Foods from Africa found throughout the region include *callaloo* (a dish of taro or malanga greens cooked with okra), dried salt cod fritters (called *bacalaitas* in Puerto Rico, these cakes have a different name on nearly every island, from *arcat de marue* to "stamp and go"), *foofoo* (okra and plantain), and *coocoo* (cornmeal-okra bread). Dishes from India and Asia are also common on many islands, although they are better known in the areas where cheap labor was most needed: the French-, British-, and Dutch-dominated islands (few Asians immigrated to Puerto Rico, Cuba, or the Dominican Republic). Curried dishes, called *kerry* in the Dutch-influenced islands and *colombo* on the French-influenced islands, and variations of pilaf are considered Caribbean foods. Chinese cuisine is also popular and Chinese-owned restaurants are ubiquitous.

The black beans and rice popular in Cuba are called *Moros y Cristianos* (Moors and Christians), a reference to Spanish history.

Pickled fish, called *ceviche,* is popular throughout Latin America. Believed to have originated in Peru, it features scallops or cubes of raw fish marinated in salted lemon or lime juice mixed with chiles and onions until "cooked," meaning the fish becomes opaque and flaky.

The most popular beverage in the Caribbean is coffee. It is often mixed with milk and is consumed at meals, as a snack, and even as dessert, flavored with orange rind, cinnamon, whipped cream, coconut cream, or rum. Some of the most expensive coffee in the world is produced in the Blue Mountains of Jamaica, where the cool, moderately rainy climate is ideal for coffee cultivation. Most of the rich beans are exported to England and Italy, although small amounts can be found in the United States.

The most important beverage in the Caribbean, at least historically, is the spirit distilled from fermented molasses—rum. This alcoholic drink is believed to have originated on the island of Barbados in the early 1600s as a by-product of sugar cane processing. Molasses is the liquid that remains after the syrup from the sugar cane has been crystallized to make sugar. It is fermented, naturally or with the addition of yeast, then distilled to make a clear, high-proof alcoholic beverage. Rum can be bottled immediately or aged in oak casks from a few months to 25 years. Caramel is added to achieve the desired color. Nearly every island produces its own variety of rum.

The molasses produced in the West Indies was crucial to the development of the region during the seventeenth and eighteenth centuries. The Caribbean Islands were one corner of the infamous slave triangle, formed when molasses was shipped to New England for distillation into rum, rum was shipped to Africa and exchanged for slaves, and slaves were shipped to the West Indies to work in the sugar cane fields.

Many well-known mixed drinks were developed in the Caribbean with rum. Planter's punch is an adaptation of the recipe from India for *panch* (lime juice, sweetening, spirit, water, and spices) and was probably invented by the British in the eighteenth century. The *daiquiri*, a popular mix of lime juice, sugar, and rum, was created in the 1890s and named after a Cuban town. The *cuba libre* (rum and coke with a slice of lemon) is popular throughout the Caribbean and Central America.

Regional Variations

Despite the similarities in foods throughout the West Indies, most islands have their own specialties. Haiti is known for its banana-stuffed chicken dish called *poulet rôti à la créole* and barbecued goat with chile peppers (*kabrit boukannen ak bon piman*); the Dominican Republic for *sancocho,* a pork intestine stew; Jamaica for its spicy vegetable soup called pepper pot and for *"picka peppa"* sauce (a sweet mango sauce or a hot chile pepper sauce); Curaçao for its orange-flavored liqueur of the same name; Dominica for its "mountain chicken," a large, tasty frog; and Barbados for its unusual seafood dishes made with flying fish, green turtles, and sea urchins.

In addition to rice and kidney beans, Puerto Rican fare is notable for its use of *sofrito,* a combination of onions, garlic, cilantro, sweet peppers, and tomatoes that are ground together in a wooden bowl, then lightly fried in lard colored with annatto seeds. Sofrito serves as a base for many dishes, as well as an all-purpose sauce. Some foods are seasoned with *adobo,* a mixture of lemon, garlic, salt, pepper, and other spices. More pork, beef, and goat is eaten in Puerto Rico than in most Caribbean countries. Plantains are stuffed with spicy beef

TABLE 6.2
Cultural Food Groups: Caribbean Islands

Group	Comments
PROTEIN FOODS	
Milk/milk products	Few dairy products used; incidence of lactose intolerance assumed to be high.
	Infants given whole, evaporated, or condensed milk.
Meats/poultry/fish/eggs/legumes	Traditional diet high in vegetable protein, especially rice and legumes; red and kidney beans used by Puerto Ricans, black beans by Cubans.
	Pork and beef used more in Spanish-influenced countries.
	Dried salt cod preferred over fresh fish; some seafood specialties.
	Eggs are a common protein source, especially among the poor.
	Entrees are often fried in lard or olive oil.
CEREALS/GRAINS	Breads of other countries well accepted.
	Fried breads popular.
FRUITS/VEGETABLES	Starchy fruits and vegetables eaten daily; leafy vegetables consumed infrequently.
	Great diversity of tropical fruits available, eaten mostly as snacks or dessert.
	Lime juice used to "cook" (a marinating method called *escabeche* or *ceviche*) meats and fish.
ADDITIONAL FOODS	
Seasonings	Chile-based sauces often used to flavor foods.
Beverages	
Fats/oils	
Sweeteners	

mixtures or *chicharrones* (fried pork rind). Chicken is frequently prepared with rice, *arroz con pollo,* which is usually served with marinated beans or peas known as *abichuelas guisada,* or in a stew called *asopao.* Land crabs and *ostiones,* a type of oyster that grows on the roots of mangrove trees, are popular, but the fish most commonly eaten is dried salt cod, called *bacalao.* It is soaked and drained before use to remove some of the salt and then added to numerous dishes including *serenata,* a mixture of cod and potatoes. Starchy vegetables

TABLE 6.2
Cultural Food Groups: Caribbean Islands—continued

Common Foods	Adaptations in the United States
Cow's milk (fresh, condensed, evaporated), *café con lèche, café latté*); aged cheeses	More milk is consumed.
Meats: beef, pork (including intestines, organs, variety cuts), goat	More meat and poultry eaten as income increases.
Poultry: chicken, turkey	Less fresh fish consumed.
Fish and shellfish: bacalao (dried salt cod), barracuda, bonita, butterfish, crab, dolphin, flying fish, gar, grouper, grunts, land crabs, mackerel, mullets, *ostiones* (tree oysters), porgie, salmon, snapper, tarpon, turtle, tuna	Traditional entrees remain popular.
Eggs: chicken	
Legumes: black beans, black-eyed peas, garbanzo beans (chickpeas), kidney beans, lima beans, peas, red beans, soybeans	
Cassava bread; cornmeal (fried breads, *surrulitos,* puddings); oatmeal; rice (short-grain); wheat (Asian Indian breads, European breads, pasta)	Short-grain rice still preferred. More wheat breads eaten.
Fruits: acerola cherries, *akee,* avocados, bananas and plantains, breadfruit, *caimito* (star apple), cashew apple, citron, coconut, cocoplum, custard apple, gooseberries, *granadilla* (passion fruit), grapefruit, guava, *guanábana* (soursop), kumquats, lemons, limes, *mamey,* mangoes, oranges, papayas, pineapple, pomegranates, raisins, *sapodilla,* sugar cane, tamarind	Temperate fruits substituted for tropical fruits when latter unavailable. More fresh fruit eaten.
Vegetables: arracacha, arrowroot, black-eyed peas, broccoli, cabbage, *calabaza* (green pumpkin), *callaloo* (malanga or taro leaves), cassava (*yuca,* manioc), chiles, corn, cucumbers, eggplant, green beans, lettuce, *malangas,* okra, onions, palm hearts, peppers, potatoes, radishes, spinach, squashes (*chayote,* summer, and winter), sweet potatoes, *taniers,* taro (*edo, dasheen*), tomatoes, yams	Starchy fruits and vegetables still frequently consumed. Low intake of leafy vegetables often continues.
Anise, annatto, bay leaf, chiles, chives, *cilantro* (coriander leaves), cinnamon, *coui* (chiles mixed with cassava juice), garlic, mace, nutmeg, onions, parsley, scallions, *sofrito* (fried onions, garlic, sweet peppers, tomatoes, and cilantro, from Puerto Rico), thyme	
Beer, coffee (*café con lèche*), soft drinks, milk, rum	Fruit juice and soft drink consumption may increase.
Butter in French-influenced countries; coconut oil; *ghee* (Asian Indian clarified butter); lard in Spanish-influenced countries; olive oil	
Sugar cane products, such as raw and unrefined sugar and molasses	

such as potatoes and plantains are eaten almost daily; leafy green vegetables are uncommon.

Cuba is unique in the West Indies for the preferred use of black beans in its cuisine. In addition to black beans and rice, spicy black bean soup is very popular. *Picadillo* is a type of beef hash that is flavored with traditional Spanish ingredients of olives and raisins, as well as Caribbean tomatoes and chile peppers. It is served with fried plantains or boiled rice, or topped with fried eggs. Other Spanish-influenced beef dishes are *ropa vieja* ("old clothes"), which is spicy beef strips, and *brazo gitano*, a cassava pastry filled with corned beef. Roast pork is also popular. A chicken specialty is *chicharrones de pollo,* small pieces of chicken that are marinated in lime juice and soy sauce, breaded, then fried in lard. As in Puerto Rico, starchy vegetables, such as *foo-foo* (cassava balls), are preferred over leafy green vegetable side dishes.

Meal Composition and Cycle

The most typical aspect of a Caribbean meal is its emphasis on starchy vegetables with some meat, poultry, or fish. Meats are frequently fried. Leafy vegetables are often an ingredient in soups, stews, and stuffed foods; fruits are enjoyed fresh, frequently as snacks or dessert.

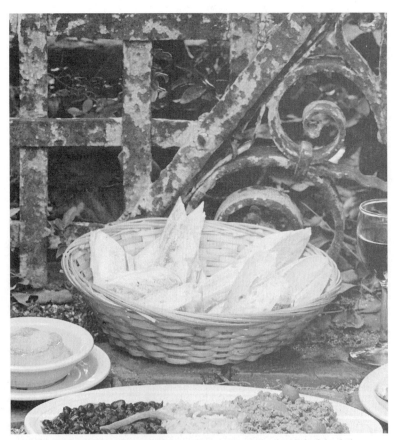

A typical Cuban meal includes savory *picadillo* (right), black beans and rice, bread, and *flan* (a Spanish-style custard) for dessert. (Courtesy of the Florida News Bureau.)

Ethnic heritage determines which dishes are served. A poor native Indian may eat mostly cassava, tomatoes, and chiles with a bit of meat or fish at every meal. An Asian Indian may serve typically Asian Indian meals adapted to Caribbean ingredients, such as a curried dish garnished with coconut, fried plantains, and pineapple. Most menus, however, consist of a multicultural mix, such as European blood sausage and *accra,* West African–style fritters made from the meal of soybeans or black-eyed peas. The list of dishes served at a meal on a French-influenced island may be identical to that on a Spanish-influenced island, yet the two meals will taste different because butter was used for cooking the former and lard the latter.

Daily Patterns

Breakfast usually consists of coffee with milk and bread. If income permits, eggs are the most common addition, then cereals and fruits. Urban residents are more likely to skip breakfast than are people in rural households.

Rice and beans with meat, if affordable, is the most popular lunch. In rural regions a starchy vegetable, such as potatoes, plantain, breadfruit, taniers, taro, or yams, with dried salt cod is also common. Meats, milk, and salad vegetables are extra items added to the basic foods whenever possible.

Dinner is similar to lunch. Rice and beans provide the core of the meal, with meats, vegetables, and milk added when available. In upper-income households the meal may consist of three or four different dishes. Milk and coffee with milk (*café con lèche*) are the preferred beverages. Soft drinks and beer are also popular. Ice cream and pastries are typical desserts for those who can afford them. Snacking is frequent among some groups, especially children. Fruits, sweetened fruit juices poured over shaved ice, and coffee with milk are common.

Special Occasions

The early European dominance in the West Indies resulted in an emphasis on Christian holidays. Christmas is important, especially in the Spanish-influenced islands that are predominantly Catholic. In Puerto Rico, *pasteles* are prepared to celebrate Christmas. Similar to Mexican *tamales,* pasteles are a savory meat mixture surrounded by cornmeal or mashed plantains, wrapped in plantain leaves, and steamed. Carolers traditionally stop at houses late at night to request hot pasteles from the occupants. Other holidays reflect the multicultural history of the islands. *Carnival* is celebrated in some Caribbean countries, such as Trinidad and Tobago, and is similar to Mardi Gras in the United States. The pre-Lenten festivities feature parades of dancing celebrants; many are elaborately costumed as traditional European or African figures. Food booths that line the parade route provide a day-and-night supply of carnival treats. Fried Asian Indian fritters are particularly popular. Examples of nonreligious events include the

On Good Friday in Trinidad and Tobago the white of an egg is added to warm water and the future is predicted by its shape.

daylong birthday open house on Curaçao for friends, relatives, and acquaintances. Thanksgiving is observed in Puerto Rico. Turkey, stuffed with a Spanish-style meat filling, is the main course.

Therapeutic Uses of Food

Some Caribbean Islanders adhere to a hot-cold classification system of diet and health similar to that found in Mexico (see previous section on Mexican therapeutic uses of foods). In addition to the categories of hot and cold, Puerto Ricans add *cool*. Imbalances in hot and cold—for example, sitting in the shade of a tree after being out in the sun—can cause illness even years after the imbalance has occurred (Spector, 1991). Haitians believe that women are warmer than men and that a person cools as he or she ages (Laguerre, 1981).

The hot-cold theory of foods practiced in the Caribbean includes not only the category of cool foods, but also those that are considered "heavy" or "light." A balance of hot-cold elements is attempted at meals, and heavy foods, such as starches, are consumed during the day, while light foods, such as soup, are eaten in the evening. Although the specific classification of items varies from person to person, one guideline for Puerto Ricans (Harwood, 1981) indicates bananas, coconuts, and most vegetables are cold; chiles, garlic, chocolate, coffee, evaporated milk and infant formula, and alcoholic beverages are hot. Cool foods include fruit, chicken, bacalao, whole milk, honey, onions, peas, and wheat. Excessive intake of cool or cold foods can make a cold condition, such as a cough, develop into a chronic illness, such as asthma.

Pregnancy, which is defined as a hot condition by most Puerto Ricans, is a time when a hot-cold balance is practiced carefully and hot foods are avoided. When infants suffer from hot ailments, including diarrhea or rash, infant formula may be replaced with whole milk, or cooling ingredients such as barley water, mannitol, or magnesium carbonate may be added to the formula. High-calorie tonics (eggnogs and malts are popular types) are taken by some Puerto Ricans to stimulate the appetite and provide strength or energy. These are considered especially appropriate for pale children and for pregnant or postpartum women.

Research with Dominican American mothers suggests that nutritional practices during lactation may sometimes include avoidance of certain protein foods and increased intake of fluids such as malt beer, milk, orange juice, chocolate milk, and noodle soup (Sanjur, 1995). Formula may be withheld from sick infants and tea provided instead.

In Haiti, pregnant women are encouraged to eat red fruits and vegetables to strengthen the blood of their babies (Laguerre, 1981). Haitians also believe that certain illnesses in infants can be caused if a nursing mother's milk is too thick or too thin. Further, if a woman is frightened while breast-feeding, her milk goes to her head, causing her a headache and diarrhea in the baby. *Gaz,* another condition, causes pain in the shoulder, back, legs, or appendix and headaches, stom-

Rum was believed to cure many types of disease and injury in the seventeenth and eighteenth centuries. As late as 1892 a physician prescribed Cuban rum for the 6-year-old future king of Spain when he suffered from a fever. The royal family was so impressed by his quick recuperation that they granted the maker of the rum, the Bacardi family, the right to use the Spanish coat of arms on their label.

achaches, or anemia. Foods such as corn or a tea made from garlic, cloves, and mint are home remedies for gaz (Unaeze & Perrin, 1995).

Contemporary Food Habits in the United States

Adaptations of Food Habits

Traditional food habits are easily maintained in the self-sustaining immigrant communities of Spanish Harlem in New York and Little Havana in Miami. Ingredients for Caribbean cuisine are readily available through Puerto Rican and Cuban American markets. Cubans, for example, consider drinking strong coffee a way to maintain their ethnic identity; by contrast, Americans drink "weak" coffee (Pasquali, 1985). Changes do occur, however, as immigrants settle into culturally mixed communities and children grow up as Americans.

One study compared the diet of three groups of women from Puerto Rico: (1) those living in New York (forward migrants), (2) those who had lived on the mainland but later returned to the island (return migrants), and (3) those who never lived on the mainland (nonmigrants). It was found that nonmigrants and return migrants ate more starchy vegetables, sugar, and sweetened foods than did forward migrants. Forward migrants ate a greater variety of foods, including more beef, eggs, bread, fresh fruit, and leafy green vegetables. Puerto Rican women who had lived on the mainland quickly reverted to their traditional food habits when they returned to the island (Immink et al., 1983).

In a study of elderly Cubans living in the United States, it was found that convenience items were sometimes used to prepare traditional foods: aluminum foil in place of banana leaves for *tamales*, and packaged crescent rolls for *pastele* dough (Pasquali, 1985).

Ingredients and Common Foods

Research on the food habits patterns of Caribbean immigrants in the United States is limited. It is thought that rice, beans, starchy vegetables, sofrito, and bacalao remain the basis of the daily diet of many Puerto Ricans who live on the mainland. Poultry is used when possible, and egg intake decreases. Because of Cuban Americans' greater discretionary income, their diet usually includes additional foods, such as more pork and beef. Recent poorer immigrants from Cuba, including the marielitos, are more restricted in what foods they purchase, however, and may follow a diet that is closer to the subsistence-level Puerto Rican regimen.

A study of Puerto Rican teenagers in New York found that, consistent with traditional food habits, there is little diversity of food items in their diet (Duyff et al., 1975). However, in the study mentioned previously, Puerto Rican women on the mainland were reported to eat a greater variety of foods than those on the island. According to marketing studies, Caribbean Islanders accept some American foods, especially convenience items, and purchase frozen and dehydrated products when they can afford to do so. The proportion of meat in the diet often increases on the mainland, as does the consumption of milk (and other dairy foods) and soft drinks (Harwood, 1981; Chávez et al., 1994; Sanjur, 1995). Intake of leafy vegetables continues to be low. Local fruits often replace the tropical fruits of Puerto Rico.

Recent data regarding Dominicans in the United States indicate that only small changes have occurred in consumption patterns. Protein and fat intake has increased slightly, mostly due to eating more meat, while carbohydrate intake has decreased. Dominican women reported that their diet was more varied and abundant than in their homeland (Sanjur, 1995).

Meal Composition and Cycle

The meals of Puerto Ricans residing on the mainland are similar to those of people on the island, with a few changes. A light breakfast of bread and coffee may be followed by a light lunch of rice and beans or a starchy vegetable, with or without bacalao. Often this traditional mid-day meal becomes a sandwich and soft drink, however. A late dinner consists of rice, beans, starchy vegetable, meat if available, or soup. Salad is included in some homes. Many researchers have reported an increase in the amount of snacking between meals, mostly on high-calorie foods with little nutritional value (Harwood, 1981; Sanjur, 1995).

Interviews with Haitians living in New York City suggest that some traditional dietary practices are discontinued; for example, the main meal is eaten in the evening instead of at noon. Although some Haitians adhere to hot-cold classifications of food, they may differ from those used in Haiti (Laguerre, 1981). Dominicans have also started eating lighter lunches (Sanjur, 1995).

One study (Haider & Wheeler, 1979) reported that many low-income Latina women living in New York did not plan menus far in advance and that this hampered their ability to add variety to their diets. It was found that food shopping serves as a social occasion for many of the women and is one of the few opportunities they have to get out of the house; thus they may go to the grocery store more often than is really necessary. The investigators reported that nearly half of the women questioned preferred to fry main dishes. Boiling was the second choice, baking third. Broiling food was a distant fourth choice. The researchers note that in many low-income households the oven or broiler element may not work, restricting food preparation methods to frying and boiling.

In Haiti, protein foods are served first to the father in the household; leftovers go to the wife and children. It is believed this pattern continues in Haitian American homes.

CENTRAL AMERICANS

The seven nations of Belize, Guatemala, El Salvador, Honduras, Nicaragua, Costa Rica, and Panama make up Central America, an isthmus connecting North America to South America. The eastern coastal region edges the Caribbean Sea. An 800-mile chain of active volcanoes and mountains, beginning at the Mexican border in the north and continuing with only one break into central Panama in the south, forms the temperate backbone of the region. Central America is similar to the Caribbean Islands in tropical climate, history of foreign intervention, and heterogeneous culture.

Cultural Perspective

History of Central America

Many native Indian civilizations thrived in ancient Central America. Most notable were the Maya, who dominated the area that is now southern Mexico, Belize, Guatemala, and Honduras from approximately 2000 BCE until the arrival of the Spanish in the sixteenth century. Intensive horticulture, advanced water management, and

Chocolate was so prized in Mayan culture that cocao beans were used as currency.

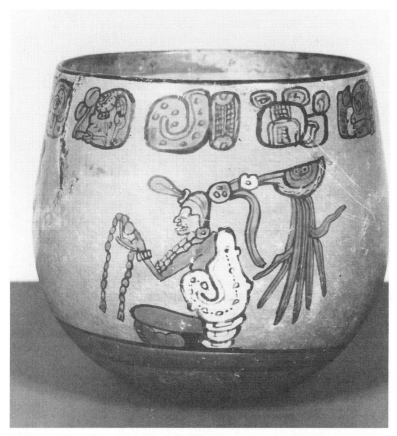

A Mayan chocolate container. (© The Bettmann Archive.)

extensive trade contributed to the success of their numerous city-states. The Maya were the first people in the Americas to keep historical records. Their descendants still live in the region today.

Spanish conquest of Central America occurred in the 1520s following the explorations of Columbus and Balboa. The Indian population of the region was devastated by disease and enslavement. Guatemala became the capital of colonial Spain. Belize (the former British Honduras) came under British influence in the 1600s when British bootleggers established strongholds in the area. Although Spain claimed sovereignty, British domination succeeded and Belize became an official colony in 1865.

Independence from Spanish control in Central America occurred in the 1820s. (Belize did not achieve independence from Great Britain until 1981.) In the nineteenth and twentieth centuries, U.S. influence increased throughout Central America with the introduction of coffee and bananas as cash crops and the construction of the Panama Canal in 1912.

Political instability has typified the region. With the exception of Costa Rica, which has maintained a democracy for most of the twentieth century, military dictatorships have most often ruled the nations. In the 1960s and 1970s, political forces, some endorsed by the United States and others supported by the then communist government of the Soviet Union, battled in El Salvador, Guatemala, and Nicaragua. Continuing conflict has led to economic decline and widespread poverty. Tenuous peace accords were signed in the 1990s, leading to free elections in some countries and a unified effort by all Central American nations to create a common market for greater economic success.

History of Central Americans in the United States

Immigration Patterns

Central American identity is sometimes more related to race and class than to country of origin. The majority of immigrants before the 1980s were white professionals; more recent refugees are predominantly *Ladino* (mixed Spanish and Indian heritage) or Indian *campesinos* (peasants).

Central American immigrants to the United States have arrived in two distinct waves. Early records are inexact because separate statistics on Central Americans were not kept until the 1960s by the U.S. Census Bureau. Even today they are usually listed with immigrants from South America in most demographic studies.

Until the early 1980s, immigrants to the United States were of two groups. The first were well-educated professional men who arrived in search of employment opportunities. The second were women, who often outnumbered the men two to one, coming in search of temporary domestic jobs. These Central American immigrants were largely urban residents and settled mostly in New York, Los Angeles, San Francisco, Miami, and Chicago, where they blended into existing Latino communities.

The second major wave began in the late 1970s and early 1980s, with the exodus of refugees from the brutal civil wars in El Salvador, Guatemala, and Nicaragua. It is estimated that millions of residents have been displaced in these countries, about one-third of whom have emigrated. Many moved to Mexico, and a substantial number have continued on to the United States. They are known as the "foot people" because many have literally walked to the United States (Melville, 1985). Less is known about this group, except that they are often younger, poorer, and less educated than the previous immigrants from the region.

Current Demographics and Socioeconomic Status

Nearly 6 percent of U.S. Latinos (approximately 1.3 million) are from the seven nations of Central America, one-half of whom arrived between 1980 and 1990. Exact figures are unknown, however, because it is believed that many Central Americans may enter the United States illegally at the border with Mexico and are undistinguished from undocumented Mexicans. Most of these recent immigrants have settled in California, Texas, and Florida. The largest known populations are the approximately 500,000 Salvadorans, 270,000 Guatemalans, and 200,000 Nicaraguans. It is believed that there may be an equal number of undocumented residents from these countries living in the United States as well. Approximately 115,000 Americans of Honduran descent were identified in the 1990 U.S. census. Immigration from the other Central American nations, Costa Rica, Belize, and Panama, is minimal.

Guatemalan Americans prefer to be called *Chapines*. The term was originally a derogatory term for residents of Guatemala City but has new meaning in the United States, reflecting ethnic pride.

Central American immigrants, even those from the first wave, are slow to naturalize; only 35 percent of Central Americans in the United States have obtained citizenship. Those who are not refugees often return to Central America for visits and maintain active contact with their homeland.

Most socioeconomic data on Central Americans are combined with statistics on South Americans and do not account for recent arrivals, many of whom may be undocumented residents. Information on the first wave of Central American immigrants suggests that they are a middle-class population with income and education levels well above most Mexican Americans and Puerto Ricans (about equal to the Cubans). American-born children of these first immigrants graduate from high school in numbers greater than whites. But these figures do not reflect the large numbers of recent immigrants employed as migrant farmworkers, gardeners, domestic cleaners, dishwashers, and foodservice workers, as well as those placed in other low-skilled jobs. Undocumented residents often face difficulties in obtaining employment and education opportunities. Disposable family income is often impacted by the money that is sent to support relatives still living in the homeland.

In 1988, Nicaraguan Americans sent between $50 and $80 million to their families in Nicaragua, second only to coffee exports as a source of foreign exchange.

Cultural Organizations

Several organizations have been founded to aid refugees and immigrants from Central America. These include the Central American Refugee Center headquartered in Los Angeles, Casa Guatemala, the Guatemala Support Network, and the Nicaraguan Interfaith Committee for Action. Other associations are committed to local support or cultural awareness, such as *Grupo Maya* and the International Maya League.

Worldview

The large numbers of recent immigrants from Central America suggest that ethnic identity is preserved by many new residents in the United States. For example, Salvadorans establish highly insular neighborhoods within the larger Latino community, where an immigrant can live and conduct business exclusively with other Salvadorans. Guatemalans are a more diverse population of immigrants, and it is the Mayan communities that are most likely to keep traditional beliefs and practices. In contrast, Nicaraguans are dispersed among other Latinos and are adapting more to the pan-Latino community than retaining their own heritage exclusively.

Religion

Most Central Americans are Roman Catholic. Some Guatemalans observe Catholic practices while adhering to Mayan religious beliefs; participation in native religions declines in the United States because they are usually dependent on sacred locations in Guatemala. Evangelical and fundamentalist denominations, such as the Pentecostal Church, have attracted many Central Americans after they arrive in the United States. Small "storefront" congregations that involve active participation and those churches that offer traditional Central American social activities in addition to worship have been especially successful.

Family

Central Americans highly value family and extended kinship. It has been noted that some apartment buildings in Latino neighborhoods are rented entirely to several families from the same village in Central America. The father is the undisputed head of the household and provider for the family. Children are carefully controlled, especially daughters.

The traditional roles of the men and women become less delineated in the United States, where women are sometimes more easily employed and husbands must take on some domestic responsibilities. Family disintegration has taken place in some refugee camps prior to immigration to the United States, where overcrowding and unemployment led to intergenerational conflict (Miralles, 1989). In other situations, family members were forced to immigrate separately. Some married outside the Central American community for immigration benefits; others found that when their families were reunited, children had become more independent (Mumford, 1995).

Communication

Guatemalans prefer a soft conversational voice and appreciate being addressed by their titles alone, without their surnames. Nicaraguans and Salvadorans like to be addressed by their titles and surnames. Guatemalans, Nicaraguans, and Salvadorans prefer a light handshake that is lingered over (a woman may have to extend her hand first before a male will shake it, however). Eye contact is direct, and smiling is expected. Touching is a way of communicating feelings; men embrace close friends and women may hug all acquaintances. Salvadorans use their hands expressively, but pointing with the fingers or feet is impolite; Hondurans clasp their hands together to indicate approval. Most Central Americans prefer to sit closely together when talking, and backing away may be seen as an affront.

Traditional Food Habits

Ingredients and Common Foods

Central American cuisine offers many of the foods common throughout Latin America. The native Indian dishes remain prominent in the highland areas, Spanish influences are found in the lowland regions, and the cooking of the multicultural eastern coast shares many similarities with Caribbean Islander fare. The northern nations have foods similar to those of southern Mexico; the southern countries have been more greatly influenced by European and African cuisines.

Staples

Early Mayan records indicate that the foundation of their diet was corn and beans, supplemented with squash, tomatoes, chiles, tropical fruit, cocoa, and some game. Indian foods were particularly important in the development of Guatemalan cuisine but gradually become less significant in the south of Central America. Rice, introduced by the Spanish, has become a staple in most regions. (See the Cultural Food Groups list in Table 6.3.)

The Mayan word for corn, *wab,* also means "food."

TABLE 6.3
Cultural Food Groups: Central Americans

Group	Comments
PROTEIN FOODS	
Milk/milk products	Milk is not widely consumed as a beverage, but evaporated milk and cream are popular in some regions.
Meat/poultry/fish/eggs/legumes	Legumes are important in the cuisine and are often served with rice. All types of meat/poultry are eaten, but pork is popular throughout the region. Eggs are commonly served. Fish and shellfish are consumed in the coastal regions. Sea turtle eggs are popular.
CEREALS/GRAINS	Rice and corn are the predominant grains of the region. Wheat flour breads are common.
FRUITS/VEGETABLES	Tropical fruits are abundant. Some temperate fruits such as grapes and apples are also available. Salads and pickled vegetables are popular.
ADDITIONAL FOODS	
Seasonings	Cilantro (fresh coriander) and *epazote* are important herbs. Sour orange juice gives a tang to some food; coconut milk flavors others. *Achiote* is used to color foods orange.
Nuts/seeds	
Beverages	Hot chocolate and coffee, grown in the region, are favorite hot beverages. *Refrescas,* cold drinks, are made with tropical fruit flavors. *Boj, chicha,* and *venado* are locally made alcoholic beverages.
Fats/oils	Lard is the most commonly used fat.
Sweeteners	Honey and sugar are used as sweeteners.

In Guatemala, refried black beans (*frijoles volteados*) are fondly called "Guatemalan caviar."

Beans are eaten daily. Black beans are especially popular in Guatemala, while red beans are common in other nations. Beans are served simmered, pureed, or fried and are often paired with rice. In Nicaragua, red beans and rice fried with onions are called *gallo pinto* ("painted rooster") due to the colors of the dish.

Corn is eaten mostly as tortillas. Enchiladas in Central America are open-faced sandwiches similar to Mexican tostadas. They typically feature meat covered with pickled vegetables such as cabbage, beets, and carrots. Known as *mixtas* in Guatemala, the tortilla is spread first with guacamole, then topped with a sausage and pickled cabbage. In El Salvador a stuffed specialty is called *pupusas.* A tor-

TABLE 6.3
Cultural Food Groups: Central Americans—continued

Common Foods	Adaptations in the United States
Milk (evaporated), cream; cheese (aged and fresh—crumbly farmer's cheese type)	Milk and hard cheeses are often disliked.
Meat: beef, iguana, lizards, pork (all parts, including knuckles, tripe, and skin), venison *Poultry:* chicken, duck, turkey *Fish and shellfish:* clams, conch, flounder, mackerel, mussels, sea snail, shark, shrimp, sole, tarpon, turtle *Eggs:* poultry, turtle *Legumes:* beans—black, chickpeas, fava, kidney, red, white Corn (tamales, tortillas), rice, wheat (bread, rolls)	
Fruits: apples, bananas, breadfruit, coconut, grapes as well as raisins, guava, *mameys,* mangoes, *nances,* oranges (sweet and sour types), papaya, passion fruit, *pejibaye,* pineapples, prunes, tangerines, *zapote* or *sapodilla* *Vegetables:* asparagus, avocados, beets, cabbage, carrots, cauliflower, chayote squash, chile peppers, corn, cucumbers, eggplant, green beans, hearts of palm, leeks, lettuce, onions, *pacaya* buds (palm flowers), peas, plantains, potatoes, spinach, sweet peppers, tomatillos, tomatoes, watercress, yams, yuca (cassava) *Achiote* (annatto), chile peppers, cilantro, cinnamon, cloves, cocoa, *epazote,* garlic, onions, mint, nutmeg, thyme, vanilla, Worcestershire sauce Palm tree nuts, *pepitoria* (toasted squash seeds)	Increased intake of potato chips has been reported.
Coffee, chocolate, tropical fruit drinks, alcoholic beverages (rum, beer, and fermented or distilled fruit, sugar cane, and grain drinks)	Increased intake of soft drinks has been noted among Guatemalan refugees in Florida.
Butter, lard, vegetable oils, shortening	
Honey, sugar, sugar syrup	Increased intake of candy.

tilla is filled with chicharrones, cheese, or black beans, then completed with another tortilla; the edges are sealed and the pupusa is then fried. They are traditionally served with pickled cabbage. Tamales are also common, often stuffed with poultry or pork. They are called *nactamal* in Nicaragua, where the dough is flavored with sour orange juice and the filling includes meat, potatoes, rice, tomatoes, onions, sweet peppers, and mint. Black tamales are served on special occasions in Guatemala, stuffed with a mixture of chicken, chocolate, spices, prunes, and raisins. *Empanadas,* small turnovers made with a wheat flour dough and filled with a savory meat mixture, are popular.

French bread, introduced from Mexico, is eaten regularly in the form of small rolls in Honduras and Guatemala. In El Salvador, French bread is used with native turkey and pickled vegetables to make sandwiches. Coconut bread is a specialty on the Caribbean seacoast. Rice is often cooked with coconut milk or fried or, in Costa Rica, served as pancakes.

Soups and stews are popular throughout Central America. Beef, plantains, and cassava in coconut milk; spicy beef stew; beef in sour orange juice; pork and white bean stew; chicken cooked in fruit wine; *mondongo* (Nicaraguan tripe soup); and *sopa de hombre* ("a man's soup") made with seafood and plantains in coconut milk are a few specialties. In Guatemala the Mayan meat stew called *pepián* is thickened with toasted squash seeds. Meat, poultry, and fish are frequently roasted as well.

Fruits and vegetables are numerous. Although bananas, coconut, plantains, yuca (cassava), tomatoes, sweet peppers, chayote squash (known as *huisquil* in Guatemala), mangoes, oranges, and avocado predominate, cabbage, cauliflower, carrots, beets, green beans, lettuce, spinach, breadfruit, passion fruit (*granadilla*), pineapples, mameys, and *nances* (similar to yellow cherries) are also common. *Pejibaye* (peach palm) is a fruit especially popular in Costa Rica. Onions and garlic flavor many dishes. Salads and pickled vegetables are very popular, as appetizers, as side dishes, and on sandwiches.

Coffee, grown throughout the region, is a popular drink, as is hot chocolate. *Refrescas,* cold beverages, are made in tropical fruit flavors, such as mango and pineapple. *Tiste,* a Nicaraguan favorite, is made with roasted corn, cocoa powder, sugar, cold water, and cracked ice. Beer is widely available. Fermented beverages like *boj* (from sugar cane) and *chicha* (a wine made from fruit or grain, fortified with rum) are consumed. *Venado* is a common distilled drink made from sugar cane. Sweets, such as the praline-like candy called *nogada,* sweetened baked plantains, ices made with fruit syrups, custards, and cakes or fritters flavored with coconut or rum, are eaten as snacks and for dessert.

Regional Variations

Although many foods of Central America are similar, they are often flavored with local ingredients for a unique taste. Coconut milk flavors many dishes in Belize and Honduras; seafood specialties include conch and sea turtle. The foods of El Salvador feature many indigenous flavors including corn, beans, tomatoes, chiles, and turkey. Achiote is common in mild-flavored Guatemalan fare. The juice of sour oranges is mixed with sweet peppers or mint in many Nicaraguan recipes. Costa Ricans prefer foods simmered with herbs and seasonings such as cilantro, thyme, oregano, onion, garlic, and pimento; rice is also frequently consumed. Panamanian fare is more international in flavor; one specialty is *sancocho,* a stew of pork, beef, ham, sausage, tomato, potato, squash, and plantains.

In Guatemala, eggs poached and served with a seasoned broth are used to treat hangovers.

Mangoes are considered an aphrodisiac in Guatemala.

Though iguana tail is eaten throughout Central America, parts of South America and the Caribbean, it is especially popular with Indians in Nicaragua.

Meal Composition and Cycle

Daily Patterns

As in other Latin American regions, beans and corn are the corner-stones of the daily diet, eaten at every meal by the poor. Rice is also common. *Queso blanco* (a fresh cheese) or meat is added whenever resources permit. Dinner in wealthier areas usually includes soup, meat or poultry (sometimes fish), tortillas or bread, and substantial garnishes such as avocado salad, fried plantains, and pickled vegetables. Appetizers, such as slivers of broiled beef, bites of meat- or cheese-filled pastry, and soft-boiled turtle eggs, are eaten in some urban regions before dinner; dessert may also be served, typically including custards, ice creams, cakes, or fritters.

Special Occasions

Celebrations in Central America are focused on Catholic religious days. Christmas, Easter and Lent, saints' days, and even Sundays may mean a change in fare. All Saints' Day is also celebrated. Special dishes include the cheese-flavored batter bread called *quesadilla* that is served in El Salvador on Sundays; *sopa de rosquillas,* a soup made with ring-shaped corn dumplings traditionally eaten on the Fridays of Lent in Nicaragua; *gallina rellena Navidena,* a Nicaraguan Christmas dish of chicken stuffed with papaya, chayote squash, capers, raisins, olives, onions, and tomatoes; and plantains served in chocolate sauce during *Semana Santa* (the Holy Week before Easter) in Guatemala.

Chicken in tomato sauce (*guisado*), chicken served with a corn-meal porridge, or stews thickened with masa harina are Indian specialties eaten at ceremonial occasions. In some areas the stews are provided by the village headman to serve the community. In Guatemala, All Saints' Day is celebrated with a unique salad called *fiambre.* As described by one author (Marks, 1985), these enormous salads are a family social event at which as many as fifty friends and relatives share the creation. They feature vegetables (e.g., green beans, peas, carrots, cauliflower, beets, radishes, cabbage) mixed with chicken, beef, pork, and sausages, then artfully garnished with salami, mortadella, cheese, asparagus, pacaya buds, and hard-boiled eggs. The dressing is either a vinaigrette or a sweet-and-sour sauce.

Therapeutic Uses of Foods

Central Americans consider a good diet essential to health, as is a balance of hot and cold. Illness can occur if one eats or touches something that is too hot or too cold. Guatemalan Americans commonly believe that diarrhea is caused by hot weather and can be alleviated by consuming cold drinks, such as Kool-Aid or Gatorade (Miralles, 1989). Herbal remedies are popular throughout Central America, including chamomile and coca leaves, the source of cocaine (Barrett, 1995).

Contemporary Food Habits in the United States

Adaptations of Food Habits

There is scant information on current Central American food habits. It is assumed that low rates of assimilation among many Central American immigrants result in preservation of many traditional food habits. Most Central American ingredients are available in the Latino communities where they settle.

Salvadoran refugees report that, in general, they believe that the quality of their diet has declined since arriving in the United States. They state that in El Salvador, more foods were made at home from fresh ingredients; they believe that in the United States, more processed items and "junk" foods are eaten, and some nutritious foods are too costly to consume (Boyle, 1989).

Health workers in Florida report that Guatemalan refugees believe that if a food is tasty and does not cause stomach discomfort, it must be "good" to eat. High intake of candy, soft drinks, and potato chips has been noted. Milk, which is often not well tolerated, is avoided. WIC (Supplemental Food Program for Women, Infants, and Children) nutritionists found that some food supplements, including milk and cheese, are disliked because of their taste or texture and are sometimes discarded (Miralles, 1989).

Lactose intolerance may be prevalent among Central Americans.

The Cooking of South America

South America is a vast land that features the rugged ridge of the Andes Mountains stretching from north to south. Highland plains, tropical rainforest, temperate valleys, and desert dunes extend from where the mountain peaks slope toward the coastal edges of the continent. Extremes in the terrain and climate limit agriculture in many areas.

The cooking of South America is similar to that of other Latin American regions in that it combines some native ingredients and preparation techniques with the foods of colonial Europeans. The diet is largely corn-based and chile pepper–spiced. Tomatoes are common and, in tropical areas, cassava (called *yuca*) is a popular tuber. Pumpkins, bananas, and plantains are consumed often. Beef, rice, onions, and olive oil, introduced by the Spanish and the Portuguese, are eaten regularly. However, South American fare also features a number of

The Cooking of South America—continued

ingredients used infrequently in the dishes of other Latin American areas. Potatoes, which were first cultivated by the Incas on mountain terraces, are particularly important in the highlands of Peru and Ecuador. Sweet potatoes (the orange-fleshed root vegetable usually called "yams" in the United States) are also native to the region. A white root similar to a mild carrot, known as *apio* or *arracacha* (*Arracacia xanthorrhiza*), is found in Colombia, Peru, and Venezuela, and the tuber known as *ahipa* (called jicama in the United States and Mexico) is native to the Amazon River basin. Beans, a foundation food in many Latin American regions, are common in most South American countries, yet not eaten at every meal. Other legumes and nuts like peanuts and cashews are used often in dishes. Local meats, including llama, deer, rabbit, wild pig, and *cuy* (guinea pigs raised for consumption), are favored in some areas. Fish, such as anchovies and tuna, and shellfish, particularly shrimp, crab, spiny lobster, oysters, clams, giant sea urchins (*evisos*), and giant abalone (*locos*), are significant foods in the extensive coastal regions.

The most popular way to prepare meats in South America is grilling. Traditionally sides of beef, whole lambs, hogs, and kids (goats) are hung over smoldering wood to slowly cook for hours in a method called *asado*. Today a grill is used more often. Steaks and marinated kebobs (which often include organ meats) are favorites. Another, even older cooking tradition is to steam foods in a pit oven. In Peru, this method is called a *pachamanca* and typically includes a young pig or goat, with guinea pigs, chickens, tamales, potatoes, and corn tucked around layers of hot stones and aromatic leaves and herbs. In Chile a *curanto* is closer to an elaborate coastal clam bake, including shellfish, suckling pig, sausages, potato patties, peas, and beans layered with seaweed.

National differences exist, although there are few clearly distinctive divisions in South American fare. Several countries share similar dishes, and only a few nations have well-developed regional cuisines.

Peru and Ecuador

The cooking of Peru and Ecuador is divided into the highland fare of the Andes and the lowland dishes of the tropical coastal regions. The cuisine of the mountain areas is among the most unique in South America, preserving many ingredients and dishes of the Inca Indians. Potatoes are eaten at nearly every meal, and often for snacks. Over 100 varieties are cultivated. *Ocopa,* boiled potatoes topped with a cheese sauce and chile peppers or peanuts, is a typical dish in Peru. In Ecuador, fried potato and cheese patties called *llapingachos* and potato cheese soup served with slices of avocado known as *lorco* are common. Traditionally the tubers are preserved by freezing in the cold night air and then drying in the hot daytime sun. *Papa seca* are boiled first, then dried until the potatoes are rocklike chunks that must be rehydrated before consumption; *chuño* are not cooked before drying and are often ground into a fine potato starch. Corn is also grown in the mountains. Some varieties have kernels the size of small strawberries that when prepared as hominy are known as *mote* and are a popular snack item. Bananas and plantains are cooked as savory chips and made into flour for breads and pastries.

The foods of Peru and Ecuador are preferred *picante* and feature abundant use of chile peppers in both the highlands and along the coast. *Salsa de ají,* a combination of fresh chopped chile, onion, and salt, is served as a condiment at most meals. Orange- or yellow-hued dishes are favored; along the coast,

continued on next page

The Cooking of South America—continued

achiote colors foods, and in the Peruvian highlands an herb known as *palillo* is used.

Charqui, dried strips of llama meat, is a specialty of the Andes. Another traditional dish is *humitas*, which are very similar to tamales but are made with fresh corn dough mixed with meats, potatoes, vegetables, and other ingredients instead of dough made from cornmeal wrapped around a stuffing. Along the coast, seafood dominates the diet. The region is famous for its *ceviches*, a method of preparing fresh fish, scallops, or crab by marinating small raw chunks in lemon, lime, or sour orange juice. The acidity of the juice "cooks" the fish and turns it opaque. At many beaches, *cevicherias* offer the dish as a snack or light meal with beer. Chopped onion, tomato, avocado, and cilantro are often added. In Peru, *ceviche* is typically garnished with sliced sweet potato.

Argentina, Chile, Bolivia, Uraguay, and Paraguay

Hearty, ample fare with an emphasis on beef exemplifies the cooking of these southern nations. Argentina is a major beef-producing region, and its people eat more beef per capita than in any other country worldwide. The temperate weather permits the cultivation of numerous fruits and vegetables, notably strawberries, grapes, and Jerusalem artichokes (known as *topinambur* in Chile). The cooking of Argentina, Chile, Paraguay, and Uruguay has been influenced more by their immigrant populations than by the numerous small Indian groups native to the area. The Spanish introduced cattle, and the Italians brought pasta. Smaller numbers of Germans, Hungarians, and other central Europeans have added their foods as well.

The national dish of Argentina is *matambre*, which means "to kill hunger." A special cut of flank steak is seasoned with herbs, then traditionally rolled pinwheel fashion around a filling of spinach, whole hard-boiled eggs, and whole or sliced carrots, and then tied with a string and poached in broth or baked. *Matambre* can be served as a main course, but it is often chilled first and offered as a cold appetizer. Grilled steaks are particularly popular in Argentina and surrounding nations. In Paraguay, steaks are typically served with *sopa Paraguay*, a cornmeal and cheese bread. In Uruguay, beef is eaten nearly as often as in Argentina, although mutton and lamb are also common.

Robust soups and stews are everyday fare. In Bolivia, beef stew is made with carrots, onions, hominy, and *chuño*. The stews of Argentina often pair meat with fruits as well as vegetables, such as *carbonada criolla* (beef cooked with squash, corn, and peaches) or *carbonada en zapallo* (veal stew cooked in a pumkin). In Paraguay, soups reveal European inspiration, such as *bori-bori*, beef with cornmeal and cheese dumplings, and *so' o-yosopy*, beef soup with bell peppers, tomatoes, and vermicelli or rice, topped with Parmesan cheese. Fish soups and stews are popular in Chile, which has an extensive coastline and plentiful seafood. Clam or abalone chowder with beans (*chupe de loco*) and *congrio* (an elongated, firm-fleshed fish that looks a little like an eel) cooked with potatoes, onions, garlic, and white wine are specialties.

Empanadas, which are pastry turnovers stuffed with various savory or sweet fillings, are found throughout South America. The traditional flaky dough used in empanada recipes brought from Spain is often enriched with indigenous ingredients, such as mashed potatoes, cassava, or corn or is flavored with achiote or other spices. The turnovers are usually baked, but sometimes they are fried. Fillings are as many as there are cooks. In Argentina, *empanadas* with Spanish flavorings are a specialty, stuffed with chopped beef,

The Cooking of South America—continued

olives, raisins, and onions. The turnovers are sometimes filled with abalone in Chile and with cheese in Bolivia, where they are called *salteñas*.

National favorites include pasta (e.g., spaghetti, ravioli, and lasagna), which is served in many homes on Sundays in Argentina. It is considered auspicious to eat it on the 29th of every month as well. In Chile, beans are especially popular, and seafood is eaten regularly. Wines from the temperate midlands of the country are considered some of the best on the continent. In Bolivia, legs from the giant frog found in the Andean Lake Titicaca are a specialty.

Although coffee is consumed throughout the area, another caffeinated beverage is equally popular in some regions. Called *maté*, it is an infusion made from the leaves of a plant (*Ilex paraguariensis*) in the holly family native to Paraguay. Served hot or chilled, *maté*, is consumed nearly every afternoon with small snacks in Paraguay and in parts of Argentina. The dried, powdered leaves are called *yerba* and are traditionally mixed in a gourd with boiling water. A special metal straw is inserted to drink the brew.

Colombia and Venezuela

The fare found in Colombia and Venezuela is colonial Spanish in character, cooked with olive oil, cream, or cheese and flavored with ground cumin, achiote, parsley, cilantro and chopped onions, tomatoes, and garlic. Yet native tastes are still evident. *Guascas,* or *huascas* (*Galinsoga parvilora Lineo*), an herb native to Colombia, provides a flavor similar to boiled peanuts in soups and stews. Hot chile pepper sauces are served on the side of most dishes. Tropical fruits and vegetables, including avocados, bananas and plantains, *naranjillo* (a small, orange fruit related to tomatoes used for its tart juice), pineapple, and coconut milk or cream are other common regional ingredients.

In Colombia, *Bogatá chicken stew* (made with chicken, two types of potatoes, and cream) and *sancocho* (a boiled dinner traditionally made with beef brisket or other roast and ample starchy vegetables like potatoes, sweet potatoes, plantains, or cassava) are typical Spanish-influenced dishes. Examples in Venezuela include *ropa vieja* ("old clothes"); shredded flank steak served in a sauce made with tomatoes, onions, and olive oil; and *pabellón caraqueño,* flank steak served on rice with black beans, topped with fried eggs, and garnished with fried plantain chips. Dishes with more indigenous flavors include *arepa*, the staple cornmeal bread of Venezuela that is formed into 1-inch thick patties and cooked on a griddle (it is sometimes stuffed with meat or cheese before it is fried), and mashed black beans, known as *caviar criollo* or "native caviar." Tropical fruits, such as guavas and pineapple, are often sweetened and dried to make fruit leathers and fruit pastes that are favorite snacks.

Brazil

The cooking of Brazil is very different from that of other South American countries due to Portuguese and African influences. The Portuguese arrived in the sixteenth century, looking for land to cultivate sugar cane. They contributed dried salt cod and linguiça to the diet, stews known as *cozidos* made with many different meats and vegetables (known as *cocido* in Portugal), and a variety of exceptionally sweet desserts based on sugar and egg yolks, such as caramel custards and coconut puddings. African slaves put to work on the sugar plantations brought foods unknown in nearby countries, such as dendê oil (a type of palm oil) and okra. Spicy dishes were preferred. In West Africa, malagueta peppercorns, a small, hot grain, was used to season foods; in

continued on next page

The Cooking of South America—continued

Brazil, Africans adopted a very small, mouth-searing chile pepper indigenous to the area and also called it malaguetal. It is typically minced and added to dendê oil, often with dried shrimp and grated ginger root, to make a hot sauce.

Although Indian, Portuguese, and African tastes and textures have influenced cooking throughout Brazil, nowhere are they more prominent than in the state of Bahia. Known as Afro-Brazilian fare, or *cozinha baiana,* it is famous for fritters made from dried shrimp, dried salt cod, yams, black-eyed peas, mashed beans, peanuts, and ripe plantains fried in dendê oil. *Vatapá,* another specialty, is a paste made with smoked dried shrimp, peanuts, cashews, coconut milk, and malaguetal chiles. It is used as a filling for fritters and sometimes served with rice as an entree.

The national dish of Brazil is *feijoda completa,* which originated in Rio. Black beans cooked with smoked meats and sausages are served with rice, sliced oranges, boiled greens, and a hot sauce mixed with lemon or lime juice. Toasted cassava meal, called *farinha,* is sprinkled over the top like Parmesan cheese. *Farinha* is served with most dishes and is often mixed with butter and other ingredients such as bits of meat, pumpkin, plantains, or coconut milk to create crunchy side dishes

called *faroja.* Rice or cornmeal porridge called *pirão* is another type of side dish. Middle Easterners who immigrated to the southeastern areas of Brazil brought the concept of couscous to the country and adapted the dish to native ingredients. *Cuzcuz paulista* is prepared with cornmeal in a *cuzcuzeiro,* which looks like a colander on legs that is inserted over a pot of boiling water to steam. The basket of the *cuzcuzeiro* is first lined with seafood or poultry and vegetables, which flavors the cornmeal as it cooks and looks decorative when the *cuzcuz* "cake" is inverted.

In the far south the cuisine has been influenced by the foods of Argentina. *Churrasco* is the Brazilian form of spit-roasting. In cities, restaurants serving grilled foods are popular. Called *churrascaria,* their diners choose their meats which are barbecued to taste. Brazilians in the south also drink *maté,* which they call *chimmarão.*

Coffee, rum, and beer are common beverages in Brazil, but several other drinks are also popular. *Guaraná* is a stimulating carbonated soft drink made from the seeds of the native *guaraná* fruit, which contain caffeine. *Cachaça* is an alcoholic beverage distilled from sugar cane that is often compared to brandy. It is used to make *batidas,* a refreshing punch made with cachaça and fruit juice.

7

Asians

Asia, one of the largest continents, is believed to have been named by the Greeks, who divided the world into two parts—Europe and Asia. It includes China (the People's Republic of China), Taiwan (Republic of China), Japan, the Democratic People's Republic of Korea (North Korea), the Republic of Korea (South Korea), the Mongolian People's Republic, and the countries of Southeast Asia, stretching from its cool northern borders with Europe to the tropical islands of the Pacific (see Figure 7.1).

Immigrants from Asia, particularly China and Japan, have been coming to the United States since the 1800s. Many settled on the West Coast, where the majority of their descendants still live. In recent years, large numbers from throughout the region have arrived in the United States; many are refugees from political oppression, while others seek education and employment opportunities. This chapter introduces the peoples and cuisines of northern and central Asia—the Chinese, Japanese, and Koreans. Southeast Asians are discussed in Chapter 8. Peoples of the Middle East and Asian Indians, who reside in parts of Asia Minor and South Asia, respectively, are considered in Chapters 9 and 10.

> Nearly half of all U.S. citizens naturalized between 1981 and 1993 were born in Asia.

CHINESE

Chinese civilization is more than 4,000 years old and has made numerous significant contributions in agriculture, the arts, religion

> Preserved ginger has been found in ancient Chinese tombs, where it was probably placed to nourish the dead.

FIGURE 7.1
China, Japan, and Korea.

and philosophy, and warfare. Silk and embroidered brocade cloth, intricate jade sculpture, Chinese porcelain and lacquerware, book printing, Confucianism, Taoism, and gunpowder are just a few examples. The name China, meaning "middle kingdom," or center of the world, is probably derived from that of a dynasty that ruled in the third century BCE.

China's landscape is dominated by the valleys of two great rivers, the Huang (Yellow) River in the north and the Chang Jiang (Yangtze) in the south. The climate is monsoonal, with most of China's rainfall occurring in the spring and summer months.

The northern plain through which the Huang River flows is agriculturally very fertile. The area is cold and sometimes the severe winter results in a growing season of only 4 to 6 months. In the south the Chang Jiang River starts in Tibet, traverses the southern provinces, and eventually empties into the China Sea near the city of Shanghai. South of the mouth of the Yangtze delta is a rugged and mountainous coastline, off which are located the islands of Hong Kong and Taiwan. The southern provinces are warmer, wetter, and have a growing season that is longer (6 to 9 months) than in the north.

The population of China is estimated to exceed 1 billion people, more than four times as large as the population of the United States. The Chinese are a heterogeneous people with numerous ethnic and racial groups. The Chinese language is equally diverse, with many dialects, some of which are incomprehensible to people of other Chinese regions.

Traditional foods of China. Some foods typical of the traditional Chinese diet include bitter melon, *bok choy,* Chinese eggplant, ginger root, long beans, lotus root, mushrooms, oyster sauce, pork, long-grain rice, shrimp, soy sauce, and water chestnuts. (Photo by Laurie Macfee.)

Cultural Perspective

History of China

China's history is generally divided into periods named for the dynasties under which it was once ruled. One of the earliest dynasties is believed to be that of Hsia (2205 to c. 1766 BCE), but it is uncertain if this dynasty actually existed. The Chou dynasty (1122–256 BCE) may have been the first to form the nation of China, although it was really only a collection of states with unstable borders. In this period the country extended south to the Chang Jiang valley and north to the Huang River.

Several schools of philosophy were established during the Chou dynasty that influenced China for centuries, such as Confucianism and Taoism, as well as the concepts of yin and yang (see the religion section of this chapter). It is believed that the philosopher Confucius lived from 551 to 479 BCE; Lao Tzu, the founder of Taoism, may have been his contemporary.

The short Ch'in dynasty (221–206 BCE) preceded the next great dynasty, Han (206 BCE–220), which lasted more than 400 years and further expanded the borders of a unified China. During this period, Confucianism became the leading philosophy of the state; its texts were studied in schools and were the basis of the civil service examination. A significant event during the Han dynasty was the introduction of Buddhism to China; it would later become one of the primary religions of the region.

Following the collapse of the Han dynasty came the period of the "Three Kingdoms," when China was divided into three major regions. It is considered the most romantic time in Chinese history, although it was also a period of political uncertainty. Buddhism spread through most of China, and Japan and Korea were brought into the sphere of China's cultural influence.

By 589, China was once again unified under the Sui dynasty, followed by the T'ang dynasty. During the T'ang dynasty (618–907), China's poetry and art attained high levels of sophistication and Buddhism reached its apex. The T'ang dynasty also pushed China's border outward to envelop Tibet, Mongolia, and southern Manchuria. Under the Sung dynasty (960–1127), China was unable to fight off Mongol invaders, and by 1279 it became part of the Mongolian empire (1280–1368) that stretched from Europe to India and Korea. Islam was introduced to China through the Mongols and there are still Muslims in China today.

The Ming dynasty (1368–1644) once again put China under Chinese rule, but it was the Manchus from Manchuria who established the subsequent Ch'ing dynasty (1644–1911), which lasted into the twentieth century. At its height, this dynasty ruled over more territory than any previous government, and in the seventeenth century, China

People from northern China often call themselves the "people of Han."

People from southern China refer to themselves as the "people of T'ang."

The most famous European traveler to China during the rule of the Mongols was Marco Polo, who is said to have brought Chinese noodles to Italy. The Italians, however, were undoubtedly making pasta long before the times of Marco Polo.

was one of the most prosperous nations on earth. The dynasty started to crumble in the nineteenth century, and by the twentieth century, it was replaced by a republic founded by Sun Yat-sen.

Japan occupied most of China during World War II. After Japan's defeat the Kuomintang (Nationalist Party) continued to rule China. In 1949 the communists under Mao Zedong ousted the nationalists, who now occupy the island of Taiwan. Today China is known as the People's Republic of China and is commonly referred to as mainland China. Taiwan is known as the Republic of China. The island of Hong Kong, which was under British control for most of the twentieth century, reverted to the People's Republic of China in 1997. In 1999, Macao, the tip of the peninsula west of Hong Kong that has been a Portuguese territory for more than 400 years, is scheduled to be restored to Chinese sovereignty.

History of Chinese in the United States

Immigration Patterns

The first major surge in Chinese immigration to the United States occurred in the early 1850s when the Chinese joined in the gold rush to California; many Chinese still refer to America as the "Land of the Golden Mountain." As mining became less lucrative, the Chinese opened their own businesses, such as laundries and restaurants, but also found employment in other occupations. The Central Pacific Railroad, which joined the Union Pacific as the first cross-country line, was built primarily by 10,000 Chinese workers.

By 1870, there were 63,000 Chinese, mostly male, in the United States, nearly all on the West Coast. It is estimated that another 120,000 Chinese entered the United States during the following decade. Racial discrimination against Asians increased as their numbers swelled. By 1880, Chinese immigration slowed to a trickle due to exclusion laws directed against Asians. The Chinese also immigrated to Hawaii, and when the islands were annexed by the United States in 1898, approximately 25,000 Chinese were living there.

Most early Chinese immigrants were from the southeastern Guang-dong province of China, usually referred to as Canton. Most were young men (94%) with no intention of staying; they came to make their fortune and then return to China and their families. Many married before coming to the United States, and more than half returned to China. By the 1920s the Chinese population in the United States had dropped to 1870 levels.

In each city where the Chinese settled, they usually lived within a small geographic area known as Chinatown. Large Chinatowns evolved in San Francisco, New York, Boston, Chicago, Philadelphia, Los Angeles, and Oakland, California. These neighborhoods offered

Chow-chow is a vegetable relish made with mustard brought to the United States by Chinese railroad workers. Its name may derive from the Chinese word for "mixed," *cha.*

In 1852, California governor John Bigler declared the Chinese in his state "nonassimilable."

It was not until 1970 that the number of Chinese American women equaled the number of men.

protection against a sometimes hostile social and economic environment; assimilation was not an option. Conditions were often crowded and unusual in the predominance of men, but were tolerated with the expectation of eventual return to China. It was not until 1943 that Chinese could become naturalized U.S. citizens.

Current Demographics and Socioeconomic Status

Early immigrants and their descendants, as well as many current immigrants from Hong Kong, speak Cantonese, a dialect that is difficult to understand by Chinese immigrants who speak Mandarin.

When the exclusion laws were repealed in 1943, people from many Asian countries once again entered the United States. Chinese immigrants who have arrived since World War II are usually not from Canton. They are urban dwellers from other regions and are generally better educated than earlier immigrants.

Political instability in the People's Republic of China has led to a recent exodus of Chinese. Following the pro-democracy uprising in Tiananmen Square in 1989, U.S. immigration laws were changed with the Chinese Student Protection Act of 1992. More than 41,000 Chinese residents were granted visas and are eligible for citizenship under the provision. Further, the return of Hong Kong to mainland China and the uncertainty of Taiwan's future have led to increased immigration from these islands.

The 1990 U.S. census reports more than 1.6 million Chinese living in the United States, with approximately two-thirds being foreign-born; nearly half arrived in the 1990s. Large numbers of Chinese Americans are found today in California, New York, Hawaii, Texas, New Jersey, Massachusetts, Illinois, Washington, and Maryland.

Four types of Chinese American households have been identified (Gould-Martin & Ngin, 1981). First are the sojourners, mostly men born in the early twentieth century, who came to the United States with the intent of returning after accumulating some wealth. Political changes in China have stranded this group in urban Chinatowns throughout America. The second type are sojourners who were successful in bringing their wives to the United States. These elderly first-generation couples still live in Chinatown neighborhoods, although their children have often moved from the area.

The third type of household is established by new immigrant families. Often one member will arrive to establish residency, and then family members will follow. These immigrants usually settle with other Asians, often in Chinatowns, where the parents speak Chinese and children learn English in school. Although many families include two wage earners or combine the incomes of extended members, they may remain poor due to low salaries, large families, and support of relatives in the homeland.

Chinese American households of the fourth type include acculturated suburban families. These families include both new immigrants who are white-collar professionals and those Americans of Chinese descent who have lived in the United States for several generations. Both parents may be college educated, often with specialization in engineering and the sciences. Unlike other immigrants of previous generations, these affluent Chinese families live in areas with university or defense research facilities, including the metropolitan areas of the Silicon Valley (California), Houston, Seattle, Pittsburgh, San Diego, and Dallas.

Chinese Americans value education, and there are disproportionately large numbers with college and graduate degrees. High levels of educational attainment often translate into well-compensated professional employment. Americans of Chinese descent are so well known for their successful transition in the United States that a stereotype has developed, obscuring what is in reality a bipolar population. Although many Chinese Americans are in the upper and middle classes, large numbers, especially recent immigrants, are poorly educated and work in low-paying service jobs.

Cultural Organizations

The early Chinese immigrants rapidly developed organizations that helped regulate their lives. Many of these groups provided jobs, acted as credit unions, resolved differences among their members, and acted as liaisons with the non-Chinese community. The primary social association for Chinese Americans is their family (clan) association, called *gongsuo*. Family associations were formed among people with the same last name. It has been estimated that there are only 438 last names in China, and everyone with the same surname is believed to be descended from the same ancestors. Chinese Americans also belong to associations known as *huiguan* that represent the district in China in which they or their family originated. The Chinese Benevolent Association represents all Chinese organizations, and each city with a considerable Chinese population usually has such an association.

In the past the Chinese Benevolent Association was a powerful institution that oversaw business transactions, arbitrated disputes, and was the unofficial voice of the Chinese community. Today its functions are primarily ceremonial. District and clan associations have become less important as Americans of Chinese descent have become more acculturated. Government social agencies have taken over many of the associations' functions, and communal organizations have little meaning for the newer immigrants from Hong Kong and Taiwan.

Other local organizations of prominence in the Chinese American community have been Christian churches, Chinese schools, and recreational groups, such as the YMCA and the YWCA. Nationally the Chinese American Citizens Alliance fights discrimination directed against the Chinese and the Chinese American Forum fosters cultural understanding.

More than 80 percent of the 1.2 billion people in China have the same last names, nearly 10 million per appellation. The government is urging adoption of combined names at marriage to lessen the confusion.

Worldview

Religion

Most Americans of Chinese descent are not affiliated with a specific church. Religious practices are often eclectic, a combination of ancestor worship, Confucianism, Taoism, and Buddhism. Many early Chinese immigrants were not formally schooled in any religion; instead, beliefs and practices were passed orally from generation to generation. Spirituality is integrated into family and community life. Daily living includes avoiding any actions that might offend the gods, nature, or ancestors.

Early Religion The ancient faith of China was probably a mixture of ancestor worship and respect for the forces of nature and the heavenly bodies. The supreme power was either *Tien* (Heaven) or *Shang Ti* (the Supreme Ruler or the Ruler Above). One gained favor with the spirits by the correct performance of ceremonies. These beliefs and practices were later incorporated into subsequent Chinese religions.

Ceremonies for the dead are a prominent Chinese religious practice. The dead are supposed to depend on the living for the conditions of their existence after death. In turn, the dead can influence the lives of the living.

Confucianism Confucius was a sage, one of many who gave order to Chinese society by defining the ways in which people should live and work together. Confucianism incorporated the ceremonies of earlier religions. Its cornerstones are

1. Fatherly love and filial piety in the son. That is, children are expected to obey their parents and adults are expected to take care of their children.
2. Tolerance in the eldest brother and humility in the younger.
3. Proper behavior by the husband and submission by the wife.
4. Respect for one's elders and compassion in adults.
5. Allegiance to rulers and benevolence by leaders.

Inherent in these relationships is the ideal of social reciprocity, which means that one should treat others as one would like to be treated. To enhance harmony in the family and in society as a whole, one must exercise self-restraint. An individual must never lose face—meaning a person's favorable name and position in society—because that would defame the whole family. Many of these values influence Chinese behavior today.

Taoism The Taoist believes, like the Confucianist, that heaven and humanity function in unison and can achieve harmony, but under Taoism, people are subordinate to nature's way. There is a fundamental duality within the universe of interacting, opposite principles or forces—the *yang* (masculine, positive, bright, steadfast, warm, hard, and dry; sometimes referred to as *Shen*) and the *yin* (feminine, negative, dark, cold, wet, mysterious, and secret; also called *Kwei*) (Figure 7.2). Everything in nature contains both yin and yang, and a balanced unity between them is necessary for harmony. This balance occurs when Tao, the way of nature, is allowed to take its course unimpeded by human willfulness. Taoism advocates a simple life, communion with nature, and the avoidance of extremes.

Buddhism Buddhism flourished during the T'ang dynasty but then suffered a slow decline. The Mahayana sect dominated in China, blending with traditional Chinese beliefs and resulting in a unique Chinese form of Buddhism. Ten schools of Buddhism flourished in China at one time, but only four were left by the twentieth century. The two dominant schools in China are Ch'an (Zen Buddhism in Japan) and Pure Land (see Chapter 2 for more information).

Chinese American Spirituality Both Catholic and Protestant churches were established in the early Chinatown neighborhoods, usually organized by the Chinese dialect spoken in the area. Few first-generation Chinese Americans joined Christian religions, but converts were found in subsequent generations.

Family

Confucian teachings about correct relationships are still important for many Chinese American families, even if they have become Christians. Chinese American families are usually patriarchal. Women are traditionally taught to be unassuming and yielding. They live by the formula of "thrice obeying": Young girls are submissive to their fathers, wives are subordinate to their husbands, and mothers obey their sons. Children are expected to be quiet, acquiescent, and deferential to their elders. Harmony in the family is the ideal, so children are taught not to fight or cry. Showing emotion is discouraged. Chinese parents may be very strict, and children are commanded to honor the family. Many of these ideas conflict with American ideals of equal rights and freedom of speech and lead to intergenerational conflict in the Chinese American home.

Communication

The Chinese have a quiet conversational approach; emotional displays are considered a sign of immaturity (Randall-David, 1989). Some speakers may pause during conversation as a sign of thoughtfulness. Interruptions should always be avoided. Many Chinese avoid confrontation and will initially say "yes" to questions that require a

FIGURE 7.2

Yin-yang symbol. This symbol represents the fundamental duality of the universe and the balance between the forces of yang (light) and yin (dark). Each force has a little of the other in it (indicated by the dot of the opposite color).

Most Chinese believe in *fengsui,* the way in which a home should be situated and its furnishings arranged to promote optimal flow of energy and personal well-being.

Confucius also developed protocols for cooking and eating that were practiced in China until the nineteenth century.

positive or negative response. Asking questions can be interpreted as disrespect, a sign that the person speaking is being unclear. Surprise or discomfort may be expressed by quickly and noisily sucking in air (Axtell, 1991). Glancing around and averted eyes are common; direct eye contact with elders is expected, however.

The traditional Chinese greeting is a nod or a slight bow from the waist while holding palms together near the chest, often without a smile. Touching between strangers and acquaintances is uncommon. Even handshaking may be inappropriate (wait for the extended hand, especially with women), except for westernized Chinese Americans and people from Hong Kong. Hugging, kissing, and backpatting should be avoided. Good posture is expected, and slouching or putting one's feet on a desk is considered rude.

Traditional Food Habits

It is said of the Cantonese that they will eat everything with four legs except a table, and anything with wings except an airplane.

The Chinese raise many kinds of insects for consumption, such as scorpions, which are prepared fried or in soups.

The Chinese eat a wide variety of foods and avoid very few. This may have developed out of necessity, as China has long been plagued with recurrent famine caused by too much or too little rainfall. Chinese cuisine largely reflects the food habits and preferences of the Han people, the largest ethnic group in China, but not to the exclusion of other ethnic groups' cuisines. For example, Beijing has a large Muslim population, whose restaurants serve lamb, kid (baby goat), horse meat, and donkey, but no pork. Foreigners have also introduced ingredients that have been incorporated into local cuisines. Some foods now common in China, but not indigenous, are tomatoes, potatoes, and chile peppers.

Ingredients and Common Foods

Staples

The Chinese, like most Asians, rinse their rice before cooking it.

The custom of throwing rice at newlyweds is believed to come from China, where rice is a symbol of fertility.

Traditional Chinese foods are listed in Table 7.1. In China, few dairy products, whether fresh or fermented, are eaten. Rice, the staple food of southern China, is used throughout Asia and is believed to have originated in India (it wasn't introduced to China until the first century BCE). There are approximately 2,500 different forms of the grain, but the Chinese prefer a polished, white long-grain variety that is not sticky and that remains firm after cooking. Sticky glutinous rice is used occasionally, mainly in sweet dishes. Although it is usually steamed, rice can also be made into a porridge called *congee,* eaten for breakfast or as a late-night snack, with meat or fish added for flavor. Congee is also fed to people who are ill. Rice flour is used to make rice sticks, which can be boiled or fried in hot oil.

Wheat is also common throughout China, although it is used more often in the north than the south. It is popular as noodles, dumplings, pancakes, and steamed bread. Thin, square wheat-flour wrappers are used to make steamed or fried *egg rolls* with a meat, vegetable, or mixed filling and *wontons* (in which the wrapper is folded over the filling), served either fried or in soup. *Spring rolls,* which are similar to egg rolls, are made with very thin, round wheat-flour wrappers. Buckwheat is grown in the north and commonly made into noodles.

The Chinese eat a variety of animal protein foods. Although they eat all kinds of meat, fish, and poultry, they eat less at any one meal than is customary in the West. In China, soybeans are known as the poor man's cow, as they are made into products that resemble milk and cheese. Soybeans are transfomed into an amazing array of food products that are indispensable in Chinese cooking:

Soy sauce, made from cooked soybeans that are first fermented and then processed into sauce. The Cantonese prefer light-colored soy sauce in some dishes over the darker, more opaque kind used in Japanese and some Chinese cooking.

Soy milk, prepared with soaked soybeans that are first pureed, then filtered, and then boiled to produce a white, milk-like drink.

Bean curd, or *tofu,* made by boiling soy milk and then adding gypsum, which causes it to curdle. The excess liquid is pressed from the curd, producing a firm, bland, custard-like product.

Black beans, made with cooked fermented soybeans preserved with salt and ginger. Black beans are usually added as a flavoring in dishes.

Hoisin sauce, a thick, brownish-red sweet-and-sour sauce that combines fermented soybeans, flour, sugar, water, spices, and garlic with chiles and is often used in Cantonese cooking.

Oyster sauce, a thick brown sauce prepared from oysters, soybeans, and brine that is also used in Cantonese fare.

Other beans are also popular, made into pastes, flour, or even thin, transparent noodles known in the United States as cellophane noodles or bean threads.

Chinese cuisine makes extensive use of vegetables. Many are those common in other regions of the world, such as asparagus, broccoli, cabbage, cauliflower, eggplant, green beans, mushrooms, onions, peas, potatoes, radish, and squash. Chinese varieties may differ, however. For instance, leafy *bok choy* and wrinkled *napa cabbage* are preferred over European types; long beans, small purple eggplant, and the large white icicle radish are featured in many dishes. One popular squash variety is called a winter melon; it is pale green and mild in flavor. Mushrooms of all types, including the tiny *enoki,* grayish oyster mushrooms, *shiitake,* straw mushrooms, and dried kinds like cloud (or wood) ears flavor numerous dishes. Lily buds, snow peas

The Chinese consider the dark meat of poultry tastier and more tender than the white meat.

The latest health food rage in China is ants, prepared as flour, paste, tea, and even wine. Ant products are a $25 million per year business.

Cabbage sales in China have plummeted as the standard of living has increased. Tomatoes, cucumbers, and celery now outsell the formerly number-one vegetable.

TABLE 7.1
Cultural Food Groups: Chinese

Group	Comments
PROTEIN FOODS	
Milk/milk products	Dairy products are not routinely used in China. Many Chinese are lactose-intolerant.
	Traditional alternative sources of calcium are tofu, calcium-fortified soy milk, small bones in fish and poultry, and dishes in which bones have been dissolved.
Meat/poultry/fish/eggs/legumes	Few protein-rich foods that are not eaten.
	Beef and pork are usually cut into bite-size pieces before cooking.
	Fish is preferred fresh and is often prepared whole and divided into portions at the table.
	Preservation by salting and drying is common.
	Shrimp and legumes are made into pastes.
CEREALS/GRAINS	Wheat is the staple in the north, white rice in the south.
	Fan (cereal or grain) is the primary item of the meal; *ts'ai* (vegetables and meat or seafood) makes it tastier.
	Rice is washed before cooking.
FRUITS/VEGETABLES	Vegetables are usually cut into bite-size pieces before cooking.
	Slightly unripe fruit is often served as a dessert.
	Both fresh fruits and vegetables are preferred; seasonal variation dictates the type of produce used.
	Many vegetables are pickled or preserved. Fruits are often dried or preserved.
ADDITIONAL FOODS	
Seasonings	
Nuts/seeds	
Beverages	In northern China the beverage accompanying the meal may be soup. In the south, it is tea.
	Alcoholic drinks, usually called wines, are rarely made from grapes. They are either beers or distilled spirits made from starches or fruit.
Fats/oils	Traditionally lard was used if it could be afforded. In recent years, soy, peanut, or corn oil is more commonly used.
Sweeteners	Traditionally sugar was not used in large quantities; many desserts were made with bean pastes.

TABLE 7.1
Cultural Food Groups: Chinese—continued

Common Foods	Adaptations in the United States
Cow's milk, buffalo milk	Most Chinese, even elders, consume dairy products, especially milk and ice cream, some cheese. Some alternative sources of calcium may no longer be used.
Meat: beef and lamb (brains, heart, kidneys, liver, tongue, tripe, oxtails); pork (bacon, ham, roasts, pig's feet, sausage, ears); game meats (e.g. bear, moose) *Poultry:* chicken, duck, quail, rice birds, squab *Fish:* bluegill, carp, catfish, cod, dace, fish tripe, herring, king fish, mandarin fish, minnow, mullet, perch, red snapper, river bass, salmon, sea bass, sea bream, sea perch, shad, sole, sturgeon, tuna *Eggs:* chicken, duck, quail, fresh and preserved *Shellfish and other seafood:* abalone, clams, conch, crab, jellyfish, lobster, mussels, oysters, periwinkles, prawns, sea cucumbers (sea slugs), shark's fin, shrimp, squid, turtle, *wawa* fish (salamander) *Legumes:* broad beans, cowpeas, horse beans, mung beans, red beans, red kidney beans, split peas, soybeans, white beans, bean paste	
Buckwheat, corn, millet, rice, sorghum, wheat	Chinese Americans eat less *fan* and more *ts'ai.* The primary staple remains rice, but more wheat bread is eaten.
Fruits: apples, bananas, custard apples, coconut, dates, dragon eyes (*longan*), figs, grapes, kumquats, lily seed, lime, litchi, mango, muskmelon, oranges, papaya, passion fruit, peaches, persimmons, pineapples, plums (fresh and preserved), pomegranates, pomelos, tangerines, watermelon	More raw vegetables/salads are eaten.
Vegetables: amaranth, asparagus, bamboo shoots, banana squash, bean sprouts, bitter melon, broccoli, burdock root, cassava (tapioca), cauliflower, celery, cabbage (*bok choy* and *napa*), chile peppers, Chinese long beans, Chinese mustard, chrysanthemum greens, cucumbers, eggplant, flat beans, fuzzy melon, garlic, ginger root, green peppers, kohlrabi, leeks, lettuce, lily blossoms, lily root, lotus root and stems, luffa, dried and fresh mushrooms (black, button, cloud ear, wood ear, *enoki, shiitake,* straw, oyster, monkey's head), mustard root, okra, olives, onions (yellow, scallions, shallots), parsnip, peas, potato, pumpkin, seaweed (agar), snow peas, spinach, taro, tea melon, tomatoes, turnips, water chestnuts, watercress, wax beans, winter melon, yams, yam beans	
Anise, bird's nest, chili sauce, Chinese parsley (fresh coriander), cinnamon, cloves, cumin, curry powder, five-spice powder (anise, star anise, clove, cinnamon or cassia, Szechuan pepper), fennel, fish sauce, garlic, ginger, golden needles (lily flowers), green onions, hot mustard, mace, monosodium glutamate (MSG), mustard seed, nutmeg, oyster sauce, parsley, pastes (*hoisin,* sweet flour, brown bean, Szechwan hot beans, sesame seed, shrimp), pepper (black, chile, red, and Szechwan), red dates, sesame seeds (black and white), soy sauce (light and dark), star anise, tangerine skin, tumeric, vinegar	Many Chinese restaurants use MSG, but it is not usually used in the home.
Almonds, apricot kernels, areca nuts, cashews, chestnuts, ginko nuts, peanuts, walnuts; sesame seeds, watermelon seeds	
Beer, distilled alcoholic spirits, soup broth, tea	
Bacon fat, butter, lard, corn oil, peanut oil, sesame oil, soybean oil, suet	
Honey, maltose syrup, table sugar (brown and white)	Sugar consumption has increased mainly because of consumption of soft drinks, candy, and American desserts.

In some regions, two longans or litchis are placed under the pillows of newlyweds because their names sound like the words "to have children quickly" (Newman, 1998b).

In China a marriage is consummated when the new in-laws officially accept a cup of tea from the bride. If the groom dies before the wedding, the bride-to-be is said to have "spilled her tea."

A *wok* is a hemispherical shell of iron or steel; some woks in the United States have nonstick finishes. The wok is placed over a gas burner or in a metal ring placed over an electric burner.

(pea pods), bamboo shoots, water chestnuts, bitter melon, and lotus root are other, more distinctively Asian vegetables found in Chinese cuisine.

The Chinese eat fresh fruit infrequently, occasionally for a snack or for dessert, and it is preferred slightly unripe or even salted. Chinese dates (*jujubes*), persimmons, pomegranates, and tangerines are favorites. A few fruits are typically preserved in syrups, such as pungent kumquats, yellow-orange loquats, longans (dragon eyes) and litchis, a tropical fruit with creamy, jelly-like flesh.

Traditionally people cooked with lard if they could afford it. In recent years, soy, peanut, or corn oil is more common. Until recently sugar was not used in large quantities; many desserts were made with sweetened bean pastes.

Hot soup or tea is the beverage that usually accompanies a meal. Tea, used in China for more than 2,000 years, was first cultivated in the Chang Jiang valley and later introduced to western Europe in the seventeenth century. There are three general types of tea: green, black (red), and *oolong* (black dragon). Green tea is the dried, tender leaves of the tea plant. It brews a yellow, slightly astringent drink. Black tea is toasted, fermented leaves that have a black color; it makes a reddish drink. Black tea is commonly drunk in Europe and America. Oolong tea is made from partially fermented leaves.

Chinese alcoholic drinks are often called wines, but they are not usually made from grapes. They are typically distilled alcohols made from grains or from fruit, like plums. A few examples are bamboo leaf-green (95 proof), *fen* (made from rice, 130 proof), *hua diao* (yellow rice wine), *mou tai* (made from sorghum, 110 proof), and red rice wine. Beer is also very popular.

Most Chinese food is cooked, and very little raw food, except fruit, is eaten. Cooked foods may be eaten cold. Common cooking methods maximize the limited fuel available, including stir-frying, steaming, deep-fat frying, simmering, and roasting. In stir-frying, foods are cut into uniform, bite-size pieces and quickly cooked in a *wok* in which oil has been heated. Food can also be steamed in the wok. Bamboo containers, perforated on the bottom, are stacked in a wok containing boiling water and fitted with a domed cover. Roasted food is usually bought from a commercial shop, not prepared in the home.

The Chinese usually strive to obtain the freshest ingredients for their meals, and in most American Chinatowns it is common to find markets that sell live animals and fish. However, because of seasonal availability and geographic distances, many Chinese foods are preserved by drying or pickling.

Regional Variations

China is usually divided into five culinary regions characterized by flavor or into two areas (northern and southern) based on climate and the availability of foodstuffs. In recent years, however, regional differences have diminished due to increased global influences, particularly television (Newman, 1998a).

Northern   This area includes the Shandong and Honan regions of Chinese cooking. The Shandong area (Beijing is sometimes included in this area, sometimes considered a third division of northern cooking) is famous for *Peking duck* and *mu shu pork,* both of which are eaten wrapped in Mandarin wheat pancakes topped with hoisin. Honan, south of Beijing, is known for its sweet-and-sour freshwater fish, made from whole carp caught in the Huang River. Much of the north is bordered by Mongolia, whose people eat mainly mutton. Grilling or barbecuing is a common way of preparing meat in this area. One specialty is the Mongolian hot pot, featuring sliced meats and vegetables cooked at the table in a pot of broth simmering over a charcoal brazier. The food is eaten first, and the broth is consumed as a beverage afterward.

Northern China has a cool climate, limiting the amount and type of food produced. In general, its staples are millet and soybeans. Winter vegetables are common, such as cabbage and onions. A delicacy from this area is braised bear paw. Hot clear soup is the beverage that usually accompanies a meal.

Southern   Southern China is divided into three culinary areas: Szechwan (Sichuan)-Hunan, Yunnan, and Cantonese (with Fukien and Hakka regional specialties). Szechwan-Hunan, which is an inland region, features fare distinguished by the use of chiles, garlic, and the Szechwan pepper *fagara.* Typical dishes include *hot and sour soup, camphor-* and *tea-smoked duck,* and an oily walnut paste and sugar dessert that may be related to the nut halvah of the Middle East. Yunnan cooking is distinctive in its use of dairy products, such as yogurt, fried milk curd, and cheese. Dishes are often hot and spicy, and some of the best ham and head cheese in China are found in this area.

Cantonese cooking is probably the most familiar to Americans, because the majority of Chinese restaurants in the United States serve Cantonese-style food. It is characterized by stir-fried dishes, seafood (fresh and dried or salted), delicate thickened sauces, and the use of vegetable oil instead of lard. The Cantonese are known for *dim sum* ("small bites," such as steamed or fried dumplings stuffed with meat or seafood) that are served with tea. Tea is the beverage served with meals. The staple foods of the south are rice and soybeans. As in the north, a variety of vegetables from the cabbage family are used, as well as garlic, melon, onions, peas, potatoes, squashes, tomatoes, and a range of rootlike crops, such as taro, water chestnuts, and lotus root. Southern cooking uses mushrooms of many types to enhance the flavor of the foods and takes advantage of an abundance of fruits and nuts. Fish, both fresh and saltwater, is popular. Also important are poultry and eggs. Pork is the preferred meat.

One hundred people were killed in China during 1995 by exploding Mongolian hot pots in restaurants. A government crackdown is addressing safety issues and the use of opium in hot pot dishes.

Dumplings shaped like animals, such as birds or frogs, are specialties in Xian.

In southern China, people greet each other by asking, "Have you had rice today?"

Bird's nest soup is served sometimes at Chinese banquets. It is made from the cleansed nests of swallows from the South China Sea. The nests are made of predigested seaweed and are bland in flavor, yet very expensive. They are reputedly an aphrodisiac.

Along the coast, Fukien provincial fare includes numerous seafood dishes and clear broths. Paper-wrapped foods and egg rolls are thought to have originated there. In the city of Shanghai, chefs specialize in new food creations and elaborate garnishes.

A southern regional specialty is Hakka cuisine, sometimes called the soul food of southern China. The Hakkas fled to the south in the fourth century BCE, when the Mongols invaded the north. They remained an insular ethnic group, preserving their traditional language, dress, and foods. Their fare is hearty and robust, featuring dishes made with red rice wine and pungent seasonings, cooked for a lengthy time, often in clay pots. Salt-baked chicken, greens simmered with pork fat, and meat-stuffed tofu are examples.

Meal Composition and Cycle

Daily Patterns

The Chinese customarily eat three meals per day, plus numerous snacks. Breakfast often includes the hot rice porridge congee, which in southern China may be seasoned with small amounts of meat or fish. In northern China, hot steamed bread, dumplings, or noodles are served for breakfast. In urban areas, lunch is a smaller version of dinner, including soup, a rice or wheat dish, vegetables, and fish or meat.

Although the Chinese are receptive to all types of food, the composition of a meal is governed by specific rules—a balance between yin and yang foods and the proper amounts of *fan* and *ts'ai*. Fan includes all foods made from grains, such as steamed rice, noodles, porridge, pancakes, or dumplings, which are served in a separate bowl to each diner. Ts'ai includes cooked meats and vegetables, which are shared from bowls set in the center of the table. Fan is the primary item in a meal; ts'ai only helps people eat the grain by making the meal more tasty. A meal is not complete unless it contains fan, but it does not have to contain ts'ai. At a banquet the opposite is true. An elaborate meal must contain ts'ai, but the fan is usually an afterthought and may not be eaten.

Etiquette

The traditional eating utensils are chopsticks and a porcelain spoon used for soup. Teacups are always made out of porcelain, as are rice bowls. At a meal, all diners should take equal amounts of the ts'ai dishes, and younger diners wait to eat until their elders have started; it is rude to reject food. It is also considered bad manners to eat rice or noodles with the bowl resting on the table; instead, it should be raised to the mouth. It is rude to pick at your food or to lick your chopsticks. Laying your chopsticks across the top of the rice bowl or dropping them brings bad luck. It is also improper to stick chopsticks

One story about the origin of chopsticks is that they were invented after an ancient Chinese emperor banned the use of cutlery at the table. More likely they were invented as an extension of the fingers. They are made from bamboo, ivory, or plastic. Chopsticks are used in most countries that have been influenced by China, including Japan (where the chopsticks are generally shorter and have rounded rather than squared sides and more pointed tips) and Korea (where the chopsticks are typically made of metal, the same length as the Japanese type, but flatter). Chopsticks are found frequently in Vietnam (the Chinese type), although forks, spoons, and fingers are also commonly used. Other Southeast Asian cultures use chopsticks occasionally, mostly for rice or noodles.

straight up in a rice bowl because in some areas this symbolizes an offering to the dead.

Special Occasions

Traditionally the Chinese week did not include a day of rest. Consequently, there were numerous feasts to break up the continuous work days. Chinese festival days do not fall on the same day each year because their calendar is lunar. Celebrations are traditionally yang occasions, because heat symbolizes activity, noise, and excitement in China (Anderson, 1987). Yang foods, such as meats, fried dishes, and alcoholic beverages, are featured at feasts (see "Therapeutic Uses of Foods").

The most important festival is New Year's, which can fall any time from the end of January to the end of February. Traditionally the New Year was a time to settle old debts and to honor ancestors, parents, and elders. The New Year holiday season begins on the evening of the 23rd day of the last lunar month of the year. At that time the Kitchen God, whose picture hangs in the kitchen and who sees and hears everything in the house, flies upward to make his annual report on the family to the Jade Emperor. To ensure that his report will be good, the family smears his lips with honey or sweet rice before they burn his picture. A new picture of the Kitchen God is placed in the kitchen on New Year's Eve.

Food preparation must be completed on New Year's Eve, as knives cannot be used on the first day of the year because they might "cut

According to the Chinese, a child is 1 year old at birth and becomes 2 years old after the New Year.

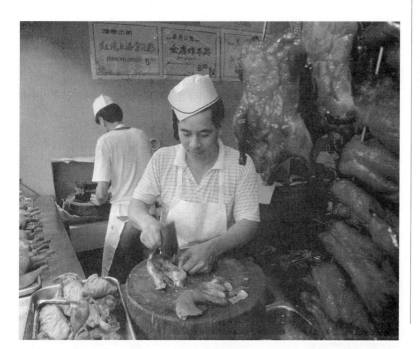

Butcher preparing meat for barbecuing in a Chinatown shop, Honolulu, Hawaii. (Corbis/Catherine Karnow.)

luck." Deep-fried dumplings, made from glutinous rice and filled with sweetmeats, and steamed turnip and rice flour puddings are usually included in the New Year's Day meal. During the New Year festivities, only good omens are permitted and unlucky-sounding words are not uttered. Foods that sound like lucky words, such as tangerine (good fortune), fish (surplus), chicken (good fortune), chestnuts (profit), and tofu (*fu* means riches), are eaten.

Friends and relatives visit each other during the first 10 days of the new year, and good wishes, presents, and food are exchanged. Children receive money in small red envelopes. Traditionally the Feast of Lanterns, the 15th day of the first month, ends the New Year's season and is marked by the dragon dancing in the streets and exploding firecrackers to scare away evil spirits.

Ch'ing Ming, the chief spring festival, falls 106 days after the winter solstice. Families customarily go to the cemetery and tend the graves of their relatives. Food is symbolically fed to the dead, then later eaten by the family. *Duan wu*, the Dragon Boat Festival, is held on the 15th day of the fifth month to commemorate the drowning death of a famous third-century BCE poet. A boat race and special dumplings are traditional. The Moon Festival occurs at the end of September on a full moon (15th day of the eighth lunar month). Because the moon is a yin symbol, this festival was traditionally for women, but today it also symbolizes the togetherness of the family. It is sometimes called the harvest festival or moon's birthday. Large round cakes filled with spices, nuts, fruit or red bean paste, called moon cakes, are typically eaten during this event.

Therapeutic Uses of Food

The Chinese believe that a good diet is critical for physical and emotional harmony and necessary to strengthen the body against disease. One study in Hong Kong reported that three-quarters of respondents listed dietary prescriptions in the prevention of disease (Koo, 1984). Health is generally maintained by eating the proper balance of yin and yang foods (see "Therapeutic Use of Foods" in Chapter 1). Hot foods generally include those that are high in calories, cooked in oil, and irritating to the mouth and those that are red, orange, or yellow in color. Examples include most meats, chile peppers, tomatoes, mushrooms, eggplant, persimmons, onions, leeks, garlic, ginger, and alcoholic beverages. Cold foods are often low in calories, raw or boiled/steamed, soothing, and green or white in color. Many vegetables and fruits are considered cold items, as are some legumes. Pork, duck, and honey also are classified as cold in some regions. Staples, such as boiled rice and noodles, are typically placed in a third, neutral category (Ludman & Newman, 1984; Anderson, 1987). Some food preparations can make foods hotter or colder by the infusion or removal of heat. Which

The New Year's dragon dance and firecrackers are thought to inhibit the yin element and promote the yang forces. Red, the color of yang, is used throughout the New Year's season.

Eating crab and persimmons together is one food taboo practiced by some elderly Chinese Americans because these foods represent extreme hot and extreme cold and may be "poisonous" if mixed.

foods are considered yin or yang varies from region to region. Chinese Americans who are acculturated may be uncertain about some categorizations and thus identify many foods as neutral.

Typically, hot foods are eaten in the winter, by menstruating, pregnant, and postpartum women (especially during the first month following childbirth), and for fatigue. Cool foods are consumed in the summer, for dry lips, and to relieve irritability. It is believed that as a person grows older, the body cools off and more hot foods should be eaten. Extra care should be taken with children's diets, because they are more susceptible to imbalance.

In addition to yin and yang, some foods are believed to affect the blood or promote wound healing and are labeled *pu,* or *bo,* meaning "strengthening." It is a classification that is separate from the concept of yin and yang but often used in conjunction with it; most strengthening foods are also categorized as hot. The yin condition of "weak" blood (most associated with pregnancy, postpartum, and following surgery) is treated with specific hot items such as protein-rich soups made with chicken, pork liver, eggs, pig's feet, or oxtail. Other health-promoting foods identified by Chinese Americans include royal jelly (made from honey), bee pollen, *lin chih* (edible fungus), rattlesnake meat, dog meat, roasted beetles, barley juice, garlic, *dong gwai* (angelica, a celery-like herb), fruit juice, and milk. Too many of certain yang items, however, can cause the blood to "thin," and these foods are avoided for conditions such as hypertension (Ludman & Newman, 1984; Anderson, 1987; Ludman et al., 1989; Sun, 1996).

Ginseng is the best-known health-promoting Chinese food. It is made from an herb (genus *Panax*) found in Asia and the Americas. The root is boiled until only a sediment remains, then powdered for use in teas and broths. Ginseng reputedly cures cancer, rheumatism, diabetes, sexual dysfunctions, and complaints associated with aging. It is most often used as a restorative tonic. Taro root is also thought to have therapeutic properties, such as improving eyesight, curing vaginal discharge, reducing weakness, and promoting multiple births—it will also bring good luck if eaten on the fourth day of the first lunar month (Newman, 1998b). Other popular remedies include deer antlers, rhinoceros horns, and pulverized sea horses (Spector, 1991). The concept of "like cures like" (sympathy healing) is seen in many food cures for specific illnesses (Koo, 1984). Hong Kong residents identify chicken with walnuts (which resemble brains) as a remedy for headaches; soups made with bones for treating broken bones; and male genital organs from sea otters, deer, or other animals to cure impotence.

Some food taboos have been noted during pregnancy. Soy sauce may be avoided to prevent dark skin, and iron supplements may not be taken because they are thought to harden the baby's bones and make birth difficult. Shellfish may also be shunned. Ginseng is used as a general tonic (Campbell & Chang, 1981).

During the postpartum period a woman is especially susceptible to disease-causing "wind." She can help prevent it from entering her body by eating chicken cooked in wine or pig's feet simmered with ginger and vinegar.

In 1718 a Jesuit missionary in Quebec discovered an American species of ginseng that is nearly identical to the Chinese variety. Growing demand in China led many Americans, including Daniel Boone, to hunt the root for export.

Contemporary Food Habits in the United States

Adaptations of Food Habits

Generally changes in eating habits correlate with increasing length of stay in the United States, particularly with subsequent generations. Dinner remains the most traditionally Chinese meal, whereas breakfast, lunch, and snacks tend to become more Americanized. Younger persons are also more likely to accept American fare.

Ingredients and Common Foods

Most Americans of Chinese descent regularly consume several Chinese foods, such as rice, soybean products, cooked vegetables, and fruit (Chau et al., 1990). One preliminary study suggests that the majority (88%) of foreign-born immigrants prefer Chinese fare at home, although younger respondents (ages 20–34) expressed preference for American foods (Sun, 1996). Meat and poultry intake increases, while some traditional protein items like pig's liver and bone marrow soup often remain popular. Traditional fruits and vegetables may be replaced by more commonly available American items, such as potatoes, lettuce, apples, peaches, and watermelon (Grivetti & Paquette, 1978; Sun, 1996). Sugar intake also increases, mainly through consumption of soft drinks, candy, and pastries.

Even though milk is not a familiar item in the typical Chinese diet, several studies suggest that milk is consumed by nearly half of Chinese Americans in the United States (Chau et al., 1990; Schultz et al., 1994; Sun, 1996). Cheese, yogurt, and ice cream have also been found to be well accepted.

One study found that U.S.-born Chinese women have a more varied diet than Chinese American women who were foreign born. They ate more breads, cereals, dairy foods, meats, vegetables and ethnic items, such as Italian and Mexicans foods (Spindler & Schultz, 1996).

Meal Composition

Surveys of Chinese elders living in northern areas of California suggest that an almost traditional diet is eaten (Chau & Lee, 1987; Chau et al., 1990). Their lunches and dinners consisted mainly of Chinese-style foods; their breakfasts varied. Approximately half of the respondents attempted to balance hot and cold foods. Other studies suggest that the use of yin and yang in the diet may diminish over time and that Chinese Americans may practice some aspects of it, but without knowledge as to why certain food combinations are preferred (Ludman et al., 1989; Chau & Lee, 1990). Stir-frying, simmering, and steaming remain the favored cooking methods (Zhou & Britten, 1994; Sun, 1996).

Americans of Chinese descent usually celebrate the major Chinese holidays of New Year's and the Moon Festival with traditional foods. Chinese American Christians sometimes combine the spring festival of Ch'ing Ming with Easter festivities. In addition, some Chinese Americans recognize the founding of the People's Republic of China (mainland China) on October 1st (on the solar calendar) or the establishment of the Republic of China (Taiwan) on October 10th with cultural performances and banquets.

JAPANESE

The multi-island nation of Japan is off the coast of East Asia and has approximately the same latitude and range of climate as the East Coast of the United States. The capital of Japan is Tokyo, located on the island of Honshu. Today Japan is a prosperous country of 125 million people that has overcome the limitations of a mountainous

Traditional foods of Japan. Some foods typical of the traditional Japanese diet include *daikon*, dried sardines, Japanese eggplant, Japanese pickles, *nori* (seaweed), red beans, *shiitake* mushrooms, short-grain rice, shrimp, soy sauce, and wheat noodles. (Photo by Laurie Macfee.)

geography, a rugged coastline, and few mineral resources. Perhaps Japan's greatest natural resource is the sea, which provides one of the richest fishing grounds in the world.

Cultural Perspective

History of Japan

It is thought that the earliest inhabitants of Japan were the Ainu, a proto-Caucasoid people who were later culturally and racially absorbed by immigrants from the mainland of Asia. Early Japanese society was organized into a number of hereditary clan units that were unified in the fifth or sixth century under the authority of the Yamato emperors.

Japan is sometimes referred to as the daughter of Chinese civilization. Contact between the two peoples dates back at least to the first century. However, it was in the sixth century that the Japanese began to absorb the Chinese knowledge of science, art, agriculture, and cooking. It was also during this period that Buddhism and Confucianism were introduced into Japan. Although the Japanese borrowed much from the Chinese, by the tenth and eleventh centuries, Japanese culture had developed a distinctive character.

By the twelfth century the emperor became a figurehead without political or economic power. Japan evolved into a feudal society whose central figure was the aristocratic fighting man on horseback (knight), managing and defending an estate in allegiance to court families or central monasteries. Although the imperial family still nominally ruled, real power was held by *shoguns* who controlled loose associations of knights by long-standing ties of friendship and loyalty.

Through the fourteenth and fifteenth centuries, warriors who had won strong local followings assumed the role of feudal lords and became increasingly powerful. They later became known as *daimyo*, and their importance grew with the rapid expansion of the Japanese economy. By the fifteenth century, Japan was an important trading partner in the East China Sea. Larger and stronger daimyo took over weaker daimyo until by the end of the sixteenth century, Japan was ruled by a single powerful overlord, Tokugawa Ieyasu. He created a political system that endured for almost 250 years. He again took the title of shogun and ruled the daimyo through strong military power and close supervision. He also controlled all cities and ports.

Tokugawa adopted the social theories of Confucianism and created a hierarchy of four social classes: the warrior/administrator, the peasant, the artisan, and the merchant. The warrior aristocrats, called *samurai,* were the most prestigious; merchants were the lowest class. A fifth social class also existed unofficially, the *eta* (which means

Heike-gani crabs are believed to be reincarnations of drowned warriors due to the facelike markings on their shells.

"much filth"), whose jobs involved killing or handling dead animals. Although Buddhism had become the dominant religion of the masses, Confucianism had become the strongest intellectual and ethical force in Japan.

Before Tokugawa came to power, Christianity had been introduced to Japan by Portuguese traders. The Jesuit missionary St. Francis Xavier had lived in Japan from 1549 to 1551 and had won converts. However, in 1587, Tokugawa expelled the missionaries and banned the practice of Christianity in Japan. His successors later banned all foreign contact, and only the Dutch were allowed a trading mission, in the port of Nagasaki.

Isolated both politically and socially, Japan remained unchanged from the sixteenth century to the mid-nineteenth century. The Japanese people became accustomed to rigid patterns of conduct. They looked to their superiors for leadership, and they followed orders without question. Eventually Japan was pressured into change by the western powers' desire to establish contact and trade. It was the U.S. government that forced the door open after Commodore Perry steamed into Tokyo Bay in 1853.

In 1868 the Tokugawa regime fell and the office of shogun was abolished. In its place a new central government revolutionized the military and social structure of Japan, ending the old feudal order. The Meiji restoration and its rulers brought Japan into the twentieth century and made the nation a world power.

In the 1930s, Japan swung violently back to authoritarian rule at home and military expansion abroad. Japan dominated Korea and large areas of northern China, and by 1941 the military controlled the Japanese government. On December 7, 1941, Japanese aircraft bombed Pearl Harbor in Hawaii, which brought the United States into World War II. Japan lost the war, but not until the United States had carried out the first and only wartime use of atomic bombs at Hiroshima and Nagasaki. Democratic rule was established after the war. Today Japan is a leading economic power.

History of Japanese in the United States

Immigration Patterns

Significant Japanese immigration to the United States occurred after 1890 during the Meiji era. The immigrants were mostly young men with 4 to 6 years of education from the rural southern provinces of Japan. Most came for economic opportunities and many eventually returned to Japan. They settled primarily in Hawaii and on the West Coast of the United States and often worked in agriculture, on the railroads, and in canneries. Like the Chinese before them, Japanese immigrants opened small businesses, such as hotels and restaurants, to

Among Japanese Americans, first-generation immigrants born in Japan are called *Issei,* second-generation Japanese Americans born in the United States are known as *Nisei,* and the third and fourth generations are known as *Sansei* and *Yonsei,* respectively.

provide services for their countrymen. In contrast to the Chinese, many Japanese became farmers, ran plant nurseries, and were employed as gardeners. The Japanese prospered within their ethnic communities.

Most Japanese women came to the United States as "picture brides": Their marriages were arranged by professional matchmakers and they were married by proxy in Japan. They did not usually meet their husbands until they disembarked from the ship in the United States.

Discrimination against the Japanese was commonplace. The Issei (first-generation immigrants) were classified as aliens who were ineligible to become naturalized U.S. citizens, and in 1913, land ownership became illegal in California. Although many bought land in the names of their children, who were Americans by birth, Japanese-owned and leased land was reduced by half in the 1920s. In 1907 the Japanese government had informally agreed to limit the number of emigrants, and in 1924 the Japanese Exclusion Act halted Japanese immigration completely.

World War II heightened the prejudice against the Japanese on the West Coast. After Japan attacked Pearl Harbor, all West Coast Japanese, even if they were U.S. citizens, were "evacuated" to war relocation camps, and many remained there for the duration of the war. Most lost or sold their businesses as a result of internment. Nevertheless, many Nisei (second generation) volunteered for combat duty and fought in Europe.

Current Demographics and Socioeconomic Status

After the war, most Japanese Americans resettled on the West Coast, and the most discriminatory laws were repealed or ruled unconstitutional. The successful postwar recovery of Japan resulted in reduced emigration to the United States, usually far below the quota allotted under current immigration laws.

According to 1990 U.S. census figures, approximately 866,000 Japanese Americans live in the United States; 70 percent of them live in California or Hawaii. Many West Coast cities have a section of town called Little Tokyo or Japantown, and a small number of older Japanese still live in these homogeneous neighborhoods. Most Japantowns contain Japanese American–owned restaurants, markets, and other small businesses, as well as Chinese churches or Buddhist temples.

More than 95 percent of Japanese Americans live in culturally mixed urban and suburban areas. Americans of Japanese descent are unique for a non-white ethnic group in the degree of assimilation and economic mobility they have experienced. Family incomes are often above the national average and only 7 percent live in poverty. Of the third-generation Sansei, many of whom were born in the relocation camps, 88 percent have attended college and most hold professional

Economic competition has renewed some anti-Japanese sentiments in the United States. In 1982 a Chinese American man was murdered in Detroit by two non-Asian autoworkers who mistook the victim for being of Japanese descent.

Japantown, San Francisco. (Photo by Pat Goyan.)

jobs. Some Japanese Americans have noted that few Asians are found in top private and public sector positions, however, and believe that they suffer from the stereotype of being too unassertive for upper management.

Cultural Organizations

The roots of the Japanese community in America lie in Japan. It is from Japan that the Issei learned the ideals of putting family and community interests ahead of personal needs. Mutual assistance groups rapidly developed in the United States to help immigrants acclimate to a new culture. Later the community institutions helped fight against discrimination.

One of the first organizations founded by the Issei was the local Japanese Association. It helped to regulate internal community affairs and served as a liaison with the outside culture. It usually had a close working relationship with the local Japanese consul, as Issei were Japanese citizens. Another important organization was the *kenjinkais* (*ken*), or prefectural association: Like the Chinese, the Japanese often belong to a group of families that immigrated from the same area in Japan and that therefore share customs and speak the same dialect. Both types of organizations are currently supported by donations and jointly sponsor the local annual Japanese picnic, which usually occurs in the summer.

A later organization was the Japanese American Citizen's League. It was formed to serve the needs of the Nisei, represent the Japanese American community, and fight discrimination. Today it is the largest national Japanese American association, with more than 100 chapters, but for many Japanese its image was tarnished during World War II when it aided the U.S. government in evacuating the West Coast Japanese.

Worldview

Religion

Early Japanese immigrants usually joined a Buddhist temple (Pure Land sect) or a Christian church after arriving in America. The church frequently provided employment and an opportunity to learn English. Today, it is thought that there are more Japanese Americans who belong to Protestant faiths than there are who follow Buddhism.

Shintoism, the indigenous religion of Japan, does not have a formal organization, but its beliefs are a fundamental part of Japanese culture. The Shinto view is that humans are inherently good. Evil is caused by pollution or filthiness, physical as well as spirtual; goodness is associated with purity. Evil can be removed through ritual purification.

Shinto deities, called *kami*, represent any form of existence (human, animal, plant, or geologic) that evokes a sense of awe. Kami are worshiped at their shrines as ritual expression of veneration and thankfulness. Prayers are also said for divine favors and blessings, as well as for avoidance of misfortunes and accidents.

Family

Until World War II the structure of the Japanese American family had its roots in Japan and was similar to that of the Chinese due to the strong influence of Confucianism. In addition, the rigid pattern of conduct that evolved in Japan during the sixteenth century resulted in the following practices among the Issei and their descendants:

1. *KoKo.* Filial piety defines the relationship between parents and children, between siblings, and between individuals and their community and rulers. (See the Chinese religion section on Confucianism in the first part of this chapter for further explanation.) One outcome is that the Issei expect their children to care for them in their old age.

2. *Gaman.* The Japanese believe it is virtuous to suppress emotions. The practice of self-control is paramount.

3. *Haji.* Individuals should not bring shame on themselves, their families, or their communities. This Japanese cultural concept exerts strong social control.

4. *Enryo.* There is no equivalent word in English, but the Japanese believe it is important to be polite and to show respect, deference, self-effacement, humility, and hesitation. Thus many older or less acculturated Americans of Japanese descent are neither aggressive nor assertive.

Japanese clan or village affiliation has traditionally been much weaker than in China, and Japanese immigrants arrived in the United States prepared to raise nuclear families similar to those in white America. Typically picture brides were trapped in unhappy marriages but persevered on behalf of their children. Most Issei women worked alongside their husbands to support the family financially.

The internment of Japanese Americans during World War II brought further changes in family structure and accelerated acculturation into mainstream society after the war. In the camps, very low wages were paid and the pay was the same for everyone; thus the father could no longer be the primary wage earner. The camps were run democratically, but positions could be held only by American citizens, so the younger generation held positions of authority. The camps also allowed the Japanese to work in a wider range of jobs than those available to them on the outside. After their internment the Nisei no longer had to follow the few occupations of their parents.

Sansei couples generally form dual-career households. Nearly 50 percent marry outside their ethnic group. The societal problems prevalent in majority American homes, such as spousal abuse, have surfaced among Japanese Americans as well (Easton & Ellington, 1995), and it is not known if the family values that have thrust Americans of Japanese descent into educational and financial success will continue in the fully assimilated fourth generation of Yonsei.

Communication

Formality and politeness are essential conversational elements in Japan. Addressing Japanese elders or Japanese American Issei, and some Nisei, by their first names is very insulting. Sansei and Yonsei are often more informal (Hashizume & Takano, 1983). Emotional displays are avoided, especially of anger. The Japanese are nonconfrontational and may be reluctant to say "no" even when the answer to a question is negative. Conversational style is often indirect, and frequent pauses are common. Direct eye contact is disrespectful; glancing around or downcast eyes are expected. Smiling can indicate pleasure but is also used to hide displeasure.

The Japanese are extremely high-context, and the slightest gesture may have meaning. (See Chapter 12 on intercultural communication for more details.) Broad hand or body gestures may be misconstrued. Touching between strangers or acquaintances is infrequent, though most Japanese Americans are comfortable with a light handshake.

The traditional greeting is a bow from the waist with palms against thighs. Slouching and putting one's feet on a desk are signs of disinterest.

Traditional Food Habits

Japanese ingredients, as well as cooking and eating utensils, are very similar to those of the Chinese, due to the strong influence China has had on Japan. Yet Japanese food preparation and presentation are unique. The Japanese reverence for harmony within the body and community and with nature has resulted in a cuisine that offers numerous ways to prepare a limited number of foods. Each item is to be seen, tasted, and relished. The Japanese also place an emphasis on the appearance of the meal so that the visual appeal reflects balance among the foods and the environment. For example, a summer meal may be served on glass dishes so that the meal looks cooler, while a September meal may include the autumn colors of reds and golds.

Ingredients and Common Foods

Japan's mountainous terrain and limited arable land have contributed historically to a less than abundant food supply. Even today much of Japan's food supply is imported.

Staples and Regional Variations

The basic foods of the Japanese diet are found in the Cultural Food Groups list (Table 7.2). Several key ingredients were adopted from China, including rice, soybeans, and tea. Rice (*gohon*) is the main staple, and it is eaten with almost every meal. In contrast to the Chinese, the Japanese prefer a short-grain rice that contains more starch and is stickier after cooking. Rice mixed with a rice vinegar (*su*) is called *sushi* and is often served with sliced raw fish (*sashimi*). Rice is also made into noodles, although those made from wheat (known as *udon, somen,* and *ramen*) or buckwheat (*soba*) are more commonly consumed.

Soybean products are an important component of Japanese cuisine. *Tofu* (bean curd), soy sauce (*shoyu*), and fermented bean paste (*miso*) are just a few. *Teriyaki sauce* ("shining broil") is made from soy sauce and *mirin,* a sweet rice wine. Sugar, shoyu, and vinegar are a basic seasoning mixture. Shoyu and mirin can vary in strength, and the amounts used depend on personal taste.

Green tea is served with most meals. Tea was originally used in a devotional ceremony in Zen Buddhism. The ritual was raised to a fine

A small grill in Japan is called a *hibachi,* meaning "fire bowl."

Gohan means cooked rice and is also the Japanese word for "meal."

In 1994, Japanese consumers took to the streets to protest the importation of rice from California needed to alleviate a crop shortage.

Red rice, made by steaming rice with adzuki beans, is often eaten at celebrations because red is considered a joyous and lucky color.

Japanese sashimi platter with salmon, octopus, and other raw seafood. (Corbis/Kelly–Mooney Photo.)

art by Japanese tea masters; as a result, they also set the standards for behavior in Japanese society. Today the tea ceremony (*kaiseki*) and the accompanying food remain a cultural ideal that reflects the search for harmony with nature and within one's self. The meal features six small courses that balance the tastes of sweet, sour, pungent, bitter, and salty. The tea that is used for the ceremony is not the common leaf tea that is usually used for meals, but rather a blend of ground dry tea or a tea powder. Hot water is added to the tea and the mixture is whipped together using a handmade whisk, resulting in a frothy green drink.

Japanese fare does not use many dairy foods. Soybean products and a wide variety of fish and shellfish (fresh, dried, or smoked) are the primary protein sources. Fish and shellfish are often eaten raw. Beef and poultry are also popular but are very expensive. Only small amounts of meat, poultry, or fish are added to the vegetables in traditional Japanese recipes.

Fresh fruits and vegetables are the most desirable and are eaten only when in season. As in China, many Asian and European varieties are consumed (see the section "Staples" in the Chinese part of the chapter). Favorites include the *daikon* radish (a long white radish

Kaiseki meals have recently become trendy in both Japan and the United States, costing up to $100 per person at restaurants featuring the ceremonial menu.

TABLE 7.2
Cultural Food Groups: Japanese

Groups	Comments
PROTEIN FOODS	
Milk/milk products	Japanese cooking does not utilize significant amounts of dairy products. Many Japanese are lactose-intolerant. Soybean products, seaweed, and small bony fish are alternative calcium sources.
Meat/poultry/fish/eggs/legumes	Soybean products and a wide variety of fish and shellfish (fresh, frozen, dried, smoked) are the primary protein sources in the Japanese diet. Fish and shellfish are often eaten raw.
	Chicken is used more often than beef; price is probably the limiting factor in meat consumption.
CEREALS/GRAINS	Short-grain rice is the primary staple of the diet and is eaten with every meal.
	Wheat is often eaten in the form of noodles, such as *ramen, somen,* and *udon.*
FRUITS/VEGETABLES	Fresh fruits and vegetables are the most desirable; usually eaten only in season.
	Many fruits and vegetables are preserved, dried, or pickled.
ADDITIONAL FOODS	
Seasonings	Sugar, *shoyu,* and vinegar are a basic seasoning mixture. *Shoyu* and *mirin* can vary in strength; amounts used will vary according to taste.
Nuts/seeds	
Beverages	Green tea is the preferred beverage with meals; coffee or black tea is drunk with western-style foods.
	Sake or beer is often served with dinner.
Fats/oils	The traditional Japanese diet is low in fat and cholesterol.
Sweeteners	

similar to the Chinese version, but longer, up to 12 inches in length), chrysanthemum leaves, and the winter tangerines called *mikan.* Pickled vegetables are available year round and are eaten extensively. Fresh fruit is the traditional dessert.

TABLE 7.2
Cultural Food Groups: Japanese—continued

Common Foods	Adaptations in the United States
Milk, butter, ice cream	First-generation Japanese Americans drink little milk and eat few dairy products. Subsequent generations eat more dairy foods.
Meat: beef, deer, lamb, pork, rabbit, veal *Poultry:* capon, chicken, duck, goose, partridge, pheasant, quail, thrush, turkey *Fish:* blowfish, bonita, bream, carp, cod, cuttlefish, eel, fllounder, herring, mackerel, porgy, octopus, red snapper, salmon, sardines, shark, sillago, snipefish, squid, swordfish, trout, tuna, turbot, yellowtail, whale *Shellfish:* abalone, *ayu,* clams, crab, earshell, lobster, mussels, oysters, sea urchin roe (*uni*), scallops, shrimp, snails *Legumes: adzuki,* black beans, lima beans, red beans, soybeans	Dried fish and fish cakes are available in the United States, but some varieties of fresh fish are not. Japanese Americans eat more poultry and meat than fish.
Wheat, rice, buckwheat, millet	Rice is still an important staple in the diet and is usually eaten at dinner.
Fruits: apples, apricots, bananas, cherries, dates, figs, grapes, grapefruits (*yuzu*), kumquats, lemons, limes, loquats, melons, oranges, peaches, pears, pear apples, persimmons, plums (fresh and pickled), pineapples, strawberries, *mikan* (tangerine) *Vegetables* artichokes, asparagus, bamboo shoots, beans, bean sprouts, broccoli, brussels sprouts, beets, burdock root (*gobo*), cabbage (several varieties), carrots, chickweed, chrysanthemum, eggplant (long, slender variety), ferns, ginger and pickled ginger (*beni shoga*), green onions, green peppers, gourd (*kanpyo,* dried gourd shavings), leeks, lettuce, lotus root, mushrooms (*shiitake, matsutake, nameko*), okra, onions, peas, potatoes, pumpkins, radishes, rhubarb, seaweed, snow peas, shiso, sorrel, spinach, squash, sweet potatoes, taro, tomatoes, turnips, watercress, yams	Fewer fruits and vegetables are eaten; freshness is less critical.
Alum, anise, bean paste (*miso*), caraway, chives, *dashi,* fish paste, garlic, ginger, mint, *mirin,* MSG, mustard, red pepper, *sake,* seaweed, sesame seeds, *shiso, shoyu,* sugar, thyme, vinegar (rice), *wasabi* (green horseradish) Chestnut, gingko nuts, peanuts, walnuts; poppy (black and white), sesame seeds	
Carbonated beverages, beer, coffee, gin, tea (black and green), *sake,* scotch	Japanese Americans drink less tea and more milk, coffee, and carbonated beverages.
Butter, cottonseed oil, olive oil, peanut oil, sesame seed oil, vegetable oil	Japanes Americans consume more fats and oils because of increased use of western foods and cooking methods.
Honey, sugar	Increased use of sugar, sweet desserts.

The Japanese use a large amount of seaweed and algae in their cooking for seasoning, as a wrapping, or in salads and soups. There are many types: *Nori* is a paper-thin sheet of algae that is rolled around rice and other ingredients. **Kombu** is an essential ingredient in *dashi,*

Kombu sounds like the word for happiness, and it is often presented as a hostess gift by guests.

Dashi is a stock made from dried bonita fish and seaweed. *Misoshiru* is a popular soup made with dashi and miso.

or soup stock. *Wakame* and *hijiki* are used primarily in soups and salads. *Aonoriko* is powdered green seaweed used as a seasoning agent.

Cooking style varies from region to region in Japan. Kyoto is known for its vegetarian specialties, and Osaka and Tokyo are known for their seafood. Nagasaki's cooking has been greatly influenced by the Chinese.

Meal Composition and Cycle

Daily Pattern

Traditionally the Japanese eat three meals a day, plus a snack called *oyatsu*. Breakfast usually starts with a salty sour plum (*umeboshi*), followed by rice garnished with nori, soup, and pickled vegetables. Some families may have an egg with their rice.

When a family moves to a new home, they give *soba* noodles to the neighbors on either side and across the street as a gesture of friendship.

Lunch is simple and often consists only of rice topped with leftovers from the previous night. Sometimes hot tea or dashi is added to the rice mixture. A bowl of noodles cooked or served with meats, poultry, or fish, and vegetables is a popular alternative to leftovers. Dinner must always include three dishes: rice, soup, and pickled vegetables. The main dish often consists of fish or shellfish, either broiled, steamed, or deep-fried. Pink pickled ginger and the very pungent green horseradish-like condiment called *wasabi* garnish many meals, and soy sauce is also usually available.

The Japanese tend not to serve meals by courses. Instead, all the dishes are presented at the same time, with each food in its own bowl or plate. The soup, however, is usually served last or near the end of the meal. Traditionally desserts were not common in Japan; meals usually ended with fruit.

Snacks include several kinds of sweets, rice crackers, or fruit. Traditional Japanese confections include *mochi gashi* (rice cakes with sweet bean paste), *manju* (dumplings), and *yokan* (sweet bean jelly). Green tea is served after all meals except when western-style food is eaten; then coffee or black tea is served. Beer or *sake* (rice wine, usually served warm) may be served with dinner.

Sukiyaki is a simmered beef dish usually prepared at the table. The name means "broiled on the blade of the plow" and probably dates back to ancient times. The current version is mislabeled, however, because it is a *nimono-*, not a *yakimono-*, style food.

Japanese dishes are classified by the way the food is prepared: *suimono*, clear soups; *yakimono*, broiled food; *nimono*, foods boiled in seasoned broth; *mushimono*, steamed foods; *agimono*, fried foods (e.g., *tempura*, adapted from a dish introduced in the sixteenth century by the Catholic Portuguese for religious fast days, consisting of shrimp and selected sliced vegetables lightly battered and deep-fried); *aemono*, mixed foods in a thick dressing; *sunomono*, vinegared salad; and *chameshi*, rice cooked with other ingredients. Foods that are cooked at the table and one-pot dishes are called *nabe*. Seafood, fish, fruits, and vegetables that are pickled in a mixture of miso, soy sauce, vinegar, and the residue from sake production are known as *tsukemono,* and they accompany nearly every meal. Japanese foods are usually cut into small pieces if the item is not naturally easy to eat with chopsticks, and dishes are frequently modified for children, as it is believed that adult recipes are too spicy for them.

Etiquette

The Japanese, like the Chinese, eat with chopsticks and follow many of the same customs regarding their use (see the section "Etiquette" in the Chinese part of the chapter); the rice bowl is not held as closely to the mouth, however. Soups are consumed directly from the bowl; the only dish eaten with a spoon is an unsweetened egg custard known as *chawanmushi.* Traditionally the Japanese eat their meals at low tables where the men sit cross-legged and women sit with their legs tucked to the side. Shoes are removed first. Dishes on the left are picked up with the right hand and dishes to the right are lifted with the left hand. It is impolite to serve sake to one's self.

Special Occasions

In Japan there are numerous festivals associated with the harvesting of specific crops or with local Shinto shrines or Buddhist temples. The most important and largest celebration in Japan is New Year's. The Japanese share many holiday traditions with the Chinese. Homes are cleaned thoroughly and all debts are settled before the New Year; food is also prepared ahead so that no knives or cooking will interfere with the 7-day event.

The Japanese celebrate New Year's on the first day of January. The New Year's foods consist of ten to twenty meticulously prepared dishes served in a special set of nesting boxes. Each dish symbolizes a specific value, such as happiness, prosperity, wealth, long life, wisdom, and diligence. For example, fish eggs represent fertility, mashed sweet potatoes and chestnuts protect against bad spirits, and black beans represent a willingness to keep healthy through hard work and sweat.

An important New Year's food is *mochi,* a rice cake made by pounding hot, steamed rice into a sticky dough. Traditionally a Buddhist *o sonae mochi* is set up in many homes. A large rice cake represents the foundation of the older generation and is placed on the bottom, and a smaller rice cake symbolizing the younger generation is placed atop it, followed by a tangerine indicating generations to come. The o sonae mochi is as meaningful to the Japanese as a Christmas tree is to Americans, preserving good fortune and happiness for future generations. Another special food is *ozoni,* a soup cooked with mochi, vegetables, fish cakes, and chicken or eggs. A special rice wine called *otoso* is consumed to preserve health in the coming year.

Teppanyaki is a Japanese term for grilling. The style familiar to U.S. diners (typified by the Benihana restaurant chain) was invented to take advantage of the tourist trade. Beef, chicken, shrimp and vegetables are cooked on a hot grill in the center of a large table, then served with *ponzu,* a soy sauce and citrus juice mixture.

At many celebrations the Japanese shout "Banzai! Banzai! Banzai!" The cheer is translated as "10,000 years!" and dates back to the third century BCE.

Rice was often in short supply in Japan, so eating the round rice cakes, *mochi,* at New Year's represented wealth and prosperity.

Obon festival, San Jose, California. Dancing and traditional foods are featured at this annual Buddhist celebration.

A crane symbolizes 1,000 years. On special birthdays, 1,000 red *origami* (folded paper sculpture) cranes are displayed as a wish for longevity.

Japanese Buddhist temples usually hold an Obon festival in the second or third week of July to appreciate the living, honor the dead, and comfort the bereaved. Food and dancing are a traditional part of the holiday.

Certain birthdays are thought to be either hazardous or auspicious in Japanese culture. When a man turns 42 or a woman becomes 33, special festivities are held to prevent misfortune. Age 61 marks the beginning of second childhood and a person dons a red cap for this honor. At age 77 a person puts on a long red overcoat, and at the most propitious birthday of all, age 88, the celebrant may begin wearing both the hat and the coat.

Sea urchin roe, called *uni,* is thought to enhance male sexual potency in Japan, where wholesalers pay up to $100 per pound for it. California imposed strict urchin harvesting laws to prevent extinction along the coast (more than 200 million pounds were gathered for export between 1985 and 1990). Maine suffers from similar overharvesting.

Therapeutic Use of Food

Although the use of yin and yang is not as prevalent among the Japanese as it is among the Chinese, there are many beliefs about the harmful or beneficial effects of specific foods and food combinations. Traditionally certain food pairs, such as eel and pickled plums, watermelon and crab, or cherries and milk, are thought to cause illness. Pickled plums and hot tea, which are customarily eaten for breakfast, are believed to prevent constipation. Both pickled plums and rice porridge are thought to be easily digested and well tolerated during recovery from sickness.

Contemporary Food Habits in the United States

Adaptations of Food Habits

In general, second-generation Japanese Americans eat a typical American diet, but they may eat more rice and use more soy sauce than nonAsians. Traditional foods are prepared for special occasions. Third- and fourth-generation Japanese Americans appear to be totally acculturated to American foodways. Even in Japan a westernized diet is increasingly followed. Bread and butter are becoming staples, and consumption of meat, milk, and eggs is increasing. One survey reported that between 1960 and 1985, fat consumption in Japan went from 11 percent of calories in the diet to more than 25 percent of calories (Lands et al., 1990).

KOREANS

The mountainous peninsula that forms Korea is suspended geographically—and culturally—between China and Japan. Korea has historically been caught in the middle of both Chinese and Japanese expansionism, yet has maintained a homogeneous population with an independent, distinctive character. Little land is arable, and the climate fluctuates between cold, snowy winters and hot, monsoonal summers that limit agriculture significantly. The peninsula is currently divided into two nations. The Democratic People's Republic of Korea (North Korea), with the capital city of Pyongyang, has a communist government. The Republic of Korea (South Korea) is a democracy supported by the United States. Seoul is the country's capital. Both nations desire the reunification of Korea through political and military domination of the other.

Cultural Perspective

History of Korea

The Korean peninsula was settled by Tungusic tribes from Mongolia in Paleolithic times. Their religion was a form of animism that operated through spiritual shamans. The first Korean kingdom, Choson, was founded in 2333 BCE. The Chinese established military outposts in 108 BCE leading to increasing Chinese control of the peninsula and

Korea is called *Choson* by Koreans, meaning "Land of Morning Calm."

Korean street vendors shredding cabbage for the preparation of the spicy vegetable pickle *kimchi*. (Corbis/Michael Freeman.)

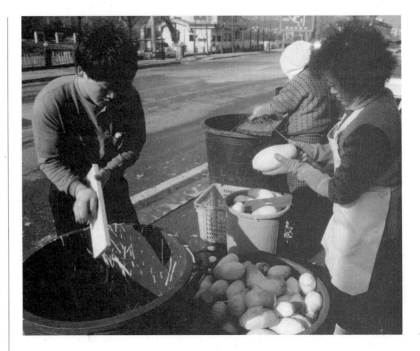

the introduction of bronze tools, agriculture, Confucianism, Taoism, Buddhism, and other aspects of Chinese culture.

Chinese domination ended in 313 with the rise and expansion of the Three Kingdoms: Silla, Koguryo, and Paekche. Silla, with Chinese assistance, destroyed the other two kingdoms in the seventh century and ruled Korea as a Buddhist state until 918, when the Koryo dynasty was founded. China once again established control of Korea in 1392 through the establishment of the Yi dynasty (aided by the Chinese Ming dynasty). Confucianism was revived and accepted throughout the nation. The modern Korean language, based on the first phonetic Asian alphabet, was invented during this period.

Roman Catholicism was introduced to Korea via China in the seventeenth century. In response a new Korean religion called *Tonghak* (Eastern Learning) emerged in 1860 and was embraced by the large peasant class. Continuous economic and political instability and repeated invasions from Japan and Manchu in the sixteenth and seventeenth centuries led to increasing anti-foreign feelings in Korea. With encouragement from China, Korea established isolationist policies so severe it became known as the "Hermit Kingdom."

Korea was finally opened to the modern world when Japan forced Korea to sign a commercial treaty in 1876; 6 years later the United

States and other western countries established relations with the nation. Korea became disputed territory during the Sino-Japanese War (1894–1895) and the Russo-Japanese War (1904–1905). Japanese victory led to annexation of Korea to Japan in 1910.

Japanese exploitation and suppression of the country continued until 1945, when the Japanese surrendered at the end of World War II. Although Korean independence was promised through a United Nations resolution, the nation was occupied in the north by military forces of the Soviet Union and in the south by U.S. troops. Each side established sovereignty in 1948 as the Republic of Korea (South Korea) and the Democratic People's Republic of Korea (North Korea). In 1950, North Korea invaded South Korea, leading to the U.S.–U.S.S.R. confrontation of the Korean War. When the war ended in 1953, little was resolved.

North Korea has remained a communist nation focused on isolationist self-sufficiency. South Korea has alternated between democratic rule and martial law, developing a successful export economy. In 1991 the two nations signed a reconciliation and nonaggression treaty. However, reunification attempts thus far have failed.

History of Koreans in the United States

Immigration Patterns

Early Korean immigration to the United States was severely restricted by the isolationist policies of Korea. A small number of Koreans arrived before 1900, most of whom were Protestants seeking to escape discrimination and further their education in America.

Between 1903 and 1905, Christian missionaries recruited more than 7,000 Korean men, women, and children to work in Hawaiian sugarcane fields. In 1905, Japan barred overseas emigration of Koreans, and in 1907 the United States entered a "Gentlemen's Agreement" with Japan limiting both Japanese and Korean immigration. During the next 17 years, only picture brides (1,000 in Hawaii and 115 in California) and oppressed political activists (just more than 500) were permitted entry. In 1924 the Japanese Exclusion Act was applied to Koreans as well, preventing all immigration. Most early Korean immigrants worked as field hands or in domestic service; many first- and second-generation Koreans living in urban areas were barred from professional jobs and established small businesses such as vegetable stands and restaurants.

Between 1959 and 1971, nearly all Korean immigrants were the wives and children of U.S. soldiers who fought in the Korean War. Following relaxation of U.S. immigration laws in 1965, the numbers of Korean immigrants increased, including many college-educated, middle-class professionals and their families.

The author Jack London contributed to anti-Asian sentiment in the United States when he wrote a newspaper article in 1904 titled "The Yellow Peril" in which he called Koreans "the perfect type of inefficiency—of utter worthlessness" (Nash, 1995).

The status of Koreans in the United States during World War II was unique. Many remained technically Japanese citizens and as such were declared enemy aliens (although none was interred). Yet many Koreans had been involved for years in anti-Japanese activities. "I am Korean" buttons were worn to distinguish themselves from Japanese residents.

Current Demographics

The Korean immigrant population has increased dramatically in recent years. As of 1993, approximately 837,000 Koreans were living in the United States; more than half have arrived since 1980. More than 80 percent of Koreans in America were born in Korea, and most do not seek U.S. citizenship. Large numbers of immigrants to the United States relocated first from North Korea to South Korea, seeking greater freedom. Koreans coming to America hope to find economic opportunity and to avoid any North Korean–South Korean conflict that may arise in the future. Large numbers of Koreans have settled in California, particularly Los Angeles. Other states with significant populations include New York, Illinois, New Jersey, Texas, Washington, Virginia, Pennsylvania, Maryland, and Hawaii.

Socioeconomic Status

The economic success of South Korea has lured thousands of second-generation Korean Americans to immigrate there, where they have taken positions in marketing, public relations, and the entertainment industry. Difficulties in adjustment have led them to form expatriate communities in many areas.

Many Koreans must accept temporary or permanent nonprofessional employment due to language difficulties or licensing restrictions. Families working together toward the success of a small business and the purchase of a home are common. Korean American descendants of the 1903–1905 immigrants to Hawaii are securely middle class. Contributing factors include high achievement in education and professionalism; quick mastery of English (faster than Japanese and Chinese immigrants of the same period); and a greater willingness to give up Korean traditions, perhaps due to their experience with nonconformity in Korea as Christians in a Confucian and Buddhist society (Kim, 1980). However, some Koreans do not find the economic prosperity they seek in the United States and so return to Korea.

There is a notable conflict in the immigrant Korean community. Korean Americans may not accept recent immigrants who demand immediate social standing based on prior status in Korea. Recent professional immigrants are sometimes contemptuous of Korean war brides, who are considered uneducated and lower class. The large numbers of new arrivals may serve to coalesce the Korean community because they share similar experiences in acculturation and are a significant percentage of the growing Korean American population.

Cultural Organizations

Early Korean immigrant organizations focused on political activism. Groups in Hawaii and California advocated independence in Korea through world pressure, military intervention, or a gradual spiritual renewal. More recent immigrants have joined other types of organizations, such as churches and alumni groups. Korean Christian churches have emerged in nearly all Korean communities, in part due to large numbers of ministers who have left Korea. Church support is highly valued by new immigrants and congregational members are involved in many activities. Alumni associations are similar to Chinese clan associations, except the "kinship" established is based on high school or college attendance rather than surname.

In each area where immigrants have settled, the largest community organization is usually the Korean Association, which is open to all Koreans. Factionalized groups active in Korean politics continue with little influence on Korea or on foreign policy decisions regarding Korea. Political organizations devoted to issues in the United States are limited due to the large numbers of noncitizens in the Korean American population.

Worldview

Religion

In South Korea, Buddhism and Confucianism are the majority religions. Approximately 28 percent of South Koreans are Christian, and smaller numbers adhere to shamanism (belief in natural and ancestral spirits) and the national Korean religion *Chundo Kyo,* formerly known as Tonghak (a mixture of Confucian, Taoist, and Buddhist concepts). In North Korea, all religious beliefs other than the national ideology of Marxism and self-reliance are suppressed.

The first Korean immigrants at the turn of the century were Christians attracted to the United States as a religious homeland. Many suffered discrimination in the largely Confucian/Buddhist society of Korea. Although specific figures are unknown, it is believed that many recent immigrants to the United States are also Christian. A study of elderly Korean immigrant women in Washington, DC indicated that 85 percent were Christian (Baptist, Methodist, Presbyterian, and Catholic), 10 percent practiced ancestor worship (veneration of ancestors often coexists with other religious practices), and 5 percent were Buddhist (Pang, 1991). Other research suggests that larger numbers of Buddhists have immigrated.

Family

Hundreds of years of Confucianism in Korea have significantly influenced family structure regardless of current religious affiliation. Family is highly valued, and loyalty to one's immediate and extended family is more important than individual wants or needs. Generational ties are more important than those of marriage, and parents are especially close to children.

In Korea a male is always the head of the family; if a father is unable to fulfill that role, the eldest son (even if still a child) takes on that responsibility. Birth sequence orders life's events within the family, and older male children are traditionally awarded privileges, such as advanced education, that younger children or daughters are denied.

Elders are esteemed and cared for in Korea. The two major birthday celebrations in Korean culture occur at age 1, and when an individual reaches age 60, meaning that the person has survived a full five repeats of the 12-year cycle of life and attained old age. The opinions of elders are respected and after age 60 a person is allowed to relax and enjoy life.

Many changes occur in the Korean family after immigration to the United States. For example, the marriage bond often becomes more important than obligations to one's parents. Few of the elderly maintain traditional arrangements of living with an eldest son's family. Some live with unmarried children or with married daughters, or live alone. Many elders feel that they are now a burden to their children and that old age is a negative experience instead of a privilege (Pang, 1991). Male dominance has declined with increased participation of women in the workplace, yet most married women assume total responsibility for home and their job and often are not paid for their work if employed in a family-owned business. Divorce rates are reportedly high, and intergenerational conflict increases with length of time in the United States.

Communication

Koreans use a quiet, nonassertive approach to conversation. Expression of emotions is avoided, and loud talking or laughing is considered impolite (although a Korean may laugh excessively when embarrassed). An indirect approach to topics is appreciated. A Korean may be hesitant to say "no" or to disagree with a statement. Instead, tipping the head back and sucking air through the teeth are often used to signal dissension. Direct eye contact is expected, and it is used to demonstrate attentiveness and sincerity. Touching is uncommon, except for a light, introductory handshake between men. Hugging, kissing, and backpatting should be avoided, as should crossing one's legs or putting feet on the furniture. It is considered respectful to rise whenever an elder enters the room and to touch the palm of the left hand to the elbow of the right arm when shaking hands or passing an item to an elder (Axtell, 1991; Morrison et al., 1994).

Traditional Food Habits

Ingredients and Common Foods

Korean cuisine is neither Chinese nor Japanese, although it has been influenced by both styles of cooking. It is a distinctly hearty Asian fare that is highly seasoned and instantaneously recognizable as Korean by its flavors and colors. Sweet, sour, bitter, hot, and salty tastes are combined in all meals, and foods are often seasoned before and after cooking. Five colors—white, red, black, green, and yellow—are also important considerations in the preparation and presentation of dishes.

Staples

Korean cooking is based on grains flavored with spicy vegetable and meat, poultry, or fish side dishes. Korean staples are listed in Table 7.3.

Rice is the foundation of the Korean diet. Short-grain varieties are usually preferred, both a regular and glutinous (sticky) type, the latter most often in sweets. Long-grain rice, called Vietnamese rice in Korea, is available but not common. Millet and barley are used, most often as extenders for rice. Noodles are also an important staple and are made from wheat, buckwheat, or mung beans. The buckwheat variety is often used in cold dishes. Fritters, dumplings, and pancakes flavored with scallions, chile pepper, and sometimes fish or meat placed directly in the batter before cooking are other popular grain dishes.

Vegetables are served at every meal. Chinese cabbage (both *bok choy* and *napa*), European cabbage, and a long, white radish (similar but not identical to the Japanese *daikon* radish) are eaten most often. Eggplant, cucumbers, perilla (a mint-like green also called shiso), chrysanthemum greens, bean sprouts, sweet potatoes, and winter melon are also very popular. Vegetables are added to soups and braised dishes and are often served individually as hot or cold side dishes. Pickled, fermented vegetables are included at every meal, usually in the form of *kimchi*. There are many types of kimchi, but most are made with shredded Chinese cabbage and white radish, heavily seasoned with garlic, onions, and chile peppers, then fermented. Cucumber, eggplant, turnip, and even fruits or fish are sometimes added. Some recipes are mild, but most are very hot. Seaweed is eaten as a vegetable, including kelp and laver (called *kim*). Kim is brushed with sesame oil, salted, and toasted to make a condiment. Fruits are eaten mostly fresh. Crisp, juicy Asian pears (known as apple-pears in the U.S.) are very popular; apples, cherries, jujubes (red dates), plums, melons, grapes, tangerines, and persimmons are also common.

Fish and shellfish are eaten throughout Korea. Fresh fish dishes are preferred near the coast or in river regions, but dried or salted fish is more common in the inland areas. *Saewujeot,* a Korean fermented fish sauce, is made from tiny shrimplike crustaceans. It flavors many dishes. Beef and beef variety cuts are especially popular in Korea. Cubes, thin slices, or small ribs of marinated beef are barbecued or grilled at the table over a small charcoal brazier or gas grill. *Bulgogi,* grilled strips of beef flavored with garlic, onions, soy sauce, and sesame oil, is best known. Another Korean specialty is the fire pot (*sinsullo*), similar to the Mongolian hot pot, featuring beef or liver, cooked egg strips, sliced vegetables (e.g., mushrooms, carrots,

Rice cooking is an important skill in Korea; the rice must be neither underdone nor overcooked and mushy.

The preparation of *kimchi* every autumn is a special family event. In the past a family's wealth was demonstrated by the ingredients in their kimchi, with rare vegetables and fruits used by the most affluent.

One of the most popular black market commodities in Korea is the diced pork and gelatin product Spam.

The Koreans say if you eat duck, your feet will become webbed.

TABLE 7.3
Cultural Food Groups: Korean

Group	Comments
PROTEIN FOODS	
Milk/milk products	Milk and milk products are generally not consumed or used in cooking.
Meat/poultry/fish/eggs/legumes	Beef and beef variety cuts are especially popular. Barbecuing is a popular method for cooking meat. Fish and shellfish, either fresh, dried, or salted, are eaten throughout Korea. Soybean products are added to many dishes.
CEREALS/GRAINS	Rice is the most important component of the Korean diet. Noodles made from wheat, mung bean, or buckwheat flours are an important staple.
FRUITS/VEGETABLES	A wide variety of fruits are consumed. Vegetables are often pickled and are eaten at every meal.
ADDITIONAL FOODS	
Seasonings	
Nuts/seeds	
Beverages	Herbal teas are popular, as well as rice tea. They are commonly served after the meal. Soup or barley water is used as a beverage with the meal.
Fats/oils	Animal fat is rarely used.
Sweeteners	Sweets are made for snacks and special occasions.

It is believed that a Portuguese Catholic priest introduced chile peppers into Korea in the sixteenth century. They were quickly adopted and have become ubiquitous in the cuisine.

bamboo shoots, onions), and nuts that are cooked in a seasoned broth heated over charcoal. After the morsels of food have been eaten, the broth is served as a soup. Chicken and poultry are not especially popular in Korea. Soybean products, however, are common, including soy sauce and soy paste. Bean curd, made from soybeans (*tobu*) or mung beans (*cheong-po*), is a favorite. Mung beans, adzuki beans, and other legumes are steamed and added to many savory and sweet dishes. Nuts, such as pine nuts, chestnuts, and peanuts, and toasted, crushed sesame seeds are frequent additions as ingredients or garnish.

Seasonings are the soul of Korean cooking. Garlic, ginger root, black pepper, chile peppers, scallions, and toasted sesame in the form of oil or crushed seeds flavor nearly all dishes. Prepared condiments,

TABLE 7.3
Cultural Food Groups: Korean—continued

Common Foods	Adaptations in the United States
Meat: beef, variety meats (heart, kidney, liver), oxtail, pork *Fish and shellfish:* abalone, clams, codfish, crab, cuttlefish, jellyfish, lobster, mackerel, mullet, octopus, oysters, perch, scallops, sea cucumber, shad, shrimp, squid, whiting *Poultry and small birds:* chicken, pheasant *Eggs:* hen *Legumes: adzuki,* lima beans, mung beans, red beans, soybeans	Milk and cheese product consumption increases. Beef, pork, and poultry consumption rises. Fish is eaten frequently. Many still consume tofu several times a week. Younger Korean Americans may consume more pork products.
Barley, buckwheat, millet, rice (glutinous and long-grain), wheat	Rice consumption declines, but it is still eaten every day.
Fruits: apples, Asian pears, cherries, dates (*jujubes,* red date), grapes, melons, oranges, pears, persimmons, plums, pumpkin, tangerines *Vegetables:* bamboo shoots, bean sprouts, beets, cabbage (Chinese, European), celery, chives, chrysanthemum leaves, cucumber, eggplant, fern, green beans, green onion, green pepper, leaf lettuce, leeks, lotus root, mushrooms, onion, peas, perilla (shiso), potato, seaweed (*kim*), spinach, sweet potato, turnips, water chestnut, watercress, white radish Chile peppers (*kochujang*—fermented chile paste), chinese parsley (fresh coriander), cinnamon, garlic, ginger root, green onions, MSG, hot mustard, red pepper sauce, pine nuts, rice wine, *saewujeot* (fermented fish sauce), sesame seed oil, sesame seeds, soy sauce, sugar, vinegar, sea salt Chestnuts, gingko nuts, hazelnuts, peanuts, pine nuts, pistachios, sesame seeds, walnuts Barley water, beer, coffee, fruit drinks, green tea, honey water, jasmine tea, magnolia flower drink, rice tea, rice water, rice wine, *soju* (sweet potato vodka), spiced teas (ginseng, cinnamon, ginger), wines made from other ingredients Sesame oil, vegetable oils Honey, sugar	Increased intake of fruits and vegetables. The majority eat *kimchi* daily. Reported that hot barley water is still the preferred beverage and that it is served after the meal.

such as soy sauce, fish sauce (*saewujeot*), hot mustard, and a fermented chile paste called *kochujang,* are also frequently added to foods. Marinades and dipping sauces are common.

Soup or a thin barley water is used as a beverage. Herbal teas are very popular; ginseng tea flavored with cinnamon is a favorite. Ginger, cinnamon, or citron can also be used separately to make a spice tea. A common drink is rice tea, made by pouring warm water over toasted, ground rice or by simmering water in the pot in which rice was cooked. On special occasions, wine might be served. Wines are made from rice and other grains; some include various flower blossoms or ginseng as flavorings. Beer is also well liked. Milk and other dairy products are generally not consumed or used in cooking.

Kochujang, a fermented jamlike chile paste, is prepared by each family on March 3rd, then traditionally stored for use throughout the year in black pottery crocks.

Korean rice wine, *mukhuli,* is customarily served with scallion-flavored pancakes as a snack.

Meal Composition and Cycle

Daily Patterns

Three small meals, with frequent snacking throughout the day, are typical in Korea. Breakfast was traditionally the main meal in Korea, but today is more likely to be something light, caught on the run. Soup is almost always served at breakfast, along with rice (usually as gruel). Eggs, meat or fish, or vegetables may top the meal. Kimchi and dipping sauces are the usual accompaniments.

Lunch is typically noodles served with broth of beef, chicken, or fish and garnished with shellfish, meat, or vegetables. Supper is more similar to breakfast, but with steamed rice. In many modern homes, it has become the main meal of the day. Snacks are widely available from street vendors, including grilled and steamed tidbits of all types. Sweets, such as rice cookies and cakes, or dried fruit (especially persimmons) are also popular snacks.

Rice is considered the main dish of each meal. Everything else is served as an accompaniment to the rice and is called *panch'an.* For dinner, at least one meat or fish dish is included, if affordable, and two or three vegetables are usually served. Kimchi is always offered. Soup is very popular and is served at most meals. Individual bowls of rice and soup are served to each diner, and panch'an dishes are served on trays in the center of the table for communal eating. Wine may be served before the meal with appetizers like batter-fried vegetables, seasoned tobu, pickled seafood, meatballs, or steamed dumplings. Dessert is seldom eaten, although fresh fruit sometimes concludes the meal. Hot barley water or rice tea is served with the meal.

Drinking is a social ritual, practiced mostly by men. Distilled beverages like *soju*, a sweet potato vodka, are consumed with snacks like spicy squid or chile peppers stuffed with beef.

Etiquette

Chopsticks and soup spoons are the only eating utensils used in Korea. In the past, seating was around a low rectangular table on the floor, and young women were assigned the awkward corner seats (today most tables are set with chairs). Traditionally elders are served first and children are served last at the meal. It is considered polite to fill the soy sauce dish of the people one is sitting beside. Food is always passed with the right hand, and a communal beverage may be passed for all to share.

Special Occasions

Korean cooking was historically divided into everyday fare and cuisine for royalty. The traditions of palace cooking and food presentation, including the use of numerous ingredients in elaborate dishes, are seen today in meals for special occasions. At a meal celebrating a

At Korean weddings, sweetened dates rolled in sesame seeds are tossed at the bride to ensure health, prosperity, and numerous children.

birthday or holiday, or one shared with guests, more dishes are served and both wine and dessert are offered. For special occasions, Koreans offer a thick drink of persimmons or dates, nuts, and spices, or a beverage made with molasses and magnolia that is served with small, edible flowers floating on top.

Both Koreans and Korean Americans celebrate several holidays throughout the year. The first is New Year's, called *Sol,* a 3-day event at which traditional dress is worn and the elders in the family are honored. Festivities include feasts, games, and flying kites. On the first full moon, in a tradition reflecting ancient religious rites, torches are lighted and firecrackers are set off to frighten evil spirits away. Shampoo Day (*Yadu Nal*) is on June 15th, when families bathe in streams to ward off fevers. Thanksgiving (*Chusok*) is a fall harvest festival; *duk,* steamed rice cakes filled with chestnuts, dates, red beans, or other items, are associated with the holiday.

A special ceremony is observed on a child's first birthday. He or she is dressed in traditional clothing and placed among stacks of rice cakes, cookies, and fruit. Family and friends offer the child objects symbolizing various professions, such as a pen for writing or a coin for finance, and the first one accepted is thought to predict his or her future career (Nash, 1995).

Therapeutic Uses of Food

Many Koreans follow the *um* (yin) and yang food classification system. Little has been reported about specific foods, although Koreans are believed to adhere to categorizations similar to other Asians: um (cold) foods include mung beans, winter melon, cucumber, and most other vegetables and fruits; meats (e.g., beef, mutton, goat, dog), chile peppers, garlic, and ginger are considered yang (hot) foods.

Preparation of healthy, tasty food is an important way that Korean women show affection for family and friends (Pang, 1991; Marks & Kim, 1993). Good appetite is considered a sign of good health. Foods that are believed health-promoting include bean paste soup, beef turnip soup, rice with grains and beans, broiled seaweed, kimchi, and ginseng tea. Ginseng products are often used to promote health and stamina and to alleviate tiredness. One very popular tonic, called *boyak,* combines ginseng and deer horn or bear gallbladder (Pang, 1989). More than one-half of Korean American respondents in one survey reported using ginseng, with older women more likely to use such products than men or younger women (Yom et al., 1995). Other home remedies commonly used include ginger tea, *yoojacha* (hot citrus beverage), bean sprout soup, and lemon with honey in hot water. Restorative herbal medicines, vitamin supplements, meat soups, bone marrow soup, and *samgyetang* (game hen soup) also were mentioned by subjects as useful when feeling weak.

Dog meat soup is eaten by men to enhance their strength and physical prowess. The South Korean government banned dog meat soup during the 1988 Olympics in Seoul in deference to outside cultural pressure.

Boyak is often given as a gift, particularly to one's parents, to promote long life.

Korean Americans celebrate *Sol,* New Year's, on the first full moon. (© Gary Conner/Photo Edit.)

Korean women traditionally consumed seaweed soup, *miyuk kook,* three times a day for 7 weeks after the birth of a child to restore their strength.

A study of pregnant Korean American women (Ludman et al., 1992) suggests that certain foods, such as seaweed soup, beef, and rice, are thought to build strength during this "difficult" time. Food taboos during pregnancy often involve the concept of like causes like. For instance, eating blemished fruit may result in a baby with skin problems. Other such items mentioned are chicken, duck, rabbit, goat, crab, sparrow, pork, twin chestnuts, and spicy foods. Although most food avoidance was attributed to personal preference and availability, many of the women acknowledged familiarity with the traditional beliefs.

Contemporary Food Habits in the United States

Adaptations of Food Habits

Ingredients and Common Foods

A survey of Korean Americans in the San Francisco area showed that many traditional Korean food habits continue after immigration to the United States. Nearly all respondents ate rice at least one meal each day, and two-thirds ate kimchi daily. Beef and beef variety cuts were consumed regularly, and fish was eaten at least once a week. Sesame oil/seeds and vegetable oils were used more often than butter or mayonnaise. Soy sauce, soybean paste, chile pepper paste, and garlic were the most popular condiments. More than 40 percent of Korean Americans surveyed consumed tobu several times a week. Pork and pork products were not commonly eaten, although younger respondents reported more frequent use of these foods than older subjects. Length of stay in the United States had little impact on diet (Yom et al., 1995).

Other preliminary research suggests that American-style food intake increases by Koreans in the United States; rice consumption declines and fruit, beef, pork, poultry, dairy, and vegetable consumption rises (Crews, 1994). Although milk and dairy products are not consumed in Korea, these foods are often well accepted in the United States. One study indicated that more than one-half of the subjects reported drinking milk or eating yogurt or cheese one or more times each week (Yom et al., 1995). Another study of pregnant Korean American women reported a similar finding that 56 percent of respondents drank milk daily.

Meal Composition and Cycle

Little has been reported regarding Korean American meal composition and cycle. It is assumed that because Korean meal and snacking patterns are similar to those in the United States, three meals a day remain common. Survey data suggest that hot barley water is still the preferred beverage of Korean Americans and that it is served after meals (Yom et al., 1995).

Korean Americans observe traditional Korean holidays (see "Special Occasions," previously in this section) as well as other events, such as Buddha's birthday on April 8th, Korean Memorial Day (June 6th), South Korean Constitution Day (July 17th), and Korean National Foundation Day (October 3rd). Fathers are honored on June 15th. In addition, Americans of Korean descent who are Christian celebrate the major religious holidays.

8

Southeast Asians and Pacific Islanders

Southeast Asians and Pacific Islanders live in similar tropical regions and it is believed that they may share some common ancestors, yet their cultures have diverged markedly over the centuries. The countries of Southeast Asia have developed under hundreds of years of Chinese domination. Spanish expansionism in the Philippines and French occupation in Vietnam were also significant. In contrast, Asian and European contact in the Pacific Islands was limited until the eighteenth century, and subsequent foreign influence almost completely overwhelmed the traditional indigenous societies.

Southeast Asians and Pacific Islanders are some of the newest, youngest, and fastest growing populations in the United States. More than 2 million mainland Southeast Asians and Filipinos have arrived since 1975; the number of Pacific Islanders has increased by 50 percent in the last decade. This section discusses the cultures and cuisines of the Southeast Asians who have immigrated in substantial numbers to the United States—the Filipinos, Vietnamese, Cambodians, and Laotians—as well as those Pacific Islander groups with significant American populations—native Hawaiians, Samoans, Guamanians, and Tongans. An introduction to the cooking of Thailand is also included.

FIGURE 8.1

Southeast Asia and the Pacific Islands.

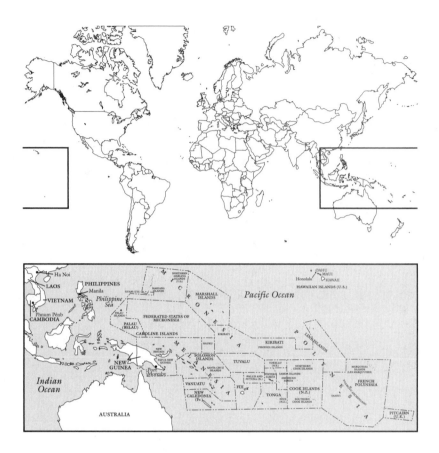

SOUTHEAST ASIANS

Southeast Asia is a subtropical region south of China and east of India whose lands straddle the equator. It includes the countries of Myanmar (formerly Burma), Thailand, the Lao People's Democratic Republic (Laos), Democratic Kampuchea (Cambodia), Vietnam, Malaysia, Brunei, Indonesia, Singapore, and the Philippines. The countries are similar in climate, flora, and fauna. Fertile deltas and river valleys are commonly separated by rugged mountains. Somewhat over half of the region is on the Asian mainland and the rest is made up of the thousands of islands that are part of Indonesia and the Philippines. (See Figure 8.1 for a map of the region.)

Cultural Perspective

History of Southeast Asia

Much of the history of Southeast Asia includes long periods of foreign domination and repeated struggles for independence. The mainland peninsula has also experienced frequent conflict between the nations of the area. National boundaries were first defined by the western nations during the nineteenth century. Conflicts with both Vietnam and Thailand have continuously influenced the politics and independence of their neighbors, Laos and Cambodia, and still do today.

The Philippines

The Philippines is an archipelago of 7,100 islands forming a nation located on the eastern edge of Southeast Asia, off the coasts of Vietnam and south of Taiwan. Manila, the trade center of the Philippines, is located on the largest island, Luzon.

The original inhabitants of the Philippines, Aetas, were short and had Negroid features. They were pushed into remote mountainous areas of the islands 30,000 years ago by successive waves of peoples from Southeast Asia, mostly Malaysians. Native society was arranged in kinship units with no centralized, unified government. Beginning in the fifteenth century, the islands developed extensive trading relations with Southeast Asia, India, China, and Japan. Numerous immigrants from these areas, particularly China, arrived to participate in the thriving economy. It was during this time that Islam was introduced to the islands.

In 1521 the Spanish explorer Ferdinand Magellan arrived in the islands and claimed them for Spain. There was little organized resistance from the inhabitants, and in 1571 the country was given a European name in honor of King Philip II—the Philippines. The Roman Catholic church sent missionaries who established rural parishes, schools, and often administered the Spanish occupation. Catholicism and Spanish cuisine became influential in the culture.

Spain ceded the Philippines to the United States at the end of the Spanish-American War in 1898. The United States accepted control of the islands but promised to prepare the nation for independence. In 1935 the Philippines became a self-governing commonwealth. During World War II the Philippines was attacked by Japan. U.S. efforts to free the region were finally successful in 1944, and on July 4, 1946 the Philippines achieved full independence. The United States maintained two military bases in the region.

The Philippine economy was in disarray. Subsequent uprisings by leftist groups, student groups, and the Muslim minority (the Moro National Liberation Front) led eventually to the establishment of martial law by then president Ferdinand Marcos in 1972. Law and order

The term *Filipino,* which originally meant a person of Spanish descent who was born in the Philippines, has come to mean any citizen of the country, many of whom are an ethnic blend of the native population, Spanish, and Chinese.

The official languages of the Philippines are Pilipino (Tagalog) and English. Although other dialects, such as Viscayan and Ilocano, are widely spoken in some regions, high literacy rates mean most Filipinos also know Pilipino or English as well.

were restored amid charges of political corruption and election fraud. Marcos was forced to flee the Philippines under pressure from Corazon Aquino and her followers in 1986. In 1992 the United States withdrew its military presence from the islands, and in 1994 an accord was signed with the Muslims, ending their 20-year guerrilla war. Economic problems continue to plague the country.

Vietnam

Vietnam, which hugs the eastern coastline of the region, borders China in the north and Cambodia and Laos on the west. The two most fertile areas of the country are along the northern Red River and the southern Mekong River deltas. The two major cities of the country are located within these regions; Hanoi is in the north and Ho Chi Minh City (formerly Saigon) is in the south.

The original inhabitants of Vietnam are thought to have been Austro-Negroid migrants who were pushed south by Mongolian tribes, then later overcome by the Chinese (207 BCE). The Chinese ruled Vietnam for 1,000 years beginning in 111 BCE. Vietnam adopted the Chinese social system (Confucianism), religious beliefs (Taoism and Buddhism), and many of their agricultural and cooking practices. However, the Vietnamese maintained their own unique culture and language; they resented Chinese rule.

Successive Vietnamese dynasties ruled after the Chinese were driven out in the tenth century. During the 1860s the French responded to attacks on Catholic Vietnamese citizens and French Catholic missionaries by seizing the southern provinces and creating the French colony of Cochinchina. By the 1880s the remaining Vietnamese court fell, relinquishing complete control of North (Tonkin), Central (Annam), and South Vietnam to the French. Vietnamese society was strongly influenced by the French presence; the language, certain foods, and Roman Catholicism were adopted, particularly by the upper classes.

France retained control into the twentieth century (except for a short period of Japanese occupation during World War II) but met with increasing resistance from the Vietnamese. The French withdrew their forces in 1954 after an 8-year-long war with the followers of the communist leader Ho Chi Minh, and the country was divided between the communist North and noncommunist South.

Democratic reunification attempts failed. South Vietnam resisted communist domination by the North, and in 1965 the United States committed troops to prevent the takeover. When the United States pulled out of Vietnam in 1975, the Saigon government fell, and the country was united under a communist government. Saigon was renamed Ho Chi Minh City and has become the national capital. Severe economic difficulties due to withdrawal of aid from the former Soviet Union prompted renewed contact between the United States and Vietnam in 1992; trade relations were subsequently restored, and in 1995, diplomatic relations began.

Cambodia

Cambodia, sandwiched between Vietnam, Laos, Thailand, and the Gulf of Thailand, was known as the Funan empire in the first century. In the fourth century an Indian Brahmin introduced Hindu customs and the legal code and alphabet to the region. The Khmer invaded from the North in the sixth century, and the height of their rule was known as the Angkorean period (802–1431), named after the massive city-state of Angkor Wat. In the twelfth century the Khmer nation gained control of a rival nation, Champa, which today is the southern province of Vietnam, as well as territories in Siam (Thailand). As the power of the Khmer nation declined, Siam encroached on the western border and Vietnam expanded on the eastern side. The capital was moved from Angkor Wat to its current location in Phnom Penh.

In 1864, Cambodia became a colony of the French and did not gain independence until 1955. In 1970, Prince Norodum Sihanouk was removed from office as chief of state and a military premier was appointed. The Khmer Rouge, a communist regime led by Pol Pot, later seized the government and renamed the nation Democratic Kampuchea. As a result of their efforts to "reeducate the masses," it is estimated that more than 3 million Cambodians were executed. In 1978 the Vietnam military removed the Khmer Rouge government and set up a puppet government that ruled Cambodia from Vietnam. Under international pressure, Vietnam withdrew its troops in 1989. The United Nations attempted to form a coalition government; in 1993 a parliamentary monarchy was established and Prince Sihanouk was elected head of state. The Khmer Rouge have refused to participate in elections and continue opposition to the new government.

> Both the people and the language of Cambodia are known as *Khmer*.

Laos

The people of Laos are believed to be descendants of southwestern Chinese and Thais. Several distinct groups exist in Laos, including the Tai, Lao Theung (a diverse group of peoples who are descendants of the earliest arrivals in the region), and the Hmong and Mien (or Yao) tribes, mountain dwellers who are more recent (1850s) migrants from southern China.

Ancient Laos was known as the Kingdom of a Million Elephants and reached its peak in the seventeenth century. Internal struggles weakened the government and left the country vulnerable to attack. Both Vietnam and Siam (Thailand) dominated portions of Laos for more than 150 years. When France claimed Vietnam and Siam as its Indo-Chinese empire in the mid-1800s, Laos also came under French colonial control until after World War II.

> The word *Hmong* means "free men."

> The Hmong are believed to have originally come to China in 2000 BCE from Siberia; some Hmong today are blond and blue-eyed.

It has been reported that the government in Laos has used biological and chemical weapons against the Hmong in an attempt to exterminate them.

In 1945, Laos declared independence under the leadership of Prince Phetsarath and was drawn into the Vietnamese struggle for freedom from French rule, as well as the subsequent U.S.-Vietnamese war. Since 1975 a communist government (Pathet Lao) strongly influenced by Vietnam has run the country, renamed the Lao People's Democratic Republic.

History of Southeast Asians in the United States

Immigration Patterns

Most Filipinos chose to come to the United States for educational and economic opportunities. In contrast, the majority of mainland Southeast Asians who have immigrated to the United States have arrived since the 1970s as refugees from the political conflicts of the region.

The Philippines   Substantial immigration from the Philippines to the United States started in 1898 after the country became a U.S. territory. Approximately 113,000 young male Filipinos traveled to the Hawaiian Islands between 1909 and 1930 to work in the sugarcane fields. Many of these immigrants later moved to the U.S. mainland. These early immigrants were considered U.S. nationals and carried U.S. passports, but most were not allowed to become citizens or own land. Most were uneducated peasant laborers from the island of Illocos. Because they were not allowed to bring their wives or families, social and political clubs replaced the family as the primary social structure.

The only Filipinos allowed to apply for U.S. citizenship prior to 1946 were those who had enlisted in the U.S. Navy, Naval Auxiliary, or Marine Corps during World War II, had served at least 3 years, and had an honorable discharge.

In 1924 the immigration of Filipinos slowed as a result of Asian exclusion laws. After World War II, it became legal for Filipinos to become U.S. citizens, and the number of immigrants increased. Significant numbers of Filipinos arrived in the United States after 1965, when the U.S. immigration laws were changed, and by 1980, more than 350,000 had emigrated to mostly urban areas. Two-thirds of the Filipinos who immigrated after World War II qualified for entrance as professional or technical workers. Yet discrimination against Asians often forced Filipinos into low-paying jobs. "Little Manilas" formed in many California cities, and similar homogeneous neighborhoods were found in Chicago, New York, and Washington, DC, where some Filipinos opened small service businesses to meet the needs of their community.

During the Marcos regime, inexpensive airfares were used to lure Filipinos in the United States (and their American dollars) to return to the Philippines for visits.

Approximately 9,000 Thais have immigrated to the United States since the 1970s; most have settled in Los Angeles, New York, and Texas. They are known for their rapid acculturation.

Vietnam   Vietnamese immigration to the United States is characterized by three distinct waves. The first occurred when South Vietnam fell to the North in 1975 and 60,000 Vietnamese left the country with the assistance of the United States. Another 70,000 managed to flee on their own. Most of these refugees had been employed by the

United States or were members of the upper classes. The latter group immigrated in intact family groups and were able to bring their property with them.

From 1975 to 1977, another wave of Vietnamese left for political or economic reasons, often escaping by sea. Many of these "boat people" left their families and what little money they had to find freedom. The third phase of immigration started in 1978, when increasing numbers of ethnic Chinese living in Vietnam fled the country. This wave of immigration was accelerated by the Chinese invasion of northern Vietnam in 1979. This second group of boat people left with no financial resources, and many lost family members escaping in unseaworthy vessels that were easy prey for pirates. After being rescued, the boat people often lived for several months, even years, in refugee camps in various Southeast Asian countries before immigrating to the United States. In addition, the United States and Vietnam developed the Orderly Departure Program (ODP) in 1979 to bring imprisoned former South Vietnamese soldiers and the approximately 8,000 Amerasians, children of U.S. fathers and Vietnamese mothers, to the United States.

Cambodia and Laos   Cambodian and Laotian immigration to the United States did not begin until the United States granted asylum to the residents of the refugee camps along the border with Thailand in 1976–1979. International concern about the large numbers of refugees and the conditions in the camps prompted accelerated admittance of Southeast Asian immigrants worldwide.

Current Demographics and Socioeconomic Status

Filipino   The Filipino American population quadrupled from 1980 to 1990. Nearly 1.5 million Filipinos now live in the United States. Almost half reside in California, with significant populations of more than 30,000 Filipinos found also in Hawaii, Florida, Illinois, New York, New Jersey, Texas, and Washington.

In general, Filipino Americans earn less than white Americans, yet as a group, they have a poverty rate (6%) that is less than half that of the general U.S. population. Many work as migrant field hands or cannery workers. Although more recent immigrants from the Philippines are better educated than those who arrived earlier, their education or professional experience is often not recognized in the United States, forcing them to accept blue-collar jobs when they first arrive. Over time, many professionals do obtain licensing or accreditation and work as physicians, nurses, or lawyers. Others are employed in the sales and service industries, and this group is economically better off than previous immigrants, many of whom are now poor, elderly single men. A schism has developed in the Filipino American community between pre-1965 immigrants who believe the newer immigrants are

During the 1920s and 1930s, Filipinos were often barred from restaurants, swimming pools (and other recreational facilities), and movie theaters because of their dark skin and heavy accents.

ungrateful for the advances achieved by the older generation and the more recent immigrants who find the older generation naive and uneducated (Melendy, 1995).

Vietnamese More than 550,000 Vietnamese have entered the United States since 1975, and the total Vietnamese population, including those born in America, was more than 614,000 in the 1990 U.S. census; the growth rate between 1980 and 1990 was more than 150 percent. Many were sponsored by American agencies or organizations, which provided food, clothing, and shelter in cities throughout the United States until the Vietnamese could become self-supporting. Many Vietnamese Americans have since relocated in the western and Gulf states, probably because the climate is similar to that of Vietnam.

Vietnamese Americans live primarily in urban areas. Many are young and live in large households with grandparents and other relatives. The first wave of Vietnamese immigrants was well educated, could speak English, and had held white-collar jobs in Vietnam. Many of them had to accept blue-collar jobs initially and had difficulties supporting their extended families. The boat people were even less prepared for life in the United States, because they often had no English language skills, were illiterate, had less job training, and did not have support from an extended family.

Language acquisition has been important in the Vietnamese community, and in 1990, nearly three-fourths of Vietnamese in the United States could speak English well (Bankston, 1995d). Many immigrants have made the decision to assimilate as quickly as possible, even changing their Asian names, such as "Nguyen," to something more Anglicized, such as "Newman." Education is highly valued, and a child's academic achievement is considered a reflection on the whole family. High school dropout rates are very low among Vietnamese Americans and almost half attend college, compared to 40 percent of white Americans.

Vietnamese have high rates of employment, but often in low-paying jobs. Nearly 25 percent lived in poverty in 1990. They are prominent in the fishing and shrimping industry in the Gulf states, and those who obtain college degrees often prefer technical professions, such as engineering.

Cambodian The 1990 U.S. census identified approximately 150,000 Americans of Cambodian descent, but it is thought that this figure may underestimate actual numbers due to a low response rate by Cambodians unfamiliar with American society in the census count. Nearly half of Cambodian Americans reside in California, with the greatest populations found in Long Beach and Stockton. Another large Cambodian community has developed in Lowell, Massachusetts.

Vietnamese immigrants are often stereotyped as either successful over-achievers or as poverty-stricken refugees.

Texas, Pennsylvania, Virginia, New York, Minnesota, and Illinois also have significant numbers of immigrants.

Adjustment to American life has been difficult for Cambodians, most of whom came from rural regions where they worked as farmers. They have a high unemployment rate (although the probability of employment increases with length of stay), and those who work have found employment mostly in service jobs and manual labor. In 1990, 42 percent of Cambodian families lived below poverty level.

Low levels of education have limited economic success for many Cambodian Americans. Approximately one-half of adult men and women have less than 6 years of formal education, and only 5 to 10 percent have graduated from high school. Low dropout rates among younger Americans of Cambodian descent may contribute to better economic outcomes in the future.

Laotian There are about 150,000 nontribal Laotians in the United States, according to 1990 U.S. census figures. Most Laotians have settled in the California cities of Fresno, San Diego, Sacramento, and Stockton. Large populations are also found in Amarillo and Denton, Texas; Minneapolis, Minnesota; and Seattle, Washington. Another 150,000 Hmong and approximately 15,000 Mien have been identified. Refugee resettlement services dispersed the Hmong, irrespective of family clan associations, in fifty-three American cities. Secondary migration of Hmong Americans has reunited clan groups, mostly in the suburban and rural communities of California's Central Valley—Fresno, Merced, Sacramento, Stockton, Chico, Modesto, and Visalia.

Poor fluency in English and low education levels have hindered economic achievement for Laotian Americans. In 1990, two-thirds reported that they did not speak English well. Only 40 percent of adults have completed high school; current Laotian students are generally believed to do well in school, but higher than average high school dropout rates and lower than average college attendance rates have been noted. Many Laotians hold jobs as machine operators, fabricators, and laborers, and the unemployment rate is high. In 1990, nearly one-third of Laotian Americans lived in poverty.

Almost two in every three Americans of Hmong descent lived below the poverty line in 1990; nearly all Hmong were employed in blue-collar jobs or manual labor. Some enterprising Hmong women have been successful in marketing the traditional Hmong needlecraft known as *paj ntaub*. The colorful wall hangings, pillows, and bedcoverings have become popular among collectors of native arts. Low levels of educational attainment have been reported for adult Hmong, but Hmong Americans born or raised in the United States show surprisingly high rates of college attendance, nearly equal to whites and surpassing African Americans.

Fresno, California, with 30,000 Hmong immigrants, is the largest Hmong community in the world.

There are five major tribes among the Hmong—the White Hmong, the Black Hmong, the Blue Hmong, the Red Hmong, and the Flowery Hmong—named according to legend by the colors of clothing they were forced to wear by the ancient Chinese for identification purposes. Most Hmong refugees in the United States come from the White and Blue tribes.

Cultural Organizations

Compared to other Asian groups, Southeast Asians have fewer organizations to serve their needs, perhaps because they have been in the United States for a relatively short time. The Filipinos have numerous regional associations (more than 400 in California alone), but they have not coalesced into a state or national group, possibly due to regional and language differences in the Philippines that prevent single, unified Filipino associations. Fraternal lodges are significant in some areas, sponsoring dances and beauty pageants. Filipinos have also been very active in the farmworkers' labor movement. The Agricultural Workers' Organizing Committee, composed primarily of Filipino farmworkers, joined with the Chicano organization the National Farmworkers' Association to initiate the successful grape strike in Delano, California, in 1965.

In some areas the social support organizations are loosely formed around the Buddhist temple or Catholic church. The largest mainland Southeast Asian organization is the National Association for the Education and Advancement of Cambodian, Laotian, and Vietnamese Americans, which works to protect the rights of its members and to provide equal educational opportunities for Southeast Asians in the schools. The Hmong National Development Association promotes Hmong interests in the United States and facilitates communication among other Hmong organizations. Other regional and statewide groups address local issues specific to each population.

Worldview

Religion

Many Southeast Asians hold beliefs dating back to the ancient religions prevalent before the introduction of Buddhism, Catholicism, and Islam. Most believe in spirits and ghosts, especially of ancestors, who have the ability to act as guardians against misfortune or cause harm and suffering. Ideas about spirit intervention have often been incorporated into eastern and western religious practices or survive as significant superstitions.

Filipino   The majority of all Americans of Filipino descent are Roman Catholics, although it is estimated that as many as 5 percent are Muslim. Religion significantly affects the worldview of Filipinos, especially the elderly. Many hold that those who lead a good life on earth will be rewarded with life after death. Human misfortunes come from violating the will of God. One should accept one's fate, because supernatural forces control the world. Time and providence will ultimately solve all problems.

Vietnamese   Nearly 70 percent of Vietnamese Americans are Buddhists, and 30 percent are Roman Catholic. Small numbers of Protestants also are found. Those who are Buddhists follow the Mahayana sect, influenced particularly by the Chinese school of Ch'an Buddhism (Zen Buddhism in Japan) called *Tien* in Vietnam. Buddhists believe that a person's present life reflects his or her past lives and also predetermines his or her own and his or her descendants' future lives. They consider themselves as part of a greater force in the universe (see Chapter 2 for more information about Buddhism).

The Vietnamese say, "Chew when you eat, think when you speak."

Cambodian   The predominant religion in Cambodia is Theravada Buddhism, which places greater emphasis on a person's efforts to reach spiritual perfection than does the Mahayana sect, which employs the help of deities. "Making merit" through good deeds, the participation in religious ritual, and the support of monks and temples is critical to one's progress through reincarnation. Although some Cambodian Americans have converted to Christian faiths, most still practice Buddhism, often in temples established in apartments or homes.

Cambodian Buddhist monks in the United States have established language classes for Cambodian children to help maintain ethnic identity.

Laotian   Almost all Laotians are also Theravada Buddhists. "Making merit" for Laotians includes the expectation that every man will devote some time in his life to living as a practicing monk, either before marriage or in his old age. In the United States, men find it difficult to fulfill their obligation to the faith. Women may become nuns for periods in their lives as well, especially if widowed. Most Laotians in the United States worship at Buddhist temples with Cambodians or Thais who share their religious practices.

About half the Hmong population in the United States is now Christian as a result of French and American missionary work in Laos and conversions after arrival. Baptists, Presbyterians, Mormons, Jehovah's Witnesses, and members of the Church of Christ have actively recruited the Hmong. The other half of Hmong Americans practice animism, shamanism, and ancestor worship. They believe that the world is divided into two spheres—that which is visible, containing humans, nature, and material objects, and that which is invisible, containing spirits. The shaman acts as intermediary between the two; some spirits, such as those of ancestors, are available to those who aren't shamans. Women are generally responsible for making contact with these more accessible spirits. A few Americans of Hmong heritage belong to a modern Hmong religion called *Chao Fa* ("Lord of the Sky"), started by a prophet in the 1960s who encouraged the Hmong to break with both Laotian and western ways.

In Thailand, miniature Thai temples are built and posted on pedestals next to a home to shelter the family ancestors. Such spirit houses are believed to prevent the ghosts from moving in with the family and causing trouble.

Hmong ancestors are fed at every festive occasion with a little pork and rice placed in the center of the feast table.

It has been suggested that many Hmong became Protestants because they believed it was necessary to gain entry to the United States or in deference to their church sponsors. Some try to combine ancestor worship with their new faiths so as not to offend the spirits (Adler, 1995).

Family

Southeast Asians share a high esteem for the family, respect for elders, and interdependence among family members. Behavior that would bring shame to the family's honor is avoided, as is direct expression of conflict. Social acceptance and smooth interpersonal relationships are emphasized.

Filipino The Filipino family is highly structured. At the center is the extended family, containing all paternal and maternal relatives. Kinship is extended to friends, neighbors, and fellow workers through the system of *compadrazgo*. Lifelong relationships are initiated through shared Roman Catholic rituals, particularly the selection of godparents and baptism of new babies. Community obligations created through this system include shared food, labor, and financial resources.

The first Filipino immigrants were single men hoping to make their fortune and return to the Philippines. They developed surrogate family systems of fellow workers who lived together, with the eldest man serving as patriarch. More recent immigrants have come as whole families and have been able to maintain much of their social organization. For example, as many as 200 sponsors may be appointed in a Filipino American baptism, although individual commitment may be less than if it were held in the Philippines (Melendy, 1995).

Filipino children are adored by the family and are typically indulged until the age of 6. At that time, socialization through negative feedback (e.g., shame) begins. Children are taught to be obedient and respectful, to contain their emotions and avoid all conflict, and to be quiet and shy. Politeness is emphasized (Anderson, 1983). A person must avoid shaming him- or herself, as well as the family; discord is minimized by the use of euphemisms and by sending go-betweens in sensitive situations.

Vietnamese The extended Vietnamese family has been modified in the United States to adapt to American norms. A nuclear family is more typical, though somewhat larger than the average family in the United States. Close relatives are encouraged to move into homes next door or in the same neighborhood.

Family values are in transition. The father is traditionally the undisputed head of the household, but patriarchy is diminishing as women attain higher levels of education and professional achievement. American-style dating has become common. Although most Vietnamese marry within their ethnic group, women are more likely than men to wed non-Vietnamese mates. Divorce rarely occurs.

The traditional Vietnamese extended family home is less common in the United States, but relatives often live near each other. (© Michael Newman/PhotoEdit.)

Intergenerational conflict is reportedly high. Children are often the first to learn English and acculturate more easily than their parents, causing value conflicts and loss of respect for elders. The role of the elderly is also changing. Old age is valued in Southeast Asia, but in the United States, older relatives are often physically isolated from their peers and even younger family members and may be linguistically isolated within the larger community.

Cambodian Large, extended families are common in Cambodia; children are considered treasures. Cambodians are notable in that their traditional kinship system was bilateral, emphasizing both the paternal and maternal lines. The family was primarily a matriarchy until the 1930s, when French influence strengthened the authority of the father. Today men are responsible for providing for their families, while women make all decisions regarding the family budget.

It has been difficult for Cambodian Americans to retain their traditional family structure in the United States. A large percentage of Cambodian homes are headed by single women, due most likely to the large numbers of men killed in recent years during conflicts in Cambodia. Further, Cambodian American women are permitted formal education and their financial contributions are needed to help support the whole family. Differences between immigrants who have lived most of their lives in Cambodia and the children of these immigrants raised in the United States (with no memory of Cambodia) can be

A Cambodian proverb states, "If you don't take your wife's advice, you'll have no rice the next year."

When Cambodians wed, a Buddhist monk cuts a lock of hair from both the bride and groom to mix together symbolically in a bowl.

enormous in terms of language, acculturation, and values. It has been noted that many Cambodian teenagers suffer from identity problems.

Laotian   Most families are agriculturally based in Laos. Extended members live and work together in the fields to support the whole family. In Laos, men represent the family in village affairs and women run the home. Great significance is given to the site of the family's house; it is believed that as long as the site exists, the family will exist.

Extended families are still important to Laotian Americans due to dependency on relatives for social and economic support. Although nuclear families have become the norm, extended members tend to live nearby each other. Women have attained nearly equal status with men in the United States, and it is not unusual for Laotian men to share responsibility for household chores. Laotians have a notably low divorce rate.

Hmong American families are among the youngest and largest in the United States. According to 1990 figures, the average age of a Hmong American is almost 13 years, compared to 30 years for other Asians combined and 34 for U.S. citizens in general (Bankston, 1995b). More than half of all Hmong are under the age of 18. Typical family size is about 6 members; the Asian average is 3.7 and the white American average is just 3.1. These large families are usually nuclear, reflecting numbers of children rather than relatives. Extended family members are often located nearby, and families frequently congregate with other families from the same traditional clan from Laos.

Men remain the heads of households in America. Women are generally held in high regard in their roles as mothers. Children are the heart of the home, and much of family life revolves around them. As in some other Southeast Asian groups, a generation gap has developed between recently arrived immigrants and their westernized children. Teenage runaways have become increasingly common among the Hmong.

Some Hmong customs have come in direct conflict with U.S. laws. Polygyny, marriage to more than one wife, is unusual but not illegal in Laos. Clan leaders might wed several women to establish political connections, and having several wives was indicative of wealth. The practice that has received the most press in the United States, however, is the kidnapping of young women and enforced marriage. Traditionally girls married between the ages of 14 and 18 after a bridal price (paid by the groom) was agreed to by both families. If no agreement was reached, the couple could elope, and a mediator would help to settle the differences. If the bride was unwilling, the groom could kidnap the girl and the marriage would be recognized after some payment to the bride's family was arranged. Men who have attempted this in the United States have been charged with abduction and sexual assault, often by the young women involved. Many Ameri-

Hmong marriages are formalized at a 2-day feast featuring a roasted pig.

By custom, Hmong men marry the widows of their deceased brothers and support their nieces and nephews.

cans of Hmong descent believe that it is best to wait until a woman is in her late teens or early twenties to wed; arranged marriages are still common.

Conversion to Christianity has been found to split many Hmong families when some members change faiths and others retain their traditional beliefs. Conflict over marriage traditions is especially prevalent.

Communication

The communication style of most Filipinos is formal and polite. Elders should never be addressed by their first names. Filipinos are often deferential and will avoid voicing disagreement. Loud talking is considered rude. Sensitive topics that might result in any embarrassment, such as how much a person earns or personal questions about looks or health, should be avoided; laughing is sometimes used to mask shame. Direct eye contact is often not made because it can be interpreted as a sign of aggression or sexual interest among Filipinos, but if eye contact is made, it is appropriate to return it. Handshaking is the common greeting, although an eyebrow "flash" (quick lifting of the eyebrows) may be used between friends and acquaintances (Axtell, 1991).

Most mainland Southeast Asians appreciate a polite, unhurried, and reserved conversational style. Excited, informal, or frank speech is often considered impolite (Rairdan & Higgs, 1992). The Vietmanese place a high value on harmony and will appear agreeable to avoid displeasing a speaker. When angry or embarrassed, Southeast Asians may laugh to hide their feelings. A handshake is common among men but not among women. Most Southeast Asians are uncomfortable with direct eye contact. Blinking may be used to indicate that a message is understood. Certain nonverbal forms of communication should be carefully observed. The head is considered sacred, and it is extremely offensive to pat or even touch the head of an adult or a child. The feet are the lowest part of the body; thus it is rude to point with the foot or show the bottoms of one's shoes. Respect is shown to elders by making a small bow from the waist in greeting and using both hands when handing any item to a person.

Traditional Food Habits

The cuisines of Southeast Asia have many ingredients in common, but food preparation methods and meal patterns reflect the foreign cultures that have influenced each nation. For example, the Vietnamese often serve cream-filled French pastries for dessert, whereas Filipinos frequently have Spanish-style custard flan. As in China and Japan, the

Traditional foods of Southeast Asia and the Pacific Islands. Some foods typical of the diets of Southeast Asians and Pacific Islanders include coconut, dried anchovies, dried mango, French bread, lemon grass, lime, *nuoc mam,* pineapple, pork, rice, rice paper, rice sticks, taro root, and water chestnuts. (Photo by Laurie Macfee.)

staple foods are rice (primarily long-grain), soybean products, and tea. A meal is not considered complete unless rice is included. Instead of soy sauce, however, Southeast Asians often season their food with strongly flavored fermented fish sauces and fish pastes.

Ingredients and Common Foods

Staples and Regional Variations

Filipino   Filipino fare has blended Malaysian, Polynesian, Spanish, and Chinese influences into a distinctive cuisine. There are three principles in Filipino cooking: First, never cook any food by itself; second, fry with garlic in olive oil or lard; and third, foods should have a sour-cool-salty taste. For example, *adobo,* a characteristic Filipino stew, combines chicken, pork, and sometimes fish or shellfish, first fried with garlic in lard and then seasoned with soy sauce and vinegar. Filipinos used a clay pot in the shape of a wok to fry, but they tend to leave the food in longer than the Chinese and allow it to absorb more fat. The common foods of the Philippines are listed in Table 8.1.

Filipinos say young persons should never sing in front of the stove or they will marry an old maid or widower.

Rice is the foundation of the diet, and the long-grain variety accompanies the meal. It is typically steamed or fried (the preferred method of serving leftover rice). Short-grain, glutinous rice is often used for sweet desserts like *puto,* a sweet, fluffy cake made from rice, sugar, and sometimes coconut milk. A favorite bread, *pan de sol,* is made from rice flour. Noodles are also used extensively. *Pancit* is a popular dish made with rice, wheat, or mung bean noodles mixed with cooked chicken, ham, shrimp, or pork in a soy- and garlic-flavored sauce.

The amount of meat, poultry, or fish a family eats depends on economic status. Pork, chicken, and fish are popular, added as available to mixed dishes such as *sinigang,* a soup of fish or meat cooked in water with sour fruits, tomatoes, and vegetables; *chicken relleño,* a whole chicken stuffed with boiled eggs, pork, sausage, and spices; *puchero,* a beef, chicken, sweet potato, tomato, and garbanzo bean stew with an eggplant sauce; *lumpia,* which are the Filipino version of egg rolls, stuffed with pork, chile peppers, and vegetables like hearts of palm; and *paella,* a Spanish recipe for saffron-flavored rice typically topped with chicken, sausage, pork, seafood, tomatoes, and peas. Filipinos use all parts of the animal in their cooking. For example, *lechon* is a whole roasted pig served on special occasions. The pig variety cuts might show up in various mixed stews, such as *dinu-guan,* consisting of diced pork, chicken, or entrails cooked in pig's blood and seasoned with vinegar and hot green chile peppers or sausage such as garlicky

In Filipino culture, sticky, glutinous rice cakes symbolize the cohesiveness of the family.

Puchero is thought to be an adaptation of the Spanish stew known as *cocido.* It is traditionally served for Sunday supper.

Two traditional Filipino dishes—*lumpia* **(similar to an egg roll) and** *pancit* **(noodles cooked with meat or shrimp in a soy- and garlic-flavored sauce).**

TABLE 8.1
Cultural Food Groups: Filipino

Group	Comments
PROTEIN FOODS	
Milk/milk products	Filipinos make one of the few native cheeses in Asia, from *carabao* (water buffalo) milk.
	U.S. influence has resulted in the availability of many western dairy products.
	Many Filipinos may be lactose-intolerant.
	In desserts, coconut milk is frequently used in place of cow's milk.
Meat/poultry/fish/eggs/legumes	The amount of protein food consumed by a family usually depends on economic status.
CEREALS/GRAINS	Rice is the main staple and is usually eaten at every meal.
FRUITS/VEGETABLES	
ADDITIONAL FOODS	
Seasonings	Food is spicy, but the variety of spices used is limited.
Nuts/seeds	
Fats/oils	
Beverages	
Sweeteners	

longaniza. The skin is commonly fried to make *sitsaron* (similar to the Mexican chicharrónes or American cracklings), which are eaten as snacks or pulverized to top noodle dishes.

The Filipinos drink *caraboa* (water buffalo) milk and use it to make one of the few native cheeses in Asia. Because of U.S. influence

TABLE 8.1
Cultural Food Groups: Filipino—continued

Common Foods	Adaptations in the United States
Evaporated and fresh milk (goat or carabao), white cheese	Consumption of milk and other dairy products has increased.
Meat: beef, goat, pork, monkey, variety meats (liver, kidney, stomach, tripe), rabbits *Poultry and small birds*: chicken, duck, pigeon, sparrow *Fish and shellfish*: anchovies, bonita, carp, catfish, crab, crawfish, cuttlefish, *dilis*, mackerel, milkfish, mussels, prawns, rock oyster, salt cod, salmon, sardines, sea bass, sea urchins, shrimp, sole, squid, swordfish, tilapia, tuna *Eggs:* chicken, fish *Legumes:* black beans, black-eyed peas, chickpeas, lentils, lima beans, mung beans, red beans, soybeans, white kidney beans, winged beans	Consumption of fish has decreased; intake of meat, poultry, and eggs has increased.
Corn, oatmeal, rice (long- and short-grain, flour, noodles), wheat flour (bread and noodles)	Rice is not usually eaten at breakfast, but is eaten at least once per day.
Fruits: apples, avocados, banana blossoms, bananas (100 varieties), breadfruit, *calamansi* (lime), citrus fruit, coconut, durian, grapes, guava, jackfruit, Java plum, litchi, mangoes, melons, papaya, pears, persimmons (*chicos*), pineapples, plums, pomegranates, pomelo, rambutan, rhubarb, star fruit, strawberries, sugar cane, tamarind, watermelon	
Vegetables: amaranth, bamboo shoots, bean sprouts, beets, bitter melon, burdock root, cabbage, carrots, cashew nut leaves, cassava, cauliflower, celery, Chinese celery, eggplant, endive, garlic, green beans, green papaya, green peppers, hearts of palm, hyacinth bean, *kamis,* leaf fern, leeks, lettuce, long green beans, mushrooms, nettles, okra, onions, parsley, pigeon peas, potatoes, pumpkins, purslane, radish, safflower, snow peas, spinach, sponge gourd, squash blossoms, winter and summer squashes, sugar palm shoot, swamp cabbage, sweet potatoes, taro leaves and roots, tomatoes, turnips, water chestnuts, watercress, yams	More green vegetables are consumed. More raw vegetables/salads eaten.
Atchuete (annatto), *bagoong, bagoong-alamang*, chile pepper, garlic, lemon grass, *patis*, seaweed, soy sauce, turmeric, vinegar Betel nuts, cashews, *kaong* (palm seeds), peanuts, pili nuts Coconut oil, lard, vegetable oil Soy milk, cocoa, coconut juice, coffee with milk, tea	Chocolate milk substituted for soy milk. Soft drinks are popular.
Brown and white sugar, coconut, honey	

in the Philippines, many western dairy products are available, but cow's milk is used infrequently. Evaporated milk is a common ingredient in *leche flan,* a custard, and in *halo-halo,* a liquid dessert that is served in a glass but is eaten with a spoon and consists of shaved ice, coconut milk, mung beans, boiled palm seeds (*kaong*), corn kernels,

It is difficult to identify a Filipino dish that is without foreign influence. Some Filipinos nominate *kari-kari,* a stew of beef, oxtails, string beans, tomatoes, onions, and ground peanuts flavored with *bagoong* and calamansi limes.

The name *coconut* comes from the Spanish, who thought the "nut" had the face of a clown *(coco).*

In the Philippines, it is considered good luck if one cleanly splits open a coconut without jagged edges.

pineapple jelly, and other ingredients. Halo-halo can be bought pre-mixed with just the shaved ice needed for completion.

A common seasoning, used instead of salt and found throughout Southeast Asia, is fermented fish paste or sauce. In the Philippines the powerful paste is called *bagoong* and tastes somewhat like anchovies, although it can be made from a variety of fish. A similar paste made of shrimp is known as *bagoong-alamang. Patis* is transparent amber fish sauce. To obtain the sour-cool taste that is popular, palm vinegar is commonly used, or a paste made from either the cucumber-like vegetable called *kamis* or the pulp of the tamarind pod. Bagoong, patis, lime *(calamansi)* wedges, and vinegar flavored with chiles are frequently placed on the table so that each diner may add saltiness or sourness to taste.

A principal food in many Pacific Islands is the coconut, and it is widely used in Filipino cooking. In addition, *copra* (dried coconut kernels used for oil extraction) is an important export crop. It takes approximately 1 year for a coconut to mature, but if picked at 6 months, the soft, jelly-like coconut meat can be eaten with a spoon and is a popular delicacy. The coconut plant provides several food products, including beverages, cooking liquids, and even a vegetable. The sweet, clear liquid found in young coconuts is the juice or water. It is consumed fresh, but is not used in cooking. Coconut cream, which is used for cooking along with coconut milk, is the first liquid extracted from grated mature coconut meat. After the cream is removed, coconut milk is made by adding water to the meat and then squeezing the mixture. Coconut milk is used primarily in special dishes. Coconut palm blossom sap can be fermented to produce a strong alcoholic drink called *tuba* in the Philippines. Hearts of palm, sometimes called palmetto cabbage, is the firm, greenish inner core of the tree; it is used as a vegetable. Bananas, durian (a large, strong-smelling, sweet fruit with a creamy texture), jackfruit, papaya, and pineapples are also popular.

Regional cooking styles are divided into four regions: Luzon (the largest group of islands, also home to the nation's capital, Manila), Bicolandia, the Viscayan Islands, and Mindanao. Luzon is made up of various ethnic groups, and the cuisine has been strongly influenced by the Spanish. Ocean fish, such as prawns, milkfish *(bangus),* and halibut, as well as the ample use of anchovy sauce and shrimp paste are preferred in the northern areas. Foods are typically boiled or steamed. *Saluyot* ("okra leaves"—not related to okra), a spinach-like green with a slippery texture when cooked, is especially popular in the north. Rice is grown in the central region of Luzon, known for its freshwater fish and richly sauced dishes flavored with onions and garlic. One delicacy is *rellenong manok,* a deboned chicken stuffed with sausage, vegetables, and ground pork mixed with raisins and spices, topped with a tangy red sauce. Stir-frying is the most common cooking technique. Beef cattle are grazed in the more southern areas;

coconut products and tropical fruits predominate. Sweetened rice dishes are a specialty, such as *bibingka,* a glutinous rice cake with coconut.

Bicolandia is an ethnically homogeneous region that came in contact with both Malaysian and Polynesian cooking. Foods are spicy hot with chile peppers, balanced by copious use of coconut milk and cream. Taro leaves cooked in coconut milk with ginger and chiles is one example of the unique blend of foods found in this area. Viscayan Islands fare also reflects its heritage: Abundant use of seafood (including a distinctive fermented shrimp paste called *guinamos*) and seaweed, as well as many dessert specialties such as candies and pastries developed due to the sugarcane plantations in the area. The Mindanao region was heavily influenced by the Indonesians and Malaysians. The many ethnic groups living there are predominantly Muslim, so little pork is consumed (see Chapter 2 for more information on Muslim food habits). Sauces made from peanuts and chiles are popular, as are curries and other spicy dishes, such as *piarun* (fish spiced with chiles) and *tiola sapi* (boiled beef curry).

Vietnamese, Cambodian, and Laotian Ingredients are similar in all the mainland Southeast Asian countries, but recipes and meal patterns vary. The French introduced and popularized such items as strong coffee, pastries, asparagus, French bread, and meat pâtés in many of the regions they occupied. The Chinese influence, seen mainly in Vietnam, resulted in the extensive use of chopsticks; stir-frying in the wok; serving long-grain rice separately at the meal, rather than mixed with other ingredients; and the more prevalent use of the yin and yang theory as applied to foods and prevention of disease. In Cambodia, Asian Indian and Malaysian influences are seen by the inclusion of curries in the fare. The common foods of mainland Southeast Asians are listed in Table 8.2.

Rice, both long- and short-grain, is the staple of the diet. Rice products, such as noodles, paper, and flour, are used extensively. In Vietnam, rice paper is used as egg roll or wonton wrappers. In the dish *cha gio,* the moistened paper is wrapped around a variety of meats, fish, vegetables, and herbs and then deep-fried. Often the rice paper is filled with meat, fresh herbs, and vegetables at the table. Dried rice noodles (sticks) are called *pho,* which is also the name of the popular noodle-based soup. In Laos the sticky, glutinous short-grain rice is more prevalent than long-grain types (traditionally formed into small balls to use as scoops for other foods), and the very thin Chinese-style rice noodles are common. Wheat is used to make French bread in Vietnam and noodles throughout the rest of the region. Fried noodles topped with meats and vegetables are a favorite.

Fish and shellfish are the predominant protein food on the mainland. Even landlocked Laos depends on freshwater varieties. Poultry

In Vietnam, *com,* meaning "cooked rice," is the same word used for "food."

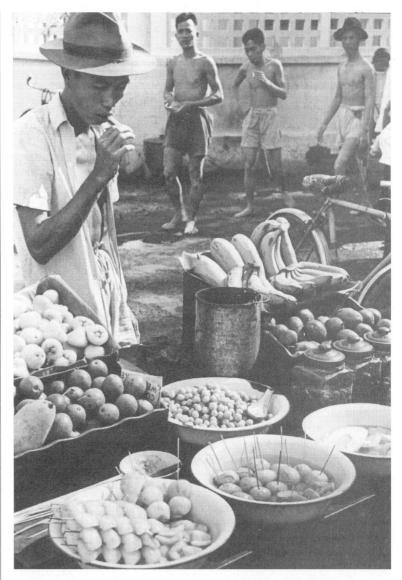

Snack vendor in Vietnam. (Courtesy of World Health Organization/P. Almasy.)

Laotians, including Hmong, often eat *lap,* raw ground pork highly seasoned with chiles, ginger, and onions.

Vietnamese Buddhists eat soybean products on the first, fifteenth, and last day of the lunar month, when meat is prohibited.

is available in many areas, and pork or goat is eaten in wealthier areas. Beef is used occasionally. Religious prohibitions often influence which meats are consumed.

Like other Asians, the people of mainland Southeast Asia do not use appreciable amounts of dairy products. However, soy milk is a common beverage. Soy products, particularly a chewier version of tofu (soybean curd) called *tempeh,* are common.

The Vietnamese serve many uncooked vegetables, often in the form of salads and pickles. A special-occasion dish is shredded chicken and cabbage salad, *goi go.* Many fresh herbs and spices, including basil, fresh coriander, chile peppers, garlic, ginger, lemon grass, and mint, give their food its distinctive flavor and add color to many dishes. Grilled lemon grass beef, *bo nuong xa,* is usually served at summer picnics and is always found at parties and celebrations. Due to the influence of the French, the Vietnamese also eat asparagus, green beans (*haricots*), and potatoes. Other mainland Southeast Asians also consume large amounts of vegetables and herbs, but usually only cucumbers are eaten raw. Fresh leafy vegetables may top rice or noodle dishes as in Vietnam, but hot broth is poured over the top.

Tropical fruits are available, although in some areas, bananas and plantains are the only fruit widely consumed. Banana leaves are used to wrap rice, vegetables, and meats for steaming in both Cambodia and Laos. Pineapple, papaya, limes, and mangoes are common, as are soursop, star fruit, custard apples, durian, jackfruit, and tamarind (a pod with very tart pulp). In Cambodia and Laos, coconut flavors many dishes. Oranges, lemons, melon, and sugar cane are also popular.

In Vietnam, foods are customarily seasoned with a sauce made from fermented fish, called *nuoc mam.* Also used in cooking, nuoc mam is a salty condiment that is often used instead of soy sauce. It can be transformed into a hot sauce, *nuoc cham,* with the addition of chiles, vinegar, sugar, garlic, and citrus fruit juice. In Cambodia the fermented fish sauce is called *tuk-trey;* a stronger fish paste is also used, known as *prahoc.* The Laotian version of fish sauce is *nam pa;pa dek* is the fermented fish paste.

Tea is the preferred beverage throughout mainland Southeast Asia. In Vietnam, it is served before and after meals, but not during the meal. Tea is often blended with flowers such as rose petals, jasmine blossoms, chrysanthemums, and lotus blossoms (which are especially popular). Coffee is popular in French-influenced areas, usually served with large amounts of sweetened condensed milk added to it. Broth is traditionally consumed at meals, and in poorer, rural regions, such as where the Hmong live, it is the only beverage besides water that is commonly available. In wealthier areas, men may drink beer, and soft drinks are consumed by women and children during meals. Soybean drinks and fruit drinks are common; rice wine is served at special occasions.

Meal Composition and Cycle

Daily Pattern

Filipino The traditional meal pattern in the Philippines is three meals a day. Breakfast is garlic fried rice with eggs or broiled fish, sausage or meat, plus coffee or hot chocolate; bread may be

Furr, a soup containing pork, noodles, garlic, and hemp (marijuana) leaves, is a Laotian specialty.

In Southeast Asia, unripe mangoes are appreciated for their crisp texture and sour flavor; they are sliced and dipped into a mixture of sugar, salt, and pulverized chiles or julienned as a main ingredient in spicy salads with shrimp or cashews.

The juicy calyces of roselle are used for jams and chutneys in parts of Southeast Asia.

TABLE 8.2
Cultural Food Groups: Mainland Southeast Asian

Group	Comments
PROTEIN FOODS	
Milk/milk products	Most Southeast Asians do not drink milk and may be lactose-intolerant.
	Sweetened condensed milk is used in coffee; whipping cream is used in pastries.
Meat/poultry/fish/eggs/legumes	The traditional Southeast Asian diet is low in protein.
	Fish, pork, and poultry are common; most parts of the animal are used (brains, heart, lungs, spleen).
CEREAL/GRAINS	Rice is the staple grain and is usually eaten with every meal.
	French bread is commonly eaten.
FRUITS/VEGETABLES	The Vietnamese eat a considerable amount of fruit and vegetables, fresh and cooked.
	Fruit is often eaten for dessert or as a snack.
ADDITIONAL FOODS	
Seasonings	Fish sauce as well as soy sauce is often used.
Nuts/seeds	
Beverages	Usually drunk after the meal or with snacks or desserts.
Fats/oils	
Sweeteners	Sweets are luxury foods.

substituted for rice. Lunch and dinner are similar in size and composition. Both are often large meals, including soup, a fish or meat dish (if affordable), rice, vegetable, and fresh fruit or dessert, served in courses (Spanish-style) or all at once (Filipino-style).

TABLE 8.2
Cultural Food Groups: Mainland Southeast Asian—continued

Common Foods	Adaptations in the United States
Sweetened condensed milk, whipping cream	It is expected that younger Southeast Asians will increase their use of dairy products. Ice cream is popular; milk and cheese are often disliked.
Meat: beef, lamb, pork	Meat, lamb, and eggs are eaten more; fish, shellfish, and duck are eaten less because of price.
Poultry and small birds: chicken, duck, quail, pigeon, sparrow	
Eggs: chicken, duck, fish	
Fish and shellfish: almost all varieties of fresh- and saltwater seafood, fresh and dried	
Legumes: chickpeas, lentils, mung beans (black and red), soybeans and soybean products (*tempeh, tofu,* soy milk), winged beans	
Rice (long- and short-grain, sticks, noodles), wheat (French bread, cakes, pastries)	Intake of baked goods increases.
Fruits: apples, bananas, cantaloupe, coconut, custard apple, dates, durian, figs, grapefruit, guava, jackfruit, jujube, lemon, lime, litchi, longans, mandarin orange, mango, orange, papaya, peach, pear, persimmon, pineapple, plum, pomegranates, pomelo, raisins, rambutan, roselle, *sapodilla,* star fruit, soursop, strawberries, tamarind, watermelon	Use of fruits and vegetables is dependent on availability and price. It is expected that use of fruits and vegetables will decline.
Vegetables: amaranth, arrowroot, artichokes, asparagus, bamboo shoots, banana leaves, beans (yard-long and string), bitter melon, breadfruit, broccoli (Chinese and domestic), cabbage (domestic, Chinese, savoy, napa), calabash, carrot, cassava (tapioca), cauliflower, celery (domestic and Chinese), chayote squash, Chinese chard, Chinese radish (*daikon*), chrysanthemum, corn, cucumber, eggplant (domestic and Thai), leeks, lotus root, luffa, matrimony vine, mushrooms (many varieties), mustard (Chinese greens), okra (domestic, lady finger), peas, peppers, potato, pumpkin (flowers, leaves), spinach, squash, sweet potatoes (tubers, leaves), taro (root, stalk, leaf, shoots), tomatoes, turnips, water lily greens, water chestnuts, wax gourd, yams	Fresh vegetables and herbs sometimes grown in backyard gardens.
Allspice, alum, black pepper, borax, cayenne pepper, chile pepper, chives, cinnamon, coconut milk, fresh coriander, curry powder, fennel, galanga root, garlic, ginger, lemon grass, lemon juice, lily flowers, lotus seed, mint, MSG, *nuoc mam,* paprika, saffron, star anise, tamarind juice, vinegar	
Almonds, cashews, chestnuts, macadamia nuts, peanuts, pili nuts, walnuts; locust seeds, pumpkin seeds, sesame seeds, watermelon seeds	Peanut butter often disliked
Coffee, tea, sweetened soybean milk, a wide variety of fruit and bean drinks, hot water, hot soup, beer	Increased use of carbonated drinks.
Bacon, butter, lard, margarine, peanut oil, vegetable oil	The Vietnamese have increased their use of butter and margarine.
Cane sugar, candy	The use of sweetened products has increased in the United States.

In addition to meals, two snacks, called *meriendas,* are consumed in the midmorning and late afternoon. Meriendas may be small or may consist of substantial amounts of food, such as fritters, pastries, fruits, *lumpia* (egg roll), or almost anything else except rice, which is served only at meals.

Turo-turo are fast-food stands in the Philippines, offering an array of hot items.

Vietnamese and Other Mainland Southeast Asians   Mainland Southeast Asians eat two or three meals a day with optional snacks; the number of meals and amount of food are often dependent on income. In Vietnam a traditional breakfast may consist of soup with rice noodles, meat, bean sprouts, and fresh coriander leaves; boiled egg with meat and pickled vegetables on French bread; and either rice and leftover meat or boiled sweet potatoes with chopped roasted peanuts. Lunch and dinner typically include rice, fish or meat, a vegetable dish, and a broth with vegetables or meat. French bread with meat or shrimp pâté may be substituted for a lunch or dinner meal. Snacks may include clear soup, fruit, or pastries. Southeast Asians do not usually associate particular foods with breakfast, lunch, or dinner; thus a variety of foods may be eaten at any meal.

In Southeast Asia, food is typically stir-fried, simmered, steamed, or boiled. Soups are common throughout Southeast Asia and often feature local ingredients. For example, in Vietnam, crab and asparagus soup is popular. Soup may accompany every meal; it is often eaten in restaurants that specialize in *pho bo ha noi* (from Hanoi), a delicate broth to which rice noodles, sliced beef, bean sprouts, herbs, and other seasonings are added immediately before serving. *Mein go* is a chicken noodle soup served in a similar manner.

Etiquette

Chopsticks are used in Vietnam and are the appropriate utensils for some foods, such as noodles, in other mainland Southeast Asian countries. Forks are common everywhere; however, in Vietnam the fingers of the right hand are used for some foods. Both hands customarily rest on the table while dining. Conversation is usually limited during a meal. It is considered polite to leave a little bit of food on the plate to indicate that hunger has been satisfied.

Special Occasions

Filipino   In the predominantly Catholic Philippines, religious festivals and saints' days are numerous (see Chapter 2). On all special occasions, it is customary to serve plenty of food buffet-style, with a roasted pig (*lechon*) as the centerpiece. The Filipinos claim to have the longest Christmas season in the world, from December 16th to January 6th. The midnight mass celebrated on Christmas Eve is usually followed by the traditional *"media noche,"* a midnight supper of fiesta foods such as roast ham, sweet potatoes, banana flower salad, and *niaga,* a dish made of boiled meat, onions, and vegetables whose name means "good life." Other specialties eaten during the Christmas season are *puto bumbong,* a rice flour delicacy cooked in a whistling bamboo kettle, and *bibingka,* a sweet roll cooked in a clay pan over hot coals.

Hospitality is very important to the Filipinos, and food gifts to express love or appreciation are common.

A midnight mass is also held on New Year's Eve, but many Filipinos attend parties to celebrate the holiday instead. Again, a midnight supper consisting of fiesta foods is traditional. There is also a superstition that eating seven grapes in succession as the clock strikes midnight will bring good luck in the coming year. For birthdays, pancit is eaten to ensure a "long life."

There are numerous Filipino practices and customs associated with Easter, beginning with observances on Ash Wednesday. Late on Easter Eve, young children are awakened to partake of special meat dishes, such as adobo and dinu-guan, in the belief that if they do not do so, they will become deaf.

Vietnamese and Other Mainland Southeast Asians   Of all Vietnamese holidays, Tet, the New Year's celebration, is the most important. It is observed at the end of the lunar year (end of January or beginning of February), just after the rice harvest. In Vietnam the first Tet ritual is an observance at the family grave sites. Offerings of cake, chicken, tea, rice, and alcohol, as well as money, are made at the graves, and then the family picnics on the offerings.

The second ritual, held on the 23rd day of the twelfth lunar month, is to celebrate the departure of the Spirit of the Hearth, Ong Tao. He is represented by three stones on which the cooking pots are placed and is honored by a small altar. Like the Chinese Kitchen God, Ong Tao returns to the celestial realm each year and reports on the family's behavior. After the family makes an offering to symbolize his departure, they share a feast including glutinous rice cakes and a very sweet soybean soup. One week later the family celebrates Ong Tao's return to their hearth. The following day is the first day of Tet. Guests (especially those with favorable names, such as Tho, meaning longevity) are entertained with tea, rice alcohol, red-dyed watermelon seeds, candied fruits, and vegetables. Special dishes prepared for the week-long celebration include *banh chung,* glutinous rice cakes filled with meat and beans and boiled in banana leaves, squid soup, stir-fried young seasonal vegetables, pork with lotus root, and sometimes a special shark fin soup.

Many Vietnamese, including those in America, celebrate the Buddhist holiday called Trung Nguyen, or Wandering Souls Day. It occurs in the middle of the seventh lunar month and is celebrated with a large banquet prepared in honor of the lost souls of ancestors.

Traditionally the Vietnamese did not commemorate birthdays but rather honored their ancestors on the anniversary of their death with a special celebration and meal. In the United States, it is now more common to celebrate birthdays.

The largest holiday of the year in Cambodia is also New Year's, *Chaul Chnam,* which begins on April 13th and lasts for 3 days. Prayers and special foods like fried coconut and fried bananas rolled in coconut are offered to the New Year Angel, who descends with

Long, uncut noodles represent a long and prosperous life.

According to legend, *banh chung* were created by the youngest son of an ancient Vietnamese king. In a contest with his siblings to prepare the best new food, God appeared in a dream and instructed him to make a simple dish of glutinous rice, meat, and mung beans formed into a round (to symbolize the universe) and a square (to represent the earth). The king was so pleased, he awarded his throne to his inventive son.

either blessings or ill will. The Water Festival, held in November after the seasonal rains have ended, features colorful floats in local rivers.

Most Laotian holidays are religious in origin and are celebrated at local temples. *Pha Vet,* which occurs in the fourth lunar month, commemorates the life of Buddha. *Boon Bang Fay,* held in the sixth lunar month, also honors the Buddha with a fireworks display. Among the Hmong and other Laotians the New Year's celebration is a major event. It begins with the first crow of a rooster on the first day of the new moon in the twelfth lunar month, usually in December. The highlight of the festivities is the world renewal ritual, which involves an elder who chants while holding a live chicken. He circles a tree three times clockwise to remove the accumulated evil of the previous year, then circles the tree three more times counterclockwise to invoke good fortune in the upcoming year. It is believed that the bad luck collects in the blood of the chicken, which is traditionally taken to a remote location and slaughtered. New Year's was the one time each year when Hmong from different clans celebrated together, and it is customarily considered a good time to meet future wives and husbands.

Therapeutic Uses of Food

Filipino

When the Spanish came to the Philippines, they introduced the Mexican hot-cold theory of health and diet (see Chapter 6, Mexican "Therapeutic Uses of Foods" section). Foods are classified as being hot or cold based on their innate qualities or their effect on the body, not on their spiciness or temperature. Although the classification of certain foods varies regionally, avocados, alcoholic beverages, coconuts, nuts, legumes, spices, chile peppers, and fatty meats are generally considered hot items; tropical fruits, vegetables, milk and dairy foods, eggs, fish, and lean or inexpensive meats are thought to be cold (Orque, 1983a; Claudio, 1994). A balance is attempted at meals between hot and cold elements. It has been suggested that the reason Filipino dishes contain so many ingredients is to ensure this balance.

Some illnesses are characterized as hot or cold and are treated with foods of the opposite category. Diarrhea and fevers are hot; colds and chills are cold. Other food beliefs are based on imitative qualities (like causes like); for instance, pregnant women may avoid dark foods to prevent their babies' skin from being too dark. Sometimes the meaning behind a therapeutic food use is more obscure; horseradish leaves and broth seasoned with ginger are believed to promote milk production in nursing mothers, and fish heads and onions are considered brain food by some Filipinos. Honey, as well as certain herbs

The Laotian word for holiday is *boon,* meaning "good deed" or "merit." Most festivals are associated with Buddhist rites.

A feast is held by the Hmong following the birth of a child. Included are two chickens representing the parents, a boiled egg signifying the child, and a small lit candle symbolic of the ancestor spirits whose blessing and protection are sought.

Filipinos believe it is inadvisable to eat oranges at the same time as drinking milk because the combination will curdle in the stomach.

like thyme, marjoram, and chamomile, is used to treat diabetes. Licorice root is considered a general tonic, especially beneficial during times of stress. Some elderly Filipinos have adopted the Asian Indian practice of chewing betel nuts, which is believed to prevent tooth decay, although it leaves permanent stains.

Licorice root, which contains *glycyrrhizin,* can cause fluid retention and increase blood pressure if consumed in large amounts.

Vietnamese and Other Mainland Southeast Asians

Many Vietnamese follow the Chinese yin-yang theory of health and diet (see Chapter 7, Chinese "Therapeutic Uses of Foods" section). As in the hot-cold system, classification is based on intrinsic characteristics rather than temperature or spiciness. Examples of yang (hot) foods are unripe fruit, coffee, and alcoholic beverages. Yin (cold) items include noodles, bananas, oranges, gelatin, and ice cream (Orque, 1983b). Some foods, such as rice, eggs, chicken broth, teas, and sweets, are classified as "neutral" (Muecke, 1983b). Not only must a balance be maintained within a meal, but extremes are also avoided during certain conditions, such as pregnancy. As with Filipinos and other Asians, illnesses are defined as yin and yang, and are sometimes caused by eating too many yin or too many yang foods. Equilibrium is restored by eating foods of the opposite type; during the postpartum period, which is yin, cold drinks are avoided. Yin and yang concepts are less prevalent among Cambodians and Laotians, although some hot and cold beliefs exist regarding specific foods and certain conditions.

Some young Hmong women avoid eating gizzards because it is believed they cause the placenta to toughen and make birth difficult.

The Chinese medical system details other influential elements in health, including the five flavors of sour, bitter, sweet, pungent, and salty; these tastes are harmonized in many Vietnamese dishes.

Vietnamese believe that ingestion of specific organ meats will benefit the like internal organs. For example, consumption of liver will produce a stronger liver. Some Vietnamese believe that eating gelatinous tiger bones (produced by prolonged cooking) will make them strong. Concurrently, some foods may be injurious because they resemble certain disorders. Pregnant women may refuse to eat ginger because the multilobed root is thought to cause polydachtyly (too many digits) in babies.

The therapeutic value of some foods is unrelated to yin or yang or how they look. Some Vietnamese eat chile peppers to get rid of worms, or noodles with roasted rice paper and shrimp sauce for curing the flu (Orque, 1983b). Vietnamese women may also consume large amounts of salty foods during pregnancy (Nguyen, 1985). Hmong women eat a diet of rice, chicken broth, black pepper, and herbs for a month after giving birth (Ikeda, 1992), and some clans have specific taboos against eating certain foods, such as heart (Rairdan & Higgs, 1992).

Thai Cuisine

There are seven times more Vietnamese Americans and sixteen times more Filipino Americans than there are Thai Americans in the United States. Yet Thai cooking is more familiar to the general population than either Vietnamese or Filipino fare. Thai restaurants have introduced the distinctive cuisine in many parts of the United States, and dozens of cookbooks published in recent years have further popularized the food.

The country of Thailand is located on the southern end of the archipelago that is Southeast Asia. The hot, monsoonal climate is ideal for rice cultivation. Long-grain rice is the foundation of the diet, and short-grain glutinous rice is used for snacks and desserts. Noodles made of rice, wheat, or mung beans are also common. Tropical fruits and vegetables, such as bananas and plantains, cassava, coconuts, durian, mangoes, pineapple, rambutan, rose apples, sapodilla, taro, and yams, and temperate produce, including carrots, cucumbers, melons, and strawberries, are prominent in the cuisine. Seafood from the lengthy coast, especially shrimp, is popular. Dried herring-like fish (which are sometimes smoked as well) are often flaked into rice for added flavor. Beef, chicken, and pork are common. Duck is a favorite.

Thai food differs from that of its Southeast Asian neighbors because of its flavors. It is one of the hottest cuisines in the world, with lavish use of chile peppers. Several varieties of basil, fresh coriander leaves (cilantro) and root, garlic, ginger root, lemon grass, and tamarind are typical seasonings. In addition, curried dishes are eaten daily. There are three types of curry sauces: yellow, which are smooth, mild, Indian-like sauces that include spices like cardamon and turmeric; red, which are chunkier, hotter, and typically include ample fresh red chiles and coconut milk; and green, which are prepared with fresh green chiles whose heat is excruciating for all but the most experienced palates. The curry sauces are used with beef, pork, chicken, duck, and seafood. Fermented fish products, such as *nam pla* (similar to the Vietnamese sauce called *nuoc mam*) and *kapi* (a paste made from fish or shrimp), are added to most dishes. *Nam prik*, a sauce that combines *nam pla* or *kapi* with other ingredients like garlic, chile peppers, shallots, lime juice, tamarind, palm sugar, and peanuts, complements dishes like *yam* (fresh vegetables rolled up into a leafy package and dipped into the *nam prik*), salads (*nam prik* is the dressing), noodle dishes, dumplings, fried or grilled foods, and highly spiced raw pork called *nam*.

Noodle dishes are usually eaten for breakfast and lunch. *Phad Thai*, stir-fried noodles cooked with bits of meat, seafood, and vegetables bound with eggs, then topped with peanuts and *nam prik*, is an example. Sweets like coconut custards and fruit jellies are preferred snacks. Thai cooking began as a court cuisine, and this heritage is most obvious in the evening meal. Dinner often includes appetizers, such as deep-fried chicken wings stuffed with ground pork and shrimp, or pastries shaped like delicate flowers. The main meal traditionally features steamed rice; soup; a curried dish, a fried dish; and a salad of raw vegetables and grilled poultry, beef, or seafood. *Mee krob*, a volcanic-looking mound of stir-fried noodles and meats or seafood cooked with sugar until carmelized and garnished with egg lace (beaten egg drizzled into hot oil), bean sprouts, scallion tassels, and fringed chile peppers, is a favorite addition. Various *nam prik* accompany the dishes. All dishes are served at the same time, traditionally on low tables surrounded by pillows; fingers and spoons are the usual implements, and forks are available for pushing food into the spoon. The meal usually concludes with elaborately carved fruits.

Contemporary Food Habits in the United States

Adaptations of Food Habits

Filipino

Little current information on the food habits of Filipino Americans has been reported. Most are able to obtain traditional foodstuffs without much difficulty, although some of the familiar tropical fresh fruits and vegetables are not available. It is believed that most Filipinos still eat rice every day, but not with every meal, and their diets tend to contain a greater variety of foods, especially more milk, green vegetables, meat, and sweets than they did in the Philippines (Lewis & Glaspy, 1975). Meriendas tend not to be eaten as often.

Filipinos born in the United States frequently consume a typically American diet. Breakfast consists of cereal, toast, eggs or meat, juice, and coffee; sandwiches, salads, and sodas are common at lunch; and dinner is usually a meat or fish dish served with rice or potatoes, followed by dessert. Traditional Filipino items may appear at some meals, such as eating longaniza sausage at breakfast or eating halo-halo (sometimes topped with vanilla ice cream) for dessert (Dirige, 1995).

Vietnamese and Other Mainland Southeast Asians

A study (Tong, 1986) conducted in Washington, DC, found that 30 percent of the Vietnamese households surveyed had changed their eating habits since coming to the United States. Although most continued to eat rice at least once a day, they ate more bread or instant noodles at lunch and more cereal at breakfast. Respondents also reported consuming more meat and poultry and less fish and shellfish than in Vietnam, mainly because of cost. Pork and pork products were still preferred to beef. They also reported consuming fewer bananas and more oranges, fruit juices, and soft drinks. These findings are similar to those reported in a survey conducted in the 1970s among Vietnamese living in northern Florida (Crane & Green, 1980). More than 90 percent of Vietnamese American adolescents in another study were found to prefer their native diet, although a majority listed items such as steak and ice cream as being among their favorite foods. Soft drinks and milk were well liked; cheese and peanut butter were strongly disliked. Only a small percentage of the teens snacked regularly (Story & Harris, 1988).

A survey of Cambodian and Hmong families indicated some similar trends. While traditional items were preferred by the adults, both American and native foods were acceptable to the children. Most-liked items among the adults included steak, oranges, candy, and soft drinks, all of which are prestige foods in Cambodia and Laos.

Vietnamese restaurants, especially those featuring the noodle soups called *pho,* have become popular in many communities where Vietnamese immigrants have settled. (© David Weintraub/Stock, Boston.)

Least-liked items included cheese, chocolate milk, and milk (Story & Harris, 1989). A detailed study of poor Hmong immigrants in California revealed that the majority of adults (52%) consumed two meals each day of rice, greens, and meats. Pork was the preferred meat, although chicken, turkey, fish, and eggs were also eaten. The adults were mostly unfamiliar with baked products, such as bread or cookies, and most strongly disliked both milk and cheese. It was found that many Hmong grow their own vegetables and seasonings (especially varieties difficult to obtain from grocery stores) in backyard gardens. Most children ate three meals, often including a free lunch at school. Snacking was uncommon, although more prevalent among children (Ikeda et al., 1991).

Food purchasing and preparation as well as meal patterns are also changing. Southeast Asian American women report that men frequently help with shopping or cooking. Vietnamese, Cambodian, and Laotian adolescents often are involved in food purchases, and surveys indicate as many as 60 percent of girls and 35 percent of boys have total responsibility for fixing dinner each evening. Southeast Asian women living in the United States are more likely to have a job or to attend adult education classes than in their homeland, relinquishing some household responsibilities to other family members. Further, many families report a significant decline in eating meals together (Story & Harris, 1988, 1989; Ikeda et al., 1991).

PACIFIC ISLANDERS

Pacific Islanders are the peoples inhabiting some of the 10,000 islands of Oceania. Polynesia, Micronesia, and Melanesia are the three areas that make up the Pacific region. Polynesia includes the major islands and island groups of Hawaii, American Samoa, Western Samoa, Tonga, Easter Island, and Tahiti and the Society Islands. The 2,000 small islands of Micronesia include Guam, Kiribati, Nauru, the Marshall and Northern Mariana islands, Palau, and the Federated States of Micronesia. Although the boundaries of Melanesia are not exact, it includes the nations of Fiji, Papua New Guinea, Vanuatu, the Solomon Islands, and the French dependency of New Caledonia.

Although the area is geographically similar, consisting of mostly small, tropical coral or volcanic islands, the Pacific Islanders are a racially and culturally diverse population. European, American, and Japanese influences have been extensive. Today there are greater numbers of some Pacific Islander groups living in the United States than in their native homelands.

Cultural Perspective

History of the Pacific Islands

Little is known about the prehistory of the Pacific Islands. Current theory suggests that Melanesia was populated first, by people from the Indonesia and Malaysia region (racially Pacific Islanders vary in heritage, suggesting Asian, Australoid, and/or Negroid ancestry). Micronesia was colonized later, followed by Polynesia. The Pacific Islanders are renowned for their boat building and navigational expertise, which permitted extensive exploration and expansion. Breadfruit, taro, and most likely pigs and poultry were introduced as the Pacific Islanders spread through Oceania; most populations were supported by sophisticated horticultural practices and fishing. Pacific Island cultures share extended family systems, and the social order was maintained mostly through the concept of duty to the family. Complex hierarchies based on kinship, clans, birth order, class, or control of land developed on each island; each imposed differing degrees of structure on the culture.

Seafaring Pacific Islanders would spit chewed ginger root at approaching storms to protect their ships.

Hawaii

The state of Hawaii includes 130 islands, of which 7 are currently inhabited. The area was originally settled sometime between 400 and 900 by Polynesians from the Marquesa Islands and Tahiti. A hereditary class system and an economy based on land were established. Adherence to the religious concepts of *mana* (potency) and *kapu* (taboos) supported the social structure. Chiefs derived their power from the deities and this mana was inherited. Obedience to those with mana and observance of taboos regulated individual actions. Violations were punished with both supernatural and social sanctions.

The British explorer James Cook landed in Hawaii in 1778, naming it the Sandwich Islands after the head of the British Admiralty and opening the islands to traders and Protestant missionaries. In 1792, Kamehameha I unified the warring factions of the islands and founded the Kingdom of Hawaii. The Kamehameha dynasty ruled until 1872. King Kamehameha II outlawed the traditional Hawaiian religion and the kapu system in 1819, and land ownership reform followed in 1839.

The kapu system was abandoned in 1819, after King Kamehameha II committed a serious breach of conduct by dining with women.

During the late nineteenth century, Hawaii became a major supply site for U.S. whaling ships, bringing an increased American presence to the region. In addition, significant numbers of Japanese, Chinese, and Polynesian (from other islands) immigrants came to Hawaii to work in sugarcane fields. Asian Indians followed. By 1894, U.S. business interests (primarily in sugar cane and pineapple plantations) dominated the Hawaiian economy, and Hawaii became a U.S. territory in 1900. Military bases were established, including Pearl Harbor, site

A rendering of the *Resolution,* the ship used by James Cook to explore Polynesia. Many Pacific Islander cultural traditions disappeared after European discovery of the islands in the eighteenth century. (© Corbis-Bettmann.)

of the Japanese attack on the United States in 1941 that prompted U.S. involvement in World War II. Hawaii became the fiftieth state in the nation in 1959.

Samoa

The islands of Samoa, located southwest of Hawaii, are politically divided into American Samoa and Western Samoa. The seven islands of American Samoa are a U.S. territory, meaning that its citizens are considered American nationals with the right of free entry into the United States. Western Samoa comprises four inhabited islands and is an independent nation.

The islands were first settled by Melanesian peoples from Papua New Guinea between 800 BCE and 500 BCE. Over time the farming and fishing culture of Polynesia evolved out of these Melanesian roots. Dutch and French explorers visited the islands in the early eighteenth century and were so impressed with the Samoan outrigger canoes that they named the archipelago the Navigator Islands. A reputation for savagery was established when a misunderstanding led to the killing of eleven French sailors by Samoans.

Samoans have been stereotyped as aggressive and even violent since the time French sailors were killed in the eighteenth century. Discrimination is especially acute in Hawaii and other areas where large numbers of Samoans have immigrated.

British missionaries successfully introduced Christianity to Samoa in 1830. The impact on Samoan culture was immediate, and within a decade the Samoans rejected their traditional religion and many central cultural practices as well. British interests in the islands collided with U.S. whaling and German trade in copra in the 1880s, leading to a partitioning of the islands into those under American control and those called German Samoa. The eastern islands were ceded to the United States by the ruling Samoan chiefs and American Samoa became a U.S. territory. Administration of German Samoa was transferred to New Zealand as a League of Nations Trust Territory after World War I. Although a Samoan movement for nationalism was quashed by New Zealand, Western Samoa eventually attained independence in 1962. Today it is governed by a parliament and prime minister, with a chief monarch serving as ceremonial head of state.

Guam

Guam is the largest inhabited island of the Mariana Islands in the mid-Pacific. It is an unincorporated U.S. territory, and in 1950 the U.S. Congress conferred full American citizenship on all Guamanians. Guam is currently seeking commonwealth status from the U.S. government.

The original settlers were the Chomorro people, who now make up one-third to one-half of the population on the island. Little is known about their arrival or subsequent culture. The Spanish explorer Magellan was the first European to visit the island, and in 1668 a Spanish mission was established. The majority of Chomorros converted from their indigenous religion to Catholicism. Guam remained under the control of Spain until 1898, when the island became a U.S. dependency. Japan captured Guam in 1941 and surrendered it 3 years later at the end of World War II. It has remained strategically important to U.S. defense of the Pacific, and American military installations cover nearly one-third of the island. Most Chomorros today speak English.

Tonga

The Kingdom of Tonga is an archipelago of more than 150 islands in the South Pacific. The islands were first populated at approximately the same time as Samoa. Its highly structured Polynesian culture was divided into three hereditary classes of royalty, nobility, and commoners. Social status was dependent on land ownership, and there was little socioeconomic mobility. British explorer James Cook arrived in Tonga in 1773, naming it the Friendly Islands. Tonga became a British protectorate in 1900 and in 1970 was granted independence and membership in the British Commonwealth of Nations. Mormon missionaries have been very active in Tonga, and many Tongans have joined the Church of Jesus Christ of Latter Day Saints. Tonga is ruled by an elected legislature and executive monarchy.

History of Pacific Islanders in the United States

Immigration Patterns

Since the first settlement of the islands in Oceania, the migration of population groups has been very fluid between Polynesia, Micronesia, and Melanesia. As conditions on one island grew too crowded, colonization of surrounding islands occurred. That trend continues, with greater economic opportunity the primary motivation for Pacific Islander immigration to the United States and other countries.

Hawaiians   When Cook first arrived in Hawaii, there were approximately 300,000 native Hawaiians living on the islands. European diseases introduced by the explorers and missionaries decimated the population, and by 1910, only a little more than 38,500 persons of Hawaiian ancestry remained. A high rate of intermarriage has resulted in a population with few Hawaiians of full native heritage. A large number of Hawaiians have migrated to the mainland United States, but the census figures do not reflect such interstate relocations.

Samoans   In 1951 the Pago Pago naval base that employed many Samoans moved to Hawaii, and many Samoans followed. Increasing population pressures and a deteriorating economy encouraged further immigration. Once in Hawaii, Samoans sometimes move to the mainland United States in search of broader job availability and for wider educational opportunities for their children. A chain of immigration between Hawaii and the West Coast was created, with Samoans established in the mainland helping extended family members to settle nearby.

Guamanians   Following attainment of citizenship in 1950, many Guamanians enlisted in the U.S. armed forces seeking better employment and higher wages. Many moved to Hawaii and the West Coast of the U.S. mainland. By the early 1970s, approximately 12,000 Guamanians had immigrated, mostly Chomorros. Major populations have settled in San Diego, Los Angeles, San Francisco, the Seattle area, and Hawaii.

Tongans   The immigration of Tongans to the United States did not begin until population pressures in the 1960s decreased economic opportunities in Tonga. Under the strict hereditary social structure, only the eldest son in a family may inherit land, leaving younger men with little economic mobility. Unlike most other Pacific Islanders, Tongans usually immigrate directly to the U.S. mainland, rather than settling first in Hawaii.

Hansen's disease (leprosy) was one of the illnesses introduced to Hawaii by the Europeans. In the mistaken belief that the disease was transmitted sexually, the afflicted were ostracized and exiled on the island of Molokai during the nineteenth century.

Current Demographics and Socioeconomic Status

Hawaiians   More than 256,000 U.S. citizens were self-identified as Hawaiians or part Hawaiians in the 1990 U.S. census. A little over half (135,231) live in Hawaii: 20 percent of the total state population is part Hawaiian, and about 1 percent is full Hawaiian. The remaining Hawaiians live primarily on the West Coast, mostly in California. Scant socioeconomic data are available, but reports indicate that Hawaiians occupy the lowest economic strata in the state of Hawaii, along with other Pacific Islander immigrants, living mostly in rural and semirural regions. Hawaiian heritage is less of a handicap on the mainland, where Hawaiians have a cultural advantage over other Pacific Islanders (through extensive exposure to American society) and often enter the middle class.

Nearly 7,500 Fijians live in the United States, primarily in California. Most are of Asian Indian descent, were originally indentured laborers in Fiji, and follow the Islamic or Hindu faith.

Samoans   There are probably more Samoans living outside Samoa than in American and Western Samoa combined. The 1990 U.S. census figures showed between 55,000 and 57,000 Samoans living in the United States, three-quarters of whom were born in America. The largest groups are found in Honolulu, Los Angeles, the San Francisco Bay area, and Salt Lake City. Smaller numbers have settled in Laie, Hawaii; Oakland, California; and Independence, Missouri. Religion is a factor for some immigrants: Samoan Mormons tend to migrate to Mormon centers such as Salt Lake City when they move to the United States. Although most Western Samoans emigrate to New Zealand, approximately 15–20 percent of Samoan immigrants come from the independent nation.

Samoans in the United States are often employed in unskilled or semiskilled labor such as assembly line jobs, construction, janitorial or maintenance jobs, or security guards. Low pay (per capita income is half that of the national average), large immediate families, and responsibilities for extended family members in Samoa often translate into a poor standard of living. In 1989, one-quarter of Samoan American families were living below the poverty line. Unemployment is thought to be high, perhaps 25 to 30 percent of men on the mainland and as high as 50 percent of men in Hawaii (Howard, 1980; Fitzpatrick-Nietschmann, 1983). Twenty-five percent of young men and 33 percent of young women do not complete high school. Samoans often find social adjustment difficult because their titled rank from Samoa is unrecognized in the United States.

Guamanians   The 1990 U.S. census statistics indicate 47,750 Guamanians residing in the United States. Many are Chomorros, although self-identification figures are unclear on the exact percentage. The Chomorros often become part of Pacific Islander communities (with Samoan and Tongan immigrants) and are believed to suffer the same discrimination and economic hardships as other Pacific Islanders.

Tongans   Nearly 17,000 Tongans live in the United States according to U.S. census figures. Many are Mormons and are aided in their immigration by their church, and most move to communities of other Pacific Islanders on the West Coast and in Salt Lake City. A small community of Tongans has also located in Hawaii.

Cultural Organizations

Many Pacific Islander Americans seek ways to maintain their ethnic identity in the absence of village associations. The church is of particular importance to both Samoans and Tongans, providing continuity between the islands and the United States and, in many cases, exposure to the traditional language.

Social, political, and welfare groups have formed as well. Hawaiians may belong to the Hawaiian Interclub Council or Hawaiians United Incorporated. The Congress of the Hawaiian People and the Daughters of Hawaii work to preserve the traditional culture. Samoans have chiefs' councils in many cities where immigrants have settled in large numbers, as well as the Samoan Civic Organization, the United Samoan Community Organization, the Samoan Community Organization, and the American Council of Samoan Communities. The National Office of Samoan Affairs, headquartered in the Los Angeles area, was founded to gather data, provide services, and promote Samoan recognition. Chomorros have established numerous local associations, such as the Sons and Daughters of Guam and the Chomorro Organization.

Worldview

Religion

Pacific Islanders follow a wide variety of religions, mostly according to which missionary groups were active in their homeland. Hawaiians practice mostly Protestantism, Buddhism, or Shintoism. Samoans are largely Methodist, Catholic, Mormon, and Anglican. Chomorros are primarily Catholic, and Tongans in the United States are mostly Mormon. Religion is often prominent in the lives of Pacific Islanders, and ministers usually are held in high esteem. In Samoa, nightly readings from the Bible are common in most homes, and prayers are offered at every meal (Cox, 1995).

Family

Although most native religions were abandoned, many concepts central to Pacific Islander culture remained within the structure of families. For example, on many islands, social rank and power were established by birth order within the extended kinship system or clan, and even within families, younger siblings deferred to their older brothers and sisters. Elders were respected. The senior male in the group, whether in the village or in a family, managed all group matters. In Hawaii, women and men were segregated under the kapu system, each with specific roles and responsibilities. Extended families were the foundation of society, and children were raised usually by grandparents, aunts and uncles, and even remote kin rather than by just the parents. Household composition was flexible, and all members were obligated to support the extended family, resulting in substantial redistribution of resources. Generosity and sharing were highly valued. Any social transgressions committed by the individual were the responsibility of the whole family. In Samoa, if the violation was severe, the family could be disinherited from their land and stripped of any social title.

Some of these same practices are continued by Pacific Islanders today. Unlike many immigrant groups, they maintain extended families in the United States. Responsibility for childrearing is shared among family members (children may move freely between homes), and household chores are assigned according to age and gender. The oldest man (or occasionally the oldest woman) in the home assumes control, collecting everyone's paycheck (or weekly contribution) and providing for the household needs. The good of the whole family is considered before the benefit to the individual, and most Pacific Islanders are guided by their desire to avoid bringing shame on their family.

The stresses of acculturation in the United States usually occur due to moving from a society in which there is little anonymity (with individual behavior reflecting on the whole family or village) to a society in which Pacific Islanders are often marginalized or even invisible if misidentified as Asians or Filipinos. Most Pacific Islanders maintain close contact with their homeland and fulfill their obligation to family by sending financial support. Trips back to the islands for political and social events are common.

In Samoa a serious offense by an individual can be ameliorated by an *ifoga* (literally "a lowering"). The extended family positions themselves in front of the victim's home and remains there until invited in and forgiven. They formally apologize through the presentation of gifts and cash.

Communication

Samoans expect exceptional politeness in all interactions; showing irritation, anger, or other hostile emotion is considered particularly rude and a sign of personal weakness (Cox, 1995). Direct eye contact is the norm. When entering a room, Samoans walk around to greet each person with a smile and a handshake. Both Samoans and Tongans are concerned that all participants in a conversation be at an equal level; for example, everyone should be sitting on chairs. It is offensive to stand while speaking to someone who is sitting. When seated, legs should be crossed or kept close to the body. Extending the legs or pointing one's feet at a person is poor manners.

Traditional Food Habits

The cooking of the Pacific Islands developed without benefit of metal pots, pans, and utensils, and many foods were eaten raw. The indigenous cuisine was probably based on breadfruit, taro, cassava, yams, and perhaps pigs and poultry. Fruits were also widely available, although those often associated with the Pacific region, such as coconuts and bananas, were not introduced from Indonesia until approximately 1000 CE. Other items, including sugar cane and pineapple, were brought by European plantation owners. Pacific Islander fare, especially in Hawaii, has been influenced by European missionaries and traders, as well as by the significant numbers of Japanese, Chinese, Korean, Filipino, and Asian Indian agricultural workers who arrived in the eighteenth and nineteenth centuries. Each group added its own cooking to that of the Pacific Islanders, but these foods did not meld into a single cuisine. Instead, each recipe retains its traditional character, and dishes from several different cultures may be served at each meal (see also Chapter 11, "Regional Americans"). Foreign flavors are less noteworthy outside Hawaii and are sometimes limited to only a few influences.

Ingredients and Common Foods

Staples

Starchy vegetables are the mainstay of the traditional Pacific Islander diet (Table 8.3). These include the root vegetable *taro,* which is a little denser and more glutinous than the white potato; breadfruit, with a fluffy, breadlike interior; cassava; and yams. These foods were often cooked, then pounded into a paste. In Hawaii, taro root paste eaten fresh, or partially fermented, is called *poi* (a word that originally referred to the pounding method). When food was scarce, the Hawaiians survived on the purplish-colored poi, sometimes with a little seaweed or fish added to it. Although taro root is also a staple in Samoa, it is usually boiled, but not pounded. Arrowroot is used to thicken puddings and other dishes. The Europeans introduced wheat, and bread is eaten in some areas; for instance, Portuguese sweet bread is known as Hawaiian bread in Hawaii. Asian settlers popularized both short- and long-grain rice, as well as noodles.

More than forty varieties of seaweed are consumed. Cooked greens, including the leaves of the taro root, yam, *ti* plant, and sweet potatoes, are very popular.

Fish and seafood are abundant in the Pacific Islands and in some regions were eaten at every meal. Mullet is one of the most popular fish, but many others, including *mahimahi* (dophinfish, not related to the mammal), salmon, shark, tuna, and sardines, are also consumed. A tremendous variety of shellfish is available, such as clams, crabs, lob-

Fish hooks are symbolic of good luck in Hawaii.

ster, scallops, shrimp, crawfish, and sea urchins, as well as many local species. Eel, octopus, and sea cucumbers are also eaten. Although some fish and seafood was stewed or roasted, some was also eaten uncooked, marinated in lemon or lime juice, which turns the fish opaque much the same as cooking it. A popular Hawaiian specialty is *lomi-lomi,* made with marinated chunks of salmon, tomatoes, and onions, served with or without poi as an appetizer.

Pork is the most commonly eaten meat, especially for ceremonial occasions. Traditionally it was cooked in a pit called an *imu* in Hawaii, a *hima'a* in Samoa, and an *umu* in Tonga. A fire was built over the stones lining the pit, and when the coals were hot, layers of banana leaves or palm fronds were added. The pig and other foods, such as breadfruit and yams, were placed on the leaves, then covered with more leaves and sealed with dirt. In some cases, water was poured over the rocks just before the pit was closed, steaming the foods instead of baking them. The pit was left sealed for hours until the food was completely cooked.

Chicken is widely available, as are eggs. Limited grazing land kept beef from becoming a frequently eaten item. Milk and other dairy products are also uncommon. Soybean products are used by Asian residents, and winged beans are a popular legume on some islands.

Fruits and nuts are important ingredients in Pacific Islander cuisine. Bananas, candlenuts (*kukui nuts*), citrus fruits, coconuts, pineapples,

Hawaii is a leader in aquaculture. As early as 1778, Captain Cook reported 360 fish farms on the island of Kauai, producing an estimated 2 million pounds of fish annually.

Lomi-lomi was adapted from the technique used to prepare the dried salted fish introduced to Hawaii by New England whalers. *Lomi* means "massage," and the slices of dried fish were rubbed under water to remove some of the salt and to tenderize it.

Certain fish in Hawaii were reserved for royalty, and women rarely consumed fish, although they were permitted to eat shellfish.

Pork was traditionally the most commonly eaten meat, particularly for ceremonial occasions. The pig and other foods were cooked in a stone-lined pit over coals. (© Porterfield/Chickering/Photo Researchers, Inc.)

TABLE 8.3
Cultural Food Groups: Pacific Islanders

Group	Comments
PROTEIN FOODS	
Milk/milk products	Milk and other dairy products are uncommon. Many Pacific Islanders are lactose-intolerant.
Meat/poultry/fish/eggs/legumes	Pork is the most commonly eaten meat. Soybean products are used by Asian residents. Winged beans are a popular legume on some islands.
CEREAL/GRAINS	Europeans introduced wheat bread, and Asians brought rice and noodles.
FRUITS/VEGETABLES	Starchy vegetables are the mainstay of the diet. They were often cooked and pounded into a paste. More than forty varieties of seaweed are eaten. Cooked greens are popular. Fruits are an important ingredient. Immature coconuts are considered a delicacy. Arrowroot is used to thicken puddings and other dishes.
ADDITIONAL FOODS	
Seasonings	Food is not highly seasoned but often flavored with lime or lemon juice and coconut milk or cream.
Nuts/seeds	Nuts are a core ingredient.
Beverages	Coconuts provide juice for drinking and sap for fermentation.
Fats/oils	Coconut oil and lard are the preferred fats.
Sweeteners	

The enzyme papain, extracted from papayas, is used in some meat tenderizers. In Hawaii, papaya juice is applied to jellyfish stings to reduce the pain.

Macadamia nuts, for which Hawaii is famous, were introduced from Australia less than 100 years ago.

guavas, litchis, jackfruit, mangoes, melons, papayas, and passion fruit are a few of the widely available varieties. Coconuts provide juice for drinking, sap for fermentation, and milk or cream used in numerous stewed dishes (coconut milk can also be made into foods resembling cheese and buttermilk). Immature coconuts are considered a delicacy throughout the Pacific. *Haupia,* a traditional gelatin-like Hawaiian dessert, is made from coconut milk sweetened with sugar.

Traditional Pacific Islander fare was not highly seasoned. The flavors of lime or lemon juice, coconut milk or cream, and salt predominate, with occasional use of ginger, garlic, tamarind, and scallions or onions. Coconut oil and lard are the preferred fats, providing a distinctive taste to many dishes. Foreign spices, such as Asian Indian

TABLE 8.3
Cultural Food Groups: Pacific Islanders—continued

Common Foods	Adaptations in the United States
	Increased intake of milk.
Meat: beef, pork *Poultry and small birds:* chicken, duck, squab, turkey *Eggs:* chicken, duck *Fish and shellfish: ahi,* clams, crabs, crawfish, eel, lobster, *mahimahi,* mullet, octopus, salmon, sardines, scallops, sea cucumber, sea urchin, shark, shrimp, swordfish, tuna, turtle, whale *Legumes:* beans (long, navy, soy, sword, winged), cowpeas, lentils, pigeon peas	Dietary changes often occur before immigration. Many are dependent on imported foods like canned meats and fish.
Rice, wheat	Increased intake of bread and rice.
Fruits: acerola cherry, apples, apricot, avocado, banana, breadfruit, citrus fruits, coconut, guava, jackfruit, kumquat, litchis, loquat, mango, melons, papaya, passion fruit, peach, pear, pineapple, plum, prune, soursop, strawberry, tamarind *Vegetables:* arrowroot, bitter melon, burdock root, cabbage, carrot, cassava, cauliflower, *daikon,* eggplant, ferns, green beans, green pepper, horseradish, jute, kohlrabi, leeks, lettuce, lotus root, mustard greens, green onions, parsley, peas, seaweed, spinach, squashes, sweet potato, *taro, ti plant,* tomato, water chestnuts, yams Curry powder, garlic, ginger, mint, paprika, pepper, salt, scallions or green onions, seaweed, soy sauce, tamarind Candlenuts *(kukui),* litchi, macadamia nuts, peanuts	Decreased use of the traditional starchy vegetables. May only be consumed at special occasions.
Cocoa, coconut drinks, coffee, fruit juice, *kava* (alcoholic beverage made from pepper plant), tea	Increased consumption of sweetened fruit beverages and soft drinks.
Butter, coconut oil or cream, lard, vegetable oil and shortening, sesame oil	Increased use of vegetable oils and mayonnaise.
Sugar	

curry blends, and sauces like soy sauce have been incorporated into some dishes.

Samoan women are traditionally treated to a rich coconut drink called *vaisalo* after childbirth.

Meal Composition and Cycle

Daily Patterns

Traditional meals included poi or boiled taro root, breadfruit, or green bananas; fish or pork; and greens or seaweed. In Samoa, Guam, and Tonga, most dishes are cooked in coconut milk or cream. Although the evening supper was generally the largest meal, little distinction was made between the foods served at the two or three daily meals.

When drinking *kava,* it is considered polite to drip a few drops onto the ground and say *"manuia"* as a blessing before quaffing.

Kava is made from the chewed or ground root of the native pepper plant, mixed with water in a stone bowl. It looks like dishwater and reputedly tastes a little like dirt or licorice.

When food was pit-cooked, amounts suitable for 2 or 3 days at a time would be prepared. Fresh fruit was eaten as snacks. Beverages made from coconut juice or sap were common. The Asians introduced various teas, including those made from lemon grass and orange leaves. In Samoa a drink made from cocoa was traditional. *Kava,* a bland-tasting but mildly intoxicating beverage made from the pepper plant, remains a popular drink in many regions.

Etiquette

Most Pacific Islanders consider hospitality an honor, and outsiders are usually exempt from traditional manners. In Samoa, for example, it is considered rude to eat in front of someone without sharing. When eating a meal, respect should be shown for the food, because it represents the host's generosity; this includes not talking during the meal. Most hosts will not eat until a guest is satisfied. As in many societies, it is impolite to refuse food, although a guest is not obligated to eat every morsel served.

Special Occasions

Throughout the Pacific Islands, special events were commemorated with feasting, often including pit-roasted foods. In Hawaii, weddings, childbirth, completion of a canoe or house, or a prolific harvest or abundant catch was celebrated with a *luau,* featuring a whole pig, poultry, fish, and vegetables cooked in the imu. In Samoa the feast is sometimes preceded by a kava ceremony, in which the beverage is distributed ritualistically to guests who are expected to drain the cup in one gulp. Traditionally kava was offered as a gesture of hospitality and for occasions such as the ordination of a new chief. In Tonga, where umu-cooked food accompanies celebrations like the commemoration of a royal birthday, special coconut frond stretchers are woven for transporting the massive amounts of food prepared for the occasion.

Holidays celebrated in the Pacific Islands are usually those associated with religious affiliation. Hawaiians also honor Prince Kuhio on March 26th and the Kamehameha Dynasty on June 11th. Samoans feast nearly every Sunday, and almost all denominations celebrate "White Sunday" on the third Sunday of October, venerating children. After a special service featuring religious recitations by children, a festive meal is served and children are waited on by the adults in their extended family (Cox, 1995).

Role of Food

Food holds particular importance within most Pacific Island cultures. Sharing food is a way of demonstrating generosity and support for family and village. It is also a way of expressing prosperity or social standing. Many events are celebrated with feasting, and food is eaten to excess as part of the ceremony in some regions. Traditionally gender roles were defined by food interactions. Boys and girls were often raised similarly until the ages of 8 or 9, at which time they were separated for training in food procurement (farming and fishing) or food preparation (cooking and food storage). Throughout the Pacific Islands, gifts of food are given often. Because the gifts are given without expectation of reciprocity, it is a serious affront to reject any item presented.

Therapeutic Uses of Foods

Hawaiians practice many home remedies. For example, drinking seawater followed by freshwater is believed to be a general tonic. Numerous botanicals are used as cures, and it is estimated that traditionally over fifty-eight different herbal remedies were available for respiratory ailments (Winters & Swartz, 1995). Most notable is the pepper plant (*Piper methusticum*—related to the betel vine), which is used to make kava. It is sometimes used medicinally as an analgesic or narcotic. In diluted form it is used as a sedative and given to teething infants.

Samoans believe a good diet is essential to good health. Eating the wrong foods can result in dislocation of the *to'ala* (the center of one's being located just below the navel) to another part of the body, where it induces pain, poor appetite, or other symptoms. Treatment requires the restoration of balance (Kinloch, 1985; Howard, 1986).

Utah is the first state in the United States to prosecute drivers under the influence of kava. A special blood screening is necessary to detect the substance.

Contemporary Food Habits in the United States

Adaptations of Food Habits

Ingredients and Common Foods

The dietary changes made by many Pacific Islanders begin before immigration to the mainland United States. Most Pacific Islanders in their homelands are highly reliant on imported foods, particularly processed items like canned meats and fish, cooking oil, mayonnaise, cookies, breakfast cereals, and soft drinks. One study on Samoa indicated that 80 percent of all foods found in one market were from the United States, New Zealand, or Australia (Shovic, 1994). Consumption of native foods, such as taro and coconut, increases on Sundays (Hanna et al., 1986). In Guam a high intake of meats, fried foods, foods cooked in coconut milk, white rice, and sweetened beverages and a low intake of produce have been noted (Pobocik & Shovic, 1996). Traditional starches, such as taro root and cassava, are often reserved for special-occasion feasts (Fitzpatrick-Nietschmann, 1983).

Little has been reported on Pacific Islander food habits in the United States. Limited studies on Samoans who have moved to Hawaii show diets with greater variety of foods; traditional foods only contribute minimally to daily intake and items such as rice, bread, sugar, beef, canned fish, milk, soft drinks, and sweetened fruit beverages make up most of the diet (Hanna et al., 1986). It is assumed from available health statistics that a diet substantially higher in fat and simple carbohydrates and lower in fruits, vegetables, and fiber has been adopted by many immigrants.

Meal Composition and Cycle

Three meals each day are common for most Pacific Islanders. Breakfast is most often cereal with coffee. More traditional meals may be eaten for lunch and dinner; a few Hawaiians still eat poi once or twice a day. Fruit appears more often as part of the meal, rather than a snack. It is believed that Sunday feasting among Samoans is still prevalent.

9

The People of Greece and the Middle East

Greece and the countries of the Middle East are considered the cradle of western civilization and democracy. Geographically the Middle East is in close proximity to Africa, Europe, and Asia. It has traditionally been a cultural crossroads; ideas and products of the region, including food, have influenced all western societies. Many immigrants from the Middle East have come to the United States in search of economic opportunity and political stability. Most immigrants in the United States retain a strong ethnic identity, exhibited in their religious faith and in their maintenance of many traditional food habits. This chapter examines the cuisine of the Middle East, its role in the culture, and the changes that have occurred in the United States.

Cultural Perspective

The countries of the Middle East include Bahrain, Egypt, Iran, Iraq, Israel, Jordan, Kuwait, Lebanon, Oman, Saudi Arabia, Syria, Turkey, the United Arab Emirates, and Yemen. In addition, there are the Palestinians (an Arab ethnic group) and the Kurds (an Indo-European ethnic group), each without a homeland. Although Greece is considered a European country, its cuisine resembles that of the Middle East; the geography and climate are also similar. (See Figure 9.1 for a map of the region.) Greece dominated or greatly influenced its Middle Eastern neighbors in ancient times, and in turn was conquered and ruled by the Turkish Ottoman empire for four centuries in the modern era. Several states and countries previously under domination of the former Soviet Union and the nations of North Africa also share certain commonalities with the Middle East, especially fare. Some notable

FIGURE 9.1

Greece and the Middle East.

immigrant populations in the United States are the Croatians and Serbians from the war-torn region of Croatia, Serbia, and Bosnia-Herzegovina (former states in the united Yugoslavia), Slovenians, and Armenians from the newly independent Republic of Armenia and from Turkey.

Populations within the nations of the Middle East are diverse in religious affiliation. Judaism, Christianity (particularly Eastern Orthodox), and Islam all have substantial numbers of followers in the region; religious faith often directs daily life.

Traditional foods of Greece and the Middle East. Some foods typically included in the diets of people in Greece and the Middle East include almonds, chickpeas (garbanzo beans), *couscous,* **cracked wheat, dates, eggplant, Feta cheese, figs,** *filo* **dough, garlic, lamb, lemon, olives,** *pita* **bread, and yogurt. (Photo by Laurie Macfee.)**

Geographically most of the area is considered sandy and arid, but distinct units of arable land exist along the seacoasts and in some plains and valleys, such as the Fertile Crescent (a plain in Iraq fed by the Euphrates and Tigris rivers) and the Nile River valley of Egypt.

History of Greece and the Middle East

Two ancient centers of political power developed in the Middle East—one in Egypt and the other in Mesopotamia (Iraq). Egypt was ruled by a succession of kings, called pharaohs, from approximately 4000 to 1200 BCE. They are known today for their monuments, pyramids, palaces, and temples. Agriculture, masonry, glass making, and metal smelting may all have developed in Egypt. In Mesopotamia the city of Babylon became the capital of the Hammurabi dynasty (1728–1686 BCE). The Hammurabi were later overthrown by the Hittites (1800–1200 BCE), who were the first to use horses in warfare and who dominated the area now known as Turkey, Lebanon, Syria, and Iraq. They were eventually deposed by the Assyrians from the city of Assur. By the seventh century BCE the Assyrian empire included most of the Middle East, with the exception of Persia (Iran).

The next hegemony to emerge in the Middle East was the Persian empire (550 BCE), which ruled until the rise of Alexander the Great from Macedonia (Greece). Greece had been divided into independent and mutually competitive city-states that were unified by Alexander in 335 BCE. Alexander extended his empire until he controlled the area that today includes Egypt, Turkey, Lebanon, Israel, Syria, Iraq, and Iran. Although Alexander's empire did not last long after his death (323 BCE), Greek cultural influence in these areas remains to this day.

The Romans were the next dominant power in the Middle East. Trading and manufacturing flourished under their rule, and many merchants grew rich from trade among Europe, Asia, and East Africa. In addition to the movement of material goods, religious ideas (especially Christianity) spread throughout the Roman empire. In 324 CE the emperor Constantine, who had become a Christian, chose the ancient city of Byzantium to be his new capital, later renamed Constantinople in his honor (now called Istanbul, Turkey).

As Constantinople rose in authority to become the center of the Byzantine empire, Rome weakened. It was sacked in 475 by Germanic barbarian tribes. The Byzantine empire, which included Greece, was Greek in language and religion (Eastern Orthodox). It ruled what is now Turkey for centuries, but its dominance over the rest of the Middle East waned by the seventh century due in part to conflicts with a powerful Persian dynasty, the Sasanid empire (226–651).

The rise of Islam in the Arabian peninsula in the seventh century radically changed the course of history in the Middle East (see Chapter 2 on religion). It ended the dominance of Greco-Roman politics and culture, introduced a new monotheistic religion, and spread a new language, Arabic, which is still spoken today in most Middle Eastern countries. After Islam had become established on the Arabian peninsula, primarily by military conquest, its influence continued to expand. Muslims conquered most of the Middle East (except Constantinople), North Africa, Sicily, Spain, Portugal, and western India by the early eighth century and in the process converted many of the inhabitants of these areas to Islam.

The height of Islamic rule came under the two great caliphate dynasties: the Umayyads and Abbasids, from 685 to 945. During this time, Islam attained its greatest literary and scientific achievements, and the Arabs were both feared and courted by the Europeans and the Chinese. Between the tenth and thirteenth centuries the Islamic community declined in power as a result of conflict among the various Islamic religious sects, rebellion in previously conquered nations (Spain and Portugal), and outside attacks by Asian Turks, Mongols, and the European Christian Crusaders.

The invading Turks adopted the Islamic religion and eventually settled in the area now known as Turkey. They rose to power and toppled the weakened Byzantine empire. By the fifteenth century the Turkish Ottoman empire controlled Greece, most of the other Balkan states (Croatia and Slovenia were able to repel the Turkish incursions), and parts of Hungary. By the sixteenth century the Turks also dominated Egypt, Syria, Lebanon, Israel, and parts of Saudi Arabia, Iraq, and North Africa.

In 301, Armenia became the first nation to adopt Christianity as its state religion.

An Arab is commonly defined as a person who speaks Arabic; the term does not refer to a particular religious belief. Iranians speak Farsi and call themselves Persians.

A *caliphate* is a Muslim community led by a civil and religious leader known as a *caliph*.

Although the Ottoman empire existed into the twentieth century, by the early eighteenth century the West (Europe, Russia, and later the United States) achieved and maintained military, political, and economic superiority in the Middle East. By 1920, France ruled Morocco, Algeria, Tunisia, and Syria (which then included the area now called Lebanon). Britain governed Egypt, Sudan, Palestine (Israel), Transjordan (Jordan), Iraq, and parts of the Arabian peninsula.

Greece became a sovereign nation in 1832, but its resentment against Turkish rule is still evident in the animosity over the now independent island of Cyprus. Iran, although influenced by the West, remained an independent nation and today is an Islamic republic. The remaining Arab nations gained their independence after World War II. Israel was established as a Jewish nation in 1948.

The region is in continuous political turmoil. Long-standing ethnic and religious hostilities regularly erupt into conflict as one group seeks independence from or dominance over another. Recent conflicts between Iraq and Iran; Iraq and Kuwait; Serbia, Croatia, and Bosnia-Herzegovina; Armenia and Azerbaijan; Israel and the Palestinians; and among Iran, Iraq, Turkey, and the Kurds have occurred during attempts to stabilize relations.

The Socialist Federated Republic of Yugoslavia, a communist satellite of the former Soviet Union, consisted of six states—Serbia, Croatia, Slovenia, Bosnia-Herzegovina, Montenegro, and Macedonia. In 1992, Serbia and Montenegro became the Federal Republic of Yugoslavia, and the remaining four states became independent republics.

History of Greeks and Middle Easterners in the United States

Immigration Patterns

Statistics on immigration from the Middle East are inexact. Until 1900, all immigrants from the area were called "Egyptians." Later arrivals were typically termed "Syrians" or "Turks from Asia." More specific nationalities have been recognized since the 1930s, yet it has only been in recent years that "Palestinian" has been defined as an immigration category.

Immigration from Greece and the Middle East has occurred primarily in two waves. The first lasted from the late 1800s to the 1920s, when the restrictive Immigration Act of 1924 was imposed; the second wave started after World War II and has not yet ended. The early Greek and Arab immigrants were mostly young men from rural agricultural areas who came to America primarily for economic opportunities. The Arabs were mainly Christians from the area that is today Lebanon and Syria, although small numbers of Turkish Armenians and Muslims also arrived during this period. Most settled in New England and the Midwest and were employed in the textile, shoe, and wire factories. Many came to make their fortune and go back to their homeland; approximately 30 percent of early Greek immigrants returned to Greece.

During the 1850s and 1860s, numerous Croatian immigrants from the area of Dalmatia arrived in the United States. Most migrated to the

Around the turn of the twentieth century an elite group of Arab artists, writers, and poets settled in New York City. They called their literary circle the Pen League; the best-known member was Kahlil Gibran, author of *The Prophet*.

So many Dalmatian farmers settled in the Pajaro Valley of northern California that Jack London called it "New Dalmatia."

southern and western regions, where they had a substantial impact on the oyster fisheries of Mississippi and the fig, apple, grape, and plum horticulture of northern California. The many Serbs who immigrated to the United States in this period were unskilled laborers who obtained industrial jobs in the Northeast. Slovenian immigrants in the nineteenth century were mostly farmers seeking economic opportunity. They settled initially in the rural Midwest, forming self-sustaining ethnic communities with Slovenian churches, schools, businesses, and social organizations.

Immigration from Greece and the Middle East after World War II reflected political unrest in the area. In Greece a bitter civil war from 1946 to 1949 and a military coup in 1967 resulted in numerous refugees who sought asylum in the United States. While most settled in New York, Detroit, Chicago, and other cities of the Midwest, a large community developed in Tarpon Springs, Florida, supported by diving for sponges. Some Greeks were attracted to mining and railroad work in the West.

A high percentage of immigrants from Jordan, Egypt, Lebanon, Iraq, and Syria were Palestinian refugees who initially fled Israel when it was declared a state. After first settling in refugee camps, many later emigrated to the United States when Israel won the 1967 war against neighboring Arab countries. Political unrest and Islamic revolution in Iran led to a large exodus of Persians beginning in 1976. Many were members of the wealthy Iranian elite; others were Jewish and Christian minorities. In addition, many Arabs who were sent to the United States for education and training remained for economic reasons.

Turkish, Croatian, and Serbian immigration also increased following World War II, including professionals, such as engineers and physicians, seeking better job opportunities. More than 60,000 Armenian refugees have arrived since 1980, settling primarily in Los Angeles, with small numbers joining the older Armenian American communities in Boston, New York, Chicago, Detroit, and the agricultural region of Fresno, California.

Current Demographics and Socioeconomic Status

More than 1 million persons claimed Greek heritage in the 1990 U.S. census. New York City has the largest concentration of Greek Americans, followed by California, Illinois, Massachusetts, and Florida. In recent years, Greek Americans have moved increasingly south and west in the United States.

Demographic figures for Middle Easterners are more problematic. It is believed that many deny their Arab ancestry due to discrimination, and others refuse cooperation with government-sponsored surveys due to negative experiences in their homelands. The census reports nearly 400,000 self-declared Americans from Lebanon; 308,000 from Armenia; 236,000 from Iran; 130,000 from Syria;

127,000 listed as Arab; 83,000 from Turkey; 80,000 from Israel; 79,000 from Egypt; 48,000 Palestinians; 23,000 Iraqi; 20,000 from Jordan; 7,600 miscellaneous Middle Easterners; 4,500 from Saudi Arabia; and 4,000 from Yemen. Unofficial estimates of these populations are often two to three times larger. Most Middle Easterners are located in the Northeast and Midwest, although significant populations are found in California, particularly in Los Angeles. Smaller communities are developing in Texas, Georgia, Alabama, and other areas of the South.

There are more than 500,000 Croatian Americans and 100,000 Americans of Serbian descent in the United States. Most originally settled in the mining regions of Pennsylvania, Ohio, and other Midwestern states; mining also attracted sizeable populations to Colorado, Nevada, Arizona, and California. Nearly 125,000 Slovenian Americans were identified in the 1990 U.S. census. Although many Slovenian immigrants also became involved in mining, others moved to industrial urban areas in search of jobs. Forty percent live in Ohio; Cleveland has the largest Slovenian community in the nation. Other states with notable Slovenian populations include Pennsylvania, Minnesota, Wisconsin, California, Colorado, Michigan, Florida, and New York.

Early Greek and Arab immigrants preferred to live in urban areas. The Arabs often became peddlers and later opened family businesses, usually dry goods or grocery stores. Many recent Arab immigrants are well-educated professionals. The Greeks sought economic independence by opening small businesses, especially in candy production

Some Arab Americans face significant discrimination due to ongoing tensions between the United States and countries in the Middle East. The media, especially movies, have recently vilified Middle Easterners and inflamed anti-Arab sentiments.

A large Greek community developed in Tarpon Springs, Florida, based on diving for sponges. (© Van Bucher/Photo Researchers, Inc.)

and restaurants. A tradition of entrepeneurship among Middle East-erners continues; Iranians are frequently involved in real estate development and Armenians often open their own businesses. Rates of self-employment among Greeks and Middle Easterners are very high, between 12 and 36 percent of all workers, compared to 7 percent for the national average.

Recent immigrants are often well educated, and there is an admitted "brain-drain" in the Middle East that has occurred since the mid-1970s. Even families that started with unskilled employment or small businesses have made substantial economic progress through schooling. Second- and third-generation Americans of Greek and Middle Eastern heritage attend college and graduate in professional fields such as engineering, medicine, pharmacy, dentistry, and law at rates far higher than the national average. Greek Americans and Middle Eastern Americans are among the most prosperous of all ethnic groups in the United States.

Cultural Organizations

Religion has played a significant role in the support of Greek and Middle Eastern immigrants to the United States. Local churches and mosques have provided cultural activities and in many cases have started parochial schools for the children of their members. Mutual assistance leagues and benevolent associations have been prominent in some cities.

The Order of American Hellenic Educational Progressive Association is one of the largest national organizations of Greek Americans. Before the 1967 Arab-Israeli War the early and late Arab immigrant groups tended not to associate with each other; after 1967, perceived American hostility toward Arabs drew the two groups closer together. The aims of the American Arab Anti-Discrimination League, the Association of Arab American University Graduates, the Arab American Institute, and the Arab Women's Council are to correct misinformation about Arabs, improve the image of Arab Americans, and influence American Middle East policy. Other groups represent the needs of specific groups, such as the Bethlehem Association (Palestinians), the Armenian Assembly of America and the Armenian Network of America, the Assembly of Turkish American Associations and the Federation of Turkish-American Associations, and the Slovene National Benefit Society.

Worldview

Religion

Religion is often the defining factor in Greek and Middle Eastern life. Although affiliation varies, strong devotion is common. Many congregations remain very insular in the United States, serving the needs of a specific ethnic group, and there is little interest in proselytizing to outsiders.

The ethnicity of Greek immigrants was affirmed mostly by religion; it was said that a person was not Greek by birth, but through the active affiliation with the Greek Eastern Orthodox Church. The first Greek Orthodox Church in America was founded in New Orleans in 1864.

Most Greek Americans today still belong to the church, which continues to be the center of Greek community life. The word "orthodox" comes from the Greek for "correct" (*orthos*) and "worship" (*doxa*). A fundamental belief of the Greek Orthodox faith is that an individual attains complete identification with God through participation in the numerous religious services and activities sponsored by the church. Although the Greek Orthodox Church is conservative and traditionally resistant to change, some accommodations have been made in the United States; for instance, the service typically is conducted both in Greek and English, and modern organ music accompanies the liturgy (see Chapter 2 for more information about Greek Orthodoxy).

Early Arab immigrants were primarily Christians belonging to the Eastern Orthodox or the Latin rite Maronite, Melkite, or Chaldean churches. Although Christian Arabs are still a majority in America, more recent immigrants follow Islam, and the number of Arab Muslims in the United States is growing rapidly. Most belong to the Sunni sect. Many Arab Muslims in the United States have made several adaptations to accommodate their religious practices to American society. Most significantly, the Friday Sabbath prayer has been moved to Sunday, and many Muslims cannot fulfill their obligation to five daily prayers due to work or school limitations (see Chapter 2 for more information about Islam).

Though the vast majority of Iranians in the United States are members of the Muslim Shi'ite sect, small numbers of Iranian religious minorities have come to the United States seeking freedom from persecution, including Jews, Catholics, Anglicans, Protestants, and members of the Baha'i faith (a Muslim offshoot that has renounced its ties to Islam and preaches gender equality, world brotherhood, and pacifism). Most Armenians are members of the Armenian Apostolic Church (an Eastern Orthodox faith noted for allowing its members to make decisions on issues such as birth control and homosexuality without religious influence), although some Americans of Armenian descent are Protestants or members of the Armenian Rite of the Roman Catholic Church. A majority of Croatians and Slovenians are devout Roman Catholics, and most Serbs belong to the Serbian Orthodox Autonomous Church.

Family

Traditionally both Greek and Arab cultures center around a strong patriarchal family whose honor must be maintained. The family demands conformity and subordination of individual will and

Greeks traditionally considered educational or career achievement among women to be unfeminine, or even un-Greek.

In some Arab American homes, girls are not allowed to play certain sports or ride bicycles.

Muslims often have serious concerns about raising their children in America. Permissive attitudes about dating and drinking and pressure to practice self-reliance and independent thought prompt some immigrants to send their children, especially their daughters, to the Middle East for schooling.

interest, but in return the members of the family are protected and can identify with the family's status. The Greek term for this pride and obligation to family is *philotomo,* meaning "love of honor." Families often live with extended members in a single home or, for well-to-do Middle Easterners, in a family compound. Elders traditionally live with the families of their sons.

Children are valued in both Greek and Arab families, and sacrifice for the good of the children is common. In Islam the teachings of the Koran state that men and women are considered equal, but different. Although men are expected to provide economic security for children, it is the role of women to socialize the children, including the preservation of religious and cultural values. Due to the strict patriarchy, women are expected to provide the love and comfort in a home as well. The relationship between mothers and daughters is very intimate. There is also a strong bond between mothers and sons, especially the first-born son (Luna, 1994). Generally, formal schooling is not considered as important for girls as for boys among Arabs. Education for women is encouraged by some Middle Easterners, such as Iranians and Armenians.

Marriage contracts in the Middle East are often arranged between children to establish political and business alliances. The wealth and status of a family may be dependent on the expansion of kinship. Among Arabs there is a preference for marriage between cousins, except among Egyptians and some Arab Christians. Only after an engagement announcement is made are young men and women allowed to "date," and then only when chaperoned. A family's honor is related to the modesty and chastity of the women in the home: A woman is chaste before her wedding and faithful after. Actual or alleged violations of moral codes by a young woman are considered evidence that her mother has failed in her responsibilities; inappropriate sexual conduct also brings shame on her male relatives.

Although Islamic law allows a man to take four wives, most only wed once. Interethnic marriages are strongly discouraged by both Muslims and Christians, especially for women. It is preferable, however, to marry someone of a different ethnic group and the same religious affiliation than to marry outside the religion.

One of the first effects of immigration to the United States is the breakdown of the extended family and reduction of the father's authority, although filial respect is retained. Family ties are still very strong among Greeks and Arabs, and it is still common for elderly parents to live with the family. Some Arab women in the United States have gradually rejected certain Middle Eastern customs, such as veils for Muslim women. Dating is becoming more prevalent as segregation of the sexes cannot be maintained in the American workplace. Interethnic and interreligious marriages are on the rise, particularly among Greek Americans. Yet, for many Middle Eastern women, their traditional roles in the home tend to isolate them from contact with much of American culture; among Iranian immigrants, women feel that their limited authority has decreased since arriving in the United States, that they spend more time on household chores, and that they are less involved in family decisions (Gillis, 1995). More acculturated Arab women also believe that they face serious setbacks in acceptance of their Americanized conduct every time a large influx of new and traditionally minded Middle Eastern women settle in their area. Intergenerational conflict is less than that seen in other ethnic immigrant groups, although second- and third-generation Greeks and Middle Easterners in America are likely to think that their parents are old-fashioned.

Croatian and Serbian families are also traditionally patriarchal. Extended families are the norm, often including friends as well as relatives. Among Croatians, communal living may involve the taking in of boarders. Both Croatians and Serbians have become well acculturated in the United States. The tradition of older generations caring for children has allowed many Croatian and Serbian women to take advantage of educational and career opportunities, and the authority of the father has lessened. Slovenian Americans also are usually acculturated. The extended family structure typical in Slovenia is rarely found among Slovenians in the United States, who prefer nuclear families. American women of Slovenian descent are active in the home, church, and Slovenian schools and are increasingly involved in politics.

Growing drug and gang problems among Armenian youth have stressed relations between recent immigrants and immigrants who have lived successfully in the United States for many years without significant social problems.

Communication

Greece and the nations of the Middle East are very high-context cultures. Body language and general atmosphere are as important to a conversation as are words. (See Chapter 12 for details.) People in the Middle East spend time getting to know one another before any business is conducted. Direct eye contact is expected and necessary to interpret meaning, so Middle Easterners usually sit or stand quite close when conversing. Greeks may smile when angry. Nodding one's head up and down or back and forth can be very confusing. Traditionally moving the chin up and down meant "no," and back and forth meant "yes" or "I don't understand." But many Greeks and Middle Easterners use the American protocol, so it is difficult to know if the gesture is affirmative or negative.

Touching between members of the same sex is frequent, including handshaking, patting, shoulder slapping, hugging, and kissing. Contact between members of the opposite sex is prohibited in some Middle Eastern Muslim cultures, and extended eye contact between men and women can be considered a sexual overture (staring between members of the same sex is acceptable). The left hand is not used for any social purposes. In general, it is best to wait for Middle Easterners to extend their hand in greeting before making any unwanted contact: Follow their lead. Proper posture is a sign of respect, and crossing one's legs, pointing with the foot, or showing the sole of the shoe is considered impolite. In Turkey, one should stand when an elder enters a room.

Traditional Food Habits

Certain common foods in Greece and the Middle East, such as wheat, olives, and dates, are indigenous to the region. Yet most countries in the area claim one dish or another prepared by all ethnic groups to be their own invention. It is doubtful if the source of any Middle Eastern dish will ever be known, as the political and economic history of the region has resulted in very similar foods and food habits.

Ingredients and Common Foods

Staples

The common ingredients used in Greek and Middle Eastern cooking are listed in Table 9.1. Numerous food items, such as wheat, rice, legumes, and lamb, are eaten in most countries.

Wheat, thought to have been cultivated first in this region, is usually eaten as leavened bread loaves in Greece and leavened flat bread in the Middle Eastern countries. One example is the thin round Arabic bread with a hollow center called *pita* (or *pida* in Turkey); another is *lavosh,* which is Armenian cracker bread. Bread traditionally accompanies every Greek and Middle Eastern meal.

Besides bread, wheat doughs are also used to make pies, prepared in a variety of sizes and shapes. Savory pies may contain meat, cheese, eggs, or vegetables. Desserts are usually filled with nuts and covered in a thick sugar and honey syrup. Pie pastry, flaky pastry, paper-thin pastry called *filo* (or *phyllo*), and bread dough can all be used. An example of a meat- or cheese-filled pastry that can be served hot or cold is *sanbusak*. Traditionally half-moon shaped and 3 inches long, it is popular in Syria, Lebanon, and Egypt. A similar pie is called *boereg* by Armenians. *Fatayeh* is another specialty served as a snack, featuring bread dough topped with cheese, meat, or spinach and baked like a pizza. Throughout the Middle East and Greece the dessert made with filo dough, *baklava,* is served at every special occasion. No café or bakery would be without it. Baklava contains numerous alternating sheets of filo dough and a walnut, almond, or pistachio filling, which is soaked in a sweet syrup flavored with honey, brandy, rose water, or orange blossom water. It is frequently cut into diamond shapes.

Raw kernels of cracked whole wheat are also used in a number of Middle Eastern dishes. When the kernels are first steamed and then

The tall white hats worn by professional chefs are thought to have originated with the tall black hats worn by Eastern Orthodox priests.

The diet of the common people in ancient Greece was wheat, legumes, fruit, vegetables, olive oil, milk, cheese, and small amounts of meat and fish.

The traditional recipe for *sanbusak* dough calls for one coffee cup each of oil, melted butter, and warm water combined with 1 teaspoon of salt and enough flour to make the mixture stiff.

Pastilla is a Moroccan dish with Middle Eastern origins featuring filo dough filled with cinnamon-scented chicken.

At ancient Greek weddings the bride and groom were showered with wheat kernels.

Muslim women purchasing sweets for Ramadan from an Iraqi street vendor. (Corbis & AFP.)

dried and crushed to different degrees of fineness, the cracked wheat is called *burghul* or *bulgur*. Unripened wheat kernels that are dried but not cracked are known in Arabic markets as *fireek*. All varieties of wheat kernels are typically cooked as side dishes or made into *tabouli*, a popular salad containing onions, parsley, mint, and a variety of fresh vegetables. *Kibbeh*, one of the national dishes of Lebanon and Syria, is a mixture of fine cracked wheat, grated onion, and ground lamb pounded into a paste. This mixture can be eaten raw or grilled, and with a great deal of dexterity it can be made into a hollow shell, then filled with a meat mixture and deep-fried.

In addition to wheat, rice is also a staple item in Greek and Middle Eastern cuisine. The long-grain variety is used to make *pilaf*, a dish that commonly accompanies meat. The rice is first sautéed in butter or oil in which chopped onions have been browned. It is then steamed in chicken or beef broth. Occasionally saffron or turmeric is added to give the dish a deep yellow color. *Polo* is the Iranian version of pilaf, but a final step in its preparation produces a rice with a crunchy brown crust that is known as the *tah dig*. A more fragrant variety of rice (*basmati*) is used in Iran to make the national dish, *chelo kebab*, which is thin pieces of marinated, charcoal-broiled lamb served over rice.

Couscous, fine granules of semolina wheat flour (like a very small pasta), is steamed in a *couscousier* (a pan with boiling water and a colander insert that holds the granules) and served with stews throughout North Africa.

The Syrians blend bulgar with yogurt, dry the mixture in the sun, then grind it into a powder to prepare *kish'ka*. It is combined with a little water and onions to make a filling for pita bread or thinned further to make soup.

TABLE 9.1
Cultural Food Groups: Greek and Middle Eastern

Group	Comments
PROTEIN FOODS	
Milk/milk products	Most dairy products are consumed in fermented form (yogurt, cheese). Whole milk is used in desserts, especially puddings.
	High incidence of lactose intolerance.
Meat/poultry/fish/eggs/legumes	Lamb is the most popular meat.
	Pork is eaten only by Christians; not by Muslims or Jews.
	Jews do not eat shellfish. In Egypt, fish is generally not eaten with dairy products.
	Legumes are commonly consumed.
CEREALS/GRAINS	Some form of wheat or rice usually accompanies the meal in Greece and the countries of the Middle East.
FRUITS/VEGETABLES	Fruits are eaten for dessert or as snacks. Fresh fruit and vegetables are preferred, but if they are not available, fruits are served as jams and compotes and vegetables as pickles. Eggplant is very popular.
	Vegetables are sometimes stuffed with rice or a meat mixture.
ADDITIONAL FOODS	
Seasonings	Numerous spices and herbs are used.
	Lemons are often used for flavoring.
Nuts/seeds	Ground nuts are often used to thicken soups and stews.
Beverages	Coffee and tea are often flavored with cardamom or mint, respectively.
	Aperitifs are often anise-flavored.
Fats/oils	Olive oil is generally used in dishes that are to be eaten cold. For most deep-frying, corn or nut oil is used; olive oil is preferred for deep-frying fish. Sheep's tail fat is a delicacy.
	Coffee is heavily sweetened.
Sweeteners	Dessert syrups are flavored with honey or rose water.

A large variety of legumes are another important ingredient in Middle Eastern cooking. Cooked pureed chickpeas (garbanzo beans) are the base for the salad called *hummus,* which is often used as an appetizer or as a dip. Ground chickpeas or fava beans are sometimes formed into small balls, then fried and served as a main course (*ta'amia*) or in a pita bread with raw vegetables (*falafal*). A common breakfast food is *foul,* slowly simmered fava or black beans topped

TABLE 9.1
Cultural Food Groups: Greek and Middle Eastern—continued

Common Foods	Adaptations in the United States
Cheese (goat's, sheep's, and cow's), milk (goat's, sheep's, camel's, and cow's), yogurt	More cow's milk and less sheep's, camel's, and goat's milk is drunk. Ice cream is popular. *Feta* is the most common Middle Eastern cheese available in the United States. Lamb is still very popular. More beef and fewer legumes are eaten.
Meat: beef, kid, lamb, pork, rabbit, veal, some varietal cuts	
Poultry: chicken, duck, pigeon, turkey	
Fish and shellfish: anchovies, bass, clams, cod, crab, crawfish, flounder, frog legs, halibut, lobster, mackerel, mullet, mussels, oysters, redfish, salmon, sardines, shrimp	
Eggs: poultry, fish	
Legumes: black beans, chickpeas, fava (broad) beans, horse beans, lentils, navy beans, red beans	
Bread (wheat, barley, corn, millet), barley, corn, cornstarch, farina, oatmeal, pasta, rice (long-grain and *basmati*), wheat (*bulgur, couscous*)	Bread and grains eaten at most meals. *Pita* bread is commonly available. Fewer fruits and vegetables are consumed. Olives still popular.
Fruits: apples, apricots, avocado, bergamots, cherries, currants, dates, figs, grapes, lemons, limes, melons (most varieties), oranges, peaches, pears, plums, pomegranates, raisins, strawberries, tangerines	
Vegetables: artichokes, asparagus, beets, broad beans, broccoli, brussels sprouts, cabbage, carrots, cauliflower, celeriac, celery, corn, cucumbers, eggplant, grape leaves, green beans, green peppers, greens, leeks, lettuce, mushrooms, okra, olives, onions, parsley (flat-leaf), peas, pimientos, potatoes, spinach, squashes, tomatoes, turnips, zucchini	
Ajowan, allspice, anise, basil, bay leaf, caraway seed, cardamom, chervil, chives, chocolate, cinnamon, cloves, coriander, cumin, dill, fennel, fenugreek seeds, garlic, ginger, gum arabic and mastic, lavender, linden blossoms, mace, *mahleb,* marjoram, mint, mustard, nasturtium flowers, nutmeg, orange blossoms or water, oregano, paprika, parsley, pepper (red and black), rose petals and water, rosemary, saffron, sage, savory, sorrel, sumac, tarragon, thyme, turmeric, *verjuice,* vinegar	
Almonds, cashews, hazelnuts, peanuts, pine nuts, pistachios, walnuts; poppy, pumpkin, sunflower, sesame seeds	
Coffee, date palm juice, fruit juices, tea and herbal infusions, yogurt drinks, wine, brandy, aperitifs	
Butter (often clarified), olive oil, sesame oil, various nut and vegetable oils, rendered lamb fat	Olive oil is still popular.
Honey, sugar	

with chopped tomato, garlic, lemon juice, olive oil, and cilantro (fresh coriander leaves). The national dish of Egypt is *ful medames,* cooked fava beans seasoned with oil, lemon and garlic, sprinkled with parsley, and served with hard-boiled eggs. Lentils and peanuts are also eaten.

Fresh fruits and vegetables are preferred, but if they are not available, fruits are served dried or as jams and compotes; fruit syrups also flavor many savory dishes. Vegetables are preserved as pickles. Fruits,

Date trees were an ancient symbol of fertility.

In Tunisia, vegetables such as tomatoes, peppers, onions and garlic are grilled, then served as a salad dressed with olive oil and lemon juice in the dish called *mechouia*.

Athens is named after the Greek goddess Athena because she gave the city the olive tree.

The term *yogurt* is Turkish. In Syria and Lebanon the fermented milk product is called *laban;* in Egypt, *laban zabadi;* and in Iran, *mast.*

Béchamel, a white sauce used in French cuisine, is thought to have originated in Greece.

many first cultivated in the region, are eaten for dessert or as snacks. Figs, dates, grapes, and pomegranates are favorites. Lemons are often used for flavoring. Although many vegetables are used, eggplant is the most popular. A common cooking method for vegetables (the Greek term is *yiachni;* the Arabic word is *yakhini*) is to combine them with tomatoes or tomato paste and sautéed onions together with a small amount of water, then cook until the vegetables are soft and very little liquid remains. Eggplant and other vegetables are sometimes stuffed with rice or a meat mixture. *Moussaka* is a Greek specialty made with minced lamb, eggplant, onions, and tomato sauce baked in a dish lined with eggplant slices. The Turks prefer *imam bayildi* (meaning "the priest fainted"), eggplant filled with tomatoes, onions, and garlic, stewed in olive oil and served cold. A delicacy favored throughout the region is stuffed grape leaves, *dolmas* or *dolmades*. Vegetables are frequently enjoyed raw, mixed together in a salad.

The olive tree contributes in many ways to Greek and Middle Eastern cooking. Olives prepared in the Middle Eastern way have a much stronger flavor than European or American olives; they often accompany the meal or are served as an appetizer. There are two basic types of olives in Greece and the Middle East. Black olives are ripe when picked; they are small, round, wrinkled, and taste slightly bitter and salty. Green olives are picked unripe, having an oblong shape, firm flesh, smooth skin, and tart flavor. Greek *kalamata* olives are a favorite; they are large and oblong, with soft flesh and smooth purplish skin.

The olive is also a source of oil, which is frequently used in food preparation, although both Greeks and Arabs also use clarified butter (*samana*) and most vegetable oils as well as rendered lamb fat and margarine. Olive oil is generally used in dishes that are to be eaten cold. For most deep-frying, corn or nut oil is used, but olive oil is preferred for deep-frying fish.

Fresh milk is not widely consumed in Greece or the Middle East, although it is used in dessert puddings. Dairy products are usually fermented into yogurt or processed into cheese. Yogurt is often eaten as a side dish and is served plain (unsweetened) or mixed with cucumbers or other vegetables. It is even diluted to make a refreshing drink. Cheese is usually made from goat's, sheep's, or camel's milk. The most widely used Middle Eastern cheese is the Greek *Feta,* which is a salty, white, moist cheese that crumbles easily. Another is *Kaseri,* a firm, white, aged cheese, mild in flavor and similar to Italian provolone. Armenian string cheese is a mild cheese sold in small logs; long "strings" can be peeled off it, and it forms mozzarella-like strands when melted. *Lebneh* or *Labni* is a fresh cheese made by draining the whey from salted yogurt overnight.

Almost all meats and seafoods are eaten in Greece and the Middle East, with the exception of pork in Muslim countries and pork and shellfish among observant Jews in Israel. Lamb is the most widely used meat. Grilling, frying, grinding, and stewing are the common ways of preparing meat in the region. A popular dish is *shish kabob,* marinated pieces of meat threaded onto skewers with pieces of raw tomatoes, onions, and sweet peppers and then grilled over a fire. *Souvlaki* or *shawarma* is very thin slices of lamb (or chicken) layered onto a rotisserie with slices of fat (resulting in one roast), grilled, then carved and served. Meatballs, called *kofta,* are eaten as snacks or served with stewed vegetables. A whole roasted lamb or sheep is a festive dish prepared for parties, festivals, and family gatherings.

Numerous spices and herbs are used in Middle Eastern seasoning as a result of a once thriving spice trade with India, Africa, and Asia. Common spices and herbs are dill, garlic, mint, cardamom, cinnamon, oregano, parsley, and pepper. *Sumac,* ground red berries from a nontoxic variety of the plant, is sprinkled over salads to give a slightly astringent flavor. Other typical Middle Eastern spices include *mahleb,* made from the ground pits of a cherry-like fruit, and *ajowan,* small, black carom seeds with a thymelike flavor. The juice of unripe lemons, *verjuice,* is used to provide a sour taste to dishes.

Ground nuts are often used to thicken soups and stews. Sesame seeds are crushed to make a thick sauce, *tahini,* which is used as an ingredient in Arabic cooking and in a sweet dessert paste known as *halvah.*

Although observant Muslims do not drink alcohol, several nations in the region (e.g., Greece, Iraq, Israel, Turkey) produce wines and spirits. Best known in the United States are the Greek specialties *Retsina* (white wine with a resinous flavor) and *Metaxia* (orange-flavored brandy). Aperitifs are particularly popular. Many are anise-flavored, such as *Arak* and *Ouzo* from Greece and *Raki* from Turkey.

Regional Variations

There are two schools of thought about the number of regional cooking areas in the Middle East. One identifies three culinary areas: Greek/Turkish, Iranian, and Arabic. The other makes five divisions: Greek/Turkish, Arabic, North African, Iranian, and Israeli. Certainly every region has some unique recipes and cooking methods, but the similarity in fare throughout the region is striking. Israel probably has the most different foods and food habits because its cuisine blends the indigenous Middle Eastern cooking with that of the many Jewish immigrant groups (Russians, Germans, Austrians, and eastern Europeans) who have settled in the area since the turn of the century. Furthermore, many of Israel's citizens adhere to the kosher laws of the Jewish religion (see Chapter 2 for more information on Jewish dietary practices). More generally, Arabic foods feature more grains, legumes, and vegetables than the Greek, Turkish, Armenian, or Iranian diet. Conversely, meats, cheeses, and oils are more prominent in the cuisines of Greece, Turkey, Armenia, and Iran.

Dill was a sacred plant in ancient Egypt.

The Arabs were the first to mix gum arabic with sugar to produce chewing gum. The Greeks prefer to chew on the licorice-flavored resin *mastic* (source of the verb *masticate).*

A Serbian specialty, popular throughout the former Yugoslavia, is *sljivovica,* a very high-proof brandy distilled from plums.

Preparing Middle Eastern coffee. The coffee of Greece and the Middle East is made in a long-handled *briki*. It is preferred strong, thick, and sweet and is often flavored with cardamom.

The cooking of Croatia, Slovenia, and Serbia has strong Middle Eastern elements due to more than 400 years of Turkish influence. Grilled meats, especially lamb, are popular. Kabobs and ground lamb meat patties are skewered and cooked over grapevine branches or charcoal. Eggplants, tomatoes, and onions are frequently consumed. *Musaka,* a minced meat and vegetable dish, is similar to the Greek version. Large, flat wheat breads are made in the countryside, and *potica,* the national bread of Slovenia, is flavored with nuts, raisins, or tarragon. Wheat kernels are cooked with sugar, dried fruits, and ground nuts to make the Serbian dish called *koljivo.* Pastries similar to Arab sanbusak are called *burek* in Slovenia. Filo dough, known as *pita* in the region, is used in numerous recipes, especially desserts; *baklava* is a favorite. Goat and sheep cheeses and fermented dairy products are common. Turkish coffee, and a variation known as Serbian coffee, is consumed at the end of nearly every meal and accompanies snacks. Croatian, Slovenian, and Serbian fare also features many foods found in central Europe, such as paprika-flavored stews, dumplings, and roast pigs and hams, as well as stuffed cabbage (*sarma*) and sauerkraut dishes (see Chapter 4 for more information about central European cuisine).

Meal Composition and Cycle

Daily Patterns

People in Greece and other Middle Eastern countries eat three meals a day. The main meal is at midday, and in the hotter climates a short nap follows. Dinner is lighter and is served in the cooler evening hours. In addition, a wide variety of bite-size snacks, *mezze,* are available in cafés and served at home throughout the day for friends and relatives, either as appetizers or as a meal in themselves.

In Greece the traditional breakfast may consist of a slice or two of bread with cheese, olives, or jam, accompanied by coffee or tea. The main meal, eaten at around 2:00 PM, might include a meat stew, meatballs, or vegetables stuffed with chopped meat or baked beans, a salad of raw seasonal vegetables, yogurt or cheese, and fruit as dessert. Roasted or baked whole meats are served on weekends, accompanied by cooked vegetables, salad, and dessert.

In other Middle Eastern countries, coffee or tea is often served first for breakfast, followed by a light meal that might include cheeses, eggs, olives, jam and bread, and plain yogurt. Lunch is the main meal of the day, eaten between noon and 2:00 PM. It is typically a meat and vegetable stew served with rice and bread. Supper is light, like breakfast, but it may also include sandwiches.

Throughout Greece and the Middle East, coffee and tea are the common beverages consumed after the meal. Frequently coffee is flavored with cardamom and tea is flavored with mint. Coffee is also served in cafés. Traditionally the drink is made in a long-handled metal *briki,* producing a strong, very thick, and often sweet brew that is served in small cylindrical cups.

In Turkey, tripe soup with vinegar and garlic is customarily eaten after dinner and is served with alcoholic beverages.

In the Middle East, coffee is consumed sweetened at happy occasions; it is drunk black and bitter at funerals.

Early Turkish immigrants to the United States were mostly young men without families; their social lives were centered around coffeehouses.

"Give the guest food even though you yourself are starving" is an Arabic saying.

Iranians say *"Namek geer,"* meaning "I have eaten your food, now I am your slave."

Unlike most Middle Easterners, Turks consider it rude to eat with your fingers; a fork and knife are preferred.

Etiquette

Throughout the Middle East, hospitality is a duty and a family's status is measured by how guests are treated. Guests, even uninvited ones, are made to feel welcome and are automatically offered food and drink. Even if they refuse at first, they must eventually accept, as refusal is considered an insult. Invited guests bring a gift, often candy or other sweets, and the host must open it immediately and serve them some. One is obligated to feed a guest, but which pieces of certain foods the guest is given and in what order the food is served express the recipient's status. Status is based on sex, age, family, and social rank. For example, a dignitary or head of the family is served the best portion first. In some areas, it is customary for women to eat separately from men.

Guests are traditionally entertained in a separate room before the meal, at which time scented water is provided so they may wash their hands. The dining table might be a large round metal tray, resting on a low stool or platform, and the diners sit around it on cushions. In Iran, food is traditionally served on a rug. The meal is set out in several bowls placed on the table or rug and then shared by the diners. After the meal the guests leave the table, wash their hands, and then have coffee or tea.

Several rules of etiquette apply to eating. One should always wash one's hands before eating, eat with three fingers (usually on the right hand), and lick the fingers after eating. It is considered polite to con-

Assorted Egyptian pastries made with filo dough, couscous, and nuts. (Corbis/Dave Bartruff.)

tinue eating until everyone else is finished, because if one person stops eating the others feel compelled to stop too. One should leave a little food on one's plate to indicate satisfaction with the abundance of the meal. Only pleasant and joyful things are discussed while dining, and one must compliment the host and hostess.

Special Occasions

In Greece and the Middle Eastern countries, food plays an important role in the celebration of special occasions (often religious) and in the observance of certain events like weddings and births.

In the Eastern Orthodox Church there are numerous feast and fast days (see Chapter 2). The most important religious holiday for the Greeks is Easter. Immediately after midnight mass on Holy Saturday the family shares the first post-Lenten meal. It traditionally begins with red-dyed Easter eggs and continues with *mayeritsa,* a soup made of the lamb's internal organs, sometimes flavored with *avgolemono,* a tart egg and lemon sauce used throughout the Middle East. The Easter Sunday meal ususally consists of roast lamb, rice pilaf, accompanying vegetables, cheese, yogurt, and a special Easter bread called *lambropsomo* that is decorated with whole, dyed eggs. Dessert usually includes sweet pastries made with filo dough and *koulourakia,* a traditional Greek sweet bread cookie, sometimes shaped into a hairpin twist or wreath or coiled in the shape of a snake (which the pagan Greeks worshiped for its healing powers).

In addition to religious holidays, Greek Americans typically celebrate Greek Independence Day on March 25th. It is commemorated with parades in traditional dress, folk dancing, songs, and poetry readings.

There are also feasts and fasts connected with Islamic religious observances. Traditional festive foods vary from country to country. *Iftar* is the meal that breaks the fast during Ramadan, the month in which Muslims fast from sunrise to sunset; it is common to dine with relatives and neighbors. The meal usually starts with a beverage, preferably water, followed by an odd number of dates and coffee or tea. A large meal, served after prayers, includes dishes that are moist and hearty. Regular items eaten during Ramadan include soups, fruit juices, fresh or dried fruit, and *kataif,* a sweet, stuffed pancake. The dawn meal is usually light, and salty foods are avoided because water is not allowed during the fast. The holiday Eid al-Fitr follows the end of Ramadan and is described as a cross between the feasting of Thanksgiving and the festivity of Christmas. Typically family, friends, and neighbors gather to celebrate; in areas with large Muslim populations, Eid al-Fitr may be held at the local fairgrounds with games, rides, and many food vendors. The other major holiday observed by Arab Muslims is Eid al-Adha, the Feast of Sacrifice, which is held in conjunction with the annual pilgrimage (Hadj) to Mecca (see Chapter 2).

At Greek baptisms the infant is first rubbed in olive oil, then immersed three times in the baptismal font to represent the 3 days Jesus was entombed.

For New Year's the Greeks prepare a sweet spicy bread called *vasilopitta* that has a coin baked into it. The person who gets the piece with the money has good luck in the upcoming year. The Serbs have the same tradition for Christmas Day.

In Greece and the Middle East, sugared almonds (Jordan almonds) are served at weddings to ensure sweetness in married life.

Some non-Christian Arab Americans celebrate the birth of Jesus on Christmas; Christ is considered a prophet in Islam.

On the tenth day of the first lunar month of the Islamic calendar, Turks celebrate the martyrdom of Mohammed's grandson and the day Noah was able to leave the ark. They prepare *aşure,* or Noah's pudding, made from the ingredients remaining after the flood waters receded: fresh and dried fruits, nuts, and legumes.

In Iran the most significant holiday of the year is Muharram, which commemorates the martyrdom of the grandson of Mohammed in the seventh century. It is a time of communal mourning and penitence for Shi'ites. Another celebration marking the spring equinox is Nau Roz, which features a meal that must include seven foods that start with the letter "s." The number seven probably relates to the seven days of the week or the seven planets of the ancient solar system. On the thirteenth day of Nau Roz it is customary to have a picnic.

A special occasion in Turkey is National Sovereignty and Children's Day on April 23rd. It commemorates the establishment of the Grand National Assembly in 1923 and specifically honors all children. The following day has become Turkish American Day in the United States, featuring parades in traditional dress and other festivities.

In addition to traditional Orthodox holidays, Armenians commemorate the martyr St. Vartan on February 10th and on September 23rd celebrate their declaration of independence from the former Soviet Union in 1991. In Croatia, Christmas Eve features a meal of cod, and a stuffed cabbage and sauerkraut dish is customary on Christmas. The Easter meal is typically lamb or ham and *pogaca,* an Easter bread that is similar to the Greek lambropsomo with painted eggs on top. Slovenians celebrate St. Nick's Feast. Gifts are distributed to children by St. Nick, dressed as a bishop, who admonishes the youngsters to be good. The grape harvest and winemaking are traditionally commemorated with numerous vintage festivals and St. Martin's Feast. Among Serbians the most auspicious day of the year is Krsna Slava, Patron Saint's Day. This holiday dates back to the worship of protective spirits in pagan times; today each family honors its self-chosen patron saint with a sumptuous feast and dancing that may last for 2 to 3 days. The family customarily announces the annual open house with a small advertisement in the local newspaper. *Krsni kolac* is a ritual bread prepared for the occasion, decorated with the religious Serbian emblem Samo, Sloga, Srvina, Spasava ("Only Unity Will Save the Serbs") as well as grapes, wheat, birds, flowers, barrels of wine, or other representations made in dough.

Contemporary Food Habits in the United States

Adaptations of Food Habits

There is scant information on the adaptation of Greek and Arab diets in the United States. It is assumed that, as in other immigrant groups, increasing length of stay is correlated with some Americanization of the diet, with traditional dishes prepared and eaten only for the main meal or for special occasions.

Ingredients and Common Foods

It has been reported that Greek Americans still use olive oil extensively, although they use less of it than their immigrant relatives (Valassi, 1962). Salads still accompany the meal, and fruit is often served for dessert. Vegetables are prepared in the traditional manner. Lamb is still very popular; for special occasions, roasted leg of lamb is substituted for the whole animal. Consumption of beef and pork has increased, whereas consumption of legumes has decreased. Cereal and grain consumption among Greek Americans remains high, and bread, rice, or cereal products are usually included in every meal. Greek Americans consume more milk than their immigrant parents, and ice cream is very popular.

Meal Composition and Cycle

Greek Americans maintain traditional meal patterns, but the main meal of the day is now dinner (Valassi, 1962). They prefer an American-type breakfast and lunch, but dinner is more traditional. However, they have adapted Greek recipes to make them less time-consuming to prepare and to include fewer fats and spices.

Reportedly many Arab Americans still eat their main meal at midday (Lipson & Meleis, 1983). Members of the extended family may dine together daily, with the women who stay at home cooking for employed female relatives (Packard & McWilliams, 1993).

Therapeutic Uses of Foods

The amount of food eaten is of special concern in the Middle Eastern diet. Ample meals are needed to prevent illness, and poor appetite is regarded as a disease in itself or as a generalized complaint signifying that one's life is not as it should be. Food deprivation is believed to cause illness (Meleis, 1981; Spector, 1991; Packard & McWilliams, 1993). Some Middle Easterners also believe that illness can be caused by hot-cold shifts in food or by eating incompatible foods together (Meleis, 1981; Lipson & Meleis, 1983). Examples of foods classified as hot include walnuts and honey; cucumbers and yogurt are cold foods. The temperature (not spiciness) can cause a shift in the body from hot to cold and vice versa, and it is believed the digestive system must have time to adjust to one extreme before a food of the opposite temperature can be introduced. Extreme shifts are thought to cause headaches, colds, and the flu. Furthermore, fresh foods are considered best and canned or frozen foods must be avoided to preserve health. Certain combinations of foods should not be eaten; for example, Egyptians do not consume fish at the same time as dairy products.

The demand for properly slaughtered *(halal)* meat among Muslims in the United States has led to increased numbers of Arab halal markets.

Greek weddings in the United States offer a blend of Greek and American foods; for example, the wedding cake is served along with baklava.

The Turks begin their meals with the prayer "May what you eat bring you well-being."

Eggs cooked in garlic and chicken soup are frequently consumed by Lebanese women after childbirth.

10

Asian Indians

India is a culturally complex country with a population of more than 967 million people, nearly four times that of the United States. The sophisticated civilization began approximately 4,000 years ago and is the source of some of the most influential religions, art, architecture, and foods in the world. The South Asian subcontinent contains the fertile Indus and Ganges river basins, as well as parts of the Himalayan mountain range; it varies in climate from extensive desert regions to jungle forests to the world's largest mountain glaciers. (See the map in Figure 10.1.)

The people of India are as diverse as its geography and climate. People from virtually every racial and religious group have migrated to or invaded India at some time in history, and each brought its own language and customs. As the different races and religions intermingled, other cultures were created. One result is that there are currently 15 separate languages recognized by the Indian government. Nearly 300 languages are actually spoken in India, and there are approximately 700 dialects.

It is estimated that more than 815,000 Asian Indians live in the United States today. They represent numerous racial and religious groups, yet many share high education levels and socioeconomic status. This chapter examines traditional Indian foods and food habits, as well as the dietary changes that occur when Asian Indians live in America.

The early settlers in India called the region *Bharat,* still an official name for the country.

FIGURE 10.1
India.

Cultural Perspective

History of India

The earliest civilization in India arose in the Indus valley around 2500 BCE. The largest city, Mohenjo-Daro, was a commercial trade center based on advanced metal, pottery, and cotton fabric crafts.

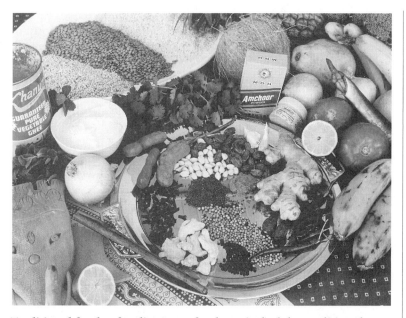

Traditional foods of India. Some foods typical of the traditional Indian diet include *amchoor* (mango powder), *basmati* rice, broccoli, coconut, cucumber, eggplant, *ghee,* herbs and spices (black pepper, cardamom, chiles, fresh coriander, cloves, coriander seeds, cumin, garlic, ginger root, mint, mustard seeds, nutmeg, tamarind, and turmeric), lentils, peas, plantains, and yogurt. (Photo by Laurie Macfee.)

Sometime between 1500 and 1200 BCE, Aryan peoples from Persia (now Iran) began to settle first in bordering Afghanistan, then in the Ganges valley. The early invaders overwhelmed the descendants of the Mohenjo-Daro culture, who are known as Dravidians. The combination of the Aryan and Dravidian cultures laid the foundation for Indian society, including the development of Hinduism and Sanskrit (the official language of India for more than 2,000 years).

The first Hindu empire was established under Chandra-Gupta Maurya, who ousted Alexander the Great (of Greece) from northern India in 320 BCE. He founded the Maurya dynasty, unifying two-thirds of the Indian peninsula. His grandson, Ashoka, was influential in the spread of Buddhism in the third century BCE. The dissolution of the Mauryan dynasty in 185 BCE resulted in numerous small regional governments. Northern India was united again 500 years later with the formation of the Gupta empire. Invasions from groups such as the White Huns terminated Gupta rule around 470.

Beginning in the tenth century, India was subjected to numerous waves of Muslim invaders from Mongolia and Afghanistan. A sultanate was established in Delhi and was extended in the fourteenth century throughout northern India. The Moghul (from the Persian word for Mongolian) empire was established in 1526 by Babar the Moghul; it was strengthened by his successors, including Akbar the Great. The Hindu rule of Vijayanagar in southern India coincided with the Moghul empire.

European contact with India began in 1497, with the arrival of Vasco de Gama from Portugal. The Dutch, French, and British were soon competing with the Portuguese for trade with India. The British East India Company rose to prominence, monopolizing European trade and subduing the Moghuls in 1757. The Hindus in central and south India were conquered in 1818. Rule passed from the British East India Company to the British government in 1858, following the massacre of British citizens in the Indian mutiny (the Sepoy rebellion of the Bengal Army) of 1857. British India was divided into sixteen provinces and included numerous states that were under British domination but governed by Indian princes.

In 1885 the Indian National Congress was formed by Indians who were discontented with British hegemony. It was followed in 1906 by the founding of the All-Indian Muslim League. Opposition to British rule grew after World War I, and a program of noncooperation was begun in 1920 by Mohandas (Mahatma) K. Gandhi. Pressure from the Indian nationalists for complete independence and from the Muslim League for a separate Muslim state resulted in limited powers being granted in 1919 and 1935. As total independence was negotiated with Britain in 1946, savage rioting erupted between Muslims and Hindus throughout northern India. When unity could not be achieved, a compromise establishing the independent nations of Pakistan (predominantly Muslim) and India (predominantly Hindu) was accepted in 1947. Violence continued during the following year as Hindus fled Pakistan and Muslims from throughout India immigrated to Pakistan.

Jawaharlal Nehru was elected the first prime minister of the democratic republic of India. Border disputes have occurred with both China, in 1962, and Pakistan, in 1965 and 1971. Nehru's daughter, Indira Gandhi, was elected prime minister in 1967. A short war with Pakistan in 1971 resulted in the formation of the nation of Bangladesh out of eastern Pakistan. Gandhi remained in power until her assassination in 1984 by members of the Sikh religion as retribution for purported government repressions. In spite of continuing tensions with neighboring nations and internal religious strife, India is currently the world's largest democracy.

The term *South Asia* is used for the nations of India, Pakistan, Bangladesh, Sri Lanka, Nepal, and Bhutan.

History of Asian Indians in the United States

Given the complexity of Indian culture, it is not surprising that the Asian Indian immigrants to the United States differ from other immigrant groups in several ways. Most significantly, the majority of Indians arriving in America are not escaping political or economic pressures in their homeland. Since 1965, when the national quota system was temporarily dropped from U.S. immigration laws, the majority of Asian Indian immigrants have been from the upper socioeconomic classes. They were somewhat acculturated at the time of arrival, often fluent in English, and acquainted with many American customs.

Immigration Patterns

The first immigrants to the United States from India were members of the Sikh religion, who arrived on the West Coast in the early twentieth century. Many were employed by the railroads and others established large farms. They faced overt discrimination and persecution. Newspapers warned of the "Hindoo invasion"; anti-Asian Indian feelings brought about the expulsion of Asian Indians from Washington logging communities and in 1907 sparked violent riots in California. Although such extreme bigotry lessened in time, the Asian Indian immigrant population remained small until after World War II.

Relaxed immigration laws encouraged Asian Indians, especially well educated urban professionals, to come to America in the 1960s and 1970s. Economic and social adjustment was a priority for this group, although many Asian Indian traditions continue within the privacy of the home. These immigrants formed a self-reliant community and discouraged comparison or identification with other ethnic groups.

Recent changes in Asian Indian immigration patterns may change this typically high degree of acculturation. Asian Indians coming to America today are more likely to be from rural towns and villages. They are less educated and have experienced less exposure to western society than previous Indian immigrants. There are also fewer professionals among them. Most recently arrived Indians are self-employed in jobs that serve their Asian Indian immigrant community, such as restauranteurs, importers, and travel agents.

As a result of the change in the Asian Indian immigrant profile, newcomers now identify more with their immediate ethnic subgroup community than with the wider, pan-Indian community. Their adjustment to American culture is more difficult. The religion, language, and social class of each cultural subgroup retain greater importance for recent immigrants than for previous immigrants from India.

Current Demographics and Socioeconomic Status

Today Asian Indians are one of the fastest growing immigrant groups in the United States. Their population more than doubled between 1980 and 1990, from 400,000 to more than 815,000. They have settled throughout the United States, but especially in the metropolitan

In the early 1900s, it was not unusual for single Sikh men living in the United States to marry Mexican American women and start families.

Small numbers of Asian Indians coming to the United States in recent years are exiles from regions where Indian immigration in the past has been substantial, such as East Africa and Fiji.

The 1990 U.S. Census reported more than 63,000 Americans of Pakistani descent.

Almost 27 percent of all hotels and motels in the United States are owned or operated by Asian Indian Americans.

Pakistani Americans are mostly well educated professionals earning middle- or upper-class incomes.

areas of California, New York, and New Jersey, as well as in Illinois, Maryland, Massachusetts, Michigan, Ohio, Pennsylvania, and Texas. There are also several Asian Indian communities in the agricultural regions of California.

The Asian Indian American community is very diverse, coming from numerous states and regions with distinctive languages and customs. The most prominent subgroups are the Gujaratis, Bengalis, Marathis, and Tamils.

The relative affluence of Americans of Asian Indian heritage is due to the large percentage of highly educated immigrants. Many were employed in professional or white-collar occupations in India, such as college professors, engineers, physicians, and scientists; most continue in their professions in the United States. Newer immigrants have found success in small business and franchise ownership involving many members of their extended family.

Many Asian Indians come to the United States to complete their college or postgraduate education. They are often unmarried or have left their spouses and children in India. It is not uncommon for the families to join the student in America after he or she has become financially established.

Cultural Organizations

In addition to small associations that serve the local needs of different Asian Indian ethnic or religious groups, three major national organizations were established in the 1970s to promote and protect pan-Asian Indian interests in the United States. They are the Association of Indians in America, the National Federation of Indian Associations, and the National Association of Americans of Asian Indian Descent.

Worldview

Ahimsa

A reverence for all life, called *ahimsa,* is fundamental to Asian Indian ideology. It is reflected in the religions native to India, as well as in the vegetarian diet that many Indians follow.

The best known example of ahimsa in the western world is the sacredness of the cow in India. It is difficult for most Americans to understand the logic of not eating beef when so many people in India exist on a subsistence level.

Anthropologists suggest that prohibitions against the slaughter of cattle serve several economic and ecological purposes in India. More than 80 percent of the Indian population lives in rural areas, and most make their living by farming. Cattle are the primary power source in this agricultural society. Animal power is required to grow the food each rural family requires; tractors and the fuels required to run them are too expensive for the average Indian farmer. Another source of energy obtained from cattle in India is dung, which is used as a clean, slow-burning cooking fuel. Because India has limited fossil fuel and forest resources, manure energy is important to both the Indian economy and the environment.

In addition to energy and power, cattle produce dung for fertilizer. Cows also provide milk for the dairy products vital to Indian vegetarian cuisine. Finally, even a dead cow serves a purpose in India. The very poor often survive through the sale of leather products crafted from salvaged hides and the consumption of needed protein gathered from carrion.

The Caste System

The traditional Indian caste system, which influences the social structure of many Asian Indian groups, is the Hindu method of ordering an individual's role in society. A more encompassing term is *jati,* which is the organization of all aspects of Hindu life, including actions, places, things, and symbols, not just people.

Caste categories are hereditary. There are four main castes associated with certain professions (although members are not necessarily employed in these jobs); the *brahmans* (priests), *kshatriyas* (soldiers), *vaisyas* (merchants or farmers), and the *sudras* (serfs). These castes are divided into more than 1,000 subcastes, usually according to occupation. Existing outside the caste system are individuals who are considered so impure that they are called "untouchables." Although the laws discriminating against untouchability were repealed in 1949, this group of the desperately poor continues to occupy the lowest stratum in Indian society.

The untouchables were considered impure because of their contact with cattle carcasses and their consumption of scavenged beef.

The caste system has permeated Indian society despite the fact that it is an exclusively Hindu classification system. Americans of Asian Indian descent often continue to identify proudly with their caste. Most come from the upper castes of brahmans and kshatriyas.

Religion

The influence of religion on Indian culture is ubiquitous. Every aspect of life and death is affected not only by individual religious affiliation, but also by the Hindu ideology that pervades Indian society.

Hinduism   Nearly 85 percent of Indians are Hindus. Hinduism is an ancient faith, believed to have developed in India between 2000 and 1500 BCE from the Aryan hymns and prayers known as the *Vedas* mixed with elements from traditional Dravidian religion (see Chapter 2 for more information about Hinduism and other major Indian religions).

The Hindu Society of India established community organizations to serve the religious needs of early Asian Indian immigrants to the United States. Many Hindu temples now exist in regions where Asian

Indians have settled, with services and religious ceremonies conducted by Brahman priests (who are often employed part-time in other occupations). However, temple attendance may be limited to significant religious events. Small shrines are often created in Asian Indian apartments or houses so that prayer and meditation may take place at home.

Islam   Today the Islamic religion is second only to Hinduism in number of followers; one in every nine Asian Indians is a Muslim. Islam was brought to India by traders from Persia, and it expanded with the Muslim invasions of the northern regions beginning about 1000. The Islamic Moghul empire dominated the country for nearly 800 years. The influence of Islam is seen today mostly in northern India.

Buddhism   Buddhism developed as a protestant revolt against Hinduism. Its founder, known as Gautama Buddha, lived in India during the fifth century BCE. Although it is a popular religion in other parts of Asia, Buddhism is followed by fewer than 1 percent of Asian Indians today.

Jainism   This branch of Hinduism developed at about the time Buddhism emerged. The Jains believed that all living things have souls. Some wear masks to prevent breathing in insects and sweep a path in front of them to prevent stepping on any creatures. Orthodox Jains are strict vegetarians. Approximately 2 percent of Indians are Jains; in the United States, Jains have established their own temples for worship.

Sikhism   The Sikh religion differs from Hinduism in its belief in a single God. It is best known for its military fraternity, although most Sikhs in India are farmers. Male Sikhs wear a turban and follow the "five Ks": uncut hair (*kes*), a comb worn in the hair (*kanga*), short pants (*kaccha*), a steel bracelet worn on the right wrist (*kada*), and use of a special saber (*kirpan*). Each has a spiritual meaning; for example, the short pants symbolize self-restraint, the bracelet obedience, and the comb purity of mind.

Syrian Christians   One form of Christianity emerged when the Syrians, who migrated to the Malabar coast of southwest India in 345, intermarried with native people. Syrian Christians do not observe Hindu dietary laws, but they do participate in the caste system. Their agricultural community is operated with farm laborers who can be described as serfs.

Nearly all Pakistani Americans are Muslim; small numbers of Hindus, Christians, and Zoroastrians are also part of the community.

It was the popularity of Buddhism that spread vegetarianism throughout India. Hinduism consequently encouraged abstinence from eating meat, a concept consistent with *ahimsa*.

Although Sikhs are only 2 percent of the population in India, it is estimated that they make up nearly one-third of Asian Indians living in California.

The *kirpan* has become a civil rights issue in some public schools, pitting religious freedom against provisions restricting "weapons" on campus.

Goan Christians Another Christian community developed at the former Portuguese colony of Goa, farther north on the southwest coast. Approximately half of the citizens are Catholic, and the city is dedicated to St. Catherine.

Zoroastrianism More than 1,200 years ago the Parsis fled from religious persecution in Persia to northern India. The religion they brought is known as Zoroastrianism, an ancient faith that venerates Ahur Mazda, the wise god of fire. The Parsis have adapted many of their practices to blend into Indian society but have maintained their faith through private schooling of their children. They are considered the most westernized of all Indians; significant Parsi communities have developed in New York and Los Angeles.

Judaism Four small Jewish communities were established in India when Jews fled persecution in Greece, Palestine (under Roman domination), Iraq, and Germany. The largest populations are found in Bombay and Calcutta.

Animism The oldest religions in India are those practiced by the small tribal populations that live in isolated regions of the Himalayas. They worship spirits associated with natural phenomena, a religious practice known as *animism*. In the past they have practiced such varied social customs as polyandry (having more than one husband) and head hunting.

Family

The husband is the head of the household in the traditional Indian family. The wife usually does not work outside the home and is expected to perform all duties related to housekeeping and child care. She obtains help in these responsibilities from the extended family and, in some homes, from servants. If the wife does hold a job, she can depend on the help of relatives. Children are expected to show respect for their elders; parents may choose what career a child should pursue. Dating is uncommon in India, and many marriages are arranged by families based on similarities in caste, education, religion, and upbringing between prospective husbands and wives.

Strains in the traditional family structure often occur in the United States. Asian Indian women are more likely to work in America than in their homeland, yet they lack the support system of an extended family. Elders may also find themselves cut off from their traditional role of advisors and may not have opportunities for involvement in certain religious activities that would fill their lives in India. Some Asian Indians, especially women raised in India, find it difficult to

It is estimated that Christians make up 3 percent of the population in India.

The sacred fires of Zoroastrianism are tended in temples protected from the sun and from the eyes of unbelievers.

Asian Indian religions, particularly Hinduism and Buddhism, have attracted some non-Indian followers in the United States.

In India, marriage is considered the beginning of a relationship from which love develops over time.

adjust to these changes. More men than women choose to become U.S. citizens.

Children who grow up in the United States usually insist on making their own career choices. Dating has become more acceptable, but most parents strongly discourage relationships with persons of other ethnic or religious backgrounds. Although most parents do not choose their child's spouse, many Asian Indian children still defer to their parents' opinion; young male students in the United States sometimes ask their families in India to find a suitable mate for them.

Asian Indian Americans who are financially secure often assume responsibility for less prosperous relatives.

The family is seen as the way to preserve Indian values and beliefs while living in America. Even after establishing permanent residence, a majority of Asian Indians regard their national identity as more Indian than American (Sodowsky & Carey, 1988). There is also strong interest in sponsoring the immigration of relatives to the United States. Most Asian Indians have found successful adjustment in the United States through educational and economic achievement in American public life, while maintaining an emphasis on Asian Indian culture within the privacy of their home life.

Communication

A leisurely, personal style of communication is preferred by most Asian Indians. Small talk is significant, and rushing is considered rude. A direct "no" is considered impolite, so an evasive negative response is the norm. Feelings and faith may be more important than objective facts. Some Indian women are less vocal than men.

Several nonverbal communication customs among Asian Indians are significant. Most Indian Hindu, Sikh, and Christian men and women avoid contact with the opposite sex in public, and contact between men and women in public is completely prohibited by Muslims. The traditional greeting is to nod with the head while holding the hands palm to palm beneath the chin and saying *namaste* (nah-mas-tay), but westernized Indians will use a handshake (it is best to wait and follow the lead). Some Asian Indians indicate agreement by shaking their head back and forth the way Americans indicate the negative. Informal smiles are used between equals only—superiors do not generally smile at subordinates or vice versa. The left hand is never used for any social purposes, including handshakes, giving an item to another person, or pointing. The head is considered the seat of the soul; patting or touching another person's head should always be avoided. Conversely, the feet and shoe soles are considered the dirtiest parts of the body, and it is impolite to point with the foot or show the bottom of one's shoe (Axtell, 1991; Morrison et al., 1994). All that said, it should be noted that most Asian Indian Americans are highly acculturated and can converse in a style comfortable for Americans.

Traditional Food Habits

It is difficult to generalize about Indian cuisine because of the diverse geography and heterogeneous population of the country. Foods vary north to south, east to west, region to region, and among religious and caste groups.

Ingredients and Common Foods

Staples

Few foods are eaten throughout all of India. Rice is the most commonly consumed. The average Indian eats one-half pound of it each day. This amount, however, varies considerably by region. Fruits and vegetables predominate in the frequently vegetarian cooking, but the types and ways in which they are prepared also depend on local customs. Dairy foods are also important in most areas. Fermented milk products such as yogurt are found throughout most of the country, as is the cooking fat *ghee,* which is pure, clarified butter (this butter, known as *usli ghee,* is too expensive for daily use in many homes, so vegetable shortening, also called ghee, is often used instead). Seasonings are distinctive. *Masalas* are mixtures of spices and herbs that can be either fresh and "wet" or dried and powdered. Coriander, cumin, fenugreek, turmeric, black and cayenne pepper, cloves, cardamom, cinnamon, and chile peppers are a common blend that is called curry in western countries. Other typical spices and herbs include *ajwain* (carom or loveage seeds), *asafetida* (a pungent powdered resin), coconut, fresh coriander, garlic, mint, saffron, and *tamarind* (the sour pulp of a bean pod). Beyond these generalities, the staples of the Indian diet are best classified by region.

The greatest division in diet is seen between northern and southern India. Northern cuisine is characterized by the use of wheat, tea, a large number of eggs, garlic, dried or pickled fruits and vegetables, and use of dry masalas that are aromatic rather than hot. These foods are typical of a cooler climate, where wheat grows better than rice and where fruits, vegetables, herbs, and spices are available only seasonally. Boiling, stewing, and frying are the most common forms of cooking.

In the South, steaming is the preferred method of food preparation. Rice, coffee, fresh pickles (some of which are known as *chutney), pachadi* (seasoned yogurt side dishes that are called *raytas* in northern India), "wet" masalas that are spicy hot, and fresh fruits, vegetables, herbs, and spices are fundamental to the cuisine. Again, these foods reflect the regional agricultural conditions.

Approximately 30 percent of Asian Indians are strict vegetarians; they use some milk products but avoid eggs. Distribution of vegetarianism ranges from 6 percent in some coastal states to two-thirds of

Ghee is sometimes poured over sacred images in the worship of certain Hindu deities.

The word *curry* is believed to be the English adaptation of a southern Indian term for sauce, *kari.* Curry powder is not a single spice, but a complex blend of seasonings that varies according to the cook and the dish. The closest Indian equivalent is *garam masala.*

the population in other states located in the northwestern regions of the country (Achaya, 1994). Pork is eaten in some communities in the West, lamb and beef are eaten in many areas of the North, and fish and poultry are eaten in several coastal regions. The Cultural Food Groups list is found in Table 10.1.

Regional Variations

Northern India In the North, rice is commonly served as a pilaf. Saffron rice with seasoned chicken, lamb, or beef, called *biryani*, is also popular, as are meatballs (*kofta*) and skewered pieces of broiled or grilled meats (*kababs*). Northern specialties include *korma*, a curried lamb dish with a nut and yogurt-thickened sauce, and masala chicken.

Bread, which is called *roti* in India, is eaten daily. Examples include whole wheat flat breads, such as *chapatis*, which are cooked on a griddle without oil, and *puris*, which are fried. *Paratha*, another fried roti, is used as a wrapping for spiced vegetable fillings; a spicy lamb, potato, or vegetable stuffing is used in the deep-fried turnovers called *samosas*. Milk desserts are favored, such as carrot pudding (*gajar halva*) and rice pudding with cardamom, called *kheer*.

In northwestern India a special cylindrical clay oven heated with charcoal and called a *tandoor* is used. *Tandoori* cooking is identified particularly with lamb and chicken dishes, although the leavened bread known as *naan* is also typically baked in a tandoor.

Coastal India The coastal regions offer a number of seafood specialties, including curried shrimp, crab, and clam dishes. Fish is prepared in a variety of ways, including fried, steamed, boiled, curried, and stuffed with herbs. Bombay, located on the west coast, boasts a dried salted fish, which is thin, bony, and strongly flavored, known as Bombay duck.

Southern India The menus of the South feature numerous steamed and fried rice dishes. Rice is even served puffed, as in a snack called *bhelpuri*. Other grains such as semolina wheat are also popular cooked as a cereal known as *uppama*, which may include vegetables. *Dals*, particularly chickpeas and lentils, accompany nearly every meal in the form of a spiced puree known as *sambar* or as a thin, crisply fried roti called *pappadams*. Fermented lentil flour is used at breakfast for *idli*, which are steamed cakes, and for *dosas*, which are spicy, fried pancakes. Fresh milk curds are also served for breakfast.

Highly spiced vegetable curries, such as *aviyal*, include such southern ingredients as bananas, bitter melons, coconut, green mango, and jackfruit seeds, in addition to potatoes, cauliflower, and eggplant. Refreshing yogurt-based pachadi and spicy pickled fruits or

Pakistani fare combines elements of Indian and Arab cooking. Halal meats (see Chapter 2) are consumed, often prepared in a *tandoor.* Flat breads and pilafs are common. Popular Asian Indian spices, such as cumin, turmeric, and chiles, are combined with more typically Arab flavors of cinnamon, cloves, and cardamom.

Dal is the Hindu word for grains, legumes, or seeds (called *pulses* in India) that have been hulled and split in half—for example, split peas.

vegetables, such as chutney, accompany the main course. Deep-fried salty foods are favored snacks, as are deep-fried sweets, such as the syrup-soaked, orange-colored pretzels called *jalebis*.

Religious Variations

In addition to region, religious affiliation may greatly influence food habits in India. Religious groups have varying dietary practices, yet their cooking is Indian in flavor. Muslims, for example, avoid all pork and pork products but are not vegetarians. Orthodox Jains may only eat "innocent" foods that avoid injury to any life and are therefore strict vegetarians. In addition, there are twenty-two prohibited foods (such as fruit with small seeds or tender new greens) and thirty-two other items that may have the potential for life to exist (including root vegetables, because insects might be killed when the tubers are harvested). They also refuse to eat any blood-colored foods such as tomatoes and watermelon. Sikh cuisine is noted for its use of wheat, corn, and sugar and the complete abstinence from alcohol and beef (pork is permitted).

The Syrian Christians are renowned for their beef (tenderized by mincing or marinating), duck, and wild boar dishes. Goan Christians are unique in Indian cooking for their use of pork. They make western-style sausages and have such specialties as a vinegar-basted hog's head stuffed with vegetables and herbs. Most Jews in India keep kosher. The Parsis blend Indian and Persian elements in their cuisine, exemplified by dishes such as *dhansak,* an entree combining lamb, tripe, lentils, and vegetables. Eggs are especially popular such as *ekuri,* spicy scrambled eggs.

Meal Composition and Cycle

Daily Patterns

Meal patterns in India, though not consistent across regions and classes, vary less than the foods served. Two full meals with substantial snacks are typical. A rich coffee or tea made with milk and sugar is enjoyed by early risers. Breakfast is usually eaten between 9:00 and 11:00 AM, consisting of rice or roti, a pickled fruit or vegetable, and a sambar, or lentil stew, which may be left over from the previous evening. At 4:00 or 5:00 PM, similar foods or snack items are eaten with coffee or tea. The main meal of the day follows between 7:00 and 9:00 PM.

Texture, color, and balance of seasoning are all important factors in an Indian meal. A menu customarily includes at least one rice dish; a curried vegetable, legume, or meat dish; a vegetable legume side dish; a baked or fried roti; a fruit or vegetable pickle; and a yogurt rayta

The English words "pepper," "sugar," and "orange" are all derived from Asian Indian terms for those foods.

Honey is prohibited by Jains because bees might be killed when it is gathered from the hive.

A French Christian colony on the east coast of India at Pondicherry introduced baguettes, croissants, pâté, and French-style desserts into the regional fare.

Traditionally six tastes (sweet, sour, salty, bitter, pungent, and astringent) and five textures (foods that need to be chewed, those that need no chewing, those that are licked, those that are sucked, and those that are drunk) were balanced in an Indian meal.

TABLE 10.1
Cultural Food Groups: Asian Indian

Group	Comments
PROTEIN FOODS	
Milk/milk products	In general, milk is considered a beverage for children. Fermented dairy products popular.
Meats/poultry/fish/eggs/legumes	Sophisticated vegetarian cuisine; legumes primary protein source.
	Eighteen varieties of beans, peas, and lentils commonly used.
	Hulled, split legumes, grains, and seeds, such as lentils, are known as *dals*.
	Legumes are typically prepared whole or pureed, or used as flour to prepare baked, steamed, or fried breads and pastries.
CEREALS/GRAINS	More than 1,000 varieties of rice are cultivated.
	Wheat used mostly in the North; rice in the South.
	Most breads (*roti*) are unleavened.
FRUITS/VEGETABLES	More than 100 types of fruit and 200 types of vegetables are commonly used.
	Fruits and vegetables may be used in fresh or preserved pickles, called *rayta* (northern), *pachadi* (southern), or chutney.
ADDITIONAL FOODS	
Seasonings	Aromatic (northern) and hot (southern) combinations of fresh or dried spices and herbs accentuate or complement food flavors.
Nuts/seeds	Nuts and seeds of all types popular. Used to thicken *korma* sauces.
Beverages	Tea common in the North; coffee in the South. Coffeehouses are favored meeting places.
Fats/oils	
Sweeteners	

or pachadi. Sometimes a dessert is served, usually fruit. Courses are not presented sequentially in Indian meals; they are placed on the table all at once. Savory dishes are eaten at the same time as sweets.

TABLE 10.1
Cultural Food Groups: Asian Indian—continued

Common Foods	Adaptations in the United States
Fresh cow's, buffalo's, ass's milk; evaporated milk; fermented milk products (yogurt, *lassi*); fresh curds very popular; milk-based desserts, such as *kheer, khir, kulfi, barfi*	More cheese consumed, ice cream popular..
Meats: beef, goat, mutton, pork *Poultry:* chicken, duck *Fish and seafood:* Bombay duck, carp, clams, crab, herring, mackerel, mullet, pomfret, sardines, shrimp, turtle *Eggs:* chicken *Legumes:* beans (kidney, mung, etc.), chickpeas, lentils (many varieties and colors), peas (black-eyed, green)	Consumption of legumes decreases; meat intake increases. Meat may be added to traditional vegetarian dishes. Fast foods popular.
Buckwheat, rice (steamed, boiled, fried, puffed), millet, wheat	Use of American-style breads in place of *roti;* breakfast cereals popular.
Fruit: apples, avocados, bananas (several types), coconut, dates, figs, grapes, guava, jackfruit, limes, litchis, loquats, mangoes, melon, *nongus,* oranges, papaya, peaches, pears, persimmons (*chicos*), pineapple, pomegranate, pomelos, raisins, starfruit, strawberries, sugar cane, tangerines, watermelon *Vegetables:* agathi flowers, amaranth, artichokes, bamboo shoots, banana rhizome, beets (leaves and root), bitter melon, brussels sprouts, cabbage, carrots, cauliflower, collard greens (*haak*), corn, cucumbers, eggplant, lettuce, lotus root, manioc (tapioca), mushrooms, mustard greens, okra, onions, parsnips, plantain flowers, potatoes, radishes (four types, leaves and roots), rhubarb, sago palm, spinach, squash, sweet potatoes (leaves and roots), tomatoes, turnips, yams, water chestnuts, water lilies	Decreased variety of fruits and vegetables available; decreased vegetable intake. More fruit juice consumed. Salad is well accepted. Use of canned and frozen produce increases.
Ajwain, amchoor, asafetida, bay leaf, cardamom (two types), chiles, cinnamon, cloves, coconut, fresh coriander, coriander seeds, cumin, dill, fennel, fenugreek, garlic, *kewra,* lemon, limes, mace, mint, mustard, nutmeg, pepper (black and red), poppy seeds, rose water, saffron, tamarind, turmeric	Spice use dependent on availability.
Almonds, betel nuts and leaves, cashews, peanuts, pistachios, sunflower seeds, walnuts	*Paan* tray may be limited to betel nuts and spices.
Coffee, tea, water flavored with fruit syrups, spices, or herbs; alcoholic beverages such as fermented fruit syrups, rice wines, beer	Increased consumption of soft drinks and coffee. Alcoholic beverages widely accepted (women may abstain).
Coconut oil, *ghee* (clarified butter), mustard oil, peanut oil, sesame seed oil	Purchased *ghee* often made from vegetable oil instead of butter.
Sugar cane, *jaggery* (unrefined palm sugar), molasses	Candy and sweets enjoyed, but not over-consumed.

Diners may combine tastes and textures according to personal preference. The meal concludes with the passing of the paan tray. *Paan* is a combination of betel (*areca*) nuts and spices, such as anise seed,

Samosas, **spicy deep-fried turnovers.**

It is illegal to bring betel leaves into the United States. There is a black market for *paan* obtained in Canada and other countries.

cardamom, and fennel, wrapped in large, heart-shaped betel leaves secured with a clove. It is chewed to freshen the breath and to aid digestion.

Snacking is very popular in India. In cities and small towns, snacks are sold in numerous small shops and by street vendors. In villages, they are prepared at home. A clear distinction is made between meals and snacks. Many Indian languages have specific words to define each form of eating. In southern India the word *tiffin* is used to distinguish a snack from a meal. The coffee or tea drunk before breakfast or in the late afternoon is considered tiffin. A meal is not a meal unless the traditional staple prepared in the traditional manner, such as boiled rice in southern India (or roti in northern India) is served. This means that no matter how substantial the snack—and some include more food than a meal—it is still called tiffin. Spicy snacks served with chutney often consist of batter-fried vegetables, pancakes with or without a filling, or fried seasoned dough made from wheat or lentils. Snacks sweetened with sugar cane, molasses, or jaggery are usually milk-based, such as the saffron-spiced *khir,* the Indian ice cream called *kulfi,* and the candy *barfi,* although nuts, coconut, sesame seeds, or lentils are also used. A snack may also include a cooling beverage, such as the sweetened, diluted yogurt drink called *lassi* or the fruit juice known as *shurbut.*

Etiquette

The most important aspect of Indian manners is that food is eaten with the hands. Food is served in small individual bowls from serving trays called *thalis*. The thalis may be silver or brass, with matching bowls. Originally the thalis were simply banana leaves and the bowls were earthenware; these are still used today in some rural areas or when disposable trays and bowls are desired.

Rules of etiquette are important for food that is eaten by hand and prepared with little or no means of refrigeration. Food spoilage and contamination are problems, especially in the warmer regions of the country. Cleanliness is imperative, and many Indian manners clearly support this need. Ancient rules of etiquette promoted healthy food preparation. They included the following: Everyone must clean their hands, feet, and mouth before and after eating, both morning and evening; servants who worked with food had to shave their beards and heads, cut their nails, and bathe before entering the kitchen; food that was cooked the previous night, that turned sour, or that was cooked twice must be discarded; and all grains, vegetables, and meat had to be washed thoroughly before cooking.

During the Buddhist period, other rules were added. Dating from 300 BCE, they recommended that one should not talk with food in one's mouth; stuff one's mouth full of food; shake one's hands while eating, as one would scatter rice all over; put one's tongue out while eating; make hissing sounds while eating; lick one's finger or bowl; or accept a drinking cup with hands that are soiled with food. Finally, everyone should start eating at the same time.

Other etiquette rules state that food should be discarded if it comes in contact with the hem of one's gown, if it has been touched by animals, or if it is contaminated by insect or rodent droppings. Indians customarily never serve themselves (especially after their hand is soiled from eating), never offer food from their plates to another person, and rarely save leftovers. Such manners are essential to maintaining sanitary conditions in rural homes. These rules of etiquette may be practiced in even the most westernized families, however, and they remain important symbols of the Indian relationship with food.

Special Occasions

Another aspect of Indian culture that affects daily diet is the concept of feasting and fasting. As with other Indian food habits, feasting and fasting activities are complex and vary greatly from person to person and group to group. No occasion passes in India without some special food observance: regional holidays, community celebrations, and personal events such as births, weddings, funerals, and illness. A

As in other cultures in which the hands are used instead of utensils, it is an unforgivable breach of manners to eat with the left hand; one eats with the right hand and takes care of all other personal needs with the left.

Traditionally it was the responsibility of the male head of the household to see that any guests, pregnant women, or elderly persons were well fed before he could sit down to eat.

devout Hindu may feast or fast nearly every day of the year (see Chapter 2).

Feasting   Feasts serve as a method of food distribution throughout the community. They are generally observed by presenting large amounts of everyday foods and sweets of all kinds to the appropriate holy figure; all members of the community then eat the food. Feasts may be the only time that the poor get enough to eat.

Some foods are associated with certain concepts. Rice and bananas both symbolize fertility, for example. Betel leaves represent auspiciousness; ghee, purity; salt, hospitality and pleasantness; mango, hospitality and auspiciousness; and betel nuts and coconuts, hospitality, sacredness, and auspiciousness.

Most festivals are Hindu in origin, and although many are observed nationwide, each is celebrated differently according to the region. *Holi* is a spectacular holiday in the North, featuring reenactments of Krishna's life, fireworks, and colored powders and waters. Celebrants snack at bazaar booths. *Dussehra* is a 10-day holiday observed in both the North and the South. A special dish is prepared each day, and every day that dish is added to those prepared the previous days, culminating in an enormous feast on the last evening, after a torchlight parade of ornamented elephants. *Divali,* the "festival of lights," is the New Year's holiday celebrated everywhere with gifts of sweets.

Non-Hindu harvest festivals also feature feasts. They are dedicated to wheat in the North and rice in the South. At the 3-day rice festival in Pongal, dishes made from the newly harvested rice are ceremonially "fed" to the local cows. The 10-day festival of Onam in Kerali culminates with a feast served by the local women, including thirty to forty dishes ranging from fiery curries to foods sweetened with a combination of molasses, milk, and sugar.

Asian Indian Muslims may dine with friends on Eid al-Fitr at the end of Ramadan and Eid al-Azha (see Chapter 9). Christians celebrate Christmas and Easter in India.

Fasting   Fasting is also associated with special occasions in India. It accompanies both religious and personal events. An orthodox Hindu may fast more days a week than not. However, the term "fast" includes many different food restrictions in India, from avoidance of a single food item to complete abstinence from all food. A person might adopt a completely vegetarian diet for the day or eat foods believed to be spiritually "purer," such as those cooked in milk (see the section "Purity and Pollution" in this chapter). Individuals rarely suffer from hunger because of fasting in India. In fact, more food may be consumed on fast days than on a nonfast day.

Muslims in India also fast, notably during the month of Ramadan. No food or drink is consumed between sunrise and sunset (see Chapter 2 for more information).

Sweets represent prosperity because they often include costly ingredients and may be decorated with silver or gold leaf.

Another holiday, *Janmashtami,* commemorates the birth of Krishna. As a boy, Krishna and his friends would steal butter or curds hung high in earthen containers. This story is recreated during the celebration as young boys attempt to break elevated clay pots full of curds.

The decorative red or yellow dot that Hindu Asian Indian women apply to their foreheads represents joy or prosperity. It is omitted during fast days.

Role of Food in Indian Society

The importance of food in Indian culture goes far beyond mere sustenance. Sanskrit texts describe how

> From earth sprang herbs, from herbs food, from food seed, from seed man. Man thus consists of the essence of food. . . . From food are all creatures produced, by food do they grow. . . . The self consists of food, of breath, of mind, of understanding, of bliss.

(Achaya, 1994, p. 61)

In a society that traditionally experienced frequent famines and chronic malnutrition, food is venerated. Complex traditions have developed around when, how, and why foods are prepared, served, and eaten.

The Sanskrit scriptures state, *"Annam Brahma"*—"Food is God."

Purity and Pollution

Many Hindu dietary customs are meant to lead to purity of mind and spirit. Pollution is the opposite of purity, and polluted foods should be avoided or ameliorated. To be pure is to be free of pollution.

The Hindu classification system of *jati* is used to evaluate the relative spiritual purity of all foods. Purity is determined by the ingredients, how they are prepared, who prepares them, and how they are served. Some foods, such as milk, are inherently pure. Raw foods that are naturally protected by a husk or a peel are less susceptible to pollution. Fried foods (*pakka* foods) are more pure than baked, boiled, or steamed foods (*kaccha* foods), especially if they are fried in ghee. Food that is served in brass dishes is also less vulnerable to pollution than is food in clay dishes. Some foods, such as alcohol and meat, are *jhuta,* meaning that they are innately polluted.

Traditionally only foods cooked and served by a member of an equal or superior caste could be consumed by any Hindu. Only members of the same caste will eat together. Untouched leftovers can be given to a member of a lower caste, such as servants, but polluted leftovers are eaten only by scavengers of the lowest caste. Asian Indians adhere to these commensal rules to various degrees, however. An orthodox Hindu would attempt to follow them at all times. A more modern Hindu might adhere to them only during holy services and holidays. Most westernized Indians eat in restaurants and use convenience products in cooking, ignoring how and by whom the food was prepared.

The consumption of jhuta foods also varies among Hindus. Historically laborers and warriors were allowed to eat meat to help keep up their strength. Some Brahman subcastes permit consumption of impure foods that happen to be plentiful in their region, such as fish (referred to as "fruit of the sea") in the coastal areas and lamb in the North. Other sects are so rigid that even inadvertent intake of

Pakka (meaning "cooked") foods are those that are fried or fat-basted during preparation, preferably in ghee. Pakka foods are relatively unrestricted due to their high degree of purity.

Kaccha (meaning "undercooked") foods are those that are boiled in water, baked, or roasted. Kaccha foods are more susceptible to pollution than pakka foods and must therefore be treated carefully during serving and consumption.

Jhuta foods are those that are inherently polluted and impure. All leftovers, unless completely untouched by the consumer or by other foods that have been eaten, are jhuta. Those foods that are innately jhuta vary according to religious sect. The term jhuta is also used for garbage and offal.

polluted food results in spiritual disaster. Members of the International Society for Krishna Consciousness (see Chapter 2) believe that if they accidentally eat a prohibited animal food, they will lose human form in their next life and assume the form of an animal that is the prey of the animal they ate.

Asian Indian Women and Food

The role of women in food preparation is extremely important throughout Indian culture. Feeding the family is an Indian woman's primary household duty. She is responsible for overseeing the procurement, storage, preparation, and serving of all meals. Because arranged marriages are common, training in kitchen management is considered essential for a Hindu woman in obtaining good marriage offers.

It is generally believed that a woman cannot be completely substituted for in the kitchen, for she imparts a special sweetness to food. If the wife is unable to perform food-related duties, a daughter or daughter-in-law may substitute. If servants help in meal preparation, it is still important for the woman of the house to serve the food directly from the *chula* (stove) to the table. This often requires many trips. Customarily the wife serves the men and guests first, then the children.

> Women never taste the food they are preparing to prevent possible pollution.

> A Hindu woman is considered impure during her menses and is prohibited from cooking or touching any food that is to be consumed by others.

> The kitchen is considered sacred in many Hindu homes. By custom, no one may enter with shoes on, all who come in must bathe and put clean clothes on first, and children with questionable hygiene are prohibited, to preserve purity.

> A person's constitution, including temperament and preferences in food, is believed to be determined at birth.

> Raw foods are considered difficult to digest.

Therapeutic Uses of Food

Ayurvedic medicine, which developed into its current form between 500 BCE and 500 CE, has had a significant impact on concepts of diet and health in India. It is based on the premise that each human is a microcosm of the universe and that three of the fundamental elements—fire, water, and wind—have their counterparts in the humors of the body—bile (*pitta*), phlegm (*kapha*), and wind (*vata*). Pitta regulates metabolic activities and resulting heat. Kapha provides structure and support through bone and flesh, and vata represents movement, of muscle and semen. Health is maintained through a careful balance of humors and substances in the body according to each person's internal constitution and external experiences. When pitta is in balance, digestion is comfortable and a person is content; balanced kapha produces physical and emotional stability, strength, and stamina; vitality and creativity are the results of balanced vata (Larson-Presswalla, 1994). Good digestion is critical because food is transformed into the body humors and substances when it is cooked by the digestive *agnis* ("fires") producing food juices and wastes. Food that is indigestible is harmful because it is believed to accumulate in the intestines and decompose, sending toxins into the bloodstream;

excessive waste or too little waste is an imbalance that causes illness (Sheikh & Sheikh, 1989; Ramakrishna & Weiss, 1992).

The hot-cold classification system is used for foods, depending on how they affect the body. The specific identification of an item as hot or cold varies regionally; for example, lentils and peas are considered hot in western India, but cold in northern India. Generally wheat, spices and seasonings (except mustard and sesame seeds), chicken, and oils are classified as hot; rice, leafy vegetables, fruits (except mango, papaya, and jackfruit), dairy products, honey, sugar, pickles, and condiments are considered cold (Achaya, 1994). The hot or cold nature of a food can be altered through the method of preparation. The use of hot spices or roasting may make a cold food hot; conversely, soaking a hot food in water or blending it with yogurt can change it into a cold food (Ramakrishna & Weiss, 1992). Although a balance of hot and cold foods is essential to health, the exact proportions of each change with age, gender, physical condition, and the weather. Traditionally six seasons are recognized, each with certain dietary recommendations. During winter, when digestion is thought to be strongest, roasted or sour and salty dishes are preferred as well as sweets; in summer and during the monsoons, when digestion is thought to be weak, salty, sour, and fatty foods are avoided (Achaya, 1994).

The way foods are eaten is as important as which foods are consumed. To maximize digestion of foods, a person should eat in a quiet atmosphere, sip warm water throughout the meal, and sit for a short while after dining (Larson-Presswalla, 1994).

Pregnancy is considered to be a normal and healthy condition; however, certain food taboos are sometimes followed. Women especially avoid extremes in foods that are too hot or too cold. Lime juice with honey is a general tonic, believed to prevent excessive bleeding at birth, while cow's milk (particularly with almonds and saffron) and rice porridge are thought to ensure proper development of the fetus. Fenugreek seeds in buttermilk are given for nausea and butter or ghee is believed to make the body supple and ease delivery of the baby.

> Cow's milk is thought to increase intelligence; buffalo's milk is believed to strengthen the body.

Numerous dietary remedies are listed for minor illness. Barley water is consumed for a fever; vomiting is treated with milk. Coconut water, buttermilk, anise seed oil, and pomegranate flowers are all considered helpful for diarrhea. A powder called *ashtachooran* (a mixture of asafetida, salt, ginger, pepper, cumin, and ajwain) is added to honey for indigestion. Ginger tea or garlic soup is used to treat colds. Gooseberries and hibiscus flower tea are considered general tonics (Khanna, 1986; Achaya, 1994).

> In parts of India, garlic is believed to excite the passions and may be avoided.

It is widely believed that a highly spiced diet is necessary in the tropical Indian climate to stimulate the liver. One food habit that may result in ill health is the common practice of disguising otherwise undrinkable water with flavorful herbs and spices. Cholera, dysentery, and typhoid are endemic in many regions.

Contemporary Food Habits in the United States

Adaptations of Food Habits.

Americans of Asian Indian descent have usually been exposed to American or European lifestyles in India and may be familiar with a westernized diet before immigration to the United States. Yet even the most acculturated Asian Indian Americans continue some traditional food habits. Most accept American foods when eating out but prefer Asian Indian foods when at home (Sodowsky & Carey, 1988).

Ingredients and Common Foods

Very little research has been conducted on the food habits of Asian Indians in the United States. One study of Asian Indians in Pennsylvania suggested that acculturation takes place in two phases (Gupta, 1976). Typically the first lasts for 2 to 3 years, often while the immigrant is a student. Interaction with mainstream American society may be limited during this period. The recent immigrant prefers to associate with members of the same caste, regional, or linguistic group; experience with American foods often includes only fast foods. Male Asian Indian students are often unable to cook and may rely heavily on purchased meals. Many Asian Indian immigrants will eat hamburgers because of their availability and low cost.

Sometime during the next 10 years, Asian Indians who stay in the United States longer than 4 years enter the second phase of acculturation. They are usually employed by American businesses and are raising families. They keep their social interactions with Americans separate from those with other Asian Indian Americans. They might serve meat and alcohol to American guests, for example, and vegetarian dishes to Indian guests.

A study of Indians living in Cincinnati found several changes in the types of foods they ate (Karim et al., 1986). Foods that subjects used frequently in India but that were in only "low moderate" use in the United States were ghee, yogurt, dal, roti, rice dishes, and tea. Foods that were in "low moderate" use in India but in frequent use in the United States were fruit juice, canned or frozen vegetables, American bread, dry cereals, cheese and cheese dishes, and soft drinks. Coffee consumption also increased.

Variables that affect acculturation include gender (men tend to change their food habits more readily than women because women are the traditional food preparers in Indian society), age (children raised in the United States prefer American foods), marital status (single unmarried men are the most acculturated, married men with families in India next, and married men with families in the United States are least acculturated), caste (depending on whether caste members used meat or alcohol in India), and region (Asian Indians from rural areas are often stricter vegetarians than those from the cities).

A majority of Americans of Asian Indian descent make an effort to obtain traditional food products. Many markets in the United States specialize in Indian canned and packaged food products, including spices, and many stores provide mail orders. Fresh foods are more difficult to find. Some fruits and vegetables can be bought at Asian specialty markets, and Indian bakeries featuring sweets and tiffin items have opened in some areas. In Cincinnati, 100 percent of Indians interviewed reported that their traditional foods were available (Karim et al., 1986).

Vegetarianism

Asian Indian vegetarians sometimes become nonvegetarians when living in America. In one study, one-third of those who were vegetarians in India became nonvegetarians in the United States (Karim et al., 1986).

Three types of nonvegetarian Asian Indian Americans have been identified: (1) "eggetarians," or those who eat eggs only; (2) semivegetarians, who eat meat, poultry, and fish at restaurants and on social occasions but not in their own homes; and (3) full nonvegetarians, who eat meat, poultry, and fish at any time (Gupta, 1976). Asian Indian

Traditional Indian *thali* (individual silver serving tray), featuring a selection of *roti* (flat breads), fruit and vegetable pickles, like chutneys, and yogurt-based *pachadi* or *rayta*.

vegetarians may pass through all these phases in becoming nonvegetarians. Eating eggs begins soon after arrival in the United States, progressing to chicken, and finally to beef. It is estimated that nonvegetarian Asian Indians take between 2 months and 1 year to accept beef. One survey on acculturation patterns revealed that nearly 75 percent of Asian Indian Americans believe it is acceptable for nonvegetarians to eat beef; 44 percent indicated that it is acceptable for vegetarians to eat beef (Sodowsky & Carey, 1988). It may take vegetarian Indians 7 years to complete the transition to beef consumption, if it occurs.

As yet, the reasons vegetarians become nonvegetarians have not been stated conclusively. It has been suggested that vegetarianism may lose its social and cultural significance in the United States. Data regarding the influence of factors like gender, income, region of origin in India, and length of stay in America have been contradictory.

Asian Indians who are practicing Muslims rarely begin eating pork in the United States. They may drive long distances to purchase halal or kosher meats to fulfill traditional Muslim dietary restrictions.

Meal Composition and Cycle

Asian Indian eating patterns may become more irregular in the United States, possibly because of the pressures of a faster paced lifestyle. Breakfast is the meal most commonly omitted; snacking occurs between one and three times per day (Karim et al.,1986; Yagalla et al.,1996). Many Americans of Asian Indian descent eat American foods for breakfast and lunch. Traditional Indian evening meals are preferred, if native foods and spices are available. Yet dinners at home may also be influenced by U.S. food habits in that more meat may be eaten and American breads served in place of roti.

Pakistani Americans generally eat at least one traditional meal each day.

11

Regional Americans

In Boston they eat beans. In Philadelphia they eat cheesesteak. In Kansas City they eat barbecue, and in Seattle they drink café lattes. A person from Montana is no more likely to eat grits (ground hominy) than a person from Mississippi is likely to eat Rocky Mountain oysters (deep-fried beef testicles). Just as certain fare is associated with ethnicity and religious affiliation, local food preferences are elemental to American regional identity.

While most Americans expect uniformity in some food products, such as the breakfast cereal they buy in the grocery or the burger they purchase at a fast-food franchise, American cuisine is anything but homogeneous. Consumption data illustrate many differences. People in the Northeast spend the most annually on poultry, bakery products, butter, wine, and tea. Those in the South spend more on pork, sugar, and whiskey. Mutton and beer are above average sellers in the Midwest; eggs, cream, frozen meals, condiments, and coffee are purchased more often in the West. Conversely, westerners spend the least on pork chops and sausages; wine is unpopular in the Midwest; southerners buy fewer frozen juices than average; and bacon is purchased less frequently in the Northeast.

These figures reflect regional tastes and specialties. Tea in the Northeast dates back to colonial times. Pork has long been a foundation of southern fare. Lager-style beer was created in the Midwest, and the ethnic diversity of the West is suggested by the variety of mustards, salsas, soy sauces, fish sauces, and chutneys consumed. This chapter will examine the traditional fare of the Northeast, South, Midwest, and West, noting significant culinary variations and trends in American regional food habits.

Clinton, Montana hosts the Testicle Festival each September: 2 days of feasting on *Rocky Mountain oysters* (marinated, sliced, breaded, and deep-fried) on toasted bread and enjoying live country music. Over 4,500 pounds of beef testicles are consumed annually at the event. Vinita, Oklahoma sponsors a Calf Fry Festival on the first Saturday after Labor Day, featuring *Prairie oysters* and fries.

American Regional Food Habits

What Is Regional Fare?

Regional fare has traditionally been home-style food prepared with local ingredients, dependent on the seasons and on storage conditions. Most families made do with what they could grow, gather, or barter.

During colonial times, only 15 percent of the American population lived in cities. The remaining 85 percent were self-sufficient on rural farms.

Available indigenous and introduced foods are the most significant of several factors that influence the development of a particular regional cuisine. The spicy cooking of the Southwest with its emphasis on corn, beans, and chiles could not have been created in the upper Great Lakes area, which produces wheat, fish, and dairy foods. Before the advent of food preservation and refrigerated shipping, local items were not only freshest and tastiest, but also most economical. Strong associations with place and food suggest the importance placed on the superior quality of local items. Even today, with a global assortment available, there is a certain cachet to Maine lobsters, Vermont maple syrup, Georgia peaches, Florida oranges, Idaho potatoes, and Washington apples (see Figure 11.1).

A study of places and foods found that Texas, California, Vermont, Oregon, and Louisiana were the states with the most food associations and that place names enhanced the perception that an item was authentic, distinctive, and high-quality (de Wit, 1992).

Ethnic and religious practices also affect the development of regional fare, particularly specialty foods. Jewish bagels in New York, German doughnuts called *Fastnachts* in Pennsylvania, Cajun French–style sausages in Louisiana, West African–influenced hoppin' John in South Carolina, southern Italian–flavored pizza in Chicago, Cornish pasties in Michigan, and Mexican-inspired chili con carne in Texas are just a few examples. Most regional cuisine is a blend of several ethnic elements, such as the British–Native American dishes of New England, the African-French-Spanish-British–Native American mélange that is southern fare, and the northern Italian–Mexican-Asian mix found in California cuisine. Religious food habits are a factor in areas where large numbers of a specific faith have congregated. For instance, the majority of Mormons live in Utah, and Mormons do not drink alcohol, tea, coffee, or other stimulating beverages. Alcohol purchases in Utah are strictly controlled through limited availability at state-run outlets. Sweets are allowed, however, and are well integrated into family activities. The people of Utah eat twice as much candy per capita as the U.S. average (Lee, 1992).

A third factor in regional foods is historical heritage. Certain dishes are linked to local tradition. A good example is the Kentucky stew called *burgoo.* Legend has it that the mixture of poultry and red meat with vegetables dates back to the Civil War, when a chef for the Confederate cavalry at Lexington created the stew from native blackbirds, game, and greens. There is no single recipe for the dish, but today it typically includes chicken; pork, beef, or lamb; and cabbage, potatoes, tomatoes, lima beans, corn, and okra. It is seasoned with cayenne. Burgoo is traditionally served at picnics, political rallies, and sporting events, including Derby Day. Current trends can be an influ-

FIGURE 11.1
Foods associated with places. (de Wit, C. W. Food-place associations on American product labels.
Geographical Review, 83, **323–330. Copyright 1992. Reprinted with permission by American Geographical Society.)**

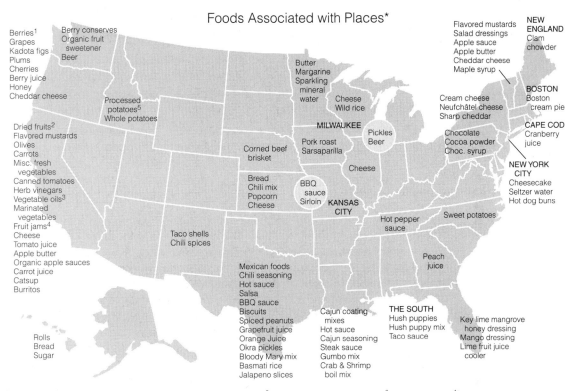

Foods Associated with Places*

Berries[1]
Grapes
Kadota figs
Plums
Cherries
Berry juice
Honey
Cheddar cheese

Berry conserves
Organic fruit
 sweetener
Beer

Processed
 potatoes[5]
Whole potatoes

Butter
Margarine
Sparkling
 mineral
 water

Cheese
Wild rice

MILWAUKEE

Flavored mustards
Salad dressings
Apple sauce
Apple butter
Cheddar cheese
Maple syrup

NEW
ENGLAND
Clam
chowder

Cream cheese
Neufchâtel cheese
Sharp cheddar

BOSTON
Boston
 cream pie

Dried fruits[2]
Flavored mustards
Olives
Carrots
Misc. fresh
 vegetables
Canned tomatoes
Herb vinegars
Vegetable oils[3]
Marinated
 vegetables
Fruit jams[4]
Cheese
Tomato juice
Apple butter
Organic apple sauces
Carrot juice
Catsup
Burritos

Corned beef
 brisket

Pork roast
Sarsaparilla

Pickles
Beer

Cheese

Bread
Chili mix
Popcorn
Cheese

BBQ
sauce
Sirloin

KANSAS
CITY

Chocolate
Cocoa powder
Choc. syrup

Hot pepper
sauce

Sweet potatoes

CAPE COD
Cranberry
juice

NEW YORK
CITY
Cheesecake
Seltzer water
Hot dog buns

Taco shells
Chili spices

Peach
juice

Mexican foods
Chili seasoning
Hot sauce
Salsa
BBQ sauce
Biscuits
Spiced peanuts
Grapefruit juice
Orange Juice
Okra pickles
Bloody Mary mix
Basmati rice
Jalapeno slices

Cajun coating
 mixes
Hot sauce
Cajun seasoning
Steak sauce
Gumbo mix
Crab & Shrimp
 boil mix

THE SOUTH
Hush puppies
Hush puppy mix
Taco sauce

Key lime mangrove
honey dressing
Mango dressing
Lime fruit juice
 cooler

Rolls
Bread
Sugar

[1]Gooseberries, boysenberries, blackberries, strawberries, blueberries, red raspberries. [2]Apples, peaches, figs, prunes, raisins. [3]Walnut, olive, pecan. [4]Black raspberry, strawberry, apricot, kiwi. [5]Hash browns, tater tots, golden fries, potatoes O'Brien, crinkle cuts, homestyle potatoes, cottage fries, shoestrings, potatoes au gratin, scalloped potatoes, instamash potatoes.

*Listed in order from most to least frequent occurrence.

ence as well. Some dishes sweep through one region but never gain national acceptance, such as caviar pie (layered hard-boiled eggs, scallions, caviar, and sour cream) in the Southeast (Anderson, 1997), or *loco moco* (a bowl with rice topped with a ground beef patty, then an egg over easy, and gravy) in Hawaii (Kelly, 1983). Other trends start out regionally and then catch on countrywide, such as the salsas of the Southwest.

Economics contribute to the popularity of certain foods. In one study, it was found that some of the best markets for beer in the country are in the poorest areas. Wine is popular in upper-income regions, which are often the worst beer markets despite the growing popularity of local brewpubs (Edmondson, 1998). Households with incomes below $20,000 a year spend about $1,400 per capita on food, buying more white bread, bacon, pork chops, luncheon meats, and eggs per person than the U.S. average. On the other end of the socioeconomic spectrum, households with incomes more than $70,000 annually spend over $2,500 per capita on food, with above average purchases in almost every category, especially expensive cuts of beef, fresh fish and seafood, dairy products, biscuits/rolls, and snack foods (Mogelonsky, 1996). Upscale consumers are more likely to be exposed to unique culinary ideas when dining out in trendy full-service restaurants and to be willing to pay for new or unusual food items.

Regional Divisions

There are many ways to divide the United States. Sometimes regions are delineated by terrain, as in the Great Plains, or marked by major rivers or mountain ranges, as in the Mississippi River Valley or the Appalachians. Sometimes areas are defined by similarities in climate, as in the Sun Belt; by economic affiliation, as in the Steel Belt and the Silicon Valley; or by the characteristics of the population, as in Indian Lands and the Bible Belt. Historical divisions, such as the Mason-Dixon line, or political divisions, including state boundaries, can also be used. The cultural geographer Wilber Zelinsky suggests that tradi-

TABLE 11.1
U.S. Regional Divisions

Northeast
New England — Connecticut, Maine, Massachusetts, New Hampshire, Rhode Island, Vermont
Mid-Atlantic — New Jersey, New York, Pennsylvania

Midwest
East North Central — Illinois, Indiana, Michigan, Ohio, Wisconsin
West North Central — Iowa, Kansas, Minnesota, Missouri, Nebraska, North Dakota, South Dakota

South
South Atlantic — Delaware, District of Columbia, Florida, Georgia, Maryland, North Carolina, South Carolina, Virginia, West Virginia
East South Central — Alabama, Kentucky, Mississippi, Tennessee
West South Central — Arkansas, Louisiana, Oklahoma, Texas

West
Mountain — Arizona, Colorado, Idaho, Montana, Nevada, New Mexico, Utah, Wyoming
Pacific — Alaska, California, Hawaii, Oregon, Washington

Source: U.S. Census Bureau/U.S. Department of Commerce.

tional regions contain elements of all these variables, characterized as a synergistic relationship between a people and the land that develops over time and is specific to the locality. He calls it *blood and soil* (Zelinsky, 1973). Such regional identity is dynamic, more of a process than a delineation, subject to changes in population, economy, and ecology. Ideally the people who live in an area, through their voluntary affiliation and their mutual agreement on group boundaries, define each region (Brown & Mussell, 1984).

Most often, however, geographic considerations are used to set arbitrary regional divisions independent of cultural relationships. The U.S. Census Bureau and the U.S. Department of Commerce list four regions with nine subdivisions for data collection purposes: Northeast, Midwest, South, and West (see Table 11.1). Although these categories group states with distinctively different cuisines together, such as Florida and Texas, or Alaska and Hawaii, most demographic and food consumption data are presented in this four-region format (see Figure 11.2). It is useful for detecting broad trends, as long as results are not overgeneralized to smaller populations who may observe alternate regional boundaries.

FIGURE 11.2
Regional divisions in the United States.

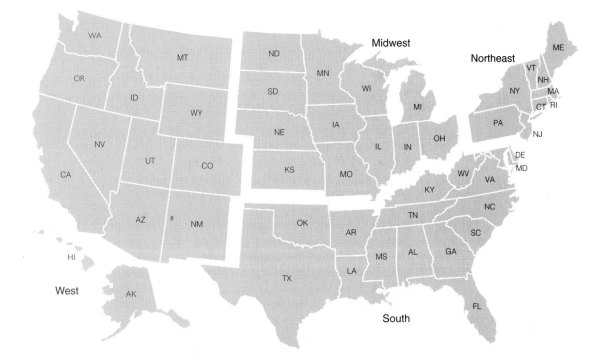

THE NORTHEAST

Regional Profile

The states of the U.S. Northeast include those of New England (Connecticut, Maine, Massachusetts, New Hampshire, Rhode Island, and Vermont) and those of the Mid-Atlantic region (New Jersey, New York, and Pennsylvania). The New England area features a rugged, irregular Atlantic coastline with many protected bays. Rolling hills and valleys that gradually become densely forested mountains extend west. The region is noted for its spectacular autumn weather and colorful fall foliage, followed by harsh winters. The Mid-Atlantic states are further south and more temperate in climate. Sandy beaches and estuaries line the long coast. The ridges, river valleys, and fertile plateaus of the Adirondack, Appalachian, Blue, Catskill, and other mountain ranges criss-cross much of the three states. Freshwater lakes dot the region and provide the northern boundary along Lake Ontario and Lake Erie.

Despite differences in climate and geography, the entire Northeast shares a common early history of sophisticated Native American societies supplanted by European settlements. The colonial immigrants from England, Germany, the Netherlands, and France were followed by newcomers from Ireland, Italy, Portugal, Poland, and other central and eastern European countries, particularly in the Mid-Atlantic states. African Americans from the South and more recent immigrants from the Caribbean, Central America, Africa, and Asia have added to the diversity of some parts of the Northeast (see each chapter on ethnic food habits for more immigration details).

Although only 19 percent of the total U.S. population is found in the Northeast, over two-thirds of Puerto Ricans living on the mainland reside there, and over one-third of all Asian Indians in the United States have settled in the region. Non-white populations total 37 percent in New York and 30 percent in New Jersey, with disproportionately large populations of blacks and Latinos. Yet the rest of the Northeast is still predominantly white (see Figure 11.3), including large percentages of the total U.S. population of Italians (51%), Ukrainians (51%), Portuguese (49%), French Canadians (45%), Russians (44%), Lithuanians (43%), Slovaks (40%), and Poles (37%). Maine, New Hampshire, and Vermont have the highest-percentage white populations in the nation, with only 2 to 3 percent non-white. Nearly half of all American Jews also live in the Northeast, primarily in New York, New Jersey, and Massachusetts.

While most of the original inhabitants and settlers of the Northeast were farmers, nearly eight in every ten persons now living in the Northeast reside in urban areas. The population of the region is also among the oldest in the nation, and the Northeast has the smallest percentage of children under age 18. A disproportionate number of persons over the age of 65 make their homes in the region, more than 11 percent above the national average, with particularly high numbers in Pennsylvania and Rhode Island.

Fiddlehead fern fronds are traditionally a harbinger of spring in the northern areas of New England. They are usually sautéed in butter.

Socioeconomically, families in both New England and the Mid-Atlantic have incomes above the 1997 U.S. median. The percentage of persons falling below the poverty level ($16,400/year for a family of four) in the Northeast was slightly below the U.S. average, with especially low rates in New Hampshire and New Jersey. New York is an exception, with a rate nearly 25 percent higher than average. More than one in every four adults over the age of 25 have a college degree in the region, 10 percent above the national average; Massachusetts and Connecticut have some of the most educated populations in the country with 33 percent and 30 percent having college degrees, respectively.

Traditional Fare

The cooking of the Northeast features the abundance of the Atlantic, the plenty of native and introduced produce, and the freshwater wealth of the many rivers and lakes (see Table 11.2). In New England, seafood, such as clams, lobster, scallops and fish, especially cod, has been prominent. Indigenous game, including wild turkey and venison, supplemented the poultry, pork, and beef brought by early immigrants. The foundation of the diet was traditionally corn, and many dishes of the region reflect its importance. Beans have also made a substantial contribution. Root vegetables (potatoes, onions, beets, turnips, rutabagas, carrots, etc.) quickly added to the vegetable selection. Wild berries, including blueberries, cranberries, gooseberries, and cloud berries (which look like bleached blackberries), grapes, and

Pickles, relishes, jams, and jellies were commonly prepared to preserve the fruits and vegetables of summer for use in winter.

Fudge was originally a maple sugar candy popular in New England in the 1800s. When cocoa became widely available, the chocolate version was developed.

Popcorn was a specialty of the Iroquois Indians of upstate New York. It was reportedly served with maple syrup.

FIGURE 11.3
Demographics in the Northeast.

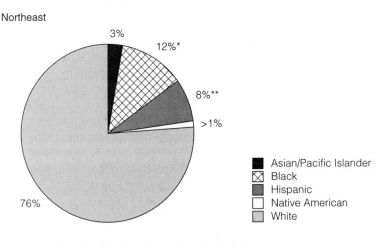

Northeast

3%
12%*
8%**
>1%
76%

■ Asian/Pacific Islander
⊠ Black
▨ Hispanic
☐ Native American
▨ White

* Mostly in New York (18%) and New Jersey (14%)
**Mostly in New York (14%) and New Jersey (11%)

TABLE 11.2
Northeastern Specialties

Group	Foods	Preparations
PROTEIN FOODS		
Milk/milk products	Cream; cheddar and cream cheese	Cream soups, sauces, puddings; ice cream
Meats/poultry/fish/eggs/legumes	Native game, particularly venison and turkey	New England boiled dinner; scrapple; red-flannel hash
	Preserved meats, such as corned beef, pastrami, salt pork, ham, bacon, sausages	
	Seafood prevalent, especially clams, lobster, oysters, scallops	Fish stews, soups; clam chowder; clam bakes; oyster or lobster loafs
	Salt and freshwater fish, such as salt cod and shad	Codcakes; shad bakes; *gefilte* fish
	Numerous beans (e.g., cranberry, kidney, lima)	Baked beans; succotash
CEREALS/GRAINS	Corn, wheat, rye	Cornmeal porridges, puddings, and breads
		Dumplings
		Baked goods, such as savory and sweet pies, cakes, doughnuts, waffles, pretzels, bagels
FRUITS/VEGETABLES	Apples, blueberries, cranberries, grapes	Applesauce, apple butter; fruit puddings, pies
	Cabbage, fiddlehead fern fronds, potatoes	Coleslaw; sauerkraut; ferns on toast; potatoes mashed, fried, creamed, baked, scalloped, hashed, as croquettes, salad
ADDITIONAL FOODS		
Seasonings	Salt, pepper, onions, saffron	
Nuts/seeds	Black walnuts, butternuts	
Beverages	Apple cider, hard cider, applejack; ale, beer; rum, whiskey; wine	New York State white, red, sparkling wines; sherry, port
Fats/oils	Lard, butter	
Sweeteners	Maple sugar; molasses	Maple sugar candies, maple syrup pie; chocolates

beach plums were the main fruits consumed until the apple orchards planted by immigrants became productive. Maple sugar sweetened many foods in New England. Even when molasses and cane sugar became widely available, maple syrup was preferred for many dishes.

The warmer weather and fertile lands of the Mid-Atlantic states have provided more native foods than New England. The coastal waters offer clams, oysters, mussels, scallops, and crabs, while the estuaries shelter ducks, geese, and turtles. Passenger pigeons once darkened the skies with their massive numbers, and bison roamed the area around Lake Erie. Freshwater fish such as catfish, eels, pickerel, salmon, shad, smelt, trout, and whitefish were plentiful; at one time, shad was the most numerous of all freshwater fish in the United States. Both the flesh and roe were commonly eaten.

Introduced foods also flourished in the region. Cabbage, potatoes, yams, carrots, peas, apples, pears, cherries, peaches, and strawberries were easily grown. Tomatoes thrived in the hot summers. Although New Jersey is now one of the most industrialized states in the nation, it is still known as the Garden State due to the success of these early agricultural efforts. Wheat, which was difficult to grow in New England, did well in the Mid-Atlantic. At one time, New York provided all the wheat consumed in the Northeast and much of the South.

New England

The cuisine of New England has been shaped predominantly by Native American preparation techniques combined with British home-style cooking. Roasting, boiling, and stewing are preferred. Dishes are often made with cream, and strong seasonings are avoided. People of the region take pride in simple fare.

The immigrants of the early seventeenth century were mostly tradespeople, inexperienced in farming and husbandry. History abounds with tales of how the first settlers were dependent on the skills and generosity of local Indians in preventing starvation (see Chapter 3 on Native Americans). Corn dishes were especially significant. Cornmeal porridge cooked into a mush-like consistency was a Native American food called *samp* by the early colonists. It was often prepared with another cornerstone of the Indian diet, beans. New Englanders used cornmeal to make an adaptation of the traditional English dish known as *hasty pudding*. The settlers would pour cornmeal porridge into a loaf pan to firm up overnight, then slice it and serve it topped with cream. This new dish, often flavored with maple syrup or molasses, was named *Indian pudding*.

Steamed, baked, and boiled puddings were eaten daily in New England homes. They were known as *grunts* (steamed dough and berries), *slumps* (baked puddings), and *flummeries* (a British molded oatmeal or custard pudding). As in England, a pudding could be savory or sweet and was generally served at the beginning of the meal. Breads were also a mainstay. Many were dense, baked without any leavening (reliable leavenings such as baking powder and baking soda were not available until the middle of the nineteenth century). Home-grown yeast from potatoes, hops, or the dregs of beer barrels

The passenger pigeon was so abundant in 1770 that a single shot from a colonial gun could bring down over 100 birds (Root & de Rochemont, 1976). Overhunting resulted in extinction. The last passenger pigeon died in an Ohio zoo in 1914.

One section of New Jersey that remains rural is the Pine Barrens, consisting of sandy soil, scrubby pines, and cedar swamplands. Many residents there depend on hunting and fishing for their daily fare. Venison and clams are specialties (Gillespie, 1984).

In the old American West, *grunt* was not a pudding, but a term for pork, as in "cluck and grunt" (eggs and bacon) for breakfast.

At what point pudding was served in the meal became a political issue during the late 1700s when conservative Federalists continued the tradition of eating it first, while more progressive Democrats (known as Republicans at the time) would eat it following the meat course (Lee, 1992).

Anadama bread is a modern-day corn bread made with mostly wheat flour, a little cornmeal, and sweetened with molasses. It is popular throughout New England. Stories about the name usually involve a woman named Anna who was either too lazy to make bread, so her husband damned her, or an outstanding baker who was damned by her husband when she died.

Boston cream pie, a favorite in New England, is not a pie. It is a custard-filled white cake covered with chocolate icing. It is probably derived from a popular colonial dessert called pudding cake that included cake, custard, and usually fruit or jam.

The *Old Farmer's Almanac,* first published in 1792, includes a recipe for New England boiled dinner and notes that it was traditionally served on Mondays and Wednesdays throughout the fall and winter months.

Boston is still known as *"Bean Town"* due to its long association with baked beans.

was used in some recipes. Corn bread cooked in a skillet over the fire was most common. Rye, which grows well in cooler climates, was often combined with cornmeal to make a popular bread called *ryan-injun* (from *"Rye 'n' Injun"*). Stewed pumpkin was sometimes added for a moister loaf. *Boston brown bread* is a traditional recipe of the region, a steamed loaf made with rye flour and flavored with molasses.

Pies made with suet pastry were served at most meals. Savory kinds included an American version of the British steak and kidney pie, chicken pot pie (later topped with biscuits instead of pie crust), a ground pork and onion pie seasoned with allspice called *tourtière* introduced by French Canadians in the region (served traditionally at Christmas or New Year's), clam pie, lobster and oyster pie, and a salt cod "pie" covered with mashed potatoes. Sweet pies were also popular, especially apple pies, made with fresh apple slices, dried rings, or even applesauce. Berry pies were common, and blueberry pie remains a specialty in Maine. Mincemeat, a traditional English treat combining savory and sweet ingredients, was featured at many meals because the filling of meat, dried fruits, nuts, and rum or other alcoholic preservative aged well, becoming tastier over time.

Pork, cod, or beef flavored most main dishes. Long winters required that most meats and fish be preserved, and few recipes called for fresh cuts. Salt pork, bacon, smoked pork, dried salt cod, corned beef, and dried beef were common, usually braised or stewed with vegetables. The *New England boiled dinner* is typical. This one-pot meal is still popular throughout the region and usually includes corned beef brisket simmered for hours with potatoes, onions, carrots, turnips and, traditionally, beets. Cabbage is added toward the end of the cooking time. Seasoning is mild, often just a little black pepper. Leftovers are often chopped up the next day and heated in a skillet with a little cream and sometimes some bacon and more onions to make another New England specialty known as *red-flannel hash,* so-called because the cooked beets would bleed into the other ingredients during frying. A dried salt cod and potato version of the New England boiled dinner is prepared in Massachusetts, called *Cape Cod turkey. Plymouth succotash* is another example. Although this Native American dish (see Chapter 3 for more information) is often associated with southern fare today, it was popular in the Northeast during colonial times. It combined corned beef, turkey or chicken, beans, corn, potatoes, and turnips. Other variations featured just vegetables, or combinations of meats, poultry, and fish.

Other popular dishes included dried beef rehydrated in boiling water and served with cream sauce over bread or potatoes (precursor to what is called *chipped beef* today), codfish cakes covered with egg-enriched cream sauce, and fried salt pork topped with cream gravy. In addition to meats and fish, beans were eaten regularly. Best known are baked beans flavored with molasses or maple syrup and salt pork, a recipe adapted from the Native American dish.

No discussion of New England fare is complete without mentioning the importance of shellfish in coastal regions. Lobster is a specialty, especially in Maine. The Indians of the area consumed the meat, used the discarded shells for fertilizer, and formed the claws into pipes. The meat was mostly added to mixed fish dishes by the British settlers. Lobster became more prestigious and more expensive in the following centuries due in part to overharvesting that resulted in scarcity and in part to the difficulty of transporting the fresh crustacean to upscale population centers inland. Clams, oysters, and scallops are also popular in New England. The clambake, in which clams, corn, and other items such as onions, potatoes, or lobster are steamed in a pit on the beach, began as a Native American tradition. Today a wood fire with large rocks stacked on top is built on the sand, and when the fire is embers and the stones are hot, the food is layered with wet seaweed, then covered with a tarpaulin until everything is cooked. Clams fill pies and are featured in the cream-based soup known as *clam chowder*. Those called *steamers* are just that—steamed and served with the broth and melted butter (a bucket of steamers is often the first course of a lobster dinner). Oysters were typically prepared with cream and breadcrumbs in a dish called "scalloped" oysters, or served in oyster stew. Today they are commonly broiled with bacon or breaded and deep-fried. Bay, sea, and Digby scallops are prepared similarly to oysters.

Development of the railways led to demand for perishables, such as shellfish, in the rapidly growing cities. The first lobster was shipped to Chicago in 1842—it made it as far as Cleveland alive on ice, at which point it was boiled before further travel (Root & de Rochemont, 1974).

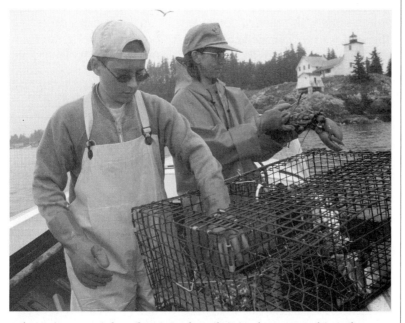

Lobster is a specialty of Maine, though it is also trapped in other New England coastal states. (Corbis/Judy Griesedieck.)

One New England dessert popular throughout the nation is chocolate chip cookies, which were created by Ruth Wakefield in 1930 at the Toll House Inn (the building dates back to 1709) in Whitman, Massachusetts.

New England desserts are mostly fruit-based. In addition to the puddings and pies already discussed, *pandowdies* (baked fruit layered with bread), shortbreads (fruit preserves, biscuits, and cream), and *roly-polys* (fruit rolled up in biscuit dough, then baked) were other favorites. Pound cakes and fruitcakes were enjoyed but were difficult to make before commercial leavening and reliable ovens were available.

Tea and apple cider were consumed daily in colonial times. Hard cider, an alcoholic beverage caused by the fermentation of sugars in apple cider, was also favored. Many New Englanders would start their day with a pint of beer or ale made from barley, corn, pumpkins, persimmons or spruce bark. Rum, as well as whiskey made from rye, was available. Wine from dandelions or gooseberries was a specialty, and an American version of the English drink called a *syllabub*, containing apple cider, sherry or wine, and whipped cream, was served at special occasions.

Mid-Atlantic

Many of the influences on New England fare are seen in the foods of the Mid-Atlantic states as well. Native American fare was combined with immigrant preferences to produce a new regional cuisine. Unlike New England, where most of the colonists were from England, many settlers in the Mid-Atlantic states came from the Netherlands and Germany. They provided a distinctively different flavor to foods, including a greater use of pork (especially sausages) and dairy products, more baked goods, and stronger seasonings. Later immigrants from southern and eastern Europe contributed many specialties. Further, the warmer climate and fertile farmlands offered a greater variety of ingredients to the cooks of New York, New Jersey, and Pennsylvania.

It was the Dutch in the mid-1600s who brought wheat to the New York area, which at the time was known as New Netherland. They also grew barley, buckwheat, and rye. Although these were preferred grains, the Dutch used what they called *turkey wheat* (corn) to make a boiled milk and cornmeal porridge known as *Suppawn* that was eaten daily at breakfast. This same porridge was topped with meats and vegetables for lunch, then baked to make the hearty dish called *Hutspot*, an American adaptation of a stew common in the Netherlands. Dairy cattle provided ample milk, butter, and cheese. The Dutch were among the first settlers wealthy enough to import sugar, brandy, chocolate, and numerous spices, including pepper, cloves, cinnamon, and saffron. Many Dutch specialties of the region have made their way into American cooking, including pickled cabbage; *Kool sla* (from the Dutch word for cabbage), now known as coleslaw; and headcheese, a ball-shaped sausage made from the head and feet of the hog. Doughnuts, crullers, pancakes, and waffles were also introduced by the Dutch.

The word "cookie" is derived from the Dutch word for a small cake, *Koeckje*.

During the same period, German immigrants arrived in the United States. Many were religious outcasts (mostly Mennonites, with smaller numbers of Amish, Schwenkfelders, and other sects) who made their home in the tolerant colony of Pennsylvania (see Chapter 4 on Europeans for more information). They became known as the Pennsylvania Dutch, a corruption of the German word *Deutsch*, which means "German." Although some German religious communities remained isolated (even to this day), many German immigrants gradually became integrated into the broader populations of Pennsylvania and surrounding states. Likewise, many German foods of the region have become an indistinguishable part of American cuisine.

Pork was the foundation of the German diet, from ham, pork chops, pork *schnitzel* (pounded into thin slices), bacon, salt pork, pickled pig's knuckles, *souse* (jellied pig's feet loaf), maw (stomach stuffed with meat and vegetables) and a German version of headcheese. Every part of the hog was used, and leftovers would be stretched with lima beans to make a Pennsylvania version of baked beans or with dried green beans and potatoes (*Bohne mit Schinken un'Grumberra*). The best-known leftovers dish is *scrapple,* still popular throughout the state. It is a combination of ground pork or sausage, cornmeal porridge, and spices that is formed into a loaf, sliced into thick slabs when firm, and fried in butter. It is typically served with fried eggs, applesauce, and maple syrup. Additionally, smoked and fresh sausages were consumed daily.

Chicken stews and soups, made substantial with home-made noodles or dumplings, were also popular with the Pennsylvania Dutch. Beef was used in the braised roast known as *Sauerbraten* and in the smoked, cured dried beef called *Bündnerfleisch*.

Asparagus, green peas, sugar peas (called Mennonite pod peas), and rhubarb are a few of the vegetables favored by the Pennsylvania Dutch. Potatoes are eaten mashed, fried, creamed, baked, scalloped, hashed, as croquettes, as dumplings, in stews and soups, and as potato salad. Cabbage is also ubiquitous, mostly as sauerkraut and slaw. Apples are particularly popular—fresh, as applesauce, in pastries, as cider, and in preserves like the thick, sweet spread known as *apple butter*. Many fruits and vegetables are pickled or preserved. Examples include spiced pears, pickled watermelon rind, sweet pickles, and corn relish. Dark rye breads, corn breads, yeast rolls, potato rolls, cinnamon rolls, *streuselkuchen* (coffeecakes with a sugar-crumb topping), doughnuts (called *Fastnachts*), and buckwheat pancakes are just a few of the baked goods found in the region. The Pennsylvania Dutch also make numerous desserts, especially pies (see Chapter 4 on Europeans for more information).

The hearty fare of the Dutch and Germans combined with many traditional items also found in New England, such as puddings, savory pies, and seafood soups and stews, to produce Mid-Atlantic cuisine. Later immigrants to the Mid-Atlantic region introduced foods that have become associated with certain cities and states (see the following

"Better a burst stomach than wasted food" is a Pennsylvania Dutch saying.

Doughnuts were traditionally dipped into milk or coffee, and the verb *to dunk* probably came from the German term *dunke* or the Pennsylvania Dutch word *tunke*.

Small half-moon pies were called *preaching pies* by the Pennsylvania Dutch because they were used to appease restless children during church services.

Angel food cake, also known as *angel cake*, is thought to be Pennsylvania Dutch in origin. It is leavened with egg whites.

"State Specialties" section). Notably, southern Italians in New York and New Jersey brought pizza and spaghetti with tomato-meat sauce; eastern European Jews introduced pastrami, smoked salmon, chopped liver, and other deli specialties.

State Specialties

Connecticut

The earliest European settlers in Connecticut were the Dutch who came from New Amsterdam (what is now New York City) and the English from the Massachusetts Bay Colony. The Dutch planted orchards and founded a dairy industry in the Hartford area, and the English established small farms. Although the state has become increasingly urbanized, some small agricultural concerns remain as a link to the past.

Fishing has provided the foods most associated with Connecticut. Shad, a flavorful relative of herring, was enjoyed by the Native Americans of the region but disdained by the earliest Europeans in the area due to its multitude of tiny, difficult-to-remove bones. Like the salmon, this ocean-dwelling fish spawns annually in freshwater rivers. Every spring the Juneberry plant, also known as the shadbush, blossoms, forecasting the arrival of the shad as they struggle up the Connecticut River. By the mid-eighteenth century, Connecticut residents had changed their opinion of shad, and by the beginning of the twentieth century, it had been fished to near extinction. River preservation programs have permitted a comeback, and the shad season is celebrated each June in the towns of the river valley. Traditionally the fish was most valued for its roe, fried quickly in butter. The Native Americans would plank the fish and slowly cook it at the edge of hot coals, a method still practiced today at shad bakes where the fillets are attached to a board with bacon, then smoked.

Lobster rolls are another Connecticut specialty. Lobster meat is mixed with mayonnaise, celery, onions, and lemon juice, then stuffed into toasted, fluffy, white bread buns. A similar dish, sautéed oysters packed into a loaf of bread, was known to the Puritans of Connecticut as *boxed oysters*.

Portuguese immigrants from the Azores arrived in the ports of Connecticut in the early nineteenth century to find work on whaling ships. They introduced their spicy sausages, such as *linguiça* and *chouriço,* to the region. Also popular are Portuguese white cornmeal breads traditional in the Azores, as well as sweet breads and other baked goods (see Chapter 4 on Europeans for more information).

Maine

While lobster is undoubtedly the food most associated with Maine, it was fishing and whaling that supported the earliest immigrants from

Connecticut is nicknamed the *"Nutmeg State"* not because it produces the spice or uses it in any specialty, but because early Yankee entrepreneurs from the region earned a reputation for selling fake wooden versions of whole nutmeg stored with the real spice so that they smelled authentic.

Some American troops of the Revolutionary War reputedly survived on barrels of shad packed in Connecticut.

England, France, and later Germany. In successive waves of popularity, cod, mackerel, herring, and sardines were harvested until the schools were fished out or tastes changed. Today commercial fishermen catch mostly haddock and hake.

Lobster was so plentiful along the Maine shoreline in the seventeenth, eighteenth, and early nineteenth centuries that it would pile up 2 feet deep after a strong storm. The Native Americans found it worthy of consumption, but Europeans used it mostly to feed pigs and as fertilizer. Commercial trapping began in the late 1800s with the advent of shipping by train and the development of the canning industry. The lobster supply diminished rapidly, and today trapping regulations are strict. Maine is also known for its mussels, providing nearly two-thirds of the shellfish consumed in the nation, and its sea urchin roe (*uni*), served at local restaurants and sushi bars or exported to Japan (Lee, 1992).

Other Maine specialties include wild or low-bush blueberries, used mostly in baked goods (Maine grows nearly 100% of this variety in the United States); potatoes (until the 1950s, Maine was the primary producer of the tuber nationally); and fiddlehead fern fronds. The ferns are eaten fresh on toast or in fiddlehead pie, similar to a quiche (Jones, 1981). They are also sold canned and frozen.

The Maine bean pot is a well-known version of baked beans. It is based on the Indian method of placing the ingredients in a pot that is then buried in a pit over embers, a so-called "bean-hole." During the winter, large vats of beans would be placed outside in the snow until frozen, then hung from the rafters of a shed so that just enough for a meal could be sliced off and reheated. Traditionalists insist that a Maine bean pot can only be made with native varieties such as yellow-eye, cranberry, or kidney beans, with one part salt pork for every three parts beans.

Lobster is now so costly that many residents of Maine resent the fact that it has become the state icon, because a majority cannot afford to eat it, even lobster trappers (Lewis, 1989).

Massachusetts

Cod is to Massachusetts what lobster is to Maine. Cape Cod, the peninsula that curls out into the Atlantic, was so named in 1602 for an abundance of the fish. Most were salt-cured for keeping, and many were exported to Europe. Dried salt cod was exchanged for temperate fruit in the Mediterranean and for molasses in the Caribbean (which was used to make rum back in the colonies). Those in charge of the cod trade became wealthy and were nicknamed the "codfish aristocracy." Numerous recipes for the fish were concocted by the Puritan immigrants, including boiled and baked dishes (see Cape Cod turkey, described previously), soups, stews, hash, pies, and, most notably, *codfish cakes*. These cakes, which are also called *codfish balls*, are a sign of regional affiliation for some residents of the Boston area. Another specialty that frequently included dried salt cod in earlier times is chowder, a cream-based soup that may also be made with corn, potatoes, salt pork, and/or seafood. One version, Boston clam chowder, is

A large wooden replica of a fish, called the Sacred Cod, hangs in the Massachusetts State House.

The name chowder may come from the French term for an iron pot, chaudière, or from the Welsh word for a fish soup, jowter.

known nationally. It is typically garnished with crackers, the slightly sweet, small, dry biscuits invented by Massachusetts sea captains for use on long journeys aboard ship. Those used in chowders were called common crackers, Boston crackers, or oyster crackers.

Baked beans are another dish well-loved in Massachusetts, especially in Boston. Traditionally the Puritans prepared a large pot of beans on Saturday morning, simmered them over the fire all day, then ate them with Boston brown bread for dinner to start the Sabbath (observed from sundown to sundown). Leftovers were kept warm on the hearth for Sunday breakfast with codfish cakes and for Sunday lunch.

Europeans first discovered Jerusalem artichokes in Massachusetts, and the state is home to the hybrid American grape named after the town of Concord. The best-known produce of the region, however, is the cranberry, called fenberry and bounce berry by the English settlers. It was the Dutch who introduced the term *Kranbeere*, meaning crane berry, because the flower resembles the head of a crane. Cranberries grow exceptionally well in the sandy peat bogs of Cape Cod, where they were first cultivated in the early 1800s. Commercial production began in the middle of the century. Most cranberry farms today are still small operations under 10 acres.

Indian names for cranberries included *sassamanesh* and *ibimi* (meaning bitter or sour). They were eaten with maple syrup or dried and added to pemmican. Cranberries were also used therapeutically and as a dye.

Over 340 million pounds of cranberries are consumed nationally each year as jellies, relishes, juice, and dried fruit.

New Hampshire

The rugged landscape and bitter winters of New Hampshire discouraged extensive farming by early European immigrants to the region. Orchards and dairying were successful, however, and the region became known for its apples and high-quality butter. Apples are still exceptionally popular in the area, made into applesauce, fried apple rings, baked apples, apple butter, cider, and apple pie (sometimes drenched in maple syrup). French Canadian settlers brought pea soup, salmon pie, and a penchant for pork dishes.

New Hampshire was the state where two crops vital to New England were introduced. The first was potatoes, planted in 1719 by Scotch Irish immigrants in Londonderry, New Hampshire. Although potatoes are a New World food (see Chapter 3), they only arrived in the United States after widespread acceptance in Ireland. The other transplant was turnips, brought by English settlers in the 1720s.

New Jersey

Over 80 percent of the large bush blueberries sold fresh in the United States are grown in New Jersey.

Over 150 crops are grown commercially in New Jersey, and it has a reputation as being the garden basket of New York City and other urban areas of the Northeast. Asparagus, peas, potatoes, tomatoes, blueberries, strawberries, and peaches are just a few of the successful fruits and vegetables in the region.

The state is famous for discoveries in agricultural research. Scientific work on hybridization has yielded new, improved varieties of peaches, tomatoes, and sweet potatoes. Food-processing techniques developed in New Jersey include condensed, canned soups (the Campbell Soup Company); inspected, bottled milk (the Borden Company); and the first application of pasteurization to milk at a small farm outside Princeton.

New Jersey is also the state where hard apple cider was first distilled to produce the apple brandy known as *applejack*. Another beverage, black tea, was introduced to the nation in the 1880s at Hoboken (the Thomas J. Lipton Company). Green tea had been the brew consumed in the colonies, but it fell out of favor following the Revolutionary War. The heartier flavor and convenience of tea bags reversed the trend.

New York

European settlers in New York discovered an abundance of native foods, such as deer, rabbits, quail, ducks, geese, and turkeys. Fish and seafood were plentiful: Oysters were eaten at every meal by the residents of New York City in the eighteenth century; littleneck and cherrystone clams were added to soups, stews, and pies; and shad was fished out of the bay, or plucked from the rivers during spawning.

The immigrants also found fertile fields and a climate conducive to many crops. Apples have been especially successful, and grapes grown in the four regions of the Finger Lakes, Lake Erie, the Hudson Valley, and Long Island support a thriving wine industry. New York is second only to California in production, including white (Chardonnay, White Riesling, and Seyval-Villard varietals), red (small amounts of Cabernet Sauvignon and Merlot), and sparkling wines as well as some fortified wines, such as Sherry and Port. Specialty vegetables like borrage, broccoli, rabe, raddichio, and baby squashes can be found on the farms of the Hudson Valley.

The cooking of New York has been forged from immigrant fare. The Dutch brought their rib-sticking porridges, stews, and baked goods. The English and Germans also settled in the region with foods similar to those in New England and Pennsylvania. In particular, the Shakers, an English religious sect, contributed savory herb seasonings; new varieties of beans, squash, and other produce; and an interest in the health-promoting qualities of whole wheat bread. French Canadians followed, bringing *cassoulet* (white beans baked with pork and goose) and onion soup. Italians introduced Mozzarella, Ricotta, tomato-meat sauces, pizza, *calzone, cannoli, gelato,* and espresso. Many central Europeans arrived during the late 1800s, including Poles who settled in the Buffalo area and Russian Jews who came to New York City. *Pierogi* (stuffed dumplings), *kielbasa* sausage, *kulich* (an

Before the advent of inspection and pasteurization of milk, it was necessary to boil it before consumption.

Applejack is sometimes called *New Jersey lightning*.

Delicately flavored Blue Point oysters are native to Long Island.

Many wines from New York are made from the native grape *Vitis labrusca*, which has a distinctive flavor often described as "foxy."

The duck that has become known nationally as Long Island duckling was first brought to the region by a Chinese sea merchant in 1873.

Buffalo wings, deep-fried chicken wings drenched in spicy (often using Tabasco sauce) seasoned butter and served with celery and blue cheese dressing, evolved in Buffalo-area bars during the 1960s. No one has established the exact origins of the appetizer.

Easter specialty cake made with sweet yeast dough) *matzah, gefilte* fish, *blintzes* (thin pancakes served with sour cream or stuffed with sweetened cheese or fruit), and *latkes* (potato pancakes) are a few foods brought by these immigrants. Bagels, introduced by the Poles, were paired with an 1872 New York invention, cream cheese; the chewy, doughnut-shaped roll was popularized throughout the nation during the 1990s. Chinese immigrants at the end of the nineteenth century brought numerous Asian specialties; Middle Easterners and Caribbean Islanders have added further spice to the cuisine (see chapters on each ethnic group).

New York is noteworthy for the influence of restaurant fare. Taverns, boarding houses, oyster houses, and coffeehouses served the needs of those eating out in the late eighteenth and early nineteenth centuries. The first European-style bakery was opened in 1825, and delicatessens serving the Jewish community were established in the 1880s. Full-service continental-style restaurants became popular in the mid-1800s. By the turn of the century, New York City had become the gastronomic center of the nation. Many dishes created for elite diners are now American specialties, such as *Waldorf salad* (originally a mixture of apples and celery in mayonnaise served at the Waldorf-Astoria), *vichyssoise* (chilled leek and potato soup from the Ritz-Carlton), and the dessert *baked Alaska* (from Delmonico's).

Vichyssoise was created by chef Louis Diat around 1917 from a recipe popular during his childhood in the Vichy region of France. American chefs sought to change the name during World War II due to collaboration of the Vichy government with the Nazis, but the new name, *crème Gauloise,* was never accepted because the soup was already too well known by its original title (Jones, 1981).

The Pennsylvania Dutch are famous for their pickles and preserves, and many Pennsylvanians eat vegetable and fruit relishes with their meals. It is fitting that the founder of Heinz catsup, pickles, horseradish, and other condiments was from a town near Pittsburgh. Henry Heinz had a reputation for honesty and quality: He and his son urged the U.S. Congress to pass the Pure Food Law of 1906 to give consumers confidence in commercial food products.

It is said that pepper pot soup was invented out of the only ingredients available by a Pennsylvania Dutch chef working for General George Washington and the American troops at Valley Forge.

Pennsylvania

Nowhere in the nation has German cooking been more significant than in Pennsylvania. Pennsylvania Dutch fare (described previously) was well accepted in the urban areas of the state, such as Pittsburgh, Allentown, Bethlehem, and Reading. Even Philadelphia, which was founded by English Quakers, favored German foods. Scrapple has become so associated with the city that it is often called Philadelphia scrapple, despite its rural origins. It is eaten for breakfast, often drizzled with catsup, and is used to make deep-fried croquettes or to stuff vegetables like green peppers and cabbage for dinner. *Lebanon bologna* is a Pennsylvania Dutch smoked beef sausage that has become a state specialty. It is traditionally sliced, battered or dipped in bread crumbs, fried, and served with sauerkraut and mashed potatoes. Other German foods of the region include sticky buns (a type of cinnamon roll); Christmas spice cookies (called *Pfeffernüsse* and *Lebkuchen*); and pretzels, which are sometimes eaten with vanilla ice cream. Although the origins are lost to history, *Philadelphia pepper pot*, a soup made with tripe, onions, potatoes, and black peppercorns, is most likely a Pennsylvania Dutch recipe and is sometimes served with dumplings. Cheesesteak (grilled strips of beef topped with American cheese and grilled onions in a toasted Italian roll), the quintessential Philadelphia sandwich, was supposedly invented during the 1930s when a hot dog pushcart vendor was accidentally sent beef instead of his standard order of frankfurters.

This is not to say that English foods have been ignored in Pennsylvania. The Quakers prepared many puddings and pies and were famous for their peach desserts. Seafood specialties included creamed oysters and delicately seasoned cream of clam soup. Poultry dishes, such as chicken with green peppers, wild birds baked with oysters, and stuffed turkey, were popular. The residents of colonial Philadelphia were criticized by some Puritans and even by a few members of their own sect for their unseemly interest in fine dining. Numerous private eating clubs opened in the city to accommodate gentlemen interested in socializing over a gourmet meal. French-influenced food was fashionable, including turtle soup (a cream-based soup sometimes flavored with Madeira), chicken or rabbit *fricassee, oeufs à la neige* (the meringue and custard dessert also known as snow eggs or floating islands), and the best cognac and fine wines of Bordeaux and Burgundy.

Pennsylvanians are fond of sweets. Philadelphia was one of the first cities in the nation to enjoy ice cream, perhaps as early as 1782. An ice cream parlor with frozen treats, cakes, syrups, and cordials was opened in 1800. The following years produced the first wholesale distributor of ice cream and the first ice cream soda. The city gained a reputation for a high-quality product made with cream, ripe fruit, and sugar, without any eggs, gelatin, arrowroot, or other thickeners. Hot chocolate and butterscotch sauces were popular toppings, and ice cream molded into flowers, fruits, animals, or holiday icons is still a specialty. Another confectionery contribution was affordable chocolate. Commercial production of chocolate for beverages and bonbons began in Pennsylvania during the late 1700s, although it was so costly it was considered a luxury item. Milton Hershey of Derry Church was the first manufacturer of chocolate for the mass market beginning in 1905, when he reduced his expenses by making uniform bars instead of fancy novelties. Two years later he introduced Hershey's Kisses.

William Penn, founder of Pennsylvania, established the first brewhouse in Philadelphia in 1685. It served what was known at the time as American beer, a heavy, top-fermented beverage similar to English ale. Two hundred years later, a German immigrant to Philadelphia founded the first brewery that made a lager-style, bottom-fermented beverage. The new, lighter beer was known as *lager*, or *pilsner* (see Chapter 4 for more information). It was an immediate success with local Germans, prompting the opening of beer halls and beer gardens that became the social centers of the immigrant community (Mariani, 1983). Lager soon became synonymous with beer in the United States.

Parisian mushrooms (the white or brown button mushrooms prevalent in modern U.S. markets) from France were introduced to America by the English in the late 1800s. They were first cultivated in 1926 in Downing, Pennsylvania. Over 75 percent of mushrooms consumed in the nation today are produced in southeastern Pennsylvania.

Milton Hershey located his chocolate factory in his hometown of Derry Church, Pennsylvania. His charitable contributions to the community included building homes, a bank, a school, stores, and a trolley system. During the depression, he employed residents of the town at hotels, gardens, museums, and other facilities. Grateful residents renamed the town Hershey.

Rhode Island

Rhode Island is the smallest state in the nation and it has always had limited arable land. Although it was self-sufficient in the 1700s, over the years it has been best known for its dairies, poultry farms (the meaty Rhode Island Red was developed in Adamsville during the 1850s), breweries, and distilleries. Famous for tolerance since its inception, the state has attracted a variety of immigrants, including English, Irish, French Canadians, Portuguese, Italians, and central Europeans. Many maintained their own food preferences, and a cuisine distinctive to Rhode Island has yet to emerge.

A few Rhode Island specialties date from colonial times. These include *Jonnycake* (often called *Johnnycake*), a fried cornmeal cake made with whitecap flint corn; and tomato-based red clam chowder, a soup that is inaccurately attributed to Manhattan. Clams and oysters were once abundant along the short Rhode Island coastline. Oysters were especially popular among the nineteenth-century elite, who served them in pies (raw oysters in cream sauce topped with biscuit dough); as patties; creamed, curried; and, for New Year's Eve pickled, with eggnog to wash them down.

Vermont

The earliest European settlers in Vermont were hardy individualists. The terrain was mountainous, the climate cold, and the territory was on the far frontier of the American colonies, claimed by surrounding Native Americans, the French, New York, and New Hampshire. In addition, Vermont was landlocked. It became much more dependent on meats and poultry than nearby states with easy access to seafood. Beef, pork, mutton (a by-product of the wool industry—today sheep are mostly raised for lamb meat), and turkey (domesticated in the early 1800s) are the foundation of Vermont fare. The New England boiled dinner made with corned beef may have originated in the state, and the accompanying fried apple rings or *Vermont fried pie* (fried applesauce turnovers flavored with cinnamon) is definitely a local touch. Ham was popular, made into turnovers, shortcakes (served on biscuits with an egg sauce), and pies.

Dairy foods were also significant in the development of the local cuisine. Cream enriches many dishes and cheese embellished other foods. Cheddar and milder Colby cheeses were most popular, and it is thought that apple pie topped with cheese originated in Vermont.

No food is as associated with Vermont as is maple syrup. The sweet sap of the sugar maple tree had long been used by Indians of the Northeast to cook beans and meats and to flavor cooked fruits and corn (see Chapter 3 for more information). The syrup was an everyday sweetener in colonial kitchens throughout the region until cane sugar became more affordable. Maple syrup production peaked in the 1880s, and the sweet has since become a costly item. Vermont

The name *Johnnycake* may have come from corruption of *journey* cake or from *Shawnee* cake. During World War II the Rhode Island legislature put an end to arguments over spelling and ingredients (yellow or white cornmeal) when it mandated that all fried corn bread in the state be spelled *Jonnycake* and contain only finely ground whitecap flint corn.

Both cattle and turkeys were herded on foot the 200 miles between the Green Mountains of Vermont and the meat markets of Boston in the fall.

The oldest continually operating cheese factory in the United States was founded in 1822 in Healdville, Vermont. Manufacturers have expanded into the European-style cheese (e.g., Brie, Camembert) market in recent years; the largest producer of Feta cheese in the nation is found in Vermont.

specialties include *sugar-on-snow* (syrup poured over fresh snow), maple sugar pie (a double-crust or single-crust, meringue-covered pie with a filling of cream, eggs, and syrup), and maple sugar candies.

THE MIDWEST

Regional Profile

The Midwest is known as the Great Plains region of the United States. The earliest American settlers and European immigrants in the area found a vast, flat terrain covered by tall prairie grasses. Oak-wooded hills and low mountain ridges ringed the territory. The rich soil irrigated by the extensive Mississippi and Missouri river systems proved ideal for wheat, corn, and numerous fruits. The region is still renowned for its agricultural productivity, which is why it is nicknamed "America's breadbasket."

The Midwest encompasses twelve states with 23 percent of the total land area and just over 23 percent of the total U.S. population. It is divided into the East North Central region (Illinois, Indiana, Michigan, Ohio, and Wisconsin) and the West North Central region (Iowa, Kansas, Minnesota, Missouri, Nebraska, North Dakota, and South Dakota).

Farming in the United States expanded from the land grant days of the 1860s until the end of World War I, when overseas demand dropped and overproduction reduced prices. By the time the Great Depression began in the 1930s, agriculture was already in a slump. Since 1935, U.S. farmers have increased efficiency and gone through a period of significant consolidation. The number of farms has gone from 6.8 million in 1935 to 1.9 million in 1994 (the lowest number since 1850); the average size of each farm has more than tripled.

Maple sap drips into a bucket positioned on a maple tree. Maple syrup is a popular sweetener in New England. (Corbis/Jonathan Blair.)

The Homestead Act and subsequent legislation provided 160 to 480 acres of land for each head of household willing to settle in the new territories. Additional property was available for from $6 to $25 per acre.

The states of the East North Central (ENC) area are bounded by the Great Lakes, which temper the climate, ensuring milder weather than that experienced by other areas of the Midwest. Although the French were the first Europeans to explore the region, it was Americans from the Northeast states, as well as Virginia and Delaware, who were the first pioneers. Later immigrants from Germany, Switzerland, Scandinavia, central Europe, and the Cornwall area of England were attracted by the fishing, dairy, mining, lumber, and meat-packing industries. The West North Central (WNC) states are geographically near the center of North America, exposed to long winters, short summers, and extreme temperatures. Most Americans who settled the territory were homesteaders, interested in the inexpensive land and farming opportunities. They came from New England and the Mid-Atlantic states, followed by new immigrants from Germany, Scandinavia, and central Europe, particularly Poland.

As suggested by the history of immigration to the area, the Midwest has the largest percentage of whites in the nation (see Figure 11.4). Over half of all U.S. citizens of Czech and Norwegian ancestry live in the Midwest, as well as large numbers of people of Finnish (47%), Croatian (43%), Swedish (40%), German (39%), and Polish (37%) heritage. There are below average numbers of blacks throughout the Midwest; the exceptions are in Ohio, Michigan, and Illinois, which have slightly above average African American populations. Native Americans, Latinos, and Asian/Pacific Islanders are also underrepresented, although there is a large population of Latinos in Illinois, approaching the national average, and above average numbers of Native Americans in the Dakotas. Over all, Illinois has the most

FIGURE 11.4

Demographics in the Midwest.

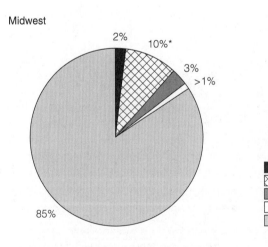

Midwest

2% 10%*

3%
>1%

■ Asian/Pacific Islander
⊠ Black
▨ Hispanic
☐ Native American
▨ White

85%

*Mostly in Illinois (15%) and Michigan (14%)

diverse population in the Midwest; nearly one in every three residents is non-white.

One immigrant group that has made the Midwest home is Laotians, including Hmong, who have arrived since the 1970s (see Chapter 8 on Southeast Asians for immigration history and food habits). Over 40 percent of all Laotians counted in the 1990 U.S. census lived in the region, with large populations in Minnesota and Wisconsin. Other Southeast Asians have not tended to settle in the area, however. Additional recent immigrant populations of note include Asian Indians in Illinois and Michigan, Koreans in Illinois, and Russians in Illinois and Ohio.

Although almost one in every four Americans lives in the Midwest, the population is not evenly distributed throughout the region: 16 percent of all Americans live in the East North Central states, and only 7 percent live in the West North Central states. The population centers in ENC states are predominantly urban, whereas more than a third of persons living in WNC states are located in rural areas, and the populations of North and South Dakota are almost equally split between urban and rural residences. The 1997 median income level in the ENC states is slightly above the national average, while that of the WNC states is slightly below average. Poverty rates are 27 percent lower in the Midwest than in the country as a whole, especially in Wisconsin, Indiana, and Nebraska, which have averages up to 40 percent below the national figures for the period 1995–1997. More people earn their high school diplomas in the Midwest than among the total U.S. population, but slightly fewer receive college degrees than the national average.

Traditional Fare

Midwestern fare is usually described as no-frills homestead and farm food, exemplifying what is typically called American cuisine. Prime meat or poultry is prepared simply, served with vegetables, potatoes, and fresh bread. Hearty breakfasts start the day, robust soups and stews replenish body and spirit, and homespun desserts round out the meal.

The Midwest is a region of food traditions maintained over generations. Beef and pork are preferred meats, although better cuts are affordable today and variety cuts may be consumed less often than in settlement days. Canning (and more recently freezing) to preserve summer's bounty is still a common activity. Bread is sometimes baked at home, and pies make use of seasonal fruits. Midwestern hospitality, which began with festive sorghum pulls, group apple peelings, and canning parties, is continued through buffets, box socials, "pitch-in" or potluck suppers, strawberry socials, corn roasts, and fish boils popular throughout the region.

The "First Law of Midwestern Dining" is: Save room for dessert (Mandel, 1996).

Although buffet dining was known in medieval times, the American buffet meal may have originated with the traditional threshers' dinner served to feed migrant farmworkers in the Midwest.

The highlight of a box social is when lunches or suppers in a basket (the "box") are auctioned off anonymously. The buyer then eats the box's contents with its preparer. In the nineteenth century, it was a way for single women and men to mingle and meet prospective partners.

TABLE 11.3
Midwestern Specialties

Group	Foods	Preparations
PROTEIN FOODS		
Milk/milk products	Milk, buttermilk, butter, cream, cheeses	Cream gravy, fondue, *rømmegrøt, skyr*
Meats/poultry/fish/ eggs/legumes	Native game, including buffalo, venison, beaver, raccoon, opossum, turkey, prairie chickens (grouse), pheasant	Jerky, *booyaw, Hasenpfeffer*
	Pork in all forms, especially salt pork, hams (country ham and Westphalian ham), and sausages (bratwurst, weinerwurst, kielbasa); beef	Ham with gravy, pork chops, barbecued pork, hot dogs, *Bubbat* Beef pot pie, stew, barbecued brisket, bierocks, pasties, Cincinnati chili
	Oysters shipped from the East Coast	
	Freshwater fish, especially smelt, sturgeon, trout, and whitefish	Fish boils, fried trout or smelt
	Dried beans	Baked beans with salt pork or bacon
CEREALS/GRAINS	Corn, wheat, rye, oats, wild rice	Corn breads, porridges; oatmeal; *bannocks;* rye breads, pumpernickel; biscuits, dumplings (including stuffed, such as pierogi and verenikas) Baked goods, especially fresh fruit pies (apple, cherry, persimmon, rhubarb), iced cakes, strawberry shortcakes, strudel, *kolaches,* butter cookies, pancakes, *aebelskivers,* Danish pastries
FRUITS/VEGETABLES	Apples, berries (blueberries, elderberries, strawberries), cherries, grapes, peaches, persimmons, rhubarb	Applesauce; apple butter, fritters, bread, salad; fried apples, candied apples; fruit jams and jellies
	Cabbage, onions, peas, potatoes, rutabagas, turnips, wild mushrooms	Sauerkraut, sauerkraut balls; coleslaw; potatoes boiled, fried, baked, as dumplings, salad; onion pie
ADDITIONAL FOODS		
Seasonings	Salt, pepper; parsley, dill; cinnamon, ginger, nutmeg, saffron; molasses	Most foods preferred mildly spiced.
Nuts/seeds	Almonds, black walnuts, hickory nuts, pecans; poppy seeds	Nut pies, almond paste; nut candies; poppy seed cakes and pastries
Beverages	Apple juice, beer, wine, apple brandy	Lager-style (American) beer
Fats/oils	Butter, lard	
Sweeteners	Sugar, honey, molasses, sorghum	

The earliest American settlement in the ENC region was in Marietta, Ohio in 1788. The people who came to the area from the original colonies were mostly farmers, who survived in their new homes on hogs, corn, beans, squash and pumpkins, cabbage, and potatoes. Corn was eaten at every meal, as porridge or as baked or fried breads. Sun-dried or smoked meat strips called *jerky* were adopted from the Indians of the region, used first for game such as venison, then later for beef. Other wild meats, such as duck, quail, rabbit, squirrel, woodchuck, and raccoon, were widely available. Meat pot pie with biscuit topping was a favorite preparation. Native fruits included persimmons, blueberries, bush cranberries, gooseberries, ground cherries, grapes, and many types of nuts. Later settlers brought wheat and oats, as well as apples, cherries, peaches, and berries. Fishing provided salmon, smelt, trout, and other freshwater fish; dairying, particularly cheesemaking, offered further food variety.

Each group of pioneers in the region brought favorite dishes. Baked beans and succotash were preferred by settlers from New England. The people from New York and Pennsylvania favored sausages, sauerkraut, pickles, and relishes. Those from southern states cooked fried chicken with cream gravy. European immigrants introduced the culinary specialties of their native lands, such as Cornish *pasties* in Michigan and Swiss cheese *fondue* in Indiana (see state specialties sections). In areas where immigrants congregated in numbers, regional ethnic fare developed, including the Michigan Dutch (actually from the Netherlands, not Germans like the Pennsylvania Dutch) and the Ohio Germans.

In the WNC states the settlers of the mid-nineteenth century came to farm the fertile land of Iowa, Kansas, Minnesota, and Missouri. Harsh winters and a scarcity of provisions limited variety in many early pioneer homes. Homemakers of the period describe burying melons in sand, which with luck would stay fresh until Christmas. Other cooks would prepare up to a hundred fresh fruit pies at a time, covering the extras with snow for use throughout the winter months. Parched corn, herbs, bark, or root brews replaced coffee (Luchetti, 1993). Prestige foods were often unavailable, so ample, even excessive, amounts of common foods became symbolic of hospitality in the midwestern frontier. The more western areas of the WNC states, which are drier and less suitable for crops, provided limited agricultural opportunities in wheat and cattle. The region attracted trappers, traders, and prospectors. Wild game, such as bear, buffalo, elk, deer, and small mammals, as well as turkeys, prairie chickens (grouse), quail, doves, and frogs, was hunted; the meat or oil was often sold in settlement towns.

As in the ENC region, pioneers from New England and the Mid-Atlantic states contributed dishes eaten frequently in their eastern homes: Baked beans and apple pies became as common as sausages and sauerkraut. One northeastern specialty that became surprisingly

John Chapman, better known as Johnny Appleseed, was born in Massachusetts but spent most of his adult life planting apple orchards throughout Ohio, Indiana, and Illinois in the early 1800s. Myth has it he traveled barefoot and wore a pan on his head while he tended the trees and preached the teachings of the Swedenborgian faith.

One of the most significant contributions to midwestern food was the founding of lager-style breweries in Cinncinati, St. Louis, Chicago, and Milwaukee by German immigrants to the region.

One source from the pioneer period commented on an exciting change in diet from "bread and bacon" to "bacon and bread" during one long winter (Luchetti, 1993).

One grizzly bear would provide 10 gallons of pure, rendered fat worth $75 in late nineteenth-century St. Louis (Luchetti, 1993).

Coon cake called for a dough made from flour, water, and raccoon fat fried in raccoon oil.

Health concerns about the meat-packing industry began with complaints about cattle driven down neighborhood streets and bad odors, prompting the Supreme Court to outlaw slaughterhouses near residences in 1873. Novelist Upton Sinclair wrote an exposé on the Chicago stockyards titled *The Jungle* in 1905, describing poor working conditions and fraud, including the use of rat meat in sausages and rendered lard that included what was left of employees who fell into the vats of boiling fat. Meat sales declined nationally, and Congress passed the Meat Inspection Act the following year.

Chemists working at Ford Motor Company in 1937 trying to create a synthetic wool discovered that soybeans could be made into analog protein products, such as bacon, by spinning vegetable protein fibers and flavoring them to taste like meat.

Deep-dish "Chicago-style" pizza is baked in a skillet. It is an American adaptation of the pizza brought to the region by Italian immigrants from Naples.

The International Horseradish Festival is held in Collinsville, Illinois each June. The highlight of the weekend is the horseradish eating contest, when timed participants eat as many hot dogs heaped with the freshly grated root as possible.

popular throughout the Midwest is oysters. By the mid-1800s the live shellfish were shipped regularly to the region packed in barrels filled with wet straw. One English visitor commented that the rich "consumed oysters and Champagne and the poor [ate] oysters and lager bier" (Mandel, 1996). One recipe from 1859 for small birds, such as magpies, suggested stuffing a breaded oyster into each bird before roasting over a hot fire (Luchetti, 1993). The new European immigrants who arrived were often scattered throughout the region due to the land grant process. Over time, foods such as Czech *kolaches*, Polish *stuffed cabbage* and *pierogi*, Hungarian *goulash,* and German Russian *bierocks* or *runsa* (also known as *pirozhki)* became familiar in midwestern cuisine.

State Specialties

Illinois

The Illinois frontier was known for corn production and hog husbandry. In the beginning of the 1800s the Chicago stockyards were built in city neighborhoods as a fattening-up rest stop for cattle being driven from Texas to the markets of the East Coast for slaughter. By the middle of the century, most beef was being butchered in Chicago for shipment to the rest of the nation. In the early 1930s a fourth major product, soybeans, was added to Illinois agriculture. Progress in soybean processing increased interest in the crop, which was used primarily for oil (to make edible products like margarine, mayonnaise, and salad dressings and for industrial use) and meal (the main source of protein in animal feed).

Meat, poultry, and cheese processing are the primary contributions of Illinois to midwestern fare, and are influential factors in American food habits. Culinary history is replete with stories about Phillip Armour, who made millions in pork sales when he founded the Chicago meat-packing industry; Gustavus Swift, who made his fortune in hams and sausages; Oscar Mayer, a German immigrant who got his start in the hot dog business as a butcher in Chicago; Louis Rich, a Russian immigrant who became involved in poultry processing and founded a turkey luncheon meat empire; and James Lewis Kraft, a grocery clerk who came up with the idea that home-delivered, uniform pieces of cheese would be more popular than freshly cut wedges from a large wheel. He later introduced processed and prepackaged cheeses, including *Velveeta.*

One, more unusual, Illinois food is horseradish. German immigrants brought the eastern European root to the Mississippi River basin area in the southern end of the state in the late nineteenth century. The pungent, gnarly root thrives in the well-drained soil of the region. Over 10 million pounds are grown each year, nearly 85 percent of the global supply.

Sausages, introduced by German and Polish immigrants, have become so much a part of the midwestern diet that they are no longer considered ethnic fare. (Corbis/Sandy Felsenthal.)

Indiana

The earliest Indiana pioneers came from Kentucky, North Carolina, and Virginia. They subsisted on acorn cakes and game meats until corn and wheat crops were established and pigs and sheep were plentiful. Agriculture was the primary industry in the state during the eighteenth and nineteenth centuries. Today Indiana is best known as the world's top popcorn producer.

Many dishes unique to Indiana feature foods from the state's early history. Whole roasted pigs, barbecued pork, pork roasts, chops, and hams are popular, as is *whole-hog sausage* made from lean cuts. Sausage patties and ham are common for breakfast, typically served with pancakes or biscuits, cream gravy, and fried apples. Batter-fried chicken is served with fried biscuits made with a yeast dough that puffs up into spheres when dropped into hot oil, then slathered with butter while still warm. Hungarians who settled in the South Bend area brought *veal paprika* and poppy seed cake. The Swiss founded the town of Vevay, where they were known for their cheese *fondue*. Vegetable pies, such as green tomato pie and onion pie, are specialties. Small, sweet, indigenous persimmons are used in steamed or baked puddings. Hickory nut cookies and sorghum fudge are other Indiana sweets. *Pork cake*, a moist dessert made with sausage or salt pork, molasses, brown sugar, flour, dried fruits, and spices, is a Christmas tradition in some Indiana homes, and *sweet cream pie*, filled with a heavily sweetened custard, is popular all year.

Popcorn dates back over 5,000 years in the Americas. It was prepared by Native Americans in New Mexico, the Caribbean, and, according to myth, at the first Thanksgiving in Plymouth.

Valparaiso, Indiana was the birthplace of gourmet popcorn promoter Orville Redenbacher. The city hosts an annual Popcorn Festival each September.

The immigrants from central Europe who grew onions in Indiana were called "knee farmers" because they crawled when planting and harvesting their crops.

A frontier recipe for *pork cake* dating from 1866 may have been the precursor to the Indiana specialty. It claimed that using lard and salted pork saves the expense of butter, milk, and eggs (Luchetti, 1993).

One Iowa specialty is *corn cream,* made by paring the kernels off the cob, then slitting each row with a sharp knife to remove the flesh and juice. The corn is combined with a little cream and cooked over very low heat until thickened.

American blue cheese was developed at Iowa State University and first produced in the 1920s at Maytag Dairy Farms in Newton, Iowa.

In 1859 a group of German Lutherans, known as True Inspirationists, settled in seven Iowa villages to form what is known as the Amana Colonies. They lived communally, with everyone eating three enormous meals and two coffee breaks each day in a large dining hall. The weekly menu was set and included *Mehlspeisen* (literally "flour desserts," such as simple puddings) on Tuesdays and boiled beef every Wednesday. The Colonies now serve German specialties to visiting tourists in several large restaurants.

The Plains Indians were wholly dependent on the buffalo, and a primary reason for exterminating the buffalo was to eliminate the Indians as well.

Iowa

Iowa is corn and pork country. Almost half of the agricultural land in the state is planted in corn, which supports the largest commercial hog production in the nation, with just over 14 million head equaling 25 percent of all U.S. pork. While some corn is exported and some is used for food products, including syrups, sugars, cornstarch, and distilled spirits, most of the grain goes for feed. It takes almost 4 pounds of corn to produce 1 pound of pork meat. Iowa is also the leading producer of soybeans.

Iowa's harsh winters and limited supplies meant that the earliest pioneers survived mostly on fried pork, boiled pork, potatoes, onions, and coffee. Milk was difficult to obtain, and one frontier woman from Norway reported in her diary that she had prepared an all-milk meal as a special treat one evening, featuring *tymelk* (clabbered, or curdled, milk sprinkled with bread crumbs and sugar) and *rømmegrøt* (a milk and flour baked pudding topped with sweetened sour cream). Those more familiar with native prairie foods, such as corn, berries, and plums, made good use of the ingredients. Once established, many settlers were self-sufficient. The Amish who settled around Kalona grew all of their own foods and butchered all of their own meat, traditions still practiced today. Corn bread with tomato juice gravy, stews or hashes with potatoes and peas, fried meats and eggs, and fresh fruit pies are common dishes in the community. The Dutch settlers of the town of Pella serve pea soup, Dutch-style bologna sausage, and special almond paste–filled cookies shaped into strips or *S* shapes. The Czechs are associated with wild mushroom dishes and *kolaches* filled with sweetened cheese, poppy seeds, or apples. The Swedes gained a reputation for "coffee," a light repast featuring fresh-brewed coffee served with butter cookies. The Germans still prepare Westphalian-style hams (brine-soaked, crusted in black pepper, then slowly smoked) and *Bratwurst.* Today the foods most associated with Iowa are the hearty farm dishes like pot roasts, hams, roasted chickens, mashed potatoes, fresh breads, and seasonal pies traditionally served at harvest meals.

Kansas

Culinary history in Kansas is dominated by the battle between indigenous buffalo herds and introduced cattle. At their peak, it is believed that over 30 million buffalo roamed the Great Plains, providing sustenance, clothing, shelter, and fuel to the Native Americans of the region. American settlers and European immigrants also ate what they called *hump-backed beef,* at least until other meats became widely available. However, the huge herds of buffalo interfered with expanding settlements, the railroads, and Texas cattlemen, who drove their longhorns through the prairie states to the slaughterhouses of the North and East. Abilene, Kansas, became the intersection between the cattle trails and the railroads. From the time the first stockyards were built in the city in the 1860s to the time the cattle drives were halted in the 1880s, over 4 million head came from Texas and were shipped from Abilene to the rest of the country. The buffalo were systematically eradicated, which provided unimpeded access to the grazing lands of the plains. Today Kansas is famous for its corn-fed beef, and cattle are the most important agricultural commodity in the state. Steaks, beef stews, barbecued beef, and hamburgers are all Kansas favorites.

Wheat is a significant crop in Kansas. The first settlers in the region were largely unsuccessful with the grain because their variety required more water than the Kansas climate provided. German Russian Mennonites, who had first migrated to southern Russia, came to the state beginning in 1874. They brought a variety of wheat they had obtained from farmers in neighboring Turkey. They called it Turkey Red and planted small fields of it near their new Kansas homes. It survived the dry conditions and provided hard wheat that was excellent for bread. Hybrids of the original grain, a red winter wheat, are grown throughout the state today.

The German Russian Mennonites also brought some German-style foods familiar in Pennsylvania Dutch areas, such as pancakes, sausages, and buttermilk pie. They introduced *bierocks* and *verenikas* served with cream gravy. Beef rolls stuffed with bacon, onions, and pickles are similar to German *Rouladen,* and sausage-filled buns called *Bubbat* are other Kansas dishes brought by the German Russians. The settlers who came from the Northeast cooked pies daily, when possible, using whatever was available for a filling. In Franklin County, French immigrants improvised with turkey stews and quail in garlic sauce (Lee, 1992).

Michigan

French explorers and traders were the first Europeans in the Michigan territory. They fished the Great Lakes for bass, trout, perch, smelt, and whitefish. The Upper Peninsula offered ample game, particularly deer. A specialty of that region with French roots is *booyaw* or *boolyaw* (perhaps from the French term *bouillon*), a game stew featuring venison or whatever else was available (including rabbit, woodchuck, squirrel, even duck), salt pork, carrots, potatoes, and onions. The French also introduced sour European cooking cherries to the state. Today Michigan is the leading producer of these tart fruits used in pies and preserves.

Pioneers from the Northeast settled in Michigan during the early 1800s. They mostly operated small farms, growing beans, corn, wheat, and garden vegetables. They raised dairy cows and kept a few hogs

The German Russian yeast dough turnover (typically filled with beef, cabbage, and onions) common throughout the Great Plains was derived from the Russian *pirozhki*. It is called a *bierock* in Kansas and the midwestern regions east and south of that state and is known as a *runsa* in Nebraska and the northern Midwest areas. There is some confusion about the dish because the name bierock sounds similar to *pierogi*, a Polish stuffed dumpling that is boiled, also called *pelmeni* by some Russians and *varenyky* by Ukrainians. German Russian Mennonites make a similar stuffed dumpling they call *verenikas* (Isern,1990).

The origins of meat loaf, the quintessential midwestern beef dish, are unknown. It may have come with German immigrants, who sometimes added rye bread as an extender or sauerkraut for moisture (Lee, 1992). It was first documented in an American cookbook in 1902. Precursors from the 1880s were made with veal and called *Cannelon* (Anderson, 1997).

Smelt must be fished at night and are most numerous after the spring ice melt. The small 4- to 5-inch fish are scooped up in baskets after being drawn to the surface by bright lights. They are traditionally dredged in seasoned flour and fried.

for meat. Michigan baked beans, which kept many families going during lean years, were topped with a layer of salt pork and baked until firm. The resulting loaf was sliced and served with catsup (Lee, 1992). Over time, farmers diversified, and Michigan became known for its agricultural variety, including celery, cucumbers (many used for pickles), berries, grapes, peaches, and pears. Apples are a significant crop, and local recipes include apple salad, apple meatloaf, apple bread, apple fritters, candied apples, and caramel apples.

In the 1840s the first U.S. mining boom began with the discovery of iron and copper in Michigan's Upper Peninsula. Miners from Cornwall who were attracted by the rush brought their unique lunch specialty called *pasties* to the region (see Chapter 4 on Europeans). The complete meal in a turnover often featured venison in the Michigan versions, and turnips were a common vegetable filling. Apples were the most popular fruit used for the dessert end of the pastry. When immigrants from Finland arrived to work the mines in the following years, they adopted the dish, which was similar to *piiraat* and *kukko*, Finnish pastries filled with meat or fish, rice, and vegetables. Local Italians also included pasties in their daily meals. The origins of the dish are sometimes claimed by Finns in the region, although those of Cornish descent point out that the Finn pasties are nontraditional because the filling is mixed instead of layered and edges are crimped instead of using a decorative pastry rope; the Finns also drink buttermilk with their pasties (Lockwood & Lockwood, 1991). Other immigrant contributions to Michigan cuisine include Dutch *Apple Kock* (a yeast-risen dough topped with apple slices, sugar, and cinnamon), Czech *kolaches* and *strudel*, Ukrainian *borscht,* and German *Hollerstriebli* (elderberry flower fritters dipped in powdered sugar).

Michigan is probably best known for its role in the development of the U.S. cereal industry. The city of Battle Creek was home to two health sanitariums during the late nineteenth century. The first was founded by Seventh-Day Adventist leader Ellen Harmon White, who advocated vegetarianism. Her medical director was Dr. John Kellogg, inventor of corn flakes (see Chapter 2 on food and religion). C. W. Post, a dissatisfied Kellogg patient, started his own health institute in Battle Creek. He created a coffee substitute, *Postum* (a blend of wheat berries, bran, and molasses) and a cereal based on his own recipe for digestive problems, called *Grape-Nuts.*

Pasties were sometimes warmed in the mines with a "Cornish stove," a shovel held over a candle flame (Lee, 1992).

Pasty shops, many with untraditional fillings (e.g., pizza ingredients), are common throughout the Upper Peninsula (U.P.) and in cities where "U.P.ers" (*Yoopers*) have settled, such as Detroit.

Grape-Nuts does not include grapes or nuts. C. W. Post invented the name because he thought slow-baking the little breadcrumbs that made up the cereal transformed the wheat starches into the sugar dextrose, which he knew as grape sugar. The resulting hard nuggets reminded him of nuts (Wyman, 1993).

Muskrat was a popular Minnesota dish at one time and was well accepted by European immigrants. One recipe, called *Swedish Muskrat,* first boils the hams, then browns them in butter.

Minnesota

Although the cooler, northern climate of Minnesota limited agricultural opportunities, white settlers in the region found game and fish plentiful: Deer, elk, moose, bear, goose, duck, trout, bass, walleye, and sturgeon are just a few examples. One pioneer commented on the bountiful, flavorful buffalo roasts and beaver tail jerky (Jones, 1981).

Some Europeans, particularly Germans and Scandinavians, were attracted to the weather, low mountains, and numerous lakes in the state. The Germans brought hogs and dairy cattle and introduced their dark rye breads, including pumpernickel. Sausages, hams, sauerkraut, and specialties like *Hasenpfeffer* (stewed rabbit), *Spätzle* (tiny dumplings), *Maultaschen* (a sort of German ravioli filled with ground ham, eggs, onions, and sometimes spinach), and *Kuchen* (thin, sweet rectangles of dough covered with fruit, cottage cheese, or streusel) were other German dishes. Preserved fish were a mainstay for the Scandinavians. Pickled fish, smoked fish, and salt-cured fish were popular, particularly the Norwegian dish known as *lutefisk* (see Chapter 4 on Europeans), served with butter and potatoes. Ham, bacon, Swedish meatballs, and Danish *fricadellar* (fried, breaded ground beef and veal patties) were consumed. Dark breads and the thin Norwegian potato pancake called *lefser* are still common, as are butter cookies (especially at Christmas) and Danish *aebelskivers*, traditionally served with chokecherry or blueberry syrup or jam. The Scandinavian concept of the smörgåsbord was introduced to the nation in Minnesota (see Chapter 4 on Europeans for more details). Scottish settlers brought shortbread, and immigrants from Croatia, Slovenia, and Serbia added the grilled meats, eggplant, and cabbage dishes familiar in their native lands. Several ethnic communities in Minnesota maintain their culinary heritage at holidays and festivals, including the German Catholic city New Ulm and the Danish town Askov.

Minnesota is famous for its high-quality hard spring wheat and flour. Minneapolis, located on the Mississippi River, became a milling center in the mid-nineteenth century. The replacement of millstones with steel rollers in 1847 increased yield, and the city became the world's largest milling center by the end of the century. It remains a major flour-producing region today. The state is also known for sugar processing, and the Red River Valley is nicknamed "America's Sugarbowl" due to the area's success in growing sugar beets. Minnesota is a major dairying region, one of the top butter and cheese producers in the nation. Wild rice, called a "grain" but actually the triangular-shaped seed of an aquatic grass found in the shallow rivers and lakes of the state, is another Minnesota specialty (see Chapter 3 on Native Americans).

Missouri

The early white pioneers who came by covered wagon to the Missouri frontier were mostly from the South. French immigrants from Canada and German settlers from North Carolina, Pennsylvania, Ohio, Louisiana, and other states followed. The southerners brought fried chicken, buttermilk biscuits, cream gravy, and long-simmered greens. The French introduced *crêpes* and *brioche* to the

The Danish community of Askov, Minnesota has an annual festival commemorating the rutabaga. Although the tuber is commonly called a *Swede* or *Swedish turnip*, it is thought that Danes introduced the rutabaga to the region.

Charles Pillsbury was one of the early flour milling innovators in Minneapolis.

Log Cabin syrup was invented in 1887 by a St. Paul, Minnesota grocer who came up with the idea of blending pure maple syrup with sugar syrup to produce a tasty, economical product.

The Minnesota Massacre occurred in 1862 when U.S. troops pushed the Ojibwa Indians out of Minnesota, in part to provide access to wild rice stands.

Smoked buffalo tongue, a dish favored by some European immigrants, contributed to the precipitous decline of the U.S. buffalo population in the mid-1800s. In 1848 alone, 25,000 buffalo tongues were shipped to St. Louis.

Anti-German sentiment during World War II led some people to rename sauerkraut "Liberty Cabbage" (Matson, 1994).

Adolphus Busch came to St. Louis in 1857. He joined in partnership with Eberhard Anheuser and established the Anheuser-Busch brewery, which has become the largest beer-producing facility in the world. Busch was the first to pasteurize beer, dramatically increasing shelf-life.

In 1910, St. Louis considered itself the U.S. spaghetti capital, due to the ten pasta factories located in the city.

Hostilities broke out between Missouri and Iowa when three hollow trees filled with honey hives were cut down on land claimed by both territories. Missouri won the Honey War and was able to extend its northern boundary into Iowa (Lee, 1992).

During the nineteenth century, Kansas City was known as *the town built on beef and bread.*

Arthur Bryant's is the most famous of the Kansas City barbecue restaurants. It was started by African American Charlie Bryant in the 1930s. He called it "a grease house" (Matson, 1994). Food writer Calvin Trillin (1974) has called it "the single best restaurant in the world." It was one of the first integrated businesses in the city.

region. They also made hard cider from apples, wine from native grapes, and brandy from peaches. German contributions included sauerkraut, pickled herring, and potato pancakes. The German settlers also established brewing and sausage making in Missouri. *Weinerwurst* (literally sausage from Vienna—probably the first hot dogs in America, also known as *weiners), Leberwurst* (liverwurst, a soft, spreadable sausage), and *Blutwurst* (blood sausage) were specialties. Smaller numbers of immigrants from Italy, Greece, Poland, Russia, and other central European countries came to Missouri in the late 1800s, forming ethnic communities throughout the state.

The hilly, wooded terrain found in much of Missouri is unsuited for grain crops or cattle, but excellent for pigs and nut trees. Pork, a meat prized by southerners and Germans alike, was used in numerous dishes. Missouri is well known for its *country hams*, which are cured with salt, then smoked, and hung to age in the cool winter months. The resulting meat is red-colored, salty-flavored, and dry in texture. It is traditionally served with biscuits and *red-eyed gravy* made from ham drippings, coffee, and flour. Eastern black walnuts are native to the region. The nuts are strongly flavored with a slightly bitter aftertaste. They are the primary ingredient in black walnut pie. Pecans, too, are indigenous to Missouri. They are popular in pies, candies, cookies, and cakes. Over 7,000 beekeepers also take advantage of the woodlands in the state to provide another specialty of the region—honey.

Some of the most isolated hill country in Missouri is found in the Ozark Mountains. Contrary to immigration trends in urban areas, the people who came to the Ozarks gradually arrived from other states in small groups and were scattered throughout the region. They were known as *backwoodsmen,* and they existed on hunting, fishing, gathering, and cultivation of corn, beans, squash, and various tubers (Matson, 1994). Hogs were let loose to forage until butchering time in December or January. The people of the Ozarks were known for their stews made from opossum, raccoon, or squirrel. Sorghum was used to sweeten foods, ginger root was brewed for beer, and sassafras was steeped for tea. Today the Ozarks are best known as a vacation and retirement destination.

Unlike most of Missouri, Kansas City is renowned for its wheat and beef. Yet its reputation was built not on agriculture, but on the numerous grain elevators, flour mills, stockyards, and meat-packing plants built to process the wheat and beef shipped to the city. It is famous for its barbecued meats, particularly beef brisket, ribs, and ham, slowly rotisseried over hickory smoke until tender, with a spicy tomato-based sauce served on the side.

Nebraska

The Lewis and Clark expedition listed game, such as buffalo, deer, elk, turkey, grouse, ducks, and numerous fish, as Nebraska food resources in 1804. They also noted wild cherries, grapes, berries, and plums.

Other explorers thought that Nebraska was more like a desert, unsuitable for agriculture. Although living off the land was possible for the nomadic Indian tribes of the region and for small groups of traders and trappers, the thousands of homesteaders who arrived with the opening of the railroad in the mid-1800s found pioneer life difficult. Corn was the most successful crop, and cornmeal replaced wheat flour in nearly all recipes. Salt pork and salted beef were staples; milk, eggs, and butter were limited until each settler could purchase livestock and poultry. Dried produce, such as apples, peaches, raisins, pumpkins, and squash, were more common than fresh fruits and vegetables. Irrigation increased agricultural variety in Nebraska. Today it is best known for livestock, including cattle, hogs, sheep, and poultry. Corn is the primary crop, but other grains, such as wheat, oats, barley, and sorghum, are also grown in significant quantities. Potatoes and sugar beets are planted in some areas, and in the driest regions, hay is produced for feed.

ConAgra, one of the world's largest food companies, got its start as Nebraska Consolidated Mills in 1919, selling 25-pound bags of flour in decorative, reusable cotton sacks.

As in other midwestern states, immigrants to Nebraska brought their favorite recipes, adapting them to available ingredients. In Nebraska the Swiss introduced plum tarts and a specialty called *Thuna*, breadsticks topped with creamed greens thickened with flour. Czech settlers brought *jaternice* (pork sausage), *jelita* (blood sausage), and *bouska* (a sweet, braided bread), as well as the popular kolaches. Swedish yeasted waffles and Hungarian chicken paprika are other examples. Meat stew with dumplings, buttermilk spoon bread, and oatmeal cookies are dishes introduced by homesteaders who came to Nebraska from the U.S. Northeast and South.

North Dakota

White settlement in North Dakota did not really begin until the 1870s, when railroads increased access and inexpensive land attracted farmers. Many immigrants came from Europe, especially Norwegians, Germans, and German Russians. They brought the dishes of their homelands, and today Norwegian food such as lefse, *spekejøtt* (smoked, dried lamb), *rullepølse* (cold, spicy rolled beef), *søtsuppe* (fruit soup) and baked goods, including the large pyramid of almond paste and meringue rings called *kransekake*. Other immigrants, such as the Scots in the northern Red River Valley, enjoyed oatmeal porridge served with fresh berries and oatmeal cakes called *bannocks*. A large population of settlers from Iceland smoked mutton, made *skyr* (a sweet, cultured milk product similar to yogurt), fried *kleinur* (doughnuts), and baked *vinarterta* (a multilayered cardamom-flavored cake with fruit fillings) for dessert. The German Russians brought *runsa,* the name for bierocks in this region. The Scotch Irish introduced *colcannon* (mashed potatoes, onions, and cabbage), and the French Canadians came with croissants and cassoulet (see Chapter 4 on Europeans).

Cream of Wheat cereal was created in 1893 by Diamond Milling Co. in Grand Forks, North Dakota to make use of the wheat hearts, or middlings, produced in processing flour.

Pierogi is a stuffed dumpling that is traditionally filled with potatoes, cabbage, onion, and/or meat. Pierogi producers in Ohio today offer such innovative fillings as taco and Cajun beef.

Cincinnati was nicknamed "Porkopolis" during the nineteenth century.

North Dakota crops are grown mostly in the eastern half of the state and include spring and winter wheat, particularly durum wheat, which is used for semolina and durum flour. Barley, sunflowers, potatoes, oats, and beans are other agricultural products. The western half of the state is mostly used for cattle ranching.

Ohio

Ohio was one of the first midwestern frontier regions settled by white pioneers, in part due to its proximity to the original colonial states and in part because land grants were offered to those who had served in the Revolutionary War (bounty lands) or whose homes had been burned by the British (the Firelands). The settlers found a wooded terrain that provided rich soil when cleared for farming. Game and fish were so plentiful that a compilation of recipes from 1880 called *Buckeye Cookery and Practical Housekeeping* included information on how to prepare raccoon, squirrel, opossum, skunks, and sturgeon, as well as how to smoke venison and roast bear meat.

The pioneers from New England brought their baked beans, chicken pot pies, and baked goods to Ohio. They used breadcrumbs to stuff meats, a practice still popular in the region (Lee, 1992). Central Europeans who immigrated contributed their specialties: The Czechs brought fish served with a black sauce made from prunes, raisins, and almonds, and the Slovenians brought *potica,* their national bread, flavored with nuts, seeds, or tarragon. The Poles, one of the largest ethnic groups to settle in the state, introduced favorites such as *kielbasa, pierogi,* and strudels. The most significant influence on Ohio cooking came from the numerous Germans who came to the state, beginning in the early nineteenth century. They popularized pork, sausage, ham, potato, and cabbage dishes, such as the unusual Ohio specialty called *sauerkraut balls,* which are deep-fried sauerkraut and ham fritters served with mustard sauce. The Germans opened beer gardens, restaurants, and bakeries throughout the region. Not only did they develop the brewing industry in Cincinnati; they also contributed to the first wine industry in the United States along the shores of Lake Erie. Many Ohio cities have retained German communities where German foods are still prevalent.

The state quickly became an agricultural center, producing corn, wheat, and more recently, soybeans. Hogs, cattle, dairy cows, and poultry are significant commodities in some regions. During the 1830s, Cincinnati produced more pork products than any other city worldwide, processing hogs from Indiana and Kentucky in addition to those from within the state. During the same period the state was also known for cheese, particularly the strong-smelling, soft, creamy cheese with a crust called *Liederkranz*. It was invented by the Monroe Cheese Company of Van Wert in 1926 as a substitute for German *Schlosskäse*, but its distinctive flavor has attracted its own devotees.

Ohio is probably best known nationally for a more recent creation, *Cincinnati chili*. In the 1920s, restaurants in the city would prepare chili with beans from the leftover meats of the day. It had a slightly unsavory reputation because one never knew what had gone into it. Tom Kiradjieff, a Macedonian immigrant, created a pure, all-beef version and started serving it over spaghetti in 1923. He boiled the beef first, then simmered it for hours in a tomato sauce flavored with a balanced blend of sweet spices (such as cinnamon, allspice, cloves, and nutmeg) and hot spices (garlic, cumin, black pepper, and chiles). It became so popular that chili parlors are commonly found throughout Ohio (and parts of nearby Kentucky) that serve the mild chili *one-way* (just the meaty stew), *two-way* (over spaghetti), *three-way* (spaghetti, chili, topped with grated cheese), *four-way* (spaghetti, chili, topped with cheese and diced onions), or *five-way* (spaghetti, chili, cheese, onions, and finished with kidney beans).

Some researchers speculate that the unique sweet-hot spicing of Cincinnati chili is a direct result of Tom Kiradjieff's culinary heritage, creating a flavor reminiscent of such eastern Mediterranean dishes as *pastitsio* or *moussaka* (Lloyd, 1981).

South Dakota

Unlike the farmers who flocked to North Dakota in search of inexpensive land, the first American settlers in South Dakota were miners and fortune hunters, who arrived after the 1870s gold strike in the Black Hills. Although there was abundant game, including deer, mountain goats, and geese, plentiful freshwater fish, and a variety of wild fruit, such as grapes, chokecherries, bush cranberries, juneberries, and buffalo berries, the miners were not hunters or gatherers. Food was scarce, and most survived on salt pork or bacon and beans. A full meal of pork roast, sourdough bread, baked potatoes, and possibly pie was a luxury.

Some immigrants noted the grazing potential of the surrounding land. Cattle ranching quickly became the primary agricultural activity in the state, and it remains so today. The first cattle were longhorns from Texas; they were soon joined by Scottish cattle, including Aberdeen, Angus, and Herefords. Immigrants from Scotland were soon exporting beef to their homeland. Hogs and sheep have also become important commodities in the state. Corn, wheat, rye, and sunflowers are grown in some sections.

Significant numbers of Swedes have settled in South Dakota, introducing the rutabaga to the region, as well as the smörgåsbord, almond cakes, and spice cookies. German Russians and Czechs brought their traditional foods. Other South Dakota specialties include lamb dishes and pheasant roasted with salt pork or prepared with onions in a casserole (Lee, 1992).

The ring-necked pheasant was introduced to the United States from China when a shipment was sent to Oregon. It has naturalized throughout much of the nation and is the state bird of South Dakota.

The largest meat-packing facility in the country is the John Morell & Co. plant in Sioux City, South Dakota.

One of the most popular cookbooks in U.S. history, and one of the first to include ethnic and religious specialties, was written by Lizzie Black Kander, president of the Milwaukee Jewish Mission. She taught cooking classes to poor immigrants at The Settlement, the mission's social house. Her compilation of recipes, called *The Settlement Cook Book*, was first published in 1901. The last revision was in 1976; it is now out of print.

Fish boils were begun by Scandinavians as an efficient way to feed the workers in lumber camps. A typical recipe includes 100 pounds of fish (usually whitefish), an equal amount of potatoes, 40 pounds of salt, onions—and a pot big enough to boil everything together. Today fish boils at the edge of Lake Michigan are annual tourist events in Wisconsin.

In 1900, nearly three in every four residents of Milwaukee were of German heritage.

Wisconsin produces over 2 billion pounds of cheese each year, 40 percent of all cheese consumed nationally.

The Great Wisconsin Cheese Festival held annually in Little Chute features cheese specialties, like *cheesewurst* (bratwurst made with added cheese) and deep-fried cheese curds (a favorite with state residents).

Wisconsin

Wisconsin fare assimilates native foods, agricultural abundance, and immigrant preferences. Although the state had been home to small numbers of trappers and traders in the eighteenth century, the first significant white settlement did not occur until the early nineteenth century, when farmers from New York, Pennsylvania, Ohio, and Indiana arrived. They established wheat as the primary crop in the region. Farming opportunities, mining jobs, and the lumber industry attracted large numbers of immigrants from Germany, Scandinavia, Great Britain (especially Cornwall, Ireland, and Wales), Poland, Russia, and Switzerland in the mid-1800s. Cities and towns were founded along Lake Michigan (including Milwaukee), many with ethnic neighborhoods. Each group contributed specialties to the cuisine, such as Cornish pasties and saffron cakes, Scandinavian fish boils, and Polish poppy seed pastries.

The Germans established the state as a major pork producer during the 1800s. Hams and sausages have become ubiquitous in the region, so much so that they have lost most of their ethnic associations, and cities such as Sheboygan call themselves the "Bratwurst Capital of the World." Today meat processing is still big business; Patrick Cudahy, Jones Dairy Farms, Hillshire Farms, and Oscar Mayer all operate in the state. Another famous Wisconsin food contributed by the Germans is beer. The first breweries were located in the southwestern section of the state and produced the ales and stouts favored by English settlers. By the middle of the nineteenth century, ten breweries producing German-style lagers had been founded in Milwaukee, including plants owned by Frederich Miller, Frederich Pabst, and Joseph Schlitz. At the beginning of the 1900s there were over 300 breweries statewide, but Prohibition and consolidation in recent years have reduced that number to 8.

Despite renown in sausages and beer, Wisconsin is reputed nationally for its dairy industry. It is the leading U.S. producer of milk, sweetened condensed milk, butter, and cheese. Dairying was sparked by the arrival of Swiss farmers to the state following the 1844 crop failure in Switzerland. They brought their expertise in breeding livestock and making cheese. *Colby*, a hard cheese similar to Cheddar, is an original Wisconsin cheese that was created in 1885. Another variety developed in Wisconsin is *Brick*, a semi-soft cheese with holes and a flavor described as sweet, nutty, and spicy. It is mild when fresh but becomes stronger with age. Italian cheeses, including Ricotta, Mozzarella, Provolone, Romano, and Parmesan, are specialties of northern Wisconsin, while blue cheese is made in the caves near Milwaukee.

Wheat has given way to vegetables throughout much of Wisconsin. Cabbage, carrots, corn, cucumbers, green beans, lima beans, and peas are significant crops in the state. One-third of the cabbage grown for sauerkraut in the United States comes from Wisconsin.

The South

Regional Profile

Most southerners say the South is more an attitude than a location. This perhaps explains why there are so many definitions of the region, such as those states below the historic Mason-Dixon line or those south of the culinary "grits" line (the divide between where grits are eaten and where they aren't). While no one questions that Alabama, Arkansas, Florida, Georgia, Louisiana, Kentucky, Maryland, Mississippi, the Carolinas, Tennessee, Virginia, and West Virginia are clearly part of the South, the borderline states of Delaware, Missouri, Oklahoma, and Texas can be argued for inclusion either way. Using the U.S. government definition, Missouri is considered part of the Midwest, while Delaware, Oklahoma, and Texas are part of the South.

The lands of the South are varied. They include the fertile coastal plains along the Atlantic and Gulf coasts, the rolling hills leading up to the mountains (called the *Piedmont* in most states), the rugged Appalachian and Ozark mountain territories, the lowlands of the Mississippi Delta, and the high desert plains of the western reaches. The climate also ranges from the warm, moderate Atlantic states to the hot, humid Gulf Coast states to the hot, dry weather in parts of Texas and Oklahoma.

The development of the South was in many ways independent from that of the northern United States. During colonial times, southern states were predominantly agricultural, growing tobacco, wheat, corn, rice, and indigo (a blue dye). The plantation system that emerged in the coastal regions was characterized by commercial farms owned by aristocratic English or French immigrants and worked by African slaves. Each plantation was a self-sufficient, independent operation providing cash crops and food products for use by each household. It was a comfortable, leisurely lifestyle for the upper classes, enlivened by occasional visits to the cultural centers of Atlanta, Charleston, or New Orleans. For the lower classes, which included the slaves and the poor farmers of the inland hill and mountain regions, it was a hand-to-mouth existence.

During the time the northern areas of the country became more urbanized and industrialized, the South remained agricultural, adding cotton as a major crop. Waves of immigrants from central, eastern, and southern Europe who arrived in the United States looking for jobs settled mostly in the North, where manufacturing opportunities existed. The South was largely isolated from changes occurring in the North. Differences of opinion regarding the role of the federal government in state issues, particularly slavery, led to the Civil War in the mid-1800s. After losing the war, the South regrouped in the late nineteenth century. The traditions and practices that give the South its character became more important than ever. The South continues to preserve its identity, in part, through its cuisine.

One song in the South goes: ". . . South is my blood and South my bone/So haply formed on pork and pone . . . You say: 'South? Where can that be?'/Chewing my sugar cane, I repeat:/'Why in all we like to cook and eat.'" (Walter, 1971, p. 19).

Over one-third (35%) of Americans make their home in the South, the highest percentage of the U.S. population in any region. It is divided into the South Atlantic states of Delaware, Florida, Georgia, Maryland, North Carolina, South Carolina, Virginia, West Virginia, and the District of Columbia; the East South Central states of Alabama, Kentucky, Mississippi, and Tennessee; and the West South Central states of Arkansas, Louisiana, Oklahoma, and Texas. Over all, the South has below average numbers of Asians and Pacific Islanders, Latinos, and Native Americans, but above average numbers of African Americans: 52 percent of all U.S. blacks live in the South (see Table 11.4). However, the very size of the southern population means that significant numbers of most ethnic groups reside in the region. For example, 30 percent of all Native Americans and Latinos live in the South; both Florida and Texas host above average populations of Latinos. While only 15 percent of U.S. Asians are found in the South, larger numbers of some groups, such as Vietnamese, Pakistanis, and Asian Indians, reside there. In addition to African Americans, groups with disproportionately large representation in the South include persons of British ancestry (39% of those in the United States), Scotch Irish ancestry (47%), Cuban ancestry (69%), and Cajun ancestry (91%) (see Figure 11.5).

Although the population of the South is now mostly urban, it ranges from the lowest national percentage of urban dwellers (in West Virginia, where only 36% of residents live in cities), to the highest percentage of urban dwellers in the country (100% in the District of Columbia, all in the city of Washington, DC). Other states with high urban populations include Florida, Maryland, and Texas. States with low rates of urban residency (where approximately half of homes are rural) are Mississippi, North Carolina, Kentucky, and South Carolina.

Median income levels in the South fall below those of the nation as a whole. Some states show particularly low median incomes, such as West Virginia (27% below average) and Arkansas (26% below average). Exceptions in the region with above average median incomes are Maryland, Virginia, and Delaware. As might be expected from these income figures, high rates of poverty exist in the South as well, 10 percent above the national average in 1995–1997. Especially high numbers of persons live below the poverty line in the District of Columbia (22%), Mississippi (20%), and Louisiana (19%).

Some of the lowest rates of educational attainment and some of the highest rates are found in the South. The lowest high school graduation rates in the nation are in Kentucky and Louisiana, with Arkansas, Alabama, South Carolina, and West Virginia not far behind. Washington, DC has the highest percentage of college completion in the country—over one in every three residents (34%) has a bachelor's degree. Maryland and Virginia also have higher than average numbers of persons with college degrees. States with particularly low percentages of college completion include Alabama and West Virginia.

South

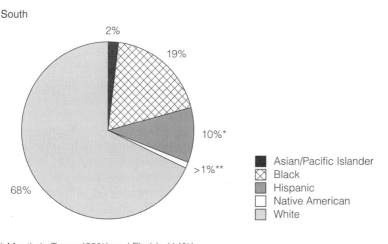

2%
19%
10%*
>1%**
68%

■ Asian/Pacific Islander
⊠ Black
▨ Hispanic
☐ Native American
☐ White

* Mostly in Texas (28%) and Florida (14%)
**Mostly in Oklahoma (8%)

FIGURE 11.5
Demographics in the South.

The population of the South is notable for its high numbers of Christians. Over half of all residents (57%) belong to a Christian faith, the highest percentage in the nation. Numbers are even higher in the East South Central States and the West South Central states: Over 70 percent of persons in Alabama, Mississippi, and Louisiana are Christian.

Traditional Fare

The foods most associated with the South reflect both the bounty of the plantation and the scarcity of the slave diet. Corn dishes, rice, all parts of the hog, sweet potatoes, and greens began as the foundation of southern fare and remain characteristic components today. (See Chapter 5 on African Americans for more information on slave foods and their influence on southern cooking.)

The southern lifestyle has fostered a culture of graciousness and cordiality. The isolation of the plantations meant socialization was limited in frequency but lengthy in duration. Hours of travel to nearby homes typically resulted in overnight visits or extended stays. Parties, balls, picnics, barbecues, and seafood feasts were all occasions for get-togethers. For the slaves, Sunday meals with extended kin were the primary way to maintain family connections. In the hills and mountains of the South the difficulties of subsistence farming necessitated friendly relationships between neighbors. Poor families often survived through regular sharing of food. As a result of these conditions, the South has become synonymous with hospitality.

"We eat everything but the squeal" is a saying in the South about pigs.

TABLE 11.4
Southern Specialties

Group	Foods	Preparations
PROTEIN FOODS		
Milk/milk products	Buttermilk, milk	Cream gravy
Meat/poultry/fish/eggs/ legumes	Native game, including buffalo, venison, raccoon, opossum, badger, squirrel, turkey, ducks, alligator, diamondback terrapin	*Brunswick stew,* squirrel stew, possum 'n' taters, turtle soup
	Pork in all forms, especially country-cured and Smithfield hams; beef, mutton, kid	Ham on beaten biscuits, sliced ham and red-eye gravy; barbecued pork; *souse* (head cheese); chitterlings; Texas-style barbecued beef, *chili con carne;* son-of-a-bitch stew; *cabrito*
	Chicken	Fried chicken with cream gravy, chicken and dumplings
	Crab (blue, stone), crawfish, conch, oysters, shrimp, spiny lobster; ocean fish, such as mullet, pompano, shad; freshwater fish, particularly catfish	Crab, shrimp, or crawfish boils; crab cakes; she-crab soup; conch chowder; oyster stew; shrimp *pilau;* shrimp Creole; jambalaya; gumbo; *étouffée;* fish muddle; fried catfish
	Chicken eggs	Scrambled eggs and brains, scrambled eggs and ramps
	Dried beans; peanuts	Baked beans, butter bean custard; peanut soup, peanut brittle
CEREALS/GRAINS	Corn, rice, wheat, buckwheat	Hominy, grits, corn pone, hush puppies, corn bread, spoon bread; rice pilaus; beaten biscuits; buttermilk or sour milk biscuits; buckwheat pancakes
FRUITS/VEGETABLES	Apples, huckleberries, key limes, oranges, mayhaw, peaches, watermelon	Preserves and pickles; fried pies; key lime pie; ambrosia; peach pie
	Wild greens (cochan, creases, dandelion, dock, lamb's quarters, poke, sorrel, and ramp), domesticated greens (e.g., mustard, turnip), black-eyed peas, cabbage, okra, ramps, sweet potatoes	Greens simmered with fat back or salt pork, consumed with pot likker; poke salad (sallet); fried ramps; hoppin' John; coleslaw, fried okra, okra stews; sweet potato pie
ADDITIONAL FOODS		
Seasonings	Chile peppers (especially bird's eye); *filé;* celery, garlic, onions, green peppers; bourbon, sherry, whiskey	Pepper sherry, chili powder, hot sauce; High Holy mayonnaise; barbecue sauce
Nuts/seeds	Black walnuts, hickory nuts, pecans; sesame (benne) seeds	Nut cakes, brittles, glazed pecans, pecan pie, pralines; sesame seed candies and cookies
Beverages	Buttermilk; bourbon, corn whiskey, Sherry, Tennessee whiskey	Whiskey and bourbon added to barbecue sauces, baked goods, candies
Fats/oils	Lard	
Sweeteners	Sorghum syrup	Used over pancakes, grits, corn bread, in coffee

The first European explorers in the South Atlantic states were the Spanish, who arrived in Florida in 1513 and founded St. Augustine in 1565. They were soon followed by the English, who started in Virginia and spread north and south along the Atlantic coastline during the seventeenth and eighteenth centuries into Delaware, Maryland, the Carolinas, Georgia, and eventually into Florida. The Native American population at the time numbered in the hundreds of thousands, includ-

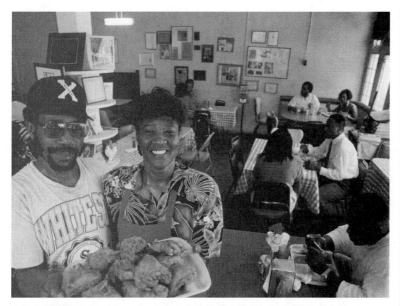

Fried chicken is the quintessential dish of the South. It is often served with cream gravy and biscuits.

ing the members of the Powhatan, Cherokee, Chickasaw, Choctaw, Creek, and Seminole tribes (see Chapter 3 on Native Americans).

The white settlers discovered a region with plentiful fruits, nuts, game, fish, and seafood. Native strawberries, blackberries, blueberries, huckleberries, ground cherries, persimmons, Scuppernong grapes, beechnuts, hickory nuts, and pecans covered the land. Bream, catfish, perch, pike, and trout filled the rivers, while oysters, clams, and crab were abundant along the coast. In Florida, pompano, red snapper, shrimp, spiny lobster, and conch were widely available. Diamondback terrapin, sea turtles, and alligators were found in many waterways, and bear, deer, opossum, rabbits, raccoons, squirrels, turkey, grouse, ducks, and quail were prevalent in woodland areas. Indians of the region grew corn, beans, pumpkin, squash, sweet potatoes, and sunflowers.

Most of the first white settlers in the region were farmers who established plantations. They brought wheat, hogs, cattle, poultry, cabbage, potatoes, and fruit trees, including apples and peaches. Africans were imported as laborers. They introduced southern staples, such as peanuts, okra, watermelon, and sesame seeds, and taught the farmers of the lowland coastal areas how to successfully grow and harvest rice (Hess, 1992).

These traditional foods of the Native Americans, the European settlers, and the African slaves combined to create the cooking of the Atlantic South. Hot breads were the cornerstone of every meal, primarily corn breads (see Table 11.5) or biscuits. Country hams, ribs, fatback, cracklings, and chitterlings were produced from hogs. A Native

South settlers liked opossum because of its fatty meat. It was typically baked with sweet potatoes, colloquially called *'possum 'n' taters*.

Many sources note that the Native Americans of the South cultivated melons. Melons are not native to the New World, although it is possible they were brought to Florida by the original Spanish explorers, in which case the Indians may have been growing them for perhaps 100 years by the time white settlers arrived from the north.

TABLE 11.5
Southern Corn Breads

Corn bread	Made with white cornmeal, eggs, and water. No sugar is added. Baked in a pan, sliced into squares, served with butter, honey, or sorghum syrup.
Cracklin' bread	Usually yellow cornmeal bread with added pork cracklings for flavor, traditionally cooked in a frying pan on the stove.
Spoon bread	Yellow cornmeal bread made with eggs and milk. Baked slowly in a pan until golden crust forms on top and center remains custard-like.
Corn pone	Yellow cornmeal and water (lard added if available) mixed into a stiff dough, formed into sticks (sometimes called *corn sticks*) or patties (sometimes called *hoecakes*) and cooked in a skillet.
Hush puppies	Yellow cornmeal and water dough, with added egg and buttermilk if available, formed into balls and deep-fried.

Pilau was probably introduced to the South by French Huguenots who settled in South Carolina during the seventeenth century.

Corn whiskey became the most popular alcoholic beverage of the Appalachians and in most areas of the South because apples for applejack were in short supply and barley for beer did not grow well in the region.

American game dish adopted by the southern settlers, *Brunswick stew*, became a mainstay throughout the region. There are many variations, but most contain chicken, ham or salt pork, corn, beans, potatoes, onions, tomatoes, and lots of black pepper. The quintessential dish of the South is chicken dredged in cornmeal or flour and fried in lard, traditionally served with cream gravy. Long-grained rice was cooked as *pilau* with meat, poultry, greens, peas, beans, or vegetables. (*Hoppin' John,* rice with black-eyed peas, is the most famous dish of this kind.) Oyster roasts (similar to a New England clam bake) and *muddle* (a stew of miscellaneous fish with potatoes and onions) capitalized on coastal resources. Fresh milk, buttermilk, coffee, and tea were the usual beverages.

Desserts have always had a place on the southern table. Tea breads and cakes (such as *Sally Lunn* cake, popular throughout the region), fruitcakes, and pies (peach, pecan, and sweet potato are most associated with the South) were common. Puddings and custards were an everyday treat. Many were made with leftover cornmeal, rice, or bread; chocolate was a favorite, but costly, so it was used only at special occasions. Candies, such as divinity with nuts and nut brittles, were specialties.

During the early 1800s, Scotch Irish immigrants searching for religious freedom began making their homes in the Blue Ridge, Cumberland and Great Smoky mountains of the Appalachians. They also spread west to the Kentucky and Tennessee frontier. English and some Welsh settlers moved from the coastal Atlantic South states inland to the Piedmont. Germans from Pennsylvania traveled south along the Shenandoah Valley into Virginia and North Carolina. "Hogs 'n' hominy" (pork and corn) kept the pioneers going until they established small farms. Frontier meals were robust. For example, the noon meal might consist of ham, bacon or sausage, chicken or grouse, game meat, dumplings or biscuits, corn bread or grits, gravy, sweet potatoes, and boiled greens served with coffee, milk, or corn whiskey.

Traditionally every bit of the pig was consumed on Appalachian farms, including the snout, or "rooter" (which was roasted), the tail (which was added to stews), and the brains (which were usually boiled, mashed, and scrambled with eggs). Most families kept a dairy cow and a breeding cow for a few calves each year. Fresh beef was preferred. When a cow was slaughtered, it would be shared with neighbors, who would later return the favor. Game of all kinds was popular, but especially squirrel, rabbit, raccoon, opossum, turtle, and frogs. Wild greens were well loved by adults in the Appalachians, but not so popular with children (Page & Wigginton, 1984). Poke, cochan (coneflower), creases (similar to watercress), dandelion, lamb's quarters, dock, sorrel, and ramp (a type of wild onion) are just a few of the varieties. Domesticated greens like mustard and turnip greens were also common. Other than greens, beans, hominy, sweet potatoes, potatoes, okra, and beets were the most frequently consumed vegetables. Corn bread (sometimes with cracklings added), biscuits, dumplings, and/or grits were served at every meal. Watermelon was a favorite, eaten fresh or preserved as pickles or jam. Honey was the most common sweetener, even consumed alone as a dessert. Sorghum syrup was also used. Many of these foods are still favored in the Appalachians today.

The early fare of the East South Central and West South Central states was similar to that of the Atlantic states, but with more significant French overtones. Immigrants from France settled in the Gulf Coast region during the seventeenth century, and at the end of the eighteenth century, French Acadians from Canada relocated to Louisiana (see Chapter 4 on Europeans for more information). They were joined by white American and English settlers arriving from the north. Plantation life in the region was similar to that of the Atlantic South, except that it was more dependent on cotton than on tobacco.

Pork and corn remained key to the cooking of the East and West South Central region. The corn bread in this area is made from white cornmeal without the addition of sugar. The French added their recipes for soups, stews, fricassees, and baked goods to the southern mix, as well as their appreciation for good eating. The resulting cuisine is found in some form throughout the Gulf Coast, from Mobile, Alabama to Beaumont, Texas. The French factor accounts for such adopted and adapted specialties as *bouillabaisse* (a French fish stew); fish cooked *en papillote* (in paper packets with a velouté sauce); and *sauce mahonaise* (homemade mayonnaise), particularly *High Holy mayonnaise* (a fanciful, Anglicized term for *aïoli*) made with fresh garlic and served with shrimp or cucumbers. Creole cuisine, a blending of French, Spanish, African, English, and Native American cooking, is unique to New Orleans. It is a complex fare with many refined dishes; celery, tomatoes, bell peppers, onions, and garlic

Poke salad is a cooked salad, which is an English tradition. Poke greens are parboiled, then fried in bacon or fatback grease until tender. They are seasoned with salt, pepper, and hot sauce or vinegar.

Leather britches were immature beans in their pods that were strung on string to dry. They would be soaked overnight before cooking, then boiled with a piece of bacon or fatback for flavoring.

are the hallmark flavorings. Cajun fare, created by the French Acadians, is mostly limited to the bayou country of Louisiana, though its gumbos, jambalayas, and étouffées have become popular throughout the region (see Chapter 4 on Europeans for more information on Creole and Cajun foods). While Oklahoma and Texas are both southern in attitude and enjoy many specialties of the South, such as grits, greens, Gulf Coast seafood, and Brunswick stews, their dishes are also influenced by Native American, central European, and Latino cooking. Beef is the dominant meat; barbecue is prevalent; and hot, spicy seasoning emboldens their dishes.

State Specialties

Alabama

The first Europeans in Alabama came by sea. In the early 1700s, France claimed the Louisiana Territory (including Alabama) and established a fort in Mobile. Young French women sent to marry the soldiers reputedly brought sophisticated culinary skills that they applied to native fish and game. Slaves imported for work on plantations and in city homes added their cooking preferences to the cuisine. Frontiersmen, most of whom were second- and third-generation Americans from Tennessee and the Carolinas, settled the inland hill country during the late eighteenth and early nineteenth centuries. The pioneers cleared substantial amounts of forested hillside in hopes of planting profitable crops, but large-scale agriculture in the area was mostly unsuccessful, and the new settlers eked out livings on small, family farms.

French influence was limited to the coast, where seafood was a primary ingredient in the cuisine. Shrimp were especially prevalent, prepared fried, boiled in seasoned water, with rémoulade sauce, and stuffed into *mirleton* (chayote squash), avocados, and other vegetables. Plump, local oysters, called Bon Secour oysters, were plentiful and popular throughout the Gulf Coast. In the 1800s, pushcart vendors sold them fresh on the streets of Mobile, and oyster bars served a dozen at a time: The first nine were eaten with lemon juice, the last three with horseradish.

The foods most associated with Alabama are traditional, inland dishes, however, such as fried chicken, chicken and dumplings, ham balls (fried fritters), Brunswick stew (made with a whole hog's head), and game dishes, especially those made with squirrels or frogs. Biscuits and corn breads were eaten daily. Sweet potato biscuits, crackling bread, and *hoecake bread* (cornmeal and water cooked in a frying pan) were everyday favorites; *beaten biscuits,* which required the dough to be hit repeatedly with a rolling pin to produce pockets of air for leavening, were prepared for special occasions. Hominy,

Oyster gumbo in Alabama includes cabbage, tomatoes, and a touch of molasses; no okra or filé is used to thicken the stew.

Beef did not become widely available in Alabama until the 1950s. The only beef dishes that were standards in traditional fare made use of inexpensive variety cuts: oxtail soup and calf's head stew (Solomon & Solomon, 1979).

greens, okra, green beans, butter beans, peas, rutabagas, and turnips were typical side dishes. Seasonal pies were popular, especially dewberry (the first ripe fruit of the summer season) and peach. Fried pies, a southern specialty, are thought to have originated in Alabama. Small circles of pie crust are filled with fruit (typically peaches or peach preserves in Alabama), then folded into a half-moon shape, crimped, deep-fried, and sprinkled with powdered sugar. Butter bean custard is an unusual dessert specialty of the region, made with mashed butter beans cooked as a sweet pudding flavored with cinnamon, cloves, and nutmeg. Buttermilk and coffee were preferred before the advent of soft drinks and iced tea—now these later beverages are common. Corn whiskey and wine from native grapes (including Scuppernongs and Muscadines) were consumed often. For parties and other social events, eggnog, punch, and *posset* (a thick eggnog served hot) were popular.

Arkansas

Arkansas is at the crossroads of the South, the Southwest, and the Midwest. The diverse terrain includes the fertile alluvial plains of the Mississippi River in the southeast of the state, the dry pasturelands of the southwest, the orchards and wheatfields of the northwest, and the rocky hills and mountains of the Ozarks in the northeast. The French established a trading post on the Mississippi River in 1686. Trappers made the post their base of operations and earned their living selling bear and buffalo products, such as meat, tallow, oil, and furs, to the residents of New Orleans. A few hardy farmers from Tennessee and Kentucky began settling in the northern parts of the state, and cotton plantations were founded in the southern region by pioneers from Mississippi. Substantial, widespread white settlement did not occur until the 1830s, however, when the Native Americans living in the area were forced into Oklahoma.

Settlers were mostly of English or Scotch Irish heritage, and they brought the foods they prepared in their home states, such as cured hams, sausages, baking soda biscuits, and molasses pies from the north, and fried chicken, buttermilk biscuits, sweet potatoes, and peach cobblers from the south. Barbecued beef and pinto beans are found in the areas of the state adjacent to Texas (Lee, 1992), and in the Ozarks the fare is similar to that found in the Missouri section of the mountains (see previous section), with pork, game meats (especially baked opossum and raccoon), corn, beans, and greens the foundation of the diet. Some Arkansas specialties are pork chops with cream gravy (sometimes made with bits of sausage in it), pan-fried chicken that is then baked with a Creole sauce, and strawberry shortcakes made with crisp biscuits drenched in strawberry juice and topped with fresh berries and whipped cream.

Peaches were brought to Arkansas by the Cherokee who had relocated in the state after being forced from their homes in the Atlantic South.

John Tyson, a pioneer in the poultry industry, got his start in the 1930s in Springdale, Arkansas when he came up with a plan for purchasing inexpensive chickens from local producers and trucking them to urban markets of Chicago, Cleveland, and Detroit, where they could be sold for a profit. Tyson is currently one of the largest poultry and pork producers in the country.

Catfish farming was started in Arkansas to control the quality of the fish (which is affected by what it eats); the Association of Catfish Farmers of America headquarters is in Little Rock.

In 1763, Delaware held one of the first agricultural fairs in the nation, featuring livestock, farm machinery, and "Ladies Work," such as quilts and needlework samplers in addition to jams, jellies, preserves, and baked goods.

Recent immigrants to Delaware include numerous Central Americans, particularly Guatemalans, who are attracted to jobs in the poultry industry.

The three original Native American groups in the region numbered over 350,000 when the Spanish arrived but were completely wiped out by the mid-1800s due primarily to disease. The Seminole, many of whom live on five Florida reservations, were originally Creek Indians who entered the state in the early 1700s.

In 1904, rice was introduced in the swampy region between the Arkansas and Mississippi rivers. German Americans from Illinois and Iowa moved into the area to establish paddies, founding cities with names like Stuttgart and Wiener. Today Arkansas leads the nation in rice production. Ducks, which make their winter homes in the dormant rice fields, attract numerous hunters to the state each year. They are a specialty in the region, roasted over a fire, baked with bacon and basted with wine or port, and prepared as gumbo. Catfish have long been an Arkansas favorite, dredged in cornmeal and fried, or in catfish stew. Catfish is traditionally served with *hush puppies* (deep-fried cornmeal biscuits) and coleslaw. The state is the second largest producer of domesticated catfish in the nation.

Delaware

The Dutch and the Swedes both established trading posts in Delaware in the early 1600s. Settlers in the region enjoyed the plentiful seafood, game, and wild fruit available. They planted gardens with vegetables and fruit trees and were particularly successful with corn. They were followed by larger numbers of English and German immigrants, whose influences on Delaware foods can be seen in some of the favorite dishes in the region. Heavily smoked and long-aged hams, sour milk biscuits, corn pudding, and cauliflower with custard sauce are a few specialties. Fish and shellfish were popular, including a local version of the fish stew called muddle, as well as steamed oysters, clams, and crabs.

Today poultry and eggs are the primary agricultural products in Delaware. The first "broilers" in the nation were marketed by Cecil Steele in Ocean View in 1923. Due to a mix-up, she received ten times more chicks than she ordered for her egg business, and she decided to sell them when they reached 2–2½ pounds at about 16 weeks. This was far younger than most chickens were sold and produced a tender bird that could be roasted or broiled instead of stewed. It was the beginning of a national industry, supported by the 1938 founding of the first large poultry processing plant in Frankfort, which made slaughtered, plucked, and cleaned chickens available. Today broiled chicken is the state dish of Delaware.

Florida

The Spanish explorers who arrived in Florida during the 1500s found a region of low rolling hills, massive marshes and swamps, numerous lakes, and dense woodlands. They established several small settlements, including the city of St. Augustine, but did not maintain a presence after the region was ceded to England. While under British rule, ambitious English immigrants came to the state in search of land for tobacco and cotton crops. One entrepreneur recruited workers from the Mediterranean, especially Greece, Italy, and the island of Minorca, to support his indigo plantation in New Smyrna. These immigrants brought eggplant, lemons, and olives to the area, all of which survived in small gardens.

Although tobacco and cotton were commercial failures, the settlers discovered that the groves of orange trees that had taken root after introduction by the Spanish provided a profitable living. Farmers from Alabama, Georgia, and the Carolinas had soon established the Florida citrus industry. Grapefruit were hybridized from pummelos that had been brought from the Caribbean, and other citrus fruits, such as tangerines, tangelos, and Persian (also known as Tahiti) limes, were introduced. Key limes, small, thin-skinned yellow limes with juicy, green flesh, were discovered in the Florida Keys. It is not known where the limes came from, but it is assumed that they drifted to the islands from the Caribbean. They are grown mostly in home gardens and are renowned for their tangy flavor. Today, 70 percent of the U.S. citrus crop is grown in Florida (nearly all the oranges are processed into juice). Florida is also known for other subtropical crops, such as avocados, guavas, kumquats, mangoes, papaya, and pineapples, as well as early ripening crops such as tomatoes and strawberries. Sugar cane is grown in the south of the state, and sabal palmetto palms grow like weeds, providing the delicacy known as hearts of palm.

The Florida waterways and coastline offered a profusion of fish and game to early settlers. Red snapper, pompano (a very large, meaty fish), mullet, and tarpon were a few of the fish commonly available; seafood included shrimp (several varieties), spiny lobster (similar to those of New England, but without claws), conch (a large mollusk), and stone crabs (only the very large claw is eaten—the claw is removed when the crab is caught, and then the crab is thrown back in the water to grow a new one). Green sea turtle and freshwater turtles, frogs, and alligators were additional game meats.

Many of Florida's specialties have developed out of this unique larder. Red snapper fillets are baked with orange juice. Pompano is stuffed with shrimp, seasoned with Sherry, and baked, or prepared *en papillote* (with a nod to the French influence of the Gulf Coast states). Spiny lobster tails are stuffed with fish and grilled, while stone crab claws are traditionally boiled and served with garlic butter or mustard sauce. Rock shrimp, a hard-shelled, white shrimp that tastes like a cross between lobster and shrimp, has become a trendy restaurant item throughout the country. Green turtle steaks are grilled or baked, and the meat is also used in stew and soups. Conch fritters and conch chowder (made with onions and tomatoes, seasoned with Worchestershire sauce, oregano, and bay leaves) are popular. Key lime pie and *ambrosia*, a dessert made from sliced oranges and grated coconut, have become favorites throughout the South.

Other Florida dishes originated with the early and later immigrants to the state. In addition to oranges, the Spanish explorers also

Before the advent of refrigerated box cars in the early 1900s, oranges were such a luxury throughout the rest of the nation that it was traditional to put an orange in children's stockings at Christmas as a special treat.

Key lime pie, which has a lime custard filling and is traditionally covered with meringue, can also be made as a chiffon pie (folding the meringue into the custard to lighten it, then topping the pie with whipped cream). Key limes must be used for an authentic pie, but imposters with the juice of other limes often borrow the name.

Palmetto palms are so prevalent in Florida they are known as "swamp cabbage."

Conchas is the Spanish word for conch mollusk, a term that has become the nickname of residents of the Florida Keys.

brought black beans and garbanzo beans (chickpeas), which were common in Cuba. Few dishes have survived in Florida fare from the Spanish period, but two soups in the region are thought to have Spanish roots: garbanzo (dried chickpeas, vegetables, and spicy Spanish chorizo sausage) and *vezada* (beans, potatoes, bell pepper, *morcilla* blood sausage, bacon, and collard greens).

At the beginning of the nineteenth century, Greek immigrants arrived in Tarpon Springs for sponge fishing jobs (see Chapter 9 on Greeks and Peoples of the Middle East). They introduced traditional dishes like *moussaka* (stuffed eggplant), *spanakopita* (spinach- or cheese-filled phyllo dough pastries), and *gyros* (pita bread sandwiches). In recent years, Cuban immigrants to the Miami area have added significant contributions to the cuisine (see Chapter 6 on Latinos for more information). *Arroz con pollo* is made with chicken and rice, flavored with the Cuban combination of tomatoes, olives, capers, raisins, and chile peppers. Black beans, traditionally prepared with rice and salt pork or ham, is common. So-called *Cuban sandwiches*, with roast pork, ham, sausage, cheese, and dill pickle filling mounded on Cuban bread, are fast-food favorites. *Flan,* a baked custard with caramel topping (sometimes flavored with orange), has become a popular dessert.

Georgia

Georgia was founded in 1733 by James Oglethorpe, who established the settlements of Savannah and Augusta as refuges for Europe's poor (particularly those in debtors' prison) and persecuted (because of political or religious beliefs). In the following years, thousands of English, Scotch, Irish, northern Italians, Swiss, German Lutherans, French Huguenots, and Sephardic Jews (from Spain and Portugal) arrived to take advantage of freedom and generous land grants. Oglethorpe expected every family to be hard-working and self-supporting, that none would be richer or poorer than another, and that slavery would be unnecessary. The settlers soon looked to the north and saw that cotton and tobacco were much more profitable than the meager food crops each small family produced, and by 1750 the ideals of Oglethorpe had been discarded in favor of the plantation system worked by slaves. Cotton, tobacco, indigo, and rice became primary crops.

The Georgia settlers quickly adopted a typically southern lifestyle. Plantation hospitality was famous in the region. A description of a company meal from the early 1800s listed turtle soup, trout, ham with sweet potatoes, turkey with a cornmeal and walnut stuffing, rice, asparagus, green beans, followed by orange sherbet to cleanse the diners' palates before continuing with cold venison, cheese, corn fritters with syrup, and sweet potato pie (Lee, 1992). Traditional southern fare was served at family meals as well, such as Georgia squirrel stew (a variation on Brunswick stew), ham, hoecakes, okra with tomatoes,

The barrier islands off the coast of Georgia and South Carolina are the last area where the Gullah dialect is spoken, a patois of English and several West African languages. The food of the islands is typically southern, with pork, greens, and sweet potatoes and specialties like broiled chitterlings (instead of boiled and fried), smoked mullet, and corn bread with sorghum syrup added to it before baking (Carlson, 1997).

and biscuits served with preserves. Mayhaw jelly, made from the cranberry-like fruit of the native mayhaw tree, is a particular favorite in Georgia and other states along the Gulf Coast.

Fish and seafood were plentiful. Seafood *pilau* (see South Carolina, following) was popular in homes along the Atlantic coast, as were oyster suppers: The informal feast featured oysters cooked over a fire in the moonlight, served with melted butter. A French nuance can be seen in the popularity of dishes such as crab soufflé. German dishes common in the region include sauerkraut and pepper pot soup; the Scots brought scones and *haggis* (hog's stomach stuffed with oatmeal—see Chapter 4 on Europeans). One unusual dish found in Georgia is *Country Captain Chicken*, invented by a sea captain from Savannah who used Indian spices to liven up his routine fare aboard ship. It is a curried dish that includes tomatoes and green peppers and is served over rice. Many southerners enjoy a bit of heat in their foods: In Georgia, bird's eye peppers, very small (¼″–½″) round, oval, or triangular chiles that are scorching hot, are sometimes crushed and placed at the bottom of a bowl before adding soup or stew.

Peaches thrived in Georgia, and at one time, Georgia was known as the "Peach State." Peach pie is the consummate Georgia dessert, although recipes vary. Some are custard pies topped with sliced peaches, others are two-crust pies, and some are individual deep-fried pies. Today peaches remain an agricultural product associated with Georgia, as do pecans and watermelon. But in recent years, they have been surpassed in economic importance by poultry, peanuts, and cattle.

Kentucky

Kentucky began as the western frontier of Virginia. Explorers had to cross the Appalachians to get into the territory and in the early eighteenth century, it was the domain of hunters and trappers, who profited from the abundant deer, elk, bear, and buffalo in the region. In 1775, Daniel Boone blazed a trail through the mountains and on the western side discovered a large, grassy plain that is now known as "Bluegrass Country." He founded Boonesborough and encouraged emigrants to make their homes in the area. By 1790 there were over 70,000 settlers in Kentucky, most of English, Scotch Irish, or German heritage from surrounding states. They planted tobacco and hemp, clearing the woodlands surrounding the central Bluegrass region.

The settlers found that wheat did not grow well in Kentucky soil, but corn was successful. Corn was used for nearly all baked goods, with the exception of biscuits and pies prepared on special occasions. Game meats were the foundation of the Kentucky diet in the early years. Bear meat was particularly popular because it could be smoked like pork and was fatty enough to provide bacon. *Burgoo*, a stew traditionally made with wild birds and game meats like squirrel, is the signature dish of Kentucky (current versions typically include

Coca-Cola was invented by an Atlanta pharmacist in 1886 as a headache remedy. "Dope" is the slang term for cola drinks in the South.

Vidalia onions are thought to be exceptionally sweet due to the mild Georgia weather and the low-sulfur soil around Vidalia, in Toombs County, Georgia. Over $50 million worth are grown there annually.

The earliest hunters in Kentucky were gone for such extended periods that they would commonly run out of provisions. They survived on game, using plain sliced meat of wild turkey as bread to make sandwiches with the moist, flavorful organ meats from bear or deer.

In Kentucky, over 1.5 million squirrels are killed each year for their meat. The brains, known as *Kentucky caviar*, are a specialty in some areas. They are usually mixed in with scrambled eggs or added to burgoo. Health officials are concerned the brains may be a source of Creutzfeldt-Jacob disease, the human version of mad cow disease.

Kentucky Fried Chicken, created by Colonel Harland Sanders in 1939, is not actually fried, but prepared in a pressure cooker. Sanders found the method ideal for cooking large quantities and invented a special seasoning mixture of eleven herbs and spices to produce the tender, juicy product familiar throughout the nation today.

Corn whiskey was often distilled illegally in the secrecy of night to avoid federal tax agents and thus became known as *moonshine*. Other names for the potent brew include "corn likker" and "white lightning"

The annual Kentucky Derby is the social event of the season. It is a week of breakfasts, luncheons, picnics, and parties, culminating in a horse race. Traditional foods include mint juleps, burgoo, bourbon-glazed ham, creamed chicken over waffles, sausage balls, beaten biscuits, Sally Lunn cake, hickory nut whiskey cake, and strawberries with fresh cream..

The term *Creole* is often used to describe Europeans born outside of Europe and is applied, for example, to the descendants of the original French and Spanish immigrants to New Orleans.

Shrimp in Louisiana are sometimes called *Cajun popcorn*.

chicken; pork, beef, or lamb; cabbage, potatoes, tomatoes, lima beans, corn, and okra; and cayenne—some variations add filé powder, curry powder, or bourbon). When supplies of game diminished, pork became the primary meat. Ham was common, and variety cuts were used to flavor vegetables, such as green beans simmered with bacon throughout the day to make a smoky, mushy stew. Root vegetables provided bulk in the winter, while fresh greens were preferred in the spring and summer. Fried chicken was a special dish prepared on Sundays.

The best known of all Kentucky food products is bourbon. The territory was especially suited for the distillation of corn whiskey due to its iron-free, limestone spring water, and some of the Scotch Irish settlers had skills in making the brew. Many farmers found corn whiskey more profitable than cornmeal. It is believed that in 1789 the Reverend Elijah Craig, of Bourbon County, Kentucky, was the first person to produce corn whiskey aged in oak barrels, producing the characteristic flavor of bourbon. In 1860 a further refinement occurred when it was accidentally discovered that charred oak barrels added not only a touch of color, but also a favorable smoky taste. The favorite bourbon drink of Kentucky is the *mint julep* (bourbon sweetened with a touch of sugar or syrup and a hint of fresh mint), traditionally served in a silver cup. Bourbon also flavors stews, hams, poundcakes, fruitcakes, and *bourbon balls* (a candy made with chocolate, crushed vanilla wafers, pecans, corn syrup, and bourbon).

Louisiana

Although Spanish explorers first claimed the Louisiana region in 1541, it was the French who first colonized the state, establishing several fortified settlements along the Gulf Coast, including Nouvelle-Orléans (New Orleans) in 1718. African slaves were brought in to work the cotton, sugarcane, and rice plantations, and thousands of French Acadians from Canada and French Creoles from Haiti seeking refuge from political persecution arrived.

It is sometimes said that Louisiana is divided by a "crawfish curtain," between the south, where the crustacean is revered, and the north, where it is scorned (Gutierrez, 1984). There is indeed a culinary difference in the foods preferred in the coastal areas and those favored in the hilly, upper reaches of the state. For example, the northern region (which was settled mostly by Americans of English, Scotch Irish, and German ancestry) has had little French influence on its cooking and the staples of traditional southern fare prevail. Notably, cornmeal is used most in breads and biscuits. In the Mississippi Delta region, where New Orleans is located, and in the southwestern portions of the state, which contain the bayou country, wheat flour has always been favored, even when it had to be imported from Europe.

Fish and seafood (including the ubiquitous crawfish) are more important than pork in the southern regions of Louisiana. The famous fish and seafood stews of the area, *bouillabaisse, gumbo,* and *jambalaya,* are examples of dishes made from coastal plenty. Shrimp is the main seafood industry in Louisiana, marketed throughout the nation fresh and frozen. It is commonly served boiled with lemon butter or with *sauce piquante* (tomatoes, green peppers, onions, bay, vinegar, and hot sauce) over rice, a dish often called *shrimp Creole*. Shrimp is also added to seafood stews and to stuffings for vegetables. Oysters are commonly served raw, on the half shell and by the dozen in the many oyster bars of New Orleans. They are traditionally slurped with a squeeze of lemon juice and a dash of hot sauce or a sauce mixed to taste by each diner with catsup, vinegar, and horseradish. Oysters, too, are added to soups and stews. Crawfish, which look like miniature lobsters, are found in the swamps, riverbeds, and rice paddies of the state. They have become the ethnic emblem of Cajuns and the regional symbol of southern Louisiana. Over 100 million pounds are produced annually. Some are harvested from the wild, but most are cultivated in the approximately 300 crawfish farms operating in the state. Crawfish are typically served at a "boil," where they are cooked in water seasoned

It is said that when a Cajun baby is 9 days old, the mother sticks his or her finger down a crawfish hole to be pinched. This is what makes a Cajun a Cajun (Gutierrez, 1984).

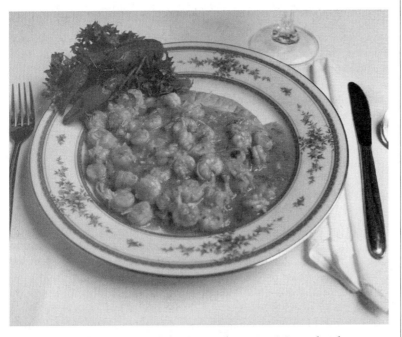

Crawfish étouffée is a specialty in southern Louisiana that has become popular in other areas of the South.

Absinthe, a liqueur made from worm-wood, was exceptionally popular in New Orleans during the nineteenth century. It was believed to be an aphrodisiac. It was later banned when it was discovered to be toxic and habit-forming.

Sandwiches with deli meats and cheese on a french bread roll are found throughout the country. In addition to being called *po' boys* and *muffeletta sandwiches* in New Orleans, they are also known as *bombers* (upstate New York), *Cuban sandwiches* (made with roast pork in Miami), *grinders* (New England), *heros* (New York City), *hoagies* (Philadelphia), *Italian meat sand-wiches* (Chicago), and *submarine sandwiches* (from a World War II naval base in Connecticut).

with cayenne, salt, and herbs. Potatoes or corn are often added for side dishes. The crawfish are placed in a gigantic mound in the cen-ter of the table, and each person takes and peels as many as desired. Only the meat in the tail and the claws is edible, along with the fat found in the head, which is extracted with a finger or sucked out appreciatively. Crawfish are also prepared fried, stuffed, as fritters, in soups and stews, in pies, and as *étouffée* (meaning smothered) in a spicy tomato sauce.

Game meats continue to be popular in some areas. Wild boar, frog's legs, and alligator are often found. Other regional specialties include rice dishes, such as the fried cakes called *calas,* red beans and rice, and dirty rice (cooked with gizzards). Rice is also the foundation of dishes like gumbo and jambalaya. Baked goods and sweets are spe-cialties, including French *petits fours, crêpes, beignets* (deep-fried squares similar to dougnuts), and pralines (pecan candies). *Café au lait*, a favorite beverage in New Orleans, is a dark roasted coffee (sometimes flavored with chicory root) prepared with equal amounts of hot milk. *Café brûlot* is a sweetened dessert coffee flavored with brandy and curaçao (orange liqueur).

Restaurant fare in New Orleans is renowned. Among the dishes created by local chefs that have obtained national recognition are *oys-ters Rockefeller* (baked on a bed of salt with a rich spinach sauce), *oysters Bienville* (baked with a béchamel sauce and green pepper, onions, pimento, and cheese), *bananas foster* (sliced bananas cooked in butter, brown sugar, rum, and banana liqueur served over vanilla ice cream—it started out as a breakfast specialty), and *Ramos gin fizz* (a shaken or blended cocktail with cream, gin, lemon juice, orange flower water, and egg whites). Street food is equally tasty in the city. Fried oysters, sliced tomatoes, and onions with tarter sauce on a french bread roll are especially popular. They are called *peacemak-ers*, from the nineteenth century when men would bring one home as a surprise for dinner after a fight with their wives. *Po' boy* (for *poor boy*) is another name for the sandwich, although a po' boy may also refer to a sandwich with deli meats, sausages, and cheeses with or without gravy or tomatoes. A *muffeletta* sandwich is yet another ver-sion, usually including a chopped olive salad with the meats and cheeses.

Maryland

In 1634, Cecilius Calvert, Lord Baltimore, was given a land grant on Chesapeake Bay to establish a refuge for 200 fellow English Catholics, many of whom were wealthy "gentlemen adventurers." They were soon outnumbered, however, by Puritan immigrants. In the early 1700s, the English settlers expanded into the inland hill country from the east, established baronial estates, and grew tobacco in the fertile lands previously cleared by the Indians. Their lavish lifestyle was supported by slave labor. Germans from Pennsylvania entered the state from the west, grew wheat in the Piedmont, and produced baked goods (particularly rye and pumpernickel breads) that were sold to markets in the east.

Wild game and pork supported the earliest immigrants. The English, who were partial to beef and mutton, soon imported cattle and sheep as supplemental meats. Herb-roasted veal; lamb stewed with exotic spices, including curry; and sweetbreads were specialties. Hams were produced in every manner: wet-cured in brine or dry-cured with a sea salt or sugar crust, then smoked. One recipe that is still popular, particularly in the southern sections of the state, is stuffed ham. It calls for inserting greens (e.g., cabbage, kale, and/or watercress) flavored with onions, mustard seeds, and cayenne into deep slits of the ham. The ham is served cold and is often the centerpiece of the Easter meal.

Maryland is best known for its seafood, however. The state is indented by the largest estuary in the nation, Chesapeake Bay, which teems with oysters, clams, scallops, and crabs. Many settlers near the bay made their living as watermen, harvesting seasonal seafood, oystering in the winter, and crabbing in summer. It was the abundance of Maryland Chincoteague and Tangier oysters that started the oyster craze in the cities of the Northeast and Midwest in the 1800s. They were eaten three times a day in the state: raw, fried, baked, fricasseed, in seafood stews, in chowder, in oyster stuffing for turkeys, and over steaks. Crabs were equally versatile. A regional specialty is blue crabs, a swimming crab so named because the underside of the large claws is blue. They are traditionally steamed over water flavored with vinegar, and seasoned with salt, pepper, ground ginger, celery and mustard seeds, and paprika. Because they are small, half a dozen or more are served to each diner, with plenty of beer to wash them down. The meat is used to make one of Maryland's most esteemed dishes, *crab cakes*. The crab is mixed with a little mayonnaise, cracker crumbs, and a spicy seasoning of cayenne, dry mustard, and hot sauce, then formed into small patties and fried. They are served with lemon wedges and tarter sauce. Crab soup (with beef stock and bacon) and deviled crabs (baked in the shell and topped with breadcrumbs) are other common preparations. Another noteworthy shellfish of the region is soft-shell crab, which is a blue crab that has shed its hard shell during a molt. The new papery shell is completely edible, but it begins to harden after only a day. Blue crabs are often kept in tanks until they shed their hard shells in order to time harvesting of the soft-shell crabs. The whole crab is served deep-fried. Clams became an important commodity when the New England supply diminished; many are shipped to the Northeast. Fried clams, deviled clams, and clam fritters are common dishes. Currently over 400 million pounds of seafood are harvested from the Chesapeake Bay each year (Lee, 1992).

Green tomato slices dipped in cornmeal and pan-fried are popular throughout the South. They are served for breakfast in Maryland.

Each female oyster releases about 5 million eggs annually, but only 15 reach maturity. Maryland produces one-third of all oysters consumed in the nation each year.

She-crab soup was a Maryland specialty before crab harvesting was regulated to prohibit keeping egg-bearing females. It included crab meat and roe in a delicate cream base. The eggs gave a slightly sour flavor to the dish. Today it is made from male meat and unfertilized roe.

In 1893 a taste test was held to determine which turtle soup was superior: the creamy Philadelphia version with turtle meat or the clear turtle consommé with a hint of Sherry preferred in Maryland. The impartial jury selected the Maryland soup as the winner (Jones, 1981).

Diamondback terrapin is another Maryland specialty found around the Chesapeake Bay. It is the turtle preferred for turtle soup. It is also the main ingredient in terrapin stew, which includes the eggs and liver, all in a gravy made from the turtle stock flavored with butter and Sherry. Beaten biscuits and a glass of Sherry are the traditional accompaniments. Atlantic fish, such as butterfish, cod, flounder, herring, mackerel, and stripped bass, are available. Poultry has always been a favorite in Maryland, even more so since broiler production became an important industry in the 1930s (see Delaware section). The early settlers prepared chicken pot pies and chicken-seafood chowders. Fried chicken with cream gravy is still served regularly.

Mississippi

The state of Mississippi is dominated by the Mississippi River, which demarcates its western boundary. Low-lying bottomlands of the Mississippi Delta form the western half of the state, with low, rolling hills found in the eastern half. The French were the first whites to settle in the region. They built forts at Biloxi in 1699, and in Natchez and Vicksburg soon after. The territory was ceded to the British in the mid-eighteenth century and became a haven for Tories escaping the impending conflict of the Revolutionary War in the Northeast. The northern half of the state was settled mostly by pioneers from Georgia.

Both the French and English influenced the cities located along the southern portion of the Mississippi River. Natchez in particular became a wealthy port city supported by the cotton plantations flourishing throughout the state. Cotton was shipped to Europe in exchange for French and English manufactured goods. The big southern breakfast and dinner were the norm for plantation owners and their city associates. Coffee and mint juleps were available for early risers. Late morning repasts included eggs, grits, biscuits, corn breads or muffins, waffles and several meats, such as ham, sausage, or even fried chicken. A large dinner with soups, stews, and dishes similar to those at breakfast was consumed in the early afternoon, Supper was a lighter version of dinner. One reason the food was so ample was that the farmers of the Midwest discovered that they could make a profit shipping flour, pork products, and perishable produce to Mississippi cities by flatboat.

Slave food on the Mississippi cotton plantations was often limited to pork variety cuts, poultry, local game and catfish, corn pone, and greens. One specialty was chicken corn bread, cooked in a fry pan in the fat remaining after the chicken was fried.

Food was not always plentiful on the plantations. During the Civil War, supplies were so short that Mississippi women prepared pie crusts from potatoes and made breads from corncob ashes (Lee, 1992).

Oysters were so prevalent in the early days of Mississippi that the streets of Biloxi were paved with oyster shells.

Local Mississippi foods include catfish, shrimp, oysters, and blue crabs. Catfish up to 100 pounds can still be caught in the rivers and lakes of the state, but most are now farmed in ponds. Although the first catfish farms were started in Arkansas, Mississippi is the leading producer in the nation, with over 250 million pounds harvested annually. Traditionally catfish is deep-fried in a cornmeal crust and served with hush puppies and coleslaw. Newer recipes include fried strips served with barbecue sauce or mustard, and catfish pâté (Carlson, 1997).

Shrimp and crab are typically boiled, served with an assortment of seasonings, such as vinegar, lemon juice, bird's eye chiles, and cloves. Oyster bakes are a popular outdoor feast. Pecans are native to the area and a Mississippi favorite, added to sausage stuffing for poultry, added to breads, sugar glazed, orange glazed, and baked in the syrupy pecan pie.

North Carolina

A rugged coast and a line of offshore sandbars known as the Outer Banks protect the state of North Carolina. The state is divided into three distinctive regions: the Tidewater coastal plain, the Piedmont hill country, and the mountainous region that includes the Blue Ridge and Great Smoky ridges of the Appalachians.

In 1663, eight British lords were granted proprietorship of the region known as Carolina (including both North Carolina and South Carolina). Settlement in the northern portion was slow but steady, attracting English, Scotch Irish, and Highland Scots, many of whom came as indentured servants. By the late 1700s, settlers from Virginia and South Carolina were streaming into the region, as well as immigrants from throughout Great Britain, Germany, and Switzerland.

At the time North Carolina was officially recognized as a state in 1789, most residents were small family farmers. Game was plentiful and corn grew easily, supporting residents until garden plots began producing other fruits and vegetables. In the Appalachians and parts of the Piedmont, bacon and cabbage, chicken pot pie, ham with cream gravy, baked beans, biscuits, hush puppies, potatoes, sweet potatoes, and poke salad were favorites. Fried squirrel and grits was a common meal. Scrambled eggs with brains were common at breakfast, and badger, considered by some a dish of last resort, became known as *bombo* in North Carolina. Barbecued pork with spicy hot sauce on the side was prepared for special occasions. *Ramp*, a particularly assertive wild onion, was added to soups, stews, potatoes, or eggs or breaded and fried as a side dish. Thick, caramel-colored sorghum syrup was poured over corn breads or used to sweeten coffee. Wealthier immigrants founded tobacco plantations and could afford roast beef, steaks, beef stew, and breaded pork chops in addition to the omnipresent ham and fried chicken. Along the coast, some residents made their living from the sea, catching mullet, shad, and rockfish and harvesting oysters and shrimp. Coastal specialties include fish muddle and corn dumplings.

One notable ethnic group in North Carolina are the German Moravians, persecuted German Protestants who had immigrated to Pennsylvania originally but moved south in the early 1700s when they discovered that much of that land was already claimed. The Moravians established an insular German community near the Winston-Salem area, founding a wholesale produce business that sold local fruits and vegetables in markets extending to Philadelphia.

Catfish consumption has more than doubled nationally since 1986. It is ranked the fifth most popular fish by Americans.

The Outer Banks were the site of numerous shipwrecks in the seventeenth and eighteenth centuries and became known as the *"Graveyard of the Atlantic."* Many North Carolinians trace their ancestry to survivors who washed up on the shore.

Early white settlements by English immigrants on Roanoke Island in the late 1500s were unsuccessful. Numerous Scuppernong grapevines brought from the mainland are a legacy of the attempts, still used by residents for jam, jelly, and pies.

An unusual Appalachian Mountain treat called a *sonker* is preserved in the annual festival named in its honor held at Mount Airy each year. It is a deep-dish fruit or sweet potato pie made with breadcrumbs or biscuit dough or pie crust—there is no agreement on how to prepare a sonker (Carlson, 1997).

The Winkler Bakery was one of the first businesses established in the Moravian community of North Carolina, and it is still operating today.

They were best known for their baked goods, such as *sugar cakes* (a yeasted, potato bread dough that is covered with brown sugar and cinnamon before baking) and *citron tarts* (tarts with lemon curd filling). Moravians commemorate special occasions with "Love Feasts." On November 17, the founding of North Carolina, the community Love Feast features wine, creamy coffee, and cakes topped with a nut frosting. At Christmas, paper-thin ginger spice cookies and a sweet bread studded with raisins and candied citron, sprinkled with sliced almonds, are specialties.

Oklahoma

Oklahoma started its U.S. history as Indian Territory, lands set aside in the 1820s for the Native American tribes that had been dispossessed of their homes in the Gulf Coast areas. Five major Indian groups lived in the region: Cherokee, Chickasaw, Choctaw, Creek, and Seminole. They were primarily agrarian, growing corn, beans, and squash. They gathered indigenous foods (including acorns, chestnuts, creases, grapes, Jerusalem artichokes, hickory nuts, persimmons, ramp, and sorghum) and hunted small game (see Chapter 3 on Native Americans). Today Native Americans make up approximately 8 percent of the total population in the state, over eight times the national average. Traditional foods, such as a Cherokee soup made with hickory nut cream, called *kanuche*, and game dishes, are served mostly at ceremonial occasions. Fry bread and adapted dishes, such as scrambled eggs with spring onions, are more common but have not been accepted into the broader Oklahoma cuisine (Milbauer, 1990).

The earliest whites in Oklahoma were fur trappers, buffalo hunters, railroad workers (including many Mexicans), and ranchers. Although the state was not officially opened up to settlement by whites until 1889, land-hungry homesteaders invaded the state before then (they were called "Sooners"), including German Russians, Italians, and central European immigrants. African Americans, many of whom had been held as slaves by the Indians, purchased land in the region after abolition. Many settlers established small family farms. Most of the plains regions in the state are arid and droughts have occurred regularly; hardship has characterized Oklahoma life.

The cooking of Oklahoma derives more from scarcity of food than from ethnic and regional preferences of the settlers. Wheat became the dominant crop in the state. Rabbit and turnip stew was flavored with a flour gravy, while beef and wheat berries are the primary ingredients of *Oklahoma Stew*. Biscuits were common, and some corn breads were prepared. *Black Blizzard Cake* (a pound cake whose name refers to the frequent dust storms in the region) was a specialty. The Indians had successfully planted watermelons, which became a popular fruit with all residents, eaten fresh and made into preserves and pickles.

Pioneers of the period lamented the monotony of eating dried apple pie; others wrote that they resorted to using sweetened crackers or potatoes to make pies when fruit was in short supply.

The southern portions of the state are called Little Dixie, and traditional foods of the South are predominant in the fare. A study of foods in the eastern portion of the state found that pork, fried chicken, catfish, biscuits and cream gravy (red-eyed gravy is not as common), corn bread, fried okra, and black-eyed peas were frequent items in local eateries. However, grits and buttermilk were rarely offered (Milbauer, 1990). Other ethnic and regional foods have had less impact over all. Authentic Mexican foods, for example, are uncommon, although a few Tex-Mex items like chili con carne have become very popular. Some dishes with Italian roots are accepted, such as spaghetti and meatballs, particularly around Krebs in the southeast. Sauerkraut, potato soup, and dark breads are evidence of German Russian influence, and central European traditions are maintained at heritage festivals.

South Carolina

Although South Carolina was part of a British land grant that included North Carolina in the seventeenth century (see North Carolina), settlement of the state was strikingly different from that of its northern neighbor. The English proprietors thought the fertile soil and warm climate would support Mediterranean fruits and vegetables. Approximately 150 white settlers from England arrived in the area in 1670 and founded Charles Town (now Charleston). They brought ginger, sugar cane, olives, and indigo; only indigo proved successful as a crop, but it was enough to begin a profitable plantation system in the region. Charleston became the primary seaport of the South.

The English were followed by thousands of French Huguenots seeking religious freedom in the 1680s. Most settled in the Charleston area, establishing indigo and later rice and cotton farms. Many who operated plantations in the coastal section also owned townhouses in Charleston. Other Europeans settled the upland Piedmont hills and Appalachian mountain areas of the state, including Germans, Welsh, Swiss, and Scotch Irish. By 1775, half of the white population in South Carolina lived in the central plains and upland regions. Unlike the coastal plains residents, most of these settlers owned small family farms. Like the Piedmont and Appalachian dwellers of North Carolina, these farmers lived on wild game and corn until their garden plots were sufficient to provide other foods.

It is the cooking of coastal South Carolina, especially Charleston, that is unique in the South. Numerous exotic foods arrived by sea, such as chocolate from Central America and bananas from the Caribbean. Unlike the English settlers in other regions of the South, large numbers of those who came to South Carolina had lived first in Barbados and other Caribbean Islands. They brought a taste for

The connection between the Caribbean and the South Carolina was so strong that, according to historian Peter H. Wood, some legal documents of the seventeenth century refer to "Carolina in ye West Indies" (Hess, 1992).

Charlotte russe was created by the great French chef Antoine Carême in honor of the Russian czar Alexander in 1815. It is a favorite special-occasion dessert in South Carolina.

Pepper sherry, made by infusing bird's eye chiles in Sherry, is a popular condiment added to shellfish, soups, and stews for zing.

The rice grown in South Carolina in the eighteenth century was of such high quality that Carolina rice was specified in the recipes of England, France, and the colonies. Thomas Jefferson tried growing Italian Piedmont rice in Virginia, but it was unsuccessful.

Hoppin' John is served on New Year's Eve in South Carolina and other parts of the South in the homes of both African Americans and whites because eating the rice and black-eyed peas is thought to bring good luck in the upcoming year.

Benne (sesame) *seeds* were introduced to the South by African slaves. In South Carolina, brown sugar benne wafers and benne brittle (made with sesame seeds instead of nuts) are popular desserts.

tropical flavors and spicy seasonings. Fruit and vegetable pickles were common, for example, mango chutney from India, which was also made with other local fruits and called *Indian pickle*. A French influence was seen in many dishes, particularly elaborate desserts like *Huguenot torte* (a sponge cake with pecans and apples) and *charlotte russe* (a special cylindrical mold lined with ladyfingers, then filled with Bavarian cream and garnished with strawberries and whipped cream).

Seafood is a specialty of the region. Shrimp was especially common in the early years of the state, featured in dishes like shrimp pâté or butter-sautéed shrimp with grits for breakfast and deep-fried shrimp and rice croquettes. Outdoor oyster roasts were the highlight of many festive occasions; they are still favorites today, served with hoppin' John, biscuits, and small sandwiches, such as a crab omelet on slices of bread. *Frogmore stew* is a spicy seafood, sausage, and corn combination similar to gumbo. *She-crab soup,* similar to that of Maryland but garnished with a spoonful of Sherry and a dollop of unsweetened whipped cream, was popular. As in other areas of the coastal South, muddle was prepared from whatever fish were available. A variation unique to South Carolina is *Pinebark stew*, a muddle flavored with bacon and the tiny roots of pine trees.

Most noteworthy are the rice dishes of the region. A variety of rice native to Madagascar was found suitable for the coastal plain climate; thousands of acres of tidal lands were diked and flooded to support the crop. By 1700, it was well established, thanks in part to the skills of slaves from the rice-growing regions of Africa. It was known as *Carolina Gold* (due to its amber color when ripe) and became the foundation of the coastal diet. The rice was traditionally boiled instead of steamed to produce individual fluffy grains that did not stick together. Numerous specialties developed with rice. *Pilau* (also spelled *purlow,* or *pullow*) "is characterized by an elegant simplicity of composition, featuring a single ingredient, that is, in addition to the rice which is the point of the dish" (Hess, 1992, p. 64). Rice is simmered in an aromatic broth (reserved from cooking the second ingredient) until dry, then mixed with the other food. Shrimp pilau and okra pilau are examples. African-influenced hoppin' John, made with black-eyed peas and rice, is also a pilau. Molded rice dishes that are baked until they form a golden crust are called rice pies or rice casseroles. Some include layers of meat or fish. Rice breads, such as *philpy* (cooked rice added to corn bread), and desserts, such as rice pudding and *Carolina snow balls* (a rice dumpling with a whole, peeled and cored apple filling), were common.

Rice production in the region was interrupted by the Revolutionary War and then again during the Civil War. After the abolition of slavery, rice farmers found the crop too labor intensive to use paid workers, and production diminished dramatically. Other crops, such as cotton, became more important in the economy. The Spanish explorers in the sixteenth century had brought peaches to the Carolinas. At one time, they were so plentiful they were used as hog feed. Today South Carolina is the largest producer of peaches in the South, second only to California in the nation.

Tennessee

At one time, Tennessee was a part of the Virginia frontier. Two waves of settlement occurred, one with families seeking safety from the turmoil of the Revolutionary War, most of whom were of English, Scotch Irish or French Huguenot heritage, and one with Germans, Scots, and Irish who sought farmland in Maryland and Pennsylvania before moving on to available properties in Tennessee. Those who settled in the western regions along the Mississippi River found fertile plains suitable for tobacco and cotton plantations. Horse ranching arose in the middle hill country. Those pioneers who settled in the east existed on subsistence farming in the rugged Blue Ridge and Great Smoky mountains of the Appalachians.

The differences between the western and eastern halves of the state were so pronounced that during the Civil War the east sided with the Union and the west joined the Confederacy. The plantation owners of the west had access to the wealthy markets of the lower Mississippi, such as Natchez and New Orleans. They developed a southern lifestyle typical of plantation life throughout the South, including large, leisurely meals. They are still known for their sumptuous breakfasts, which traditionally feature eggs, tomatoes, potatoes, and cornmeal biscuits with sorghum syrup. During the winter, thick slices of Tennessee country ham, with grits and red-eye gravy made with the ham drippings, may also be served with the meal; in the summer, fried chicken is more common. Tennessee sausages are also a specialty, as is spiced beef (marinated in vinegar, brown sugar, and seasonings, then simmered and sliced thinly). Baked sweet potatoes with butter, as well as greens, are frequent side dishes.

Settlers in the hills and mountains had a diet similar to that of other Appalachian dwellers (see also Kentucky and North Carolina). Game was the primary meat, including deer, raccoon, opossum, squirrel, and wild turkey. Those who could afford a hog would butcher it in the winter, providing fresh meats, such as ribs barbecued with a tomato-whiskey sauce, and meats for curing as hams, salt pork, and cracklings. Stews were favored. One specialty was *cabbage gumbo*, made without seafood but including country ham and Tennessee smoky sausage in a milk base. As in the wealthier western regions, corn breads, biscuits, and greens were additional core foods. Baked beans were also common. Many farms had at least one apple tree, providing fruit for apple butter and pies. Funnel cakes, undoubtedly introduced by German immigrants, were topped with sorghum syrup. Fried pies were a favorite dessert, and sassafras tea was a popular beverage.

Moon Pies are a Chattanooga, Tennessee confection that have become an obsession in the South. (Moon Pies are eaten at Mardi Gras in Mobile, Alabama, for example.) They are graham cracker sandwiches with a marshmallow filling covered in chocolate, vanilla, banana, or caramel icing. During the depression a Moon Pie and an RC Cola was called a "working-class dessert" because both could be had for a dime.

The tiny town of Lynchberg, Tennessee, where the Jack Daniels Distillery is located, has been dry since 1909.

Chuck wagon fare was a cooking style all its own, dependent on the skills and whims of the cowboy chefs called "Cookie" or "Miss Sally." Beans, corn bread, sourdough biscuits, and coffee were the staples, but some specialties were created on the trail, including son-of-a-bitch stew (known as *son-of-a-gun stew* in more genteel circles) made with beef organs, including tongue, brain, liver, heart, and kidneys.

One specialty of the northeast is rattlesnake, which is chopped into bite-size pieces, marinated in beer and vinegar, coated with cornmeal, and deep-fried.

In 1866, Jack Daniel purchased a corn whiskey still and added an extra refinement to the distillation process, using maple wood charcoal to filter the whiskey before aging it in charred oak barrels. This produced a flavor distinct from bourbon, and the liquor became known as Tennessee whiskey.

Texas

Texas is the size of New England, the Mid-Atlantic states, Ohio, and Indiana combined. Although the terrain is usually associated with desert plains, there are also wooded regions, hill country, mountains, and hot, humid lowland areas along the Gulf Coast. It was occupied by Native Americans, claimed by the Spanish and French, ruled by Mexico, and existed as an independent nation before it became part of the United States in 1846. The first American settlement was 300 families in what is now Austin on land granted by the Mexican government. Other Americans were provided land if they were Roman Catholics; thousands from the South (Catholic in name only) entered the state from the east to take advantage of the offer. Germans, Czechs, and Poles emigrated from Europe to central Texas, attracted by later land grants. In the west, small numbers of ranchers and cowboys made their living from raising and driving cattle.

Texas is divided into five culinary regions, each influenced by the available foods, proximity to other ethnic and regional fare, and the preferences of the residents. In the northeast and panhandle areas, immigrants scraped out a living on small family farms, surviving on corn, beans, and native fish and game. When wheat proved a successful crop in the region, corn breads were replaced with biscuits. In the eastern areas, foods of the South dominate. It has always been an affluent region, and meals are often opulent: Dishes frequently feature costly ingredients and tend to be richer (with extra butter, eggs, and cream) than versions from Louisiana, Mississippi, and Arkansas. Corn breads, biscuits, hominy and grits, black-eyed peas, okra, sweet potato pie, bread pudding, and pralines are a few common items. Rice is an important crop, and southern-style rice dishes are popular. Alligator, trout, catfish, and crawfish are available in local rivers. Over 100 million pounds of fish and seafood are produced along the Texas Gulf Coast each year, including shrimp, crab, and oysters (Lee, 1992). *Crab au gratin,* oyster stew, and shrimp casserole are a few specialties. Classic Creole and Cajun dishes, such as jambalaya, étouffée, and gumbo, can also be found.

There are strong German and central European influences in the central regions of the state. Common foods include sausages, ham, sauerbraten, sauerkraut, pumpernickel bread, potato salad, potato dumplings, bierocks, and strudel. Czech kolaches and Polish poppy seed cake are baked for festive occasions. One specialty is "German fried" liver (dredged in cornmeal, cooked in bacon drippings, and served with bacon strips). In the western areas of Texas, beef has always been popular. It is served traditionally as stews and steaks. Chicken-fried steak was created to treat tough cuts—the steak is cut thinly, then pounded with a mallet, coated in flour, and fried. It is traditionally served with a ladleful of gravy made with coffee. Corn bread or tortillas and pinto beans often round out the meal. Few fresh vegetables or fruits were consumed. Today Texas pasturelands are the leading producer of cattle, sheep, and lambs in the nation.

The most distinctive Texan fare evolved in the south of the state, where Mexican and Spanish influence added their flavors to dishes. Some authentic Mexican foods, such as tortillas, tamales, *chalupas*, salsas, guacamole, and *buñuelos* (see Chapter 6 on Latinos), were accepted by white settlers in the region. However, most foods in the area are adapted dishes with Mexican overtones, often referred to as

Barbecue and political events go hand in hand in many parts of the country, and especially in the South. In 1840 an Alabama plantation owner hosted 4,000 at a celebration barbecue for the election of Martin Van Buren. A German journalist at a Fourth of July barbecue in Little Rock, Arkansas in 1843 reported that two oxen and two bears, as well as numerous sheep, calves, pigs, deer, turkeys, opossums, raccoons, squirrels, chickens, geese, ducks, partridges, and prairie chickens (grouse) were prepared for the event, at which everyone ate with their hands—no plates or utensils were available. President Lyndon B. Johnson was famous for the enormous barbecues held at his Texas ranch.

Barbecue is a traditional Tex-Mex method for preparing meat.

Tex-Mex chili con carne was probably first popularized in the mid-1800s. Chili powder was invented by a German in New Braunfels, Texas in 1902. It usually includes spices like cumin in addition to ground, dried chile peppers.

The term *mop* for the sauce basted on barbecued meat may have come from the use of a clean mop to slap the sauce on whole carcasses.

Texas caviar is black-eyed pea salad, seasoned with chiles and garlic and served on tortilla chips.

Spice cookies called cry babies were made by Virginia settlers in the Appalachians to appease distressed children. Brunswick stew, *black-pot chicken* (cooked in a Dutch oven), and fried apple pies were other favorites.

Originally it was said that the Smithfield ham got its flavor from the peanuts that the pigs foraged on. It was found that the curing, not the diet, determined taste, and today's hogs are fed on grain. Although many processors in the counties surrounding Smithfield make Virginia-style hams, only those actually produced in the town can bear the Smithfield name.

Tex-Mex cuisine. Examples include tamale pie, nachos, and most tacos and enchiladas, which usually feature nontraditional fillings. One regional specialty is *chili con carne*, known in Texas as "a bowl of red," which began as beans, progressed to beans with beef, and is now typically an all-beef stew flavored primarily with hot chili powder. Barbecue is also favored. Unlike barbecue in other regions of the country (such as Kansas City), there are two sauces involved in Texas barbecue. The first, called the "mop" or "sop," is used to marinate the meat before cooking and for basting the meat on the spit or grill. The second sauce is served on the side with the cooked meat. Although barbecued beef is most associated with the state, barbecued goat kid (*cabrito*) is almost as popular in the southern sections.

The unifying element in most of these foods is that they are preferred hot and spicy. In addition to chili powder, chile peppers are used in many dishes. Numerous varieties are added, but worth mention is the *chiletepín* chile, the indigenous precursor to domesticated *pequin* chiles. They are among the hottest of all chiles (they are also called bird's eye peppers, described previously). Chiles often flavor foods in Texas not normally associated with the spice, such as corn bread, and jelly. In addition to chile peppers, other fresh fruits and vegetables are now prevalent in southern Texas due to irrigation. Cantaloupe, pink grapefruit, peaches, sugar cane, and tomatoes are a few examples of specialty crops.

Virginia

The state of Virginia is famous both for its ham and for its historic role in the development of American cuisine. Early success with tobacco and the plantation system of agriculture in Virginia established the pattern for the southern lifestyle and led to many food firsts.

The colony at Jamestown, founded in 1607 by English settlers seeking precious metals, was the first white settlement in the state. It began as a communal endeavor, but agricultural efforts were largely unsuccessful. Thousands of settlers died during the early years from starvation and disease. In 1614, land grants were made to individuals and tobacco was planted as a cash crop. Many Virginians living in the coastal Tidewater region of the state quickly made the transformation from subsistence farmers to wealthy, slave-owning plantation proprietors. Those who remained small family farmers migrated west into the hill country and Appalachian mountains, where they made do with limited supplies supplemented by game and wild fruits and vegetables.

Many of the dishes that originated in Virginia were based on Native American ingredients and preparation methods shared with the first settlers. The best known food to evolve is the *Smithfield ham*. The dry-curing process used was learned from the Powhatan Indians, who salt-cured and smoked venison. As early as 1608 the method was being used on wild razorback hogs that had been brought by the Spanish and had since naturalized throughout the South. A few years later, pigs were introduced to the region, and the process was applied to domestic hams. A Smithfield ham is similar to a country ham, but it is made with the shank end of the leg and with the bone in. It is first rubbed with salt, sugar, and pepper for curing, then smoked over hickory, then hung to age. The total processing time is 9 to 20 months. The meat differs from a country ham in that it is saltier, darker in color, and leaner. The flavor is very strong and it is traditionally eaten in very thin slices on beaten biscuits or fried with red-eye gravy and served with fried apples. Another dish adapted from the Indians was *spoon bread*, a corn bread that is enriched with eggs and milk and baked slowly until it forms a crust on the top but remains custard-like underneath.

In addition to ham, the English plantation owners favored the beef and mutton dishes familiar to them from home. Roast beef with Yorkshire pudding and mutton roasted with bacon and herbs are examples. Roasted poultry, including turkey, was common. Seafood from the Chesapeake Bay was also featured, in dishes such as deviled crab, oysters in brown butter, and shad roe sautéed in bacon fat. Soups, such as pumpkin soup or peanut soup, were offered as a first course. Elaborate desserts were the highlight of formal meals, served as a separate course. They included items such as fruitcakes, pound cakes, cheesecakes, *hedgehog* (a molded almond paste filling studded with sliced almonds to look like the English animal), pumpkin pie, and cranberry tarts. Although many plantations had numerous auxiliary buildings, including the kitchen (separate to prevent fires from spreading to the main house), smokehouses, ice houses, cellars, and spring houses (built over a running spring, where perishables like butter could be stored in cold water), the settlers were still dependent on seasonal foods. During the summer, fresh green vegetables and fruits were featured, and more preserved meats were served. In the winter, root vegetables predominated and more fresh meats were available. Virginians today often list Brunswick stew, greens consumed with the pot likker (see Chapter 4 on Africans), corn pone, black-eyed peas, pickled watermelon rind, pickled Jerusalem artichokes, and sweet potato pie as traditional specialties.

Many colonial recipes from Virginia had an everyday version and a special-occasion version with additional eggs, butter, and cream.

An elaborate Christmas dish in Virginia was Yorkshire Pie, made by baking five kinds of boned, seasoned poultry stuffed inside each other in a pastry crust—first a turkey, then a chicken inside the turkey, with pheasant or partridge in the chicken, followed by smaller game birds such as pigeon or dove. The crust was removed and the multilayered dish was served in slices (Lee, 1992).

Although most Virginian foods were Native American and English in origin, Thomas Jefferson brought many French specialties to his home in Monticello, such as *boeuf à la daube* (jellied beef) and crêpes. He also brought Italian foods, including pasta, to the United States. His daughter Mary Randolph is credited with introducing macaroni and Parmesan cheese, which became macaroni with cheddar cheese.

West Virginia

West Virginia is known as the Mountain State because it is located in the heart of the Appalachians. It was originally part of the Virginia territory. Plantation owners in the Tidewater region of Virginia encouraged settlement of the area to act as a buffer from the Native Americans and French in the region. Germans and Scotch Irish from Pennsylvania and New Jersey moved into the state, establishing small farms and orchards in the steep terrain. When Virginia joined the Confederacy during the Civil War, West Virginians voted to form a separate state aligned with the Union. Timber, salt, iron, coal, gas, and oil brought an influx of European immigrants looking for work in the late nineteenth century. Most were from Ireland, Italy, Germany, Hungary, and Poland.

The rugged landscape, damp climate, and short summers limited most agricultural endeavors. Apples and peaches were successful orchard crops, and small amounts of corn, beans, peanuts, pumpkins, and watermelon were grown in family gardens. Buckwheat was found to be an ideal, fast-growing grain, and buckwheat pancakes traditionally served with applesauce and whole-hog sausage (see Indiana) became popular. Game meats supplemented the small amounts of beef and pork available: Squirrel stew seasoned with bacon, onions, garlic, and thyme was a favorite. In ethnic communities, traditional dishes include European foods. For example, lasagna, *fagiole* (pasta with beans), *minestra* (vegetable soup), and cannoli are popular in the area around Clarksburg where more than half the population of the county is of Italian descent (Carlson, 1997). Other West Virginia specialties include pumpkin pie; eastern black walnut confections; and huckleberry muffins, cakes, and pies.

The Golden Delicious apple was hybridized in West Virginia by A. H. Mullins in 1890.

Social events in early West Virginia centered on church and civic activities. They were called "soups," because when people gathered to meet, they would all bring ingredients to make enough soup to feed the group.

The West

Regional Profile

The western United States is the largest region in the nation, encompassing an enormous diversity of lands, from the icy tundra of Alaska to the tropical volcanic islands of Hawaii. The tallest mountains in the country, vast fertile valleys and coastal plains, stretches of scenic desert, and temperate rainforest add to the variety.

It is the history of the open wilderness that links this region. Indigenous peoples adapted their lifestyles to fit each climate and terrain. Pueblo Indians made their homes in the cliffs and cultivated corn, beans, chiles, and squash; the Inuits of Alaska lived in ice igloos and hunted sea mammals and fish for food; and the native Hawaiians enjoyed such fresh abundance that they cooked few dishes (see Chapter 3 on Native Americans and Chapter 8 on Southeast Asians and Pacific Islanders for more information). The first whites in the West were explorers, trappers, miners, and traders—hardy individuals (mostly men) seeking their fortune. Emigrants came from every direction: the Spanish and Mexicans from Mexico in the south, Russians from the north, Chinese and Japanese from the west, and the numerous pioneers of northern and southern European descent (mostly English, Scottish, Welsh, Danes, Swedes, Slavs, Italians, and Greeks) from the Midwest, looking for new farming, ranching, and fishing opportunities. Not only is the West the most diverse region in climate and terrain, but also in population.

The West is divided into the Mountain states of Arizona, Colorado, Idaho, Montana, Nevada, New Mexico, Utah, and Wyoming and the Pacific states of Alaska, California, Hawaii, Oregon, and Washington. Approximately 22 percent of Americans reside in the West, and of these, over half live in California. It is a mostly urban population, with a majority of people living in cities or suburbs, ranging from a low of 52 percent in Montana to almost 93 percent in California. It is also a young population, with fewer persons over the age of 65 than the national average; the exceptions are Arizona and Montana, with slightly above average numbers of elders.

Large numbers of many ethnic groups reside in the West (see Figure 11.6). Compared to total U.S. figures, three times as many Asians and Pacific Islanders, more than twice the Latinos, and two times as many Native Americans are part of the western population. African Americans and whites fall below the U.S. average in the region. As a portion of each group nationally, 55 percent of all Asians and Pacific Islanders, 47 percent of all Native Americans, and 45 percent of all Latinos live in the West. This includes disproportionate numbers of total Inuit (89%), Japanese (72%), Aleut (72%), Filipinos (68%), Salvadorans (62%), Chinese (55%), Vietnamese (54%), Mexicans (52%), American Indians (46%), and Koreans (44%). Among whites residing

FIGURE 11.6
Demographics in the West.

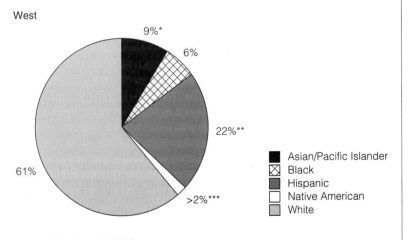

West

9%*

6%

22%**

61%

>2%***

■ Asian/Pacific Islander
⊠ Black
▨ Hispanic
□ Native American
▨ White

*   Mostly in Hawaii (63%)
**   Mostly in New Mexico (39%) and California (29%)
*** Mostly in Alaska (15%), New Mexico (9%) and Arizona (5%)

in western states, there are large numbers with Danish and Spanish ancestry (45% each), and Yugoslavian heritage (37%, including those from what are currently Croatia and Serbia). In 1991, 31 percent of immigrants to the United States settled in the West, 23 percent in California.

Further, a few individual western states report notable ethnic population figures. Asians and Pacific Islanders account for 63 percent of the population in Hawaii, for example. Latinos are 39 percent of the New Mexico population and 29 percent of the California population. Over 5 percent and 9 percent of the respective populations in Arizona and New Mexico are American Indian, and Native Americans, including Inuits and Aleuts, make up 15 percent of the population in Alaska.

Median income is a little below the U.S. 1997 average in the Mountain states and above the national average in the Pacific states: Alaska boasts the highest median income in the country, $50,829, almost 30 percent above the U.S. average. Yet, despite these figures, poverty levels in the West were approximately 10 percent above the national average. Particularly high levels are found in California and Arizona, and nearly one in every four persons lives below the poverty line in New Mexico, the highest rate in the nation. At the opposite end, low poverty rates are found in Colorado, and Utah and Alaska have the lowest numbers of persons living in poverty in the nation, around 8 percent.

Both the Mountain and Pacific states have above average numbers of high school graduates in their populations, and average and above average numbers respectively of persons over the age of 25 with college degrees. Although only 40 percent of persons living in the West adhere to a Christian faith, the highest percentage of Christians in the nation reside in Utah (80%—nearly all are Mormons) and large numbers are also found in New Mexico (58%—many are Roman Catholics).

Traditional Fare

The West was largely unknown to whites before the nineteenth century. Good maps of the region did not exist until the 1870s. Before that time, adventurous trappers and traders made their way into the territory from the Great Plains, where the buffalo was a source of jerky, pemmican, and fat for cooking. Miners who followed the strikes in the California Mother Lode, Colorado's Pike's Peak, Montana's Grasshopper Creek, and the Alaska Klondike prepared their own meals, usually pork, beans, and hardtack (tough, dry, unleavened bread or biscuits) three times a day. Some were dependent on the waystations, hotels, and boarding houses that opened to support the rush (Luchetti, 1993). Neighborly hospitality so common in the Midwest and South disappeared in the name of profit; miners were charged the maximum for supplies (e.g., eggs for a half dollar each, potatoes for a dollar a pound, and a box of apples for $500) and a meal would cost about three dollars in a local establishment. The farmers and ranchers

European visitors to the West were appalled by both the poor quality of food and the manners practiced by the inhabitants. They complained of frenzied, rushed meals eaten with knives used like forks and handkerchiefs used like napkins. The "boarding house reach" came about in response to service at the earliest waystations, where a meal was offered at one time only to any and all comers. Diners who hesitated to grab food from the single platter placed in the middle of the large table didn't eat (Luchetti, 1992).

TABLE 11.6
Western Specialties

Group	Foods	Preparations
PROTEIN FOODS		
Milk/milk products	Milk, cheese (Cheddars like Cougar Gold, Monterey Jack, Tillamook); Basque sheep's milk cheeses	
Meat/poultry/fish/eggs/ legumes	Native game, including buffalo, deer, elk, moose, antelope, mountain sheep, mountain goats, bear, *javelina* (wild pig), beaver, rabbit	Game meat steaks, roasts, stews (such as *chili con carne*), hamburger, sausages; beaver tail
	Beef, mutton and lamb, pork	Steaks; beef *enchiladas, tamales, chimichangas, pirozhki; teriyaki;* Indian tacos; *Pueblo pozole;* lamb spit-roasted or roasted with chiles; *chorizo;* luau (pit-cooked) pork
	Clams (e.g., geoducks), crab (Dungeness, king, snow), oysters, shrimp, squid	Clam chowder, Seattle clam hash; *cioppino,* steamed crab, crab cocktails, fried *calamari;* grilled or poached salmon, *lobimuhenno`s* (salmon chowder); *sushi, sashimi, teriyaki;* trout grilled with bacon
	Salmon, tuna, halibut, mackerel, sardines, anchovies, *mahi mahi,* bonito, marlin, snapper; freshwater fish, particularly trout	
	Chicken eggs	Hangtown fry
	Dried beans	Garbanzo beans with lamb, garbanzo bean pudding; Basque beans; lentil soup with lamb, lentil and sausage casserole, white beans cooked with pimento and cheese; split-pea soup
CEREALS/GRAINS	Wheat, corn	Sourdough breads, biscuits, pancakes; *sopapillas;* fry bread; *panocha; capriotada;* whole wheat Mormon bread; *bara brith; malasadas;* Hawaiian bread; tortillas (corn or wheat); *piki;* Asian noodle dishes (e.g., *saimin*) and dough-wrapped foods (egg/spring rolls, *lumpia,* wonton); fortune cookies
FRUITS/VEGETABLES	Apples, apricots, wild and cultivated berries, cactus fruit, cherries, dates, figs, grapes, kiwifruit, lemons, oranges, peaches, pears, pineapple, plums, prunes, sugar cane	Fresh fruit desserts; fruit added to roasts or poultry stuffings; preserves, jellies, wines; cold fruit soups
	Artichokes, avocados, asparagus, broccoli, breadfruit, cauliflower, chile peppers, eggplant, *jicama, nopales,* olives, onions, specialty lettuces (arugala, radicchio, rocket), tomatoes, *tomatillos,* potatoes, taro root, zucchini	Fresh vegetable side dishes; mesclun salads; *guacamole;* Basque potatoes; squash patties; *poi*
ADDITIONAL FOODS		
Seasonings	Chile peppers (especially New Mexico/Anaheim, Jalapeño/Chipolte, Serrano); cinnamon, cilantro, *epazote,* cumin, garlic, oregano, mint, safflowers (dried petals), *yerba buena;* chocolate; vanilla	Fresh chiles, dried chile powders, smoked chiles, pickled chiles; salsas; red or green chile sauces; mole sauce; fresh, dried, powdered, roasted, pickled garlic
Nuts/seeds	Almonds, hazelnuts, macadamia nuts, pine nuts (piñon seeds), pumpkin seeds	
Beverages	Varietal wines; coffee; tea (camomile, Brigham Young); hot chocolate	Coffee drinks (lattes, etc.); *picón punch*
Fats/oils	Olive oil	
Sweeteners	Sugar from beets, cane	Sugar cane eaten fresh in Hawaii

who later made their way westward survived on game, including rabbit, squirrel, beaver, bear, deer, elk, and moose. Venison, for example, was prepared as steaks, chili con carne, and even as mincemeat for pies. Corn breads and potatoes rounded out the meals. Sourdough breads and biscuits were popular with settlers in the Mountain states, California, and Alaska. Mashed potato or a milk and flour starter was left out to "catch" wild yeast and begin fermentation. Once going, the starter was kept indefinitely, replenished each time a little was used as leavening. Many supplies shipped to the West Coast, such as butter, arrived moldy or rancid.

The growth of towns and the success of irrigation increased the food supply in the West. Expensive goods like wines and chocolates became available, and eastern specialties, including Long Island duck and Smithfield ham, were offered at restaurants. Depending on the region, potatoes, corn, apples, wheat, and hops prospered; cattle, dairy cows, and sheep became plentiful. With the arrival of experienced fishermen, more of the Pacific coast seafood was utilized. Salmon, crab, oysters, and clams were especially popular. Hearty breakfasts of the time featured steak and eggs or ham and eggs, served with hash brown potatoes and buttermilk, buckwheat, or sourdough pancakes.

Many of the immigrants to the West came in search of mining and railroad jobs, including the Chinese and Mexicans. Both of these groups enjoyed highly seasoned foods and promoted the use of chile peppers in the West. Other groups, such as the Italians, Japanese, and some Greeks, became involved in the fishing industry and introduced specialties like seafood *cioppino* (a seafood stew using local fish and shellfish) and *teriyaki*. Many immigrants opened restaurants and markets to serve the needs of the booming towns. German sausages, Italian cannoli, and Chinese stir-fried dishes were all available. Still other immigrants arrived looking for farmland; they planted the fertile Pacific coastal regions and the California Central Valley with temperate fruits and vegetables, such as apples, pears, dates, grapes, plums, prunes, cherries, artichokes, avocados, broccoli, brussels sprouts, lemons, grapefruit, and oranges.

In Alaska and Hawaii, white settlers faced different challenges. Both states became dependent on whaling. In Alaska, seafood was the main food commodity, including salmon, halibut, and several kinds of crab. In Hawaii, pineapple, sugar cane, and other tropical crops were successful exports. Both states were, and still are, reliant on the mainland for the majority of other food supplies.

State Specialties

Alaska

The cooking of Alaska has been hampered in its development by the limited variety of foods. The climate and terrain are by no means uni-

One innovative seafood recipe was the *Hangtown Fry*, a platter of scrambled eggs with fried oysters, and bacon on the side, created in Placerville, California (known at the time as Hangtown) during the 1860s for a miner who had just struck it rich.

Dairying in the West has produced several Cheddar-style cheeses, such as Cougar Gold from Washington, Tillamook from Oregon, and Monterey Jack (a mild, white cheese) from California. More recently, French-style Chèvre goat cheeses have become a specialty.

form throughout the state, with warmer regions found along the coastal panhandle extending south into Canada, around the Yukon River Delta, and the protected Matanuska Valley in the south-central region, but there is little land suited for agriculture.

The Indians, Inuits, and Aleuts of the region lived primarily on seafood and game. Wild berries and roots were harvested in the short summer months (see Chapter 3 on Native Americans). The first permanent white settlement in Alaska was on Kodiak Island. The Russians arrived in 1784 to hunt fur seals. They tried to grow wheat to supply the colony, but the grain wasn't hardy enough for the cold climate. The Russians spread southward and established settlements in California to provide goods for the Alaska hunters. They brought *kasha*, a cooked buckwheat porridge, buckwheat *blini*, and soups of fish or cabbage. *Pirogs,* large filled pastries, were made with fish, game, or cabbage. At Easter, they prepared traditional dishes, such as the rich fruitcake called *kulich* (see Chapter 4 on Europeans).

In 1896, gold was discovered in the Klondike, starting a rush of prospectors to the territory. Supplies were severely limited, and most of the new settlers lived on little more than flour, bacon, salt pork, lard, and a bit of coffee or tea. Most kept a sourdough culture going to make breads and biscuits. Sourdough specialties included poppy

The Klondike prospectors were so dependent on sour yeast cultures used to make bread that they became known as "Sourdoughs."

Salmon and other seafood are favorites in Alaska and the Pacific Northwest.

Reindeer herds were imported to Alaska in the late 1800s from Siberia and Scandinavia in the hopes they would become a profitable meat source. Many starved to death when the ranges were overgrazed, and others are thought to have become part of caribou herds. Today some reindeer in the Seward peninsula are raised for meat and to supply reindeer antlers to Asia.

During the Great Depression the U.S. government supported the relocation of 200 families from Michigan, Minnesota, and Wisconsin to establish farming in the Matanuska Valley. Many were of German or Scandinavian descent.

Fresh coriander (also known as *cilantro* or *Chinese parsley*) and cumin were probably introduced to the New World by the Spanish. They were quickly accepted in Mexican cuisine and from there were brought to California with the Spanish missionaries.

seed potato bread, rye bread with caraway seeds, and whole wheat bread. Kelp was collected at the coast, and wild flowers were boiled to make syrup. Some miners hunted to supplement their diets, and game, such as deer, caribou, moose, Dall sheep, rabbits, and ptarmigan, was available. Game meats are still popular today, including steaks, roasts, and hamburgers made from moose meat, and caribou meat sausages and Swiss steaks.

Sheep are now raised on the Aleutian Islands, providing lamb for the mainland. Cattle ranches are found on Kodiak Island and in the Delta and Matanuska Valley. Hog farming is on the rise, particularly around Palmer. More important are the dairy operations, providing fresh milk, butter, and cream. Potatoes are the most successful crop, but vegetables like cabbage, cauliflower, and rhubarb also grow in the region. Many of the vegetables attain gigantic proportions in the long daylight hours of summer; for example, cabbages may reach 70 pounds and rhubarb sometimes grows 4 feet tall. Blueberries, gooseberries, lingonberries, raspberries, salmonberries, and strawberries are produced in small amounts. The primary agricultural product of Alaska is seafood, ranking first nationally in quantity and value of the yearly catch. Salmon, herring, and halibut are the most prevalent fish. Shrimp and crab, including Dungeness, Snow (also known as Tanner), and limited King crabs, are trapped during the winter months. Most are frozen or canned for export to the rest of the United States and Japan.

Arizona

The state of Arizona has some of the most scenic terrain in the nation, from the majestic Grand Canyon to the fantastic formations of Monument Valley to the broad plains of the Sonoran Desert. Despite a climate conducive to growing many fruits and vegetables, there is not enough rainfall to support much agriculture without irrigation. Arizona fare reflects the arid conditions and the preferences of the people who settled the region, especially the Native Americans, the Spanish, and the Mexicans.

Some Native Americans who lived in the state prior to European contact, particularly Pueblo peoples, cultivated small amounts of corn, beans, chile peppers, squash, and pumpkins. Pine nuts (piñon seeds) were indigenous foods. Juicy fruits (called *tunas*, or Indian figs) and the young pads (*nopales*) of the saguro and prickly pear cactus were other native items. Small game provided meat in the diet. They prepared stews flavored with chiles and very thin blue corn tortillas called *piki*. Other tribes, such as the Navajo and Apache, were initially hunters who roamed the region in search of big game and wild plants (see Chapter 3 on Native Americans for more information). When the Spanish arrived in the sixteenth century, they introduced many of the foods that became elemental in the cooking of the

Indians in both the United States and Mexico, including wheat, hogs, sheep, and cattle. The foods and flavors of the Old World and the New coalesced into a new cuisine. Wheat tortillas became a staple in parts of the American Southwest and in northern Mexico. Hearty beef or lamb stews replaced the mostly vegetarian versions, and fry bread, made with wheat flour and cooked in lard, became common. Dishes that are popular in Arizona with Native American and Spanish or Mexican roots include *menudo* (spicy tripe soup flavored with mint), *pozole* (hominy flavored with pork and chile peppers), *chimichangas* (wheat tortillas wrapped around a beef or chicken and vegetable filling, then deep-fried), beef tamales, quesadillas, burritos and *Indian tacos* (fry bread folded and filled with meats, cheeses, vegetables, and salsa).

Irrigation has provided some agricultural opportunities in the state. Grapefruit, lemons, melons, and figs flourish in the region, as do winter crops of broccoli, cauliflower, potatoes, onions, and carrots. Two vegetables popular in Mexico have found success in Arizona also. *Tomatillos*, a relative of the ground cherry that looks a little like a green tomato in a papery husk, and jicama, a crispy tuber related to the morning glory, have both been transplanted from Mexico to Arizona. Tomatillos are added to salsa verde and other green sauces, and the sweet pea–flavored jicama frequently provides a crunch in local salads. Cattle ranching and hog farms are common and the Navajo have specialized in raising sheep and goats.

The Roosevelt Dam on the Salt River in Arizona was completed in 1911. It was the first major irrigation project undertaken by the U.S. government, providing water to the Phoenix region for agriculture and housing.

California

California cuisine is a fortuitous fusion of natural resources, agricultural abundance, and a diversity of people. The physical terrain varies between Death Valley (the lowest point in the United States) to Mount Whitney (the highest point in the forty-eight contiguous states). The climate ranges from cool and moist in the redwood forests of the north to hot and dry in the southern deserts. One range of mountains edges the eastern boundary of the state, and a second runs along the Pacific, dropping down dramatically to the coastline. Seafood is prolific, and the annual catch is second only to Alaska. The state leads the country in agricultural output, however. It supplies over half of the nation's fruits and vegetables and is first in egg and milk production.

The foods of the California Native Americans depended on their location. Coastal tribes survived on clams, mussels, and fish, with local berries and greens. In inland areas, acorns were the foundation of the diet, leached of tannins and processed as a meal or flour (see Chapter 3 on Native Americans). The first whites to settle in the state were the Spanish in the eighteenth century. They built several *presidios* (forts), *pueblos* (small farms), and a series of missions (each one day apart in travel time), with the purpose of protecting their claim to the territory. The Spanish cultivated wheat, olives, grapes, tomatoes, oranges,

The earliest Spanish settlement in what is now San Francisco was named Yerba Buena (meaning good herb), after a prolific native mint-like plant, *Satureja douglasii*. The herb was used by Indians in the region as a flavoring, especially for soups and stews.

Although there are undoubtedly other incidents of cannibalism in U.S. history, one of the most famous occurred in 1846–47 when a group of eighty-seven settlers coming from Illinois to California was stranded in the mountains of the Sierra Nevada during the winter months. Almost half the people in the Donner Party perished from hunger, and those who made it survived, in part, through eating the dead.

Both San Francisco and Los Angeles claim to be the place where fortune cookies were invented. Sometime between 1907 and 1916 a Chinese chef created the popular treat, probably as a restaurant promotion. The idea of the written fortune may date back to the twelfth century, when Chinese insurgents plotting the overthrow of Mongolian rule distributed their plans inside moon cakes.

lemons, pears, apricots, figs, and pomegranates in the lands surrounding the missions and planted native foods including corn, beans, and squash as well. Cattle and hogs were raised. Many of the local Indians were forced into the missions as laborers.

Despite Spanish claims to the contrary, many other European powers sought access to California riches. Russia, in particular, established colonies in northern California to support their fur trade along the Pacific coast and in Alaska. When Mexico gained control of much of the state in the early nineteenth century, much of the mission territory was redistributed as grants to resident families, who founded wealthy *rancheros* producing mostly beef. At the same time, settlers from throughout the country were making their way across the mountains and founding farms in the fertile valleys of the state. With the discovery of gold in 1848, over 200,000 prospectors and fortune seekers arrived, followed by thousands of Chinese, Italian, and Japanese immigrants. By the beginning of the twentieth century the population had surged to over one and a half million people, many lured by jobs in farming, ranching, fishing, fish processing, meat packing, and the canning of fruits and vegetables. Agriculture continues to draw immigrants from Mexico and Central America looking for migrant farm work. Other recent immigrants who have added to the diversity of the state include Vietnamese, Cambodians, Laotians (particularly Hmong), Koreans, Asian Indians, Ethiopians, Filipinos, and Samoans.

Many California specialties are attributable to the ethnic preferences of the population. The Spanish planted the first vineyards in the state to supply wine for the Catholic sacrament. The Mexicans brought corn tortillas, refried beans, guacamole, and popular filled dishes like tacos and enchiladas. Italians introduced northern Italian favorites, such as polenta and pesto, as well as seafood dishes, such as the tomato-based fish stew made with local fish and Dungeness crab called *cioppino* and fried *calamari* (squid). They were the first to plant artichokes in the region. The Chinese offered authentic southern-style stir-fried dishes, wontons, eggrolls, and adapted dishes like chop suey and fortune cookies. The Japanese added *sukiyaki, teriyaki, tempura, sushi,* and other favorites to the mix. Armenians in the Central Valley brought flavorful lamb skewers, *dolma* (rice- and lamb-stuffed eggplant or grape leaves) and specialty desserts like baklava. Newer immigrants have popularized hot Thai dishes, Vietnamese *pho*, Filipino *lumpia,* and Indian *Tandoori* cooking and flat breads in the state (see the chapter specific to each ethnic group for more details).

The abundance of fruits and vegetables in the state has led to the creation of "Californian cuisine," dishes that emphasize what is fresh and local. California accounts for nearly the entire U.S. production of avocados, artichokes, garlic (some of which is processed as granules and powder), walnuts, almonds, apricots, nectarines, olives, dates, figs, pomegranates, prunes, and persimmons. It leads the nation in grow-

California produces more than half of the fruits and vegetables consumed in the nation and takes pride in a cuisine based on fresh, local ingredients.

ing lettuce, broccoli, celery, cauliflower, carrots, lima beans, spinach, grapes, lemons, strawberries, plums, peaches, cantaloupes, and honeydew melons. Further, 90 percent of all raisins consumed in the world are produced in California. Specialty fruits, such as kiwifruit and feijoa (a small, green egg-shaped fruit native to Brazil that tastes a little like pineapple and eucalyptus with mint nuances), are now being grown in the state. Innovative dishes like pasta with chanterelles and grilled duck breasts, goat cheese salad with arugula and radicchio (both created by Wolfgang Puck, who started two well-known Los Angeles restaurants called Spago and Chinois on Main), poached salmon with fresh basil and olive butters, and pears and figs poached in Zinfandel with Cassis cream (by Alice Waters, founder of the restaurant Chez Panisse in Berkeley) are examples of the California approach to cooking.

Seafood is also popular in the state. During the early twentieth century, sardines were the leading catch. As their numbers diminished due to overfishing, other fish, such as tuna, salmon, halibut, mackerel, and anchovies, became the predominant catch. Dungeness crab, traditionally eaten steamed with melted butter and lemon or in crab cocktails, and squid, served deep-fried or over pasta, are popular. Abalone, a large, flat-shelled mollusk that clings to rocks off the California coast, is a specialty. The tough muscle must be pounded into a thin steak to tenderize it before cooking. It has a delicate, sweet flavor and is typically lightly floured and sautéed in butter.

Luther Burbank, a native of Massachusetts, moved to California in 1875 to conduct his experiments on plant breeding. While there, he developed nearly 800 new varieties of fruits, vegetables, and flowers, including the Russet Burbank potato, the plumcot (a cross between plums and apricots), and the Santa Rosa plum.

Cultivation of dates is extremely laborious. It takes almost 20 years before the palm produces fruit, and all dates must be pollinated by hand.

Kiwifruit were first popularized by specialty produce maven Frieda Caplan of Los Angeles. In the 1960s, she imported the fuzzy-skinned, juicy green fruits known as *Chinese gooseberries* from New Zealand. When they met consumer resistance, she promoted them with the catchier name kiwifruit, and a trend was born.

Other trendy vegetable dishes started in California include *mesclun* salads (made with a mixture of baby lettuces) and roasted garlic, which can be added to salads and stews or spread on bread like butter.

By 1853 a settlement with over 500 Chinese fishermen existed at Monterey Bay (later made famous by author John Steinbeck in his 1945 novel *Cannery Row*). They fished in Chinese-style boats called junks and sold most of their catch to San Francisco markets. They were edged out by Italian fishermen after the turn of the century.

European grape varietals are very susceptible to phylloxera *(Viteus vitafolii)*, an insect indigenous to the United States. They were only successful when it was discovered they could be grafted onto native grape rootstock, which is somewhat resistant to the pest.

E. & J. Gallo, headquartered in Modesto, California, is the largest wine producer in the world. They control approximately 30 percent of the national market and over 50 percent of exported U.S. wines.

Pioneer cooks in Colorado had difficulties making some baked goods at high altitudes. It took much experimentation to determine that leavening must be reduced and oven temperatures raised to produce moist, finely crumbed cakes.

Buffalo is being raised and processed as a specialty meat at several ranches in the West, including Rocky Mountain Natural Meats in Denver.

California is probably best known for its wine. The European settlers of the mid-nineteenth century first introduced the superior varietal grapes used in French and German wine making to the region. Today there are many premier wine regions in the state, including Napa Valley, Sonoma, Santa Cruz, Monterey, San Luis Obispo, and Santa Barbara. The Central Valley accounts for most of the grapes cultivated for the bulk wine market. Successful varietals include Barbera, Cabernet Franc, Cabernet Sauvignon, Merlot, Petite Sirah, Pinot Noir, Syrah, and Zinfandel among red wines and Chardonnay, Chenin Blanc, French Colombard, Gewürztraminer, Muscat, Pinot Blanc, Sauvignon Blanc, Semillon, and White (Johannisberg) Riesling among whites. More recently wine makers have been experimenting with other varietals, such as Cinsault, Grenache, Marsanne, and Mourvedre. Sparkling wines, which may be made from red or white grapes, and dessert wines are also specialties of the state.

Colorado

Colorado is the highest state in the nation, with an average elevation of nearly 6,800 feet. The east comprises high plains and Piedmont areas, while the west is noteworthy for two parallel ridges of the Southern Rockies. Although fur trappers and traders were familiar with the mountain region, the first permanent white settlements were established in the fertile San Luis Valley by Spanish and Mexican colonists. A short time later, thousands of prospectors from the Midwest were drawn to the territory when gold was discovered in 1861. Tin miners from Cornwall also arrived. Those who were skilled at farming stayed to homestead on the plains of the east when the gold boom ended and found that wheat was successful in some areas. German and Russian immigrants with beet farming and sugar processing experience were attracted to the state when it became known for its sugar beet crop, and Mexicans moved north to work the fields. Chinese immigrants came for jobs building the railroads. A silver boom in the 1890s brought Greeks and Slavs to the area. In more recent years, immigrants from Vietnam, the former states of the Soviet Union, and Guatemala have chosen Colorado as home.

Colorado pioneer fare was similar to that in the rest of the West. Game was a significant food source; beaver tail was a specialty. Bighorn sheep, deer, javelina (wild pig), and buffalo were also prevalent. The region developed a reputation for mountain trout, still a favorite. The Germans brought dishes like sauerbraten, *Rouladen*, and sauerkraut, and the Russians introduced stuffed cabbage, pirozkis, and sliced cucumbers in sour cream. Chile peppers and other spices came with the Mexicans, and dishes like chicken or turkey cooked in *mole* sauce (a rich blend of spices, nuts, and unsweetened chocolate) became popular throughout the state. Legend is that the famous Denver (or Western) sandwich, made with an omelet containing ham, onions, and green peppers between slices of bread, was invented by a Chinese chef making *eggs foo yung* with available ingredients (Jones, 1981).

In some mountain areas and drier plains, cattle and sheep ranching proved the best agricultural use of the land. Today Colorado is the leading producer in the nation of lamb, known as Rocky Mountain lamb.

Hawaii

It is thought that the volcanic islands of Hawaii were first settled by Polynesians from the Marquesa Islands and Tahiti in the fifth century. The foundation of their diet was starchy vegetables, such as taro root (traditionally made into *poi*—boiled, pounded into a paste, and slightly fermented), breadfruit, plantains, cassava, and yams. Seafood and possibly pork and chicken were also eaten (see Chapter 8 on Southeast Asians and Pacific Islanders for more information). British explorers discovered the islands in 1778, and missionaries soon followed. The area became a major American port for whaling ships in the nineteenth century, and Japanese, Chinese, Korean, Filipino, and Asian Indian agricultural workers came to support the developing pineapple and sugarcane industries.

Hawaiian fare today is an amalgamation of traditional native dishes and foods introduced by the many immigrants to the islands. Unlike some areas of the nation, where various foreign contributions have melded into a single cuisine with occasional European or Latino overtones, many dishes in Hawaii maintain their ethnic integrity. Foods from different cultures are commonly served at the same meal, however, representing the state's diverse heritage.

Popular Hawaiian foods include those with Japanese origins, such as teriyaki-grilled meats and fish, *sashimi* (raw, thinly sliced fish), and noodle dishes like *saimin*, an island adaptation of ramen noodles, topped with pork and frequently eaten for lunch. The Chinese brought wok cooking, *dim sum*, long-grain rice, soybeans, bok choy, lotus root, kumquats, litchi, and ginger to the region. Scottish scones and shortbreads are available, and Portuguese sweet bread is so common it is often called Hawaiian bread. Another Portuguese specialty, *malasadas* (fried doughnuts without a hole), is especially popular, and local variations made with poi or macadamia nuts are novelty items. Filipino fish sauces and *lumpia* (Filipino-style egg rolls), Korean *kimchi* (hot cabbage relish) and spicy beef dishes, and Indian curries are other contributions.

Historically sugar cane is the most important crop in Hawaii, accounting for 20 percent of the raw sugar produced nationally. But soaring costs and environmental concerns have put most sugarcane plantations out of business (only three remain), and Hawaiians are working toward agricultural diversification. Pineapples have also

Coors beer (called "Colorado Kool-Aid" by some locals), made in Golden, Colorado by the Adolph Coors Company, may be the best-known product of the state. Coors is the third-largest producer of beer in the country, following Anheuser-Busch and Miller.

The *luau*, featuring pit-cooked foods such as suckling pig, is the traditional Hawaiian feast.

The Hawaiian *pupu* platter with bite-size snacks epitomizes the international nature of food in the state. Typical appetizers include lomi-lomi (Hawaiian marinated fish or scallops); *rumaki* (water chestnut–chicken liver–bacon skewers); Chinese chicken wings, spareribs, wontons, and dumplings; roast pork; poi; coconut chips; Portuguese sausage; Korean meatballs; curried fritters; or small *kumaki* skewers of meat, chicken, or fish.

Macadamia nuts are native to Australia. It took years of research to grow them commercially in Hawaii. They reputedly have the hardest shell of all nuts to crack (a job traditionally done by placing a board on top of the nut and driving a car over it) and are processed between steel rollers. They are grown on the islands of Hawaii, Maui, Oahu, and Kauai.

Maui onions are considered the sweetest in the world—by Hawaiians, that is. They are the same variety as the Vidalia onions of Georgia.

The Parker Ranch on the island of Hawaii has 60,000 head of cattle and is second only to the King Ranch in Texas in size.

Potatoes were first grown in Idaho by Henry Harmon Spaulding, a Presbyterian missionary invited by the Nez Percé Indians to bring Christianity to the region. The first commercial crops were grown by Mormons in the area.

Trout is farmed in the Magic Valley of Idaho, providing over half of all the trout consumed in the United States.

Boise is sometimes called the Basque capital of the United States due to the large numbers of businesspeople of Basque descent working in the city.

been a significant commodity, including fresh, canned, and juice products. More profitable operations developed in Asia have cut into production on the islands in recent years, however. Hawaii grows most of the world's supply of macadamia nuts and also exports famous kona coffee, which is grown on the western slopes of the island of Hawaii. Cattle ranches are found on the islands of Maui, Hawaii, and the privately owned Niihau; most provide beef for local consumption. Seafood, another Hawaiian specialty, is also mostly fished for Hawaiian markets, although some tuna is canned and exported. In addition to tuna, common food fish include mahi mahi (also called *dorado*), bonito, mackerel, marlin, scad, and both pink and red snapper.

Idaho

Potatoes are synonymous with Idaho. The blight-resistant variety developed in 1872 by horticulturist Luther Burbank (see California) called the Russet Burbank potato is so common in the state it is now legally known as the Idaho potato. They are grown primarily in the volcanic soils of the Snake River plain. Ten billion pounds are harvested annually, approximately one-third of national production. Sixty percent of the potatoes from Idaho are frozen, dehydrated, or milled into flour.

Idaho was the last state in the country to be explored by whites. The earliest adventurers in the region were trappers and Christian missionaries. Although thousands passed through the state along the Oregon Trail heading west, few settled in the area. It wasn't until the 1860s, when gold was discovered in the north of the state, that tens of thousands of fortune hunters arrived, including numerous Finnish, Welsh, and Chinese miners. The poorest lived on beans, bread, and coffee. Specialties included *lobimubenno's* (a salmon chowder) brought by the Finns and *bara brith,* a bread studded with currants favored by the Welsh. Trout, salmon, bass, and sturgeon filled the local rivers, and game, such as deer, elk, and buffalo, was available. Recreational fishing and hunting continue today. Venison with huckleberry sauce is a popular dish.

Some miners stayed and took up farming after the gold rush, joined by southern European immigrants in the north of the state. Crops like wheat, oats, barley, hops, peas, lentils, and beans grew well in the dry climate of the north. Farmers in the more southern valleys discovered that, with irrigation, potatoes, corn, broccoli, and peppermint and spearmint (grown for their oils used in flavorings) could be cultivated. Cattle ranchers and sheepherders arrived in the region, particularly Basque immigrants. They introduced sourdough bread and a pencil-thin version of the spicy Spanish sausage *chorizo*. Lamb dishes, including grilled lamb and lamb stew, were a Basque specialty. *Basque potatoes*, still a favorite in the state, is a sliced potato, onion, and bacon casserole. Many dishes in Idaho today feature local ingredients with European nuances, such as split-pea soup, lentil soup with lamb, lentil and sausage casserole, white beans cooked with pimento and cheese, and ham with apple casserole. Apple jelly is added to mayonnaise to make salad dressing. Prunes are used in preserves and desserts, like prune-whip pie and prune pudding (Lee, 1992).

Montana

Although the name Montana means "mountainous" in Spanish, two-thirds of the state is covered by the Great Plains, with Rocky Mountain ranges found only in the western region. Wheat, oats, barley, sugar beets, potatoes, beans, cherries, and apples are the primary crops. Beef, dairy goods, lamb, and pork are other agricultural commodities.

Native Americans in the state lived mostly in the plains region, surviving on buffalo and wild fruits and nuts. The first whites in the region were fur trappers and Jesuit missionaries. Major settlement did not occur until the gold rush at Grasshopper Creek began in the 1860s. The influx of people to the state provided opportunities in cattle ranching. Longhorns from Texas were driven to Montana, where they were fattened on the abundant prairie grasses before continuing on to distribution via Wyoming. Soon sheepherders of Basque, Russian, Rumanian, or Turkish heritage also made their way to the vast pasturelands. Most survived on the rudimentary meal of the prairie pioneer: salt pork and beans.

Montana specialties reflect the abundant game of the region, especially venison. It is prepared roasted or made into chili con carne or meatballs in a spicy tomato sauce. Elk, moose, and antelope are still plentiful. Wild birds include geese, ducks, pheasant, and grouse. Fish is available in the over 10,000 freshwater lakes and streams, particularly sockeye salmon and many kinds of trout. Native berries are a favorite, especially huckleberries, which are made into breads and pies, and the sour-tasting chokecherries, which are used in pies, cakes, preserves, jellies, and wine. Immigrants to the state have added their foods to the cuisine. Scandinavians who arrived from Minnesota to work in lumbering brought yellow split-pea soup, cold fruit soups, Swedish meatballs, and ham with cherry sauce. Borscht, cheese-filled pastry shells (*vatroushki*), and cherry desserts were favored by the Russians. The Scots made oatmeal porridge and Mulligatawny stew with mutton, and central Europeans brought stuffed cabbage, dumplings filled with fruit or cheese, and pancakes rolled around cherries.

Nevada

The Nevada landscape is mostly stark, arid desert. Even though early Mormon settlers from Utah were successful in setting up small farms using crop rotation and irrigation, the largest agricultural commodities

In 1923 a cloud of grasshoppers 300 miles long, 100 miles wide, and half a mile thick descended on Montana, eating every green plant down to its roots.

A Montana specialty is *Rocky Mountain oysters*, or "tendergroin," which are calf testicles. They are traditionally served with beans and grilled bread.

Deer is ranched commercially in some parts of Nevada, and venison is a specialty.

in Nevada are cattle and sheep; most crops that are grown are used for forage.

It was discovery of gold and silver at the Comstock Lode in 1859 that brought significant numbers of Europeans to the state. Before that time the region was sparsely populated by the Paiute, Shoshone, and Washoe Indians. Mining towns like Virginia City grew out of the dust into bustling urban centers, complete with theaters and operas. Food was in short supply and extremely expensive, yet wealthy prospectors and those who provided services to them supported extravagant restaurants, where internationally known chefs prepared oysters brought from San Francisco over the Sierra mountains as stews, oyster loafs, and stuffings for quail. Champagne imported from France was drunk from crystal goblets.

By 1900 the Comstock Lode was depleted and many of the mining towns disappeared. Although half the state population of the time had been born outside the United States, few of the immigrants from Asia, Europe, and India who came to work in the mines, on the railroads, or on farms and ranches had the resources to maintain their culinary traditions in the privations of the desert. The exception was the Basques, who came in large numbers to the state, at first as hired shepherds and later as land-owning sheep ranchers. Initially only men came, and then they later brought their families. Women did most of the cooking, providing meals for the ranchers such as sourdough breads and biscuits with sheep's milk cheese and coffee for breakfast, and *Basque beans* (pinto beans with lamb or pork), lamb stews, or Spanish-style potato omelets for the main meal. In the towns, Basques often established hotels, which served as meeting places for Basques doing business in the area and for new immigrants. The hotels became famous for their four- or five-course meals served family-style, and non-Basque visitors often came for the food. Garbanzo bean and meat stews, spit-roasted lamb, spicy chorizo sausages, and even traditional seafood dishes like *bacalao al pil-pil* (dried salt cod cooked with garlic and olive oil) were offered when the ingredients were available. Red wine, chamomile tea, and *picón punch* (a beverage no longer common in Spain but still available where Basques live in the United States, made from bitter-orange picón liqueur, brandy, grenadine, and soda) were popular drinks.

Basques from Nevada may have introduced sourdough bread to San Francisco, where it has become a signature item.

The Basque hotels were also where the wives of Basque sheepherders went during their pregnancies to escape the isolation of the ranches and to find help with the delivery.

New Mexico

The state of New Mexico is an arid mix of high desert plateaus, portions of the Great Plains, and sections of the Rocky Mountains. Although the Spanish had explored the region extensively looking for gold and other minerals, it was Mexican-born settlers who established small farms called *ranchos* and *estancias* along the fertile banks of the Rio Grande River beginning in 1584. Missionaries followed, and Spanish culture pervaded the region. When the Santa Fe Trail opened in the early nineteenth century, Anglo-Americans (those who spoke English) arrived, adding to the population of Spanish Americans (mostly of Mexican and Native American ancestry who spoke Spanish), and Native Americans. The ethnic heritage of the state is evident in the many Native American celebrations, adobe villages, and numerous examples of Spanish architecture that still exist.

Nowhere is the blending of Native American, Spanish American, and Anglo-American culture more evident than in the cuisine of New Mexico. The Native Americans, mostly Pueblo peoples and nomadic Apache and Navajo tribes (see Chapter 3 on Native Americans), and early settlers survived on corn, game like deer and rabbit, beans, squash, tomatoes, and chile peppers. The Mexicans brought beef, mutton, chicken, wheat, rice, chocolate, and numerous spices obtained through Spanish trade with the New World. Traditional dishes that evolved during this period are still common today. Examples include breads (corn tortillas, blue cornmeal piki, and the light, deep-fried wheat flour puffs called *sopaipillas*); soups and stews, such as *Pueblo pozole* (made with dried corn, beef or pork ribs, onions, garlic, and *epazote* or oregano), green chili stew (beef, tomatoes, onions, and a variety of green chile peppers), and garbanzo beans with lamb; and puddings, such as chile-flavored garbanzo bean pudding, *panocha* (similar to Indian pudding from the Northeast, but made with wheat kernels and flavored with cinnamon), and *capriotada* (bread pudding with pine nuts, raisins, and mild cheese, traditionally served with a caramel sauce). Indian roasted lamb with red and green chile peppers, Spanish *arroz con pollo* (updated with chiles), and Mexican *chilaquiles, enchiladas* and *flautas* are other common dishes in the region. Popular desserts include anise cookies called *biscochitos* (a Christmas specialty), sopaipillas served with honey or cinnamon syrup, and *flan*.

Chile peppers, onions, garlic, oregano, *yerba buena*, *epazote*, safflower blossoms (dried and powdered, reminiscent of saffron), and abundant amounts of mint flavor savory dishes. Sweets depend on chocolate, vanilla, cinnamon, and nutmeg. Toasted pumpkin seeds or pine nuts from the native piñon tree were added to spice blends for sauces, providing a nutty flavor to roasted meats and poultry. Today almonds are used in the same way.

Oregon

Oregon is divided by bands of the Cascade-Sierra mountains, both physically and climatically. The temperate, wet coastal weather of the west contrasts dramatically with the semi-arid plateaus in the east with their cold winters and warm summers. The coastal region is endowed with a wealth of native foods, including deer, elk, antelope, rabbits, beaver, muskrats, ducks, geese, greens, wild mushrooms, and a multitude of berries. In many eastern regions of the state, near desert conditions exist.

Hot chocolate, made from unsweetened cocoa and hot water, sweetened with honey or sugar and flavored with spices like cinnamon, was a popular beverage with settlers in New Mexico.

Chiles are native to the Americas. There are five domesticated species (*Capsicum annum, C. baccatum, C. chinense, C. frutescens,* and *C. pubescens*), but there is no consensus on the common names for the hundreds of varieties, nor is there a single heat classification system. Mild New Mexican (also called Anaheim) chiles, hotter Jalapeños (sliced, pickled Jalapeños are sprinkled on nachos; smoked Jalapeños are called *Chipoltes*), and very hot Serrano chiles are the most popular in New Mexican cuisine.

The official state question in New Mexico is "Red or green?" referring, of course, to chile pepper sauce preference.

The strings and wreaths of dried red peppers known as *ristras* in New Mexico are made from ripe New Mexican/Anaheim chile peppers.

The piñon tree is the state tree of New Mexico.

The famous American gourmand and cookbook author James Beard was born in Portland, Oregon in 1903. His father had come as a youth to the state from Iowa by covered wagon.

An adapted New England dish popular in Oregon is *Portland popovers,* essentially Yorkshire pudding batter that is flavored with herbs and baked in ramekins greased with drippings from roast beef or pork (Jones, 1981).

Schnitzel sandwiches, thin, breaded and fried veal or pork cutlets served between slices of bread, were invented in the United States and introduced to Germany by American soldiers. They are popular in some parts of Oregon (Carlson, 1997).

The state was first explored by white trappers seeking beaver pelts. Methodist missionaries who followed had little success in converting the local Native Americans but did encourage settlement of the region. Tens of thousands of pioneers from New England, the South, and the Midwest traveled the Oregon Trail in the middle of the nineteenth century to participate in the promise of the new frontier. Yankees from the east named their settlements after their hometowns of Portland, Salem, and Albany. Many also survived on the coastal seafood that was familiar in Atlantic fare, particularly clams. Over two dozen varieties (e.g., butter, horse, Japanese littleneck, Manila, razor) live in the sands of the Pacific Northwest. Clam chowder, adapted with whatever local settlers could rustle up, including rice, tomatoes, and cabbage, was common (Jones, 1981). Geoduck (pronounced *gooey-duck*) clams are a large, native bivalve that have necks (siphons) that can stretch several feet. A geoduck may weigh up to 15 pounds, although most are in the 2 to 3 pound range. The body is sliced and pounded into thin steaks (similar to abalone), and the neck is usually minced or ground up for soups or stews. Other seafood specialties of the region include salmon, shrimp, crab, squid, and flounder.

Some settlers started small farms, particularly in the fertile Willamette Valley and the northwestern areas of the state. Fruit, such as pears (mostly Bartlett, with some Anjou, Bosc, Comice, Seckel, and Winter), Hood River apples, Golden Oregon prunes, plums, cherries, and domestic berries (strawberries, raspberries, cranberries, blackberries, and blueberries), proved very successful. Much of the annual fruit harvest is canned or frozen. An Oregon specialty is hazelnuts (also called filberts). The trees were introduced by an immigrant from France in 1858, and today nearly all hazelnuts consumed in the United States are grown in the state. Dairying is an important industry, producing milk, butter, and nationally marketed cheese. In more recent years, Oregon wines have gained a reputation for quality, especially for cool weather varietals like Pinot Gris (a white wine) and Pinot Noir (a red grape used in French-style burgundies). Fruit wines, such as those made from blackberries, currants, cranberries, or peaches, are also favorites in the region.

Fresh seafood, fruits, and vegetables are featured in Oregon cuisine. Grilled and poached salmon is a specialty. Poultry stuffed with prunes is popular, as are various fruit pies, soups, preserves, jams, and jellies. Some ethnic and regional fare traced to the settlers can also be found, such as German foods (schnitzels, sauerbraten, sage sausages, stuffed cabbage, sauerkraut, and strudels), and southern fried chicken served with biscuits and hominy.

Utah

It was the isolation of Utah that attracted the first white settlers to the state. In 1847 an advance party of Mormons led by Brigham Young arrived in the Great Basin area surrounding the Great Salt Lake. He declared it the site where Mormons would found a self-sufficient community free from the persecution suffered in Ohio, Illinois, Missouri, and other states where the members of the Church of Jesus Christ of Latter-Day Saints had lived. That year, another 1,500 settlers joined his group, and by 1860, over 40,000 Mormons were living in the towns of Salt Lake City, Ogden, Bountiful, Provo, and Manti. Most came by wagon train, but nearly 3,000 walked the distance pulling all their possessions in hand trucks.

Most of Utah is scenic desert country, with the exception of the fertile valleys and foothills of the Wasatch Mountains in the northeast. Agriculture was difficult at first, and the early settlers survived on indigenous greens, weeds, and birds such as crows. The Mormons gradually created a sophisticated irrigation system that captured runoff from the mountains and were able to cultivate wheat, potatoes, onions, beans, peas, and a variety of fruit, including apples, apricots, tart cherries, peaches, and pears. Most farms in the state remain small, family-run operations, providing just what is needed for local consumption. Livestock proved a more profitable agricultural pursuit than field crops: Cattle, turkeys, eggs, and sheep became primary products. Swiss Mormon converts started dairying concerns in the Salt Lake City area.

Today approximately 80 percent of the state population are Mormon. Many were of northern European descent, particularly British and Scandinavians. Most had lived first in areas of the Midwest. They brought a preference for hearty foods. Ham, pot roast, roast beef, stews, and fried chicken remain favorite entrees, often served with homemade whole wheat bread or buttermilk biscuits. Spicing is usually mild: *Hamburger bean goulash*, a Utah specialty, is thought to be a denatured version of chili con carne (Lee, 1992). Milk gravy, made with browned flour, pork grease, milk, and seasoned with black pepper, was served with so many foods that cowboys riding through the area dubbed it *Mormon dip*. Potatoes, red cabbage, green beans, and peas are still common side dishes. The Mormons are well known for their love of sweets, and desserts are prominent in the diet. Layer cakes, fruit pies, strawberry shortcake, fruit candies, chocolates, and ice cream are commonly consumed. One notable favorite is *pepparakor,* a Scandinavian ginger cookie that is often Anglicized as *pepper cookies*. Mormons do not drink alcohol or stimulating beverages like coffee or tea; lemonade and *Brigham Young tea* (sweetened hot water with milk) are traditional beverages.

One immigrant group in Utah that has maintained many of their food traditions are the Roman Catholic Italians who came from Calabria to Carbon County in central Utah. They often grow Mediterranean vegetables and seasonings, such as eggplants, tomatoes, endive, fava beans, fennel, zucchini, garlic, parsley, and basil, in home gardens. Everyday fare includes bread sticks, pastas, minestras, salads,

Utah's nickname is the "Beehive State," denoting the industrious agricultural efforts of the first Mormon settlers. The state flower is the sego lily, which some settlers were forced to eat to survive in the first years of settlement.

A popular tale in Utah history regards a plague of crickets that threatened the Mormons' first crops in 1848. They prayed to God, and suddenly sea gulls appeared (more than 1,000 miles from the nearest ocean) and ate the insects before they could do harm.

Sour cream raisin pie is a twentieth-century recipe of undetermined origins that harkens back to the sweetened clabber, milk custards, and dried fruits of early pioneer days. It is popular in Utah.

Mormon tea, or Brigham tea, is also the name for a Native American brew common in the arid areas of the Southwest made from *Ephedra nevadenis.*

and fresh fruits for dessert. Specialties like goat meats and goat cheeses, variety meats cooked up with eggs in a *frittata* or in a spicy stew, boiled chicken's feet, and deep-fried squash patties made with chopped squash and squash blossoms are traditional favorites (Raspa, 1984).

Washington

The state of Washington has a terrain and history similar to that of Oregon. Like Oregon, the state is divided by the Cascade Mountains into the wet, fertile western coast region and the dry, prairie-like eastern plateaus. Trappers were the first whites to enter the territory, followed in the mid-1800s by other pioneers, mostly farmers seeking land grants, of English, Dutch, German, and Scandinavian descent. Unlike in Oregon, large numbers of African Americans and immigrants from China and Japan came to Washington in search of work on the railroads.

Regardless of ancestry, most settlers lived on cultivated wheat, potatoes and other vegetables, wild game, fish (particularly salmon and halibut), and berries. Few distinctively ethnic flavors are common in Washington fare. Instead, immigrants in the state adapted their cooking to the plentiful food resources of the region: produce and seafood.

In the temperate western areas, corn, asparagus, onions, peas, pears, grapes, strawberries, peaches, raspberries, and plums became important products. Washington leads the nation in the production of both apples and cherries. Apples are especially associated with the state: Grown on the eastern slopes of the Cascades, they require extensive hand-labor to thin each cluster of blossoms to a single "king blossom" and to pick any fruit that appears after the initial crop sets. This process produces exceptionally large, well-formed apples. Nearly the entire crop is devoted to Red Delicious and Golden Delicious varieties, although several other types are grown in small amounts, such as Fuji, Gala, Granny Smith, and Winesap. Hops, Walla-Walla onions (a cool weather sweet onion that is a different variety from the sweet onions grown in Georgia and Hawaii), mint, and spearmint are specialty crops. Washington is also known for its white varietal wines, such as Chardonnay, Chenin Blanc, Gewürtztraminer, and White Riesling.

Washington has an abundance of seafood. Beginning in the 1800s the five species of salmon in the region (king or chinook, sockeye, dog, humpback, and silver) were sent fresh to West Coast markets or pickled and shipped in barrels to Hawaii, South America, the East Coast, and Europe. Iced fish was also sent to Europe, where it was smoked, then returned to the United States. Washington still leads the nation in total salmon catch and products. Oysters are another specialty. Many species live in the area, but only a few are commercially viable. The small, native Olympia oyster is a favorite, but overharvest-

Legend has it that the early settlers of Seattle who came from New England longed for hash but were unable to obtain corned beef. So they substituted clams for the meat, cooking them with bits of bacon, onions, potatoes, and eggs to create a new dish. Today *Seattle clam hash* omits the eggs in favor of more traditional cream (Jones, 1981).

Floating oystering communities were established in the Puget Sound area during the late 1800s. Families would rake the mudflats at low tide for prized Olympia oysters. Steamboat merchants would later come by at high tide to purchase burlap bags full of oysters from the gatherers.

ing has greatly reduced availability. Pacific oysters, which were imported from Japan in the early 1900s, are the species consumed most often on the West Coast. They are usually named after the location where they are farmed, such as Malaspina and Willapa Bay. European flat oysters and the gigantic geoduck oysters (see Oregon) are also harvested. Oysters are typically served on the half shell in the region, although bacon-wrapped broiled oysters, oyster fritters, oyster loaf, and oyster stew are common cooked preparations. Mussels are cultivated at Whidbey Island, and Dungeness crab, named for the town of Dungeness on the Olympic Peninsula, are caught during the winter months.

Wyoming

The vast grasslands covering much of eastern Wyoming offered grazing for the cattle herds of Texas when pastureland in that state was depleted in the mid-nineteenth century. The fact that it was free added extra incentive for ranchers to move their operations north. By 1886 there were 2 million head in the state, most of which were processed through Cheyenne for East Coast markets. An exceptionally cold winter that year, followed by overgrazing, dramatically reduced the number of cattle in Wyoming. Sheep became a significant commodity, and today cattle and sheep are the main agricultural products. Most crops supply forage for livestock, although sugar cane, winter wheat, barley, beans (especially pinto and Great Northern), and potatoes are cash crops for the region.

Wyoming is best known for its wild fish and game. Some of the most famous names in the history of the West made their living as trappers in the state during the early 1800s, including Jedediah Strong Smith and Kit Carson. Wyoming is amply endowed with big game, including mule deer, white-tail deer, pronghorn antelope, elk, moose, mountain sheep, black bears, and grizzly bears. Game meat is a specialty, especially venison and antelope. Tenderloin, sirloin, and T-bone steaks are cut; the ribs and sirloin tips make roasts (which are sometimes marinated and braised in wine, vinegar, and spices); the brisket, flank, and plate are used for stews or hamburgers; the hams are smoked; and miscellaneous meat is used to make Polish sausage or salami. Game birds include grouse, pheasant, and partridge, and wild turkeys are now being raised for sport. Pheasant roasted with apples or in a pie is a favorite. Many species of trout are found in the mountain streams, and lakes host bass, crappie, and catfish.

The state attracted a diversity of European immigrants, many of whom opened bakeries, confectionery stores, and restaurants. French croissants, Middle Eastern *halvah* (sesame seed candy), German schnitzel, and Chinese wonton soup were reportedly available in southeastern Wyoming as early as 1900 (Lee, 1992).

Coffee drinks like lattes have become a specialty item associated with Seattle. The city is home to the Starbucks Corporation, which started as a coffee stand at the open-air Pike Place Market in 1971. Founder Harold Schultz almost single-handedly started the trend of U.S. coffee bars (modeled after Italian espresso bars) in 1984. There were nearly 1,400 Starbucks coffee bars throughout the nation by 1997.

Dairying is the primary agricultural activity of the Star Valley in western Wyoming. Mormons from Utah began the cooperative in the region in the late 1800s, producing mostly Swiss Emmanthaler-style cheese.

Wyoming was the first state in the nation to grant women the right to vote, own property, and receive equal wages for equal work in 1869. Legend has it that suffragist Ester Morris invited the representatives running for election to tea and "buttered them up" with her cakes and cookies as she persuaded them to support equality issues. A more likely scenario is that Wyoming passed the legislation hoping for publicity and to encourage more women to settle in the territory.

Canadian Regional Specialties

Canada is the second largest nation in the world in area, a diverse land with rainforests, vast prairies, deciduous forests, and sparse tundra regions. There are more lakes and inland waters in Canada than in any other country. It is a nation rich in natural resources, especially abundant freshwater fish and seafood, game, and fertile farmland.

The country is divided into ten provinces and three territories. Just as in the United States, Canadian regional fare reflects indigenous foods and the preferences of the groups who have significantly impacted the nation historically: Native Americans and immigrants from Great Britain and France, with added flavors from smaller populations of immigrant groups from northern Europe and Asia. A recent conference explored Canadian regional fare, and its findings were published in a book titled *Northern Bounty: A Celebration of Canadian Cuisine* (Stewart & Powers, 1995). Although the editors note that there are many nationally known foods, from apple pies and cinnamon buns to lobster and Cheddar cheese, they emphasize that much of Canadian cooking is dependent on local ingredients. They provide an overview of five culinary regions: the Atlantic Provinces, Quebec, Ontario, the Prairies, and British Columbia.

Atlantic Provinces

The cooking of the Atlantic Provinces uses seasonal ingredients prepared as dishes familiar to the Acadians and British immigrants who settled the region, with a little German influence found in Nova Scotia. Seafood is preeminent, including lobster, oysters, clams, and mussels, as well as cod, salmon, haddock, halibut, smelt, and herring. Lobster and corn boils are popular in summer, and "clamburgers" with a little fat rendered from salt pork poured over the top are an Acadian specialty. Planked salmon and *Solomon Gundy* (pickled herring, a Lund-berg County favorite) are also common. Malpeque Bay oysters and Prince Edward Island (P.E.I.) mussels are renowned worldwide. A foundation of the diet is many varieties of potatoes, such as Yukon Golds, Red Pontiacs, purple-fleshed potatoes, and Russets grown for their length (to make french fries) or their roundness (for chips). In Nova Scotia, new potatoes are combined with baby peas, beans, and carrots and flavored with butter and cream to make Scottish *Hodge Podge*. The Acadians make potato dumplings the size of baseballs (*poutine râpée*) that are served as a main course, side dish, or even as dessert with molasses. *Rappie* pie is another Acadian specialty, made from grated potatoes that are squeezed dry, then cooked with enough chicken broth to equal the extracted potato juices, until the potatoes are jellylike. It can be topped with cooked chicken, meat, or clams, flavored with molasses, and covered with bacon or salt pork before it is baked. Fish and chips (sometimes made with lobster) was a tradition in the Atlantic Provinces that is regaining popularity. Other foods of the region include fresh spring shoots of *Salicornia europaea* (crowfoot, glasswort, or samphire green) and fern fronds. Rhubarb, strawberries, saskatoonberries (also called shadbush or juneberries in the United States) and blueberries are seasonal favorites. Lamb dishes and meat pies are common British foods found in the region (Comfort, 1995; Nightingale, 1995).

Quebec

The cuisine of Quebec is influenced by the French country roots shared by many of the residents. Yet even the most traditional of dishes, such as the meat pie called *tourtière*, vary according to the area where they are prepared. In Charlevoix, *tourtière* is made with cubed meat instead of ground meat, and in Saguena-Lac-St-John, it is more of a layered dish.

Canadian Regional Specialties—continued

In the Mauricie, it is made with salmon, and in Quebec City the filling is thickened with oats instead of potatoes, a British contribution.

Specialty foods of the region include leeks, oyster mushrooms, white asparagus, endive, apples (often used to make hard apple cider), and strawberries. Lamb, rabbit, game birds, salmon, and cod are popular. Seventy percent of the world's maple syrup comes from Quebec, and it is used to flavor many products, including *viande boucanée*, salt pork smoked in the maple sugar shack so that it is sweetened by the vapors of the bubbling pots; maple sugar pickles; and even maple sugar wine. Maple sugar pie is a specialty. Dairying is significant in the region. In addition to traditional French cheeses like *Brie*, Quebec produces *Oka* (also called Trappist monk cheese), similar to Port Salut; Swiss-style Raclette; and several Chèvres (goat cheeses). Other common dishes include *cretons* (a pork pâté), *cipaille* (a layered meat pie, sometimes prepared with game), and *fèves au lard* (baked beans) (Armstrong, 1995; Burkhard, 1995).

Ontario

The cooking of Ontario originally emphasized the foods favored in Great Britain. The Scots brought scones, shortbread, and haggis, and the Irish added a love of potatoes. Cookbooks from the late nineteenth century include many recipes for game, beef, and poultry as entrees and numerous descriptions of sweet and savory pies and puddings. Two ethnic communities have influenced the cuisine of Ontario: the native Cree and Iroquois, and the German Mennonites who came to the Waterloo County from Pennsylvania (Pennsylvania Dutch). Indian foods include corn and bean soups made with venison or pork; bannocks baked in an oven, in a fry pan, or wrapped around a stick over a fire; and many game dishes. Moose muzzle was a specialty. Mennonite foods include those traditional in Pennsylvania, such as smoked hams, sausages, headcheese, dumplings, doughnuts, preserves and relishes, and numerous pies. Wild meat, fowl, and fish are often cooked by the Canadian Mennonites. Fried trout and pot pies made with pigeons or rabbit are examples (Duncan, 1995; Skye, 1995; Staebler, 1995).

Ontario is also known for its plentiful fruits. The temperate climate around the Great Lakes supports numerous varieties of apples, peaches, pears, cherries, berries, grapes, and rhubarb. Specialties include Dutch apple pies topped with streusel, apple or rhubarb coffee cakes, apple dumplings, apples baked in a crust and drenched in caramel sauce, peach crisps, and blueberry jam. Fruit is used to complement meats and poultry, and is added to cabbage salads, mashed rutabagas, and even spicy chili sauces. Wines are produced on the Niagara peninsula, Pelee Island, and the Lake Erie north shore. One unusual dessert wine that has become popular in recent years is *icewine*, similar to the German version known as *Eiswein*. It is made from White Riesling or Vital grapes that are allowed to ripen until they shrivel and the sugars become concentrated. They are harvested after they freeze; the small amounts of the intensely sweet juice that remain are pressed from the grapes and fermented. It is described as having an ambrosial flavor reminiscent of honey, apricots, peaches, oranges, tea, and toffee (Aspler, 1995; Baird, 1995; Ziraldo, 1995).

The Prairies

The Prairie provinces of Canada are red meat country. Buffalo sustained the few Native Americans and white pioneers who made their homes in the region in the early years. The meat was barbecued or dried to make pemmican. The intestines were used for sausages and to wrap a strip of meat that was then grilled

Canadian Regional Specialties—continued

over a smoky fire in the dish colorfully called *Crow-Indian-Guts*; baby bison were pit-roasted. As the buffalo herds diminished in the early nineteenth century, cattle took their place. Chuck wagon and range cooking were specialties. Although coffee, beans and sour-dough breads, biscuits, and pancakes were mainstays, fresh beef dishes were the favorites, particularly fried steaks and stews made with onions, potatoes, and canned tomatoes. *Prairie oysters* (breaded, fried beef testicles) were popular. Some of the cowboy terms applied to foods indicated their role in the diet, such as "baked wind pills" (beans), "paperweights" (hot biscuits), and "yesterday, today, and for-ever" (hash) (Barss, 1995; Schultz, 1995).

The Prairies are also the breadbasket of Canada. The first wheat crops planted by the German Mennonites, Icelanders, Scandina-vians, Americans, and British settlers often failed due to poor seed quality, droughts, fires, grasshoppers, and blizzards. But by 1904, Cana-dian flour won the Gold Medal at the St. Louis World's Fair, and wheat became a significant export crop. Foods of the Prairie farm families often included dishes from immigrant home-lands, such as roast beef and Yorkshire pud-ding, stews, pot roasts, chicken and dumplings, stuffed cabbage, sauerkraut, and perogies (like midwestern bierocks). Biscuits accompanied many meals, including bannocks, *gems* (similar to muffins, cooked in fluted cups), and fried biscuits. During the depression years, bread with gravy and bread puddings filled many stomachs. Traditional baked goods included pound cakes, tea cakes, banana bread, short-bread, chocolate cake, carrot pudding, matri-monial cake (date squares), sour cream raisin pie, cinnamon buns, strawberry shortcake, and ethnic breads like Dutch Kringle bread, French bread, and Ukrainian *paska* (Fraser, 1995).

British Columbia

The West Coast of Canada was settled by British trappers and traders, not farmers. The relatively wealthy populace quickly became reliant on imported foods. As early as 1886, fresh fruit was being shipped to the region from California. Although Chinese, Japanese, and Asian Indians began to immigrate to the West Coast in the 1880s, their ethnic fare was isolated within each of their communities, while most residents favored the mildly sea-soned foods of colonial England (Johnson, 1995). It was the globalization of cooking that brought native ingredients and Asian influ-ences to the forefront of British Columbia cui-sine. Indigenous greens, such as miner's lettuce and the new shoots of thimbleberries or salmonberries, are lightly dressed as salads; camass bulbs are served as side dishes; and the many wild berries of the region (including thimbleberries, salalberries, salmonberries, huckleberries, saskatoonberries, red elderber-ries, and soapberries) are used in savory sauces for meats, in fresh desserts, in preserves, and in juices and teas. Sushi and samosas are now available at delicatessens along with the sand-wiches and soups. Canadian native foods used in traditional Asian dishes offer new flavors, such as Filipino *sinigang* with salmon instead of pork, Chinese pork and cod braised with garlic, or Japanese geoduck sashimi. Four major varietal grape–growing regions have developed in British Columbia, producing well-respected Chardonnay, White Riesling, Pinot Blanc, and Pinot Noir wines (McWatters, 1995; Turner et al., 1995; Wong, 1995).

Contemporary Trends

The saga of American cooking is far from over. It is perhaps useful to look at the evolution of regional fare as it progressed from the first colonies of the Northeast to the Midwest, the South, and finally the West. What started out as a cuisine dependent on corn, beans, pork, seafood, and root vegetables prepared according to Native American and British traditions became increasingly diverse as it spread through the country. German and Scandinavian influences in the Midwest reinforced the role of pork (especially as sausages) and cold weather vegetables (particularly potatoes, and cabbage) in the diet, but also contributed the rich dairy products, the hearty wheat flour breads and abundant baked goods typical of the American table. In the South the Spanish, French, and Africans brought new foods, seasonings, and cooking techniques to the region. Ingredients like okra, rice, peaches, oranges, watermelon, peanuts, and sesame seeds helped redefine traditional pork, corn, and bean dishes. Indigenous ingredients, such as chile peppers, crawfish, oysters, and pecans, were appreciated for the unique flavors they added to southern fare. By the time the West was settled, many of the pioneers had lost touch with much of their European heritage, and although the foods they brought had their roots in Britain, Germany, Scandinavia, or other nations, they were considered all-American fare. Beef became the most important meat. Native game, fowl, fish, and shellfish took on added significance in a diet that was often limited to available resources. Fresh fruits and vegetables assumed prominence in regions where agriculture flourished. New influences emerged, particularly from Mexico, and more recently from Asia, which have begun to reshape American approaches to cooking and eating.

Despite this wealth of regional diversity, many people see only the uniformity in American fare. It is true that, beginning with the flatboats of the Mississippi and the cross-continental railroads, people in the United States have had unprecedented access to foods of all regions. Oysters from Chesapeake Bay could be transported fresh to Illinois, and beef from Wyoming could be shipped to Kansas City for processing before it was sent to New York. With the advent of air travel, markets have expanded further to regularly offer Alaskan king crab and Hawaiian pineapples. While such abundance offers an endless array of possible new flavors, the flip side of constant availability of foods that are not native or not in season locally can be homogeneity and blandness. If all Americans are cooking with inexpensive hamburger, canned tomato sauces, instant potatoes, and fruit picked underripe to prevent blemishes from occurring during shipping, meals are easy to prepare but creativity is limited and flavors are underdeveloped.

Uniformity in American fare can be traced, in part, to the popularity of certain cookbooks in the early twentieth century. Cooking

H. L. Mencken held a low opinion of American food and did not hesitate to express his disdain: "The national taste for bad food seems all the more remarkable when one recalls that the United States, more than any other country of the modern world, has been enriched by immigrant cuisines" (1926).

The Smith-Hughes Act of 1917 funded home economics education in U.S. high schools, furthering the scientific approach to cooking.

instructor Fannie Farmer exerted an enormous influence on cooking in the United States with the first publication of her *Boston Cooking-School Cook Book* in 1896. She eliminated the inexact system of measurements in traditional recipes, such as a teacupful of sugar or a pinch of salt, and replaced them with a "scientific" approach using exact measurements. This change, adopted by other cookbook publishers, increased the possibility that a cook in an average home kitchen could more accurately replicate a dish.

The development of convenience foods has also played a significant role in the monotony of fare:

> Many of the recipes our mothers and grandmothers loved were product-driven: canned soup casseroles, molded salads, mayonnaise cakes, graham cracker crusts, even chocolate chip cookies. We may scoff at the hokier of these today, but they belong to this century's culinary history and cannot be ignored. Moreover, as a riffle through any regional cookbook quickly proves, they remain popular over much of the country.
>
> (Anderson, 1997, p. 3)

Contributing further to the sameness in American cuisine are the omnipresent franchise restaurants. Be it homey fried chicken or trendy juice bar drinks, such establishments thrive on standardized offerings.

Yet, there have always been Americans interested in authentic ethnic and regional cooking, dating back to Thomas Jefferson, whom Patrick Henry accused of being too "Frenchified" in his food preferences. Duncan Hines, who began his career as a food critic traveling the country in search of fine dining, published *Adventures in Good Eating* in 1936. He was among the first in modern times to encourage diners to try the local specialties, from regional black-bottom pie to ethnic manicotti. He felt it was essential that diners ask about dishes they were unfamiliar with, because much of the pleasure in eating depends on knowledge of how foods are prepared (Hines, 1959).

In recent years there has been a consumer desire—even obsession—to try what is new and different in food. Ethnic cuisines continue to become more popular, especially less familiar kinds, such as Asian Indian and Central American. And regional fare is resurgent. Starting with the Cajun craze begun by Paul Prudhomme in the early 1980s, American cooking has enjoyed a new respect among chefs and diners alike. The foods of the Southwest and California have become common in many areas of the country. Now subregions are emerging, such as the Florida panhandle and coastal South Carolina.

Cultural foods researchers caution that when people explore a new cuisine through restaurants or cookbooks, the foods they encounter are in "attenuated situations, tinged with commercialism [and that] the meanings of the food and their surrounding rituals for

The first drive-through restaurant was a McDonald's that opened in 1948 in San Bernardino, California.

Regional food festivals flourishing throughout the nation are evidence of a growing pride in U.S. foods. From alligator in Florida and garlic in California to zucchini in Ohio, there are celebrations for many American ethnic and regional specialties.

the subcultural groups that consume and produce them are lost" (Brown & Mussell, 1984, p. 4). To a certain degree, this has always been the case in the evolution of American cuisine. Only in ethnic or regional enclaves largely isolated from outside influences do food traditions, and their cultural purposes, remain intact. Otherwise, even significant symbolic food use can lose meaning over time and with exposure to other cultures. For example, a study of Chinese Americans living in California found that while many subjects attempted to balance their meals with hot and cold foods, few were familiar with the yin-yang principles behind the practice (Chau et al., 1990).

In many ways, all U.S. regional cooking is founded on adaptive processes. Even foods usually identified with American cooking, such as hamburgers, hot dogs, and fried chicken, are clearly derived from other cultural fare, yet they are changed through use of native ingredients and local preferences. Cheese melted over burgers on sesame buns, chili con carne poured over frankfurters, and cornmeal-crusted chicken served with cream gravy and buttermilk biscuits are unrecognizable from their origins in Europe and Africa. And while the tamale pie found in Texas and the saimin noodles of Hawaii are not authentic ethnic fare, they are authentic American foods. The trend today in regional cooking is the same as it has always been. As stated by Southwestern chef Mark Miller, regional fare in the United States "memorializes traditional techniques and tastes. It takes folk cooking and uses it as a template, and today's regional chefs create from within that template. And there's lots of room to move around within that" (Belman, 1997). What could be more American?

12

Intercultural Communication in the Foodservice Workplace

The foodservice and hospitality industry is facing new challenges due to increasing pluralism in the workforce. Up until the late 1980s, foodservice employees were predominantly white. Dramatic changes in recent years have reduced this former majority to a minority. African Americans, Asians, and Latinos are disproportionately represented in foodservice compared to their total percentage in the U.S. population. Latinos now follow whites as the largest minority group preparing, serving, and distributing food to the public.

White Americans, however, still fill most management jobs. This mix of supervisors and employees from many ethnic backgrounds presents several impediments to effective management, from minor differences in cultural worldview to serious issues regarding employee recruitment and retention. Communication difficulties can be especially formidable. Latinos often feel that management is cold and insensitive. African Americans sometimes find that supervisors misinterpret their expressive conversational style. Asians may not be comfortable questioning or complaining to their boss and consequently feel taken advantage of when they are assigned extra work (Miller et al., 1998). Middle Easterners are offended by direct criticism (Harris & Moran, 1987). In the foodservice industry, communication is at the crux of conflict resolution and employee morale; it is also essential to successful training programs, particularly those dealing with food safety.

Intercultural Interaction in the Workplace

Communication is so associated with culture that some researchers claim they are inseparable (Ronen, 1986). The ways in which oral, written, or nonverbal messages are conveyed, received, and interpreted are almost wholly dependent on cultural upbringing (Table 12.1). Most of the time, people are on autopilot when conversing with each other, using the symbolic systems learned as children to understand messages (Gudykunst, 1994). Becoming mindful of personal verbal and nonverbal behaviors and then adjusting them as needed to interact with people from different ethnic or religious backgrounds is the foundation of successful intercultural communication.

Intercultural Challenges

Researchers use an iceberg analogy (Figure 12.1) to describe how a person's heritage can impact communication (Kreps & Kunimoto, 1994). Ethnicity, age, and gender are the most visible characteristics that affect dialogue, the so-called "tip" of the iceberg. Beneath the surface, but equally influential, may be degree of acculturation or assimilation, socioeconomic status, health condition, religion, educational background, group membership, sexual orientation, and-or political affiliation.

Most people are comfortable conversing with persons who are culturally similar to them. Communication is sometimes described as an action chain (Hall, 1977), meaning that one phrase or action leads to the next: In the United States a person who extends a hand in greeting expects the other person to take the hand and shake it, or when a person says, "Thank you," a "You're welcome" should follow. Communication is a whole series of unwritten expectations of reciprocity, and such expectations are largely cultural in origin. If a person under-

TABLE 12.1
Getting the Attention of a Waiter or Waitress

Culture	Gesture
Africa	Knock on the table.
Asia/South Pacific	Do *not* point or wave a finger, which may be considered obscene.
Colombia	Put palm on table, then make a scratching motion with index finger.
Europe	Call for attention or clink glass or cup with utensil or ring on finger.
Japan	Extend arm and hand with palm down, then wiggle the fingers.
Latin America/Spain	Extend hand palm down on table, then quickly open and close fingers.
Middle East	Clap hands.
Pakistan/Philippines	Say "pssssssst!"
Singapore/Malaysia	Extend arm and wave hand, palm down with thumb folded across palm.

Source: Adapted from data in R. T. Moran and P. R. Harris, *Managing Cultural Differences* (2nd ed.) (Houston, TX: Gulf, 1987).

FIGURE 12.1

Iceberg Model of Multicultural Influences on Communication.

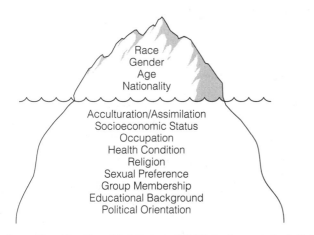

Race
Gender
Age
Nationality

Acculturation/Assimilation
Socioeconomic Status
Occupation
Health Condition
Religion
Sexual Preference
Group Membership
Educational Background
Political Orientation

Source: Adapted from Kreps, G. L. & Kunimoto, E. N. Effective Cummunication in Multicultural Health Care Settings, 6, Sage. Copyright 1994. © Reprinted with permission.

stands the communication action chain and responds as expected, a successful relationship can develop. When a person does not respond as expected, communication can break down and the relationship can deteriorate (Kreps & Kunimoto, 1994).

When meeting a person for the first time, the only information speakers usually have to work from are their own cultural norms. They use them to predict how a person will respond to their words and what conversational approaches are appropriate. They may also use social roles to determine their communication behavior. Furthermore, speakers modify their words and actions as they get to know a person individually, observing personal cues about communication idiosyncrasies that vary from cultural or social customs (Gudykunst & Nishida, 1994). An employee, for example, may make certain assumptions about a supervisor based on ethnicity, gender, or age, and especially occupational status, and then make adaptations. For example, an employee may start out calling his boss "Mrs. Smith" as a sign of respect for her position but use the more informal "Sue" when she requests that he call her by her first name.

Interpersonal relationships between two individuals are based mostly on personal communication preferences; group interactions commonly depend on cultural or social norms. There is a greater possibility for misinterpretations to occur at the cultural or social levels of communication because they are more generalized. As mentioned in Chapter 1, stereotyping occurs if a person overestimates another individual's degree of association with any particular cultural or social group. It is believed that only about one-third of the people from any given group actually behave in ways typified by the group as a whole (Gudykunst & Nishida, 1994). Assumptions about how a person of a different cultural heritage should communicate can elicit certain types of reactions based on norms in that culture: Stereotyping can become a self-fulfilling prophecy. For instance, Asians have a reputation for being restrained in conversation compared to the typical American approach. A manager may respond to more aggressive speakers during a meeting, failing to ask the opinions of a Vietnamese American employee because he interprets her silence as indifference. The Vietnamese American may begin to feel that the supervisor is uninterested in her input, becoming even less likely to offer her viewpoint, reinforcing the manager's perception that Asians are quiet.

The challenge is to increase familiarity with cultural communication behaviors, while remaining aware of personal cues and moving toward an interpersonal relationship as quickly as possible.

Intercultural communication awareness is believed to occur in four stages. The first is unconscious incompetence, when a speaker misunderstands communication behaviors but doesn't even know misinterpretation has occurred; the second stage is conscious incompetence, when a speaker is aware of misunderstandings but makes no effort to correct them. The third stage is conscious competence, when a speaker considers his or her own cultural communication characteristics and makes modifications as needed to prevent misinterpretations. The final stage is unconscious competence, when a speaker is skilled in intercultural communication practices and no longer needs to think about them during conversation (Howell, 1982). Effective intercultural communication begins when the speaker is cognizant of his or her own communication behaviors and is sensitive to misinterpretations that may result from them (Gudykunst & Nishida, 1994).

Intercultural Communication Concepts

Communication uses symbols to represent objects, ideas, or behaviors. Thoughts, emotions, and attitudes are translated into language and nonverbal actions (e.g., gestures, posture, eye contact) to send messages from one person to another. Only the person sending the message knows the exact meaning of the message: The person receiving the message must use what he or she knows about cultural norms, social expectations, and the speaker personally to interpret the message. The two components of the message are the content and the relationship between the speaker and the receiver. Depending on the situation, the content or the relationship may assume greater prominence in interpretation of meaning. Messages that violate cultural expectations may be accurate in content but have a negative impact on the relationship. If the message consistently offends the receiver, the relationship will deteriorate and the message will be disregarded. For instance, repeated memos outlining hand-washing procedures may be totally ignored by Puerto Rican employees. First, the written messages are seen as impersonal, even an insult to the desire for a family-like work environment. Further, the procedures

Only the person sending the message knows the meaning of the message—the recipient must use what he or she knows about cultural and social norms, as well as what is known about the speaker personally, to interpret the message. (© Tom McCarthy/PhotoEdit.)

may be contrary to the hot-cold concept followed by some Latinos that hands cooled by washing cannot touch hot food or surfaces for 1 hour without causing arthritis. Messages that demonstrate respect for the individuality of the receiver are called *personal messages* and improve relationships; those that are disrespectful of individuality are termed *object messages* and often degrade relationships. Communication occurs in a continuum between personal and object messages (Kreps & Kunimoto, 1994).

Verbal messages are most useful for communicating content, while nonverbal messages usually convey information about relationships. If the nonverbal message is consistent with the verbal message, it can build the relationship and help the receiver correctly interpret the meaning intended by the speaker. When the nonverbal message is inconsistent with the verbal message, both the relationship and the content are undermined. Successful communication depends on verbal and nonverbal skills, both of which are significantly impacted by cultural considerations.

Verbal Communication

The abstract nature of language means that it can only be correctly interpreted within context. The cultural aspects of context are so embedded that a speaker often believes they are innate—that is, that all other people must communicate according to the same expectations. Context includes issues common to cultural worldview, such as the role of the individual in a group and perceptions of power, authority, status, and time. Additionally, context in communication also encompasses the significance of affective and physical expression (termed low- or high-context) and level of tolerance for uncertainty and ambiguity (called uncertainty avoidance). Verbal communication occurs within these cultural premises, often operating at an unconscious level in the speaker.

Low- and High-Context Cultures

The context in verbal communication varies culturally. Conversational context can be defined as the affective and physical cues a speaker uses to indicate meaning, such as tone of voice, facial expression, posture, and gestures.

Bureaucrats operate in a low-context setting, using technical words with limited nonverbal communication.

In most western cultures, messages usually concern ideas presented in a logical, linear sequence. The speaker tries to say what is meant through precise wording, and the content of the language is more objective than personal along the continuum of personal and object messages. This communication style is termed low-context, because the actual words are more important than who is receiving the message, how the words are said, or the nonverbal actions that accompany them. Communication in a low-context culture is so dependent on words that the underlying meaning is undecipherable if wording is chosen poorly or deliberately to mislead the recipient. Nearly every American has also experienced the obtuse professional languages of attorneys or scientists who fail to convey their message in common terminology. The Swiss, Germans, and Scandinavians are considered examples of low-context cultures (Hall, 1977).

One area of conflict often found between blacks and whites is due to differences in high- and low-context communication. African Americans tend to be more high-context than white Americans, using cognitive, affective, and physical responses that may appear disruptive or overly emotional to whites (Gilbert & Gay, 1989).

In cultures with a high-context communication style, most of the meaning of a message is found in the context, not in the words. In fact, the wording used may be vague, circuitous, or incomplete. The content of the language is more personal than objective, dependent on the relationship between speaker and listener. Attitudes and feelings are more prominent in the conversation than thoughts. Communication in high-context cultures is analogous to the saying "reading between the lines." Misunderstandings easily occur if either participant is unfamiliar with the meaning of the nonverbal signifiers being used, such as small eye movements or the sounds that are made when in agreement, or disagreement, or when upset. For example, white, majority Americans tend to squirm a bit when uncomfortable with a conversation, while the Japanese will quickly suck in air. High-context cultures are most prevalent among homogeneous populations with a common understanding of the affective and physical expression used

Low-context communication is so dependent on words that the meaning is lost if obtuse language is used. (*Dilbert* **by Scott Adams. © Reprinted with permission of United Media.**)

in sending the message (see the following "Nonverbal Communication" section). Asian, Middle Eastern, and Native American cultures are very high-context. Latino societies are moderately high-context. American culture is thought to be toward the low end, but more middle-context than many European societies.

In low-context cultures, communication is usually explicit, straightforward, and unambiguous. The focus is on the speaker, who uses words to send messages that are often intended to persuade or convince the receiver. In high-context cultures, indirect communication is preferred. Implicit language is used, and many qualifiers are added; nonverbal cues are significant to interpreting the message. The locus of conversation is the receiver; the speaker makes adjustments in consideration of the listener's feelings (Gudykunst & Nishida, 1994). Low-context listeners are often impatient with high-context speakers, wondering when the speaker will get to the point of the conversation. Low-context listeners frequently miss the affective and physical expression in the message. High-context listeners may be confused by low-context speakers because the message contains mostly words or they may be offended by the impersonal, objective emphasis.

Foodservice management tends to be low-context. The dialogue is centered on the supervisor, who delivers a verbal (or written) object message to the employee with little consideration for the nonverbal personal message. The communication is high on content and low on relationship. One example is performance appraisals (see Table 12.2). American managers use direct, objective criticism and praise in their evaluation, frequently presented in written form. Managers in higher-context cultures use indirect, subtle criticism and praise with subjective examples. Connections between the supervisor and the employee may be more important than the content of the appraisal.

One way to patronize a person is to speak in a low-context mode, elaborating beyond what is needed for understanding.

The evaluation is typically verbal and may be directed at a group rather than an individual.

Interactions may range from low- to high-context depending on the situation, regardless of the overall cultural context. A white, American female executive presenting trends in MAP (modified-atmosphere package) spinach sales would be very low-context, while that same woman attempting to get her toddler to eat spinach may be very high-context. In uncomfortable or embarrassing situations a low-context communicator may be very sensitive and indirect. In high-context cultures, direct language is frequently used in intimate relationships. Identification of a culture as either low- or high-context provides a general framework for communication, but the classification may be affected by other situational factors.

Individuals and Groups

The relationship of the individual to the group is determined in part by whether a culture is low- or high-context. In low-context cultures the individual is typically separate from the group and self-realization is an important goal. Self-esteem is dynamic, based on successful mastery or control of a situation. In high-context cultures the individual is usually defined by group association and a person desires oneness with the group, not individuation. A mutual dependency exists and self-esteem is based on how well a person can adjust to a situation (Gudykunst & Nishida, 1994). Individualism is a prominent characteristic in Australia, Canada, Great Britain, New Zealand, the Netherlands, and the United States. Collectivism is especially valued in the nations of Denmark, Ghana, Guatemala, Indonesia, Nigeria, Panama, Peru, El Salvador, Sierra Leone, Taiwan, Thailand, and Venezuela. Such differences can affect job performance. For example, a foodservice manager hires a new immigrant from Egypt for a position in marketing. The manager carefully outlines his expectations for the job, then hands her the company policy manuals. The manager becomes dismayed when he observes her spending her first several days at work "socializing" with other employees. While the manager believes that she should be reading about the organization and learning the functions of her job, the Egyptian believes that the role of a new employee in a company is to be accepted by the group and feels the need to establish relationships before any individual work can be undertaken.

In societies that emphasize individuality a person must communicate to gain acceptance by the group, whether it is the family, the workplace, or the community. Communication is used to establish the self within an individual or group relationship. When meeting someone new, the action chain in the conversation is flexible, with few expectations. The two people may focus on one or the other speaker

Even within low-context cultures, intimate conversations are usually highly contextual; words and phrases may be significantly shortened or abbreviated—just a look may be enough for understanding.

It is evident that the model for food habits using Maslow's Theory of Human Maturation (see Chapter 1) is, in fact, a cultural construct. Self-realization is the pinnacle of development only in cultures that value individuality over the needs of the group.

TABLE 12.2
Cultural Variations: Performance Appraisals

General Dimensions	U.S. (Low-Context)	Saudi Arabia (High-Context)	Japan (High-Context)
Objective	Fairness, employee development	Placement	Direction of company/employee development
Who does appraisal	Supervisors	Manager—may be several layers up—appraiser has to know employee well	Mentor and supervisor; appraiser has to know employee well
Authority of appraiser	Presumed in supervisory role or position	Reputation important (prestige is determined by nationality, age, sex, family, tribe, title, education)	Respect accorded by employee to supervisor or appraiser
	Supervisor takes slight lead	Authority of appraiser important—don't say, "I don't know"	Done co-equally
How often	Once a year or periodically	Once a year	Developmental appraisal once a month
			Evaluation appraisal—after first 12 years
Assumptions	Objective appraiser is fair	Subjective appraiser more important than objective	Objective and subjective important
		Connections are important	Japanese can be trained in anything
Manner of communication and feedback	Criticism direct	Criticisms subtle; older more likely to be direct	Criticisms subtle
	Criticisms may be in writing		Criticisms given verbally
	Objective/authentic	Criticisms not given in writing	Observe formalities
Rebuttals	U.S. will rebutt appraisal	Saudi Arabians will rebutt	Japanese will rarely rebutt
Praise	Given individually	Given individually	Given to entire group
Motivators	Money and position strong motivators	Loyalty to supervisor strong motivator	Internal excellence strong motivator
	Career development		

Source: Harris, P. R. & Moran, R. T. *Managing Cultural Difference, 4th Ed.* Gulf Publishing Company. Copyright 1996. Reprinted with permission, all rights reserved.

and often delve into personal preferences, such as favorite restaurants or sports teams. When group identity is the focus of a society, there is no need for a person to seek acceptance from the group or to communicate individuality. Silence is highly valued. Interactions between strangers tend to be ritualized, and if the action chain is broken, communication cannot continue. The expectation is that each speaker will indicate group affiliation and that such identity conveys all the information that is needed to know that person.

Persons from cultures that emphasize group identity often feel uncomfortable with any communication that recognizes individual performance. Explicit praise or criticism (even bonuses or perquisites based on achievement or position) may be seen as isolating the person from the group. Evaluation and rewards based on group performance are often preferred (Scarborough, 1998).

Uncertainty Avoidance

Related to role of the individual in a group is tolerance for uncertainty and ambiguity. Some groups exhibit great discomfort with what is unknown and different; these are defined as high uncertainty avoidance cultures. People from these groups prefer greater structure and formality and are most comfortable with external supervision. They may become anxious about behavior that deviates from the norm; there is a desire for consensus in high uncertainty avoidance cultures. Argentina, Belgium, Chile, Columbia, Costa Rica, Croatia, Egypt, France, Greece, Guatemala, Israel, Japan, Korea, Mexico, Panama, Peru, Portugal, Turkey, Serbia, and Spain are stronger in uncertainty avoidance than the United States, as are most African and other Asian nations. They typically have a history of central rule and complex laws that regulate individual action on behalf of the group (Gudykunst, 1994; Scarborough, 1998).

Cultures with low or weaker uncertainty avoidance include Canada, Denmark, Great Britain, Hong Kong, India, Indonesia, Jamaica, the Netherlands, the Philippines, Sweden, and the United States. People from these nations are usually curious about the unknown and different. They are more informal, willing to accept dissent within a group, open to change, and mostly internally driven in their jobs.

It is important to distinguish the differences between risk avoidance and uncertainty avoidance. A person from a high uncertainty avoidance culture may be quite willing to take familiar risks or even new risks in order to minimize the ambiguity of a situation. But in general, risks that involve change and difference are difficult for people with strong uncertainty avoidance; this is especially a concern regarding goals or objectives that involve a "stretch" for the employee, with unknown outcomes (Scarborough, 1998). A formal, polite conversational approach, clear delineation of organizational relationships, and consistent expectations enhance intercultural communication for employees from high uncertainty avoidance cultures.

Power, Authority, and Status

The perception of power, or power "distance," can strongly influence communication patterns. In low-context cultures, and where individuality is respected, power or status is usually attributed to the role or job that a person fulfills. Power distance is small. People are seen as equals, differentiated by their accomplishments. It is common for an individual to question directions or instructions; the belief is that a person must understand "why" before a task can be completed. There is often the expectation that employees will be consulted before a major decision is made by management. In many high-context cultures, where group identification is esteemed, superiors are seen as fundamentally different from subordinates. Authority is rarely questioned. Employees expect that management will make decisions without consultation, and deference is accorded superiors. For instance, a white supervisor is planning to expand the menu cycle at his institution, so he meets with his Greek American chef. The supervisor asks the chef how long he expects it will take to develop the specifications for a new item he wants to include in the menu cycle. The chef hedges and ultimately refuses to give him a projection. The supervisor comes from a culture with small power distance, and he sincerely wants the input of the chef for accurate scheduling. Meanwhile the Greek American, who comes from a culture with a larger power distance, cannot understand why the supervisor is asking this question. He is thinking: This guy is the boss—doesn't he know his job? Better not to answer than to risk a wrong response.

Although there is usually some combination of both small and large power distance tendencies in a culture, one is predominant. Some countries with small power distance include Austria, Canada, Denmark, Germany, Great Britain, Ireland, Israel, the Netherlands, New Zealand, Sweden, and the United States. Those with larger power distance perception include most African, Asian, Latino, and Middle Eastern cultures, including (but not exclusively) Egypt, Ethiopia, Ghana, Guatemala, India, Malaysia, Nigeria, Panama, Saudi Arabia, and Venezuela (Gudykunst, 1994; Scarborough, 1998). Employee empowerment, particularly in setting goals and objectives, may be resisted by persons from groups who come from cultures with a larger power distance; persons from groups with a smaller power distance may prefer maximum autonomy and individual responsibility.

Several cultures are gender-oriented as well. In masculine cultures, power is highly valued. Some, such as Germany, Hong Kong, and the United States, are considered masculine due to their

Differences in power distance may explain why some members of an employee team may have difficulties in assuming greater responsibility for performance outcomes.

aggressive, task-oriented, materialistic culture. Others, such as Italy, Japan, Mexico, and the Philippines, are characterized as masculine because sex roles are strongly differentiated. Men are accorded more authority in masculine societies. In more feminine cultures, quality of life is important; men and women share more equally in the power structure. More feminine countries can be task-oriented and materialistic, such as Denmark, the Netherlands, Norway, and Sweden, but hard work and good citizenship are seen as benefiting the whole society, not a hierarchy of superiors within the company or nation. Workplace relationships and an obligation to others are characteristically emphasized. Nearly all other nations combine masculine and feminine power qualities. Strong gender-orientation can cause conflict. An Italian American waiter may have difficulty respecting a female supervisor, and a Dutch chocolate exporter may not understand the competitive tactics practiced by a U.S. importer. Generally, masculine-oriented American managers can communicate more successfully with most ethnic employees by using a less assertive, less autocratic approach that includes compromise and consensus (Scarborough, 1998).

Time Perception

The Inuit conception of time is governed by the tides—one set of tasks is done when the tide is out, another when the tide comes in.

Being "on time," sticking to a schedule, and not "taking too much" of a person's time are valued concepts in America that are unimportant in societies in which the idea of time is less structured. Low-context cultures tend to be monochronistic, meaning that they are interested in completing one thing before progressing to the next. Monochronistic societies are well suited to industrialized accomplishments. Polychronistic societies are often found in high-context cultures. Many tasks may be pursued simultaneously, but not to the exclusion of personal relationships. Courtesy and kindness are more important than deadlines in polychronistic groups (Hall, 1977). Exceptions occur, however. The French have a relatively low-context culture but are polychronistic; the Japanese can become monochronistic when conducting business transactions with Americans.

The Arabs say, *"Bukra insha Allah,"* which means "Tomorrow, if God wills."

To many Chinese the gift of a clock means the same as "I wish you were dead." Each tick is perceived as a reminder of mortality.

People who are single-minded often find working with those performing multiple tasks frustrating. Monochronistic persons may see polychronistic behaviors, such as interrupting a face-to-face conversation for a phone call or being late for a meeting, as rude or contemptuous. Yet no disrespect is intended, nor is it believed that polychronistic persons are less productive than monochronistic people. In fact, "multitasking," the ability to do many things simultaneously, is valued in many businesses today.

Nonverbal Communication

High-context cultures place great emphasis on nonverbal communication in the belief that body language reveals more about what a person is thinking and feeling than words do (Hall, 1977). Yet customs about touching, gestures, eye contact, and spatial relationships vary tremendously among cultures, independent of low- or high-context communication style. As discussed previously, such nonverbal behavior can reinforce the content of the verbal message being sent, or it can contradict the words and confuse the receiver. Successful intercultural communication depends on consistent verbal and nonverbal messages. During personal and group interactions, persons move together in a synchronized manner. Barely detectable motions, such as the tilt of the head or the blink of an eye, are imitated when people are in synch and communicating effectively. The ways in which a person moves, however, are usually cultural and often unconscious. Although body language is closely linked to ethnicity, most people believe that the way they move through the world is universal. Misinterpretations in the subtleties of nonverbal communication are common and often inadvertent. More than 7,000 different gestures have been identified (Axtell, 1991), and meaning is easily misunderstood when awareness of differences is limited.

Touching

Touching includes handshakes, hugging, kissing, placing a hand on the arm or shoulder, and even unintentional bumping. In China, for example, touching between strangers, even handshaking if one person is male and the other female, is uncommon in public. Orthodox Jewish men and women are prohibited from touching unless they are relatives or are married. To Latinos, touching is an expected and necessary element of every relationship. The *abrazo,* a hug with mutual back patting, is a common greeting. Touching norms frequently vary according to attributes like gender, age, or even physical condition. In the United States, it is acceptable for an adult to pat the head of a child, but questionable with another adult. Women may kiss each other, men and women may kiss, but men may not publicly kiss other men. It is admirable to take the arm of an elderly person crossing the street, but rude to do so for a healthy young adult.

Cultures in which touching is mostly avoided include those of the United States, Canada, Great Britain, Scandinavia, Germany, the Balkans, Japan, and Korea. Those in which touching is expected include the Middle East and Greece, Latin America, Italy, Spain, Portugal, and Russia. Cultures that fall in between are those of China, France, Ireland, and India (Axtell, 1991), as well as those in Africa,

It is an unwritten law in Great Britain that no one may touch the Queen in public.

Anthropologists speculate that the handshake, the hug, and bow with hands pressed together all originated to demonstrate that a person was not carrying weapons.

Russians begin with a handshake and move into a "bear hug" when meeting friends and strangers.

In Japan the small bow used in greetings and departures is a sign of respect and humility. The inferior person in the relationship always bows lower and longer than the person in the superior position.

Touching norms frequently vary according to attributes such as gender, age, or physical condition. (© Michael Newman/PhotoEdit.)

Many Asians completely avoid touching strangers, even in transitory interactions, such as returning change after a purchase. This can be offensive to persons who consider physical contact a sign of acceptance, such as African Americans and Latinos.

Some East African tribes spit at each others' feet in greeting to prevent witchcraft.

Kissing may have originated when mothers orally passed chewed solid food to their infants during weaning.

Southeast Asia, and the Pacific Islands. Foodservice workers should take careful note of cultural touching behaviors. Vigorous handshaking is often considered aggressive behavior and a reassuring hand on the shoulder may be insulting. Of special mention are attitudes about the head. Many cultures consider the head sacred, and an absent-minded pat or playful cuff to the chin may be exceptionally offensive. Conversely, persons from cultures in which frequent touching is the norm may be unaware of legal issues regarding inappropriate touching in the United States, and of potential foodservice sanitation issues.

Gesture, Facial Expression, and Posture

Gestures include overt movements like waving, signaling, or standing to indicate respect when a person enters the room, as well as more indirect motions like handing an item to a person or nodding the head in acknowledgment. Facial expression includes deliberate looks of attention or questioning and unintentional wincing or grimacing. Even smiling has specific cultural connotations.

Confusion occurs when movements have significantly different meanings to different people. Crossed arms are often interpreted as a sign of hostility in the United States, yet do not have similar negative associations in the Middle East, where it is a common stance while talking. The thumbs-up gesture is obscene in Afghanistan, Australia, Nigeria, and many Middle Eastern nations. The crooked-finger motion used in the United States to beckon someone is considered lewd in Japan; is used to call animals in Croatia, Malaysia, Serbia, and Vietnam; and summons prostitutes in Australia and Indonesia. To many Southeast Asians, it is an insolent or threatening gesture (Dresser, 1996).

Asians find it difficult to directly disagree with a speaker and may tilt their chins quickly upward to indicate "no" in what appears to Americans to be an affirmative nod. Some Asian Indians, Greeks, Turks, and Iranians shake their heads back and forth to show agreement and nod up and down to express disagreement. Puerto Ricans may smile in conjunction with other facial expressions to mean "please," "thank you," "excuse me," or other phrases. The Vietnamese may smile when displeased, and in India, smiles are used only between intimates. An Asian Indian employee may not know what to make of a manager who smiles in a friendly fashion.

Good posture is an important sign of respect in nearly all cultures. Slouching or putting one's feet up on the desk are generally recognized as impolite. In many societies the feet are considered the lowest and dirtiest part of the body, so it is rude to point the toe at a person when one's legs are crossed or to show the soles of one's shoes.

Eye Contact

The subtlest nonverbal movements involve the eyes. Rules regarding eye contact are usually complex, varying according to issues such as social status, gender, and distance apart. White, majority Americans consider eye contact indicative of honesty and openness, yet staring is thought rude. To Germans, direct eye contact is an indication of attentiveness. African Americans may be uncomfortable with prolonged eye contact but may also find rapid aversion insulting. In general, blacks tend to look at a person's eyes when speaking and look away when listening. To Filipinos, direct eye contact is an expression of sexual interest or aggression. Among Native Americans, direct eye contact is considered rude, and averted eyes do not necessarily reflect disinterest. When Asians and Latinos avoid eye contact, it is a sign of respect. Middle Easterners believe that the minute motions of the eyes and pupil are the most reliable indication of how a person is reacting in any situation.

Special eye contact taboos involve what is known as the *evil eye*. It is widely believed in parts of Africa, Asia, Europe, Greece and the Middle East, India, Latin America, and parts of the United States that an individual who stares (especially with envy) can project harm on another person, even if the gaze is unintentional. Children are believed particularly vulnerable to the evil eye, resulting in colic,

The one-finger salute is considered an insult in many cultures. This gesture dates back to Roman times, when it was called *digitus impudicus,* or the "impudent finger."

Koreans say, "A man who smiles a lot is not a real man."

The Japanese demonstrate attentiveness by closing their eyes and nodding.

Other names for the evil eye include *the bad eye, the look, the narrow eye,* and *the wounding eye.* Those who are victims have been *blinked, eye bitten, forelooked,* or *overlooked.*

Fear of the evil eye is mentioned in Talmudic writings, the Bible, and the Koran.

crying, hiccups, cramps, convulsions, and seizures. Among adults the evil eye can cause headache, malaise, complications in pregnancy and childbirth, impotence and sterility in men, and insanity (Hand, 1980).

Spatial Relationships

Each person defines his or her own "space"—the surrounding area that is reserved for the individual. Acute discomfort can occur when another person stands or sits within the space identified as inviolate. Middle Easterners prefer to be no more than 2 feet from whomever they are communicating with so that they can observe their eyes. Latinos enjoy personal closeness with friends and acquaintances. African Americans are likely to be offended if a person moves back or tries to increase the distance between them. Intercultural communication is most successful when spatial preferences are flexible.

In addition to distance, the way a person is positioned affects communication in some cultures. It is considered rude in Samoan and Tongan societies, for instance, to speak to a person unless the parties are positioned at equal levels, for example, both sitting or both standing.

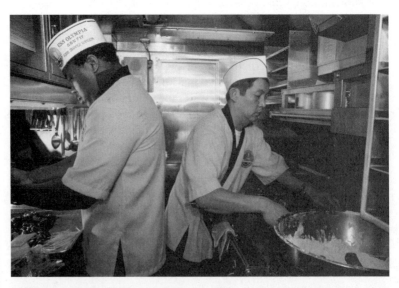

Different cultural expectations regarding nonverbal behaviors, such as eye contact and spatial preferences, can lead to misunderstandings in the workplace.

Practically Speaking: Intercultural Communication in the Workplace

Reading about culturally based communication differences is an individual, intellectual undertaking. Actually applying intercultural communication concepts in the workplace is much more challenging. Successful face-to-face interactions require understanding cultural communication expectations and being familiar with the idiosyncratic style of the other person. Often there is contradictory information to assimilate. The Japanese, for example, come from a culture that is male-dominated, assertive, and achievement-oriented, yet is also high in uncertainty avoidance, emphasizing consensus and ritualistic communication practices. Should an explicit or implicit approach be used when speaking with someone of Japanese heritage? Clearly, much depends on the circumstances surrounding the conversation and the particular people involved.

Such complexities are magnified in the multicultural group dynamics found in many foodservice organizations. Numerous books and articles provide detailed advice on managing pluralism in the workplace. In this section a limited overview of intercultural communication applications is presented, with a special focus on management strategies and training programs.

One researcher reports that the use of cultural food potlucks among hospital staff members has facilitated understanding between employees of diverse backgrounds (Burner et al., 1990).

Management Strategies

Supportive Workplace Environment

There are several steps managers can take to enhance effective intercultural communication in the foodservice setting (Harris & Moran, 1987; Usunier, 1993; Blank & Slipp, 1998; Costa, 1998; Hemphill & Haines, 1998; Miller et al., 1998):

1. *Get to know all employees.* What is their heritage? Where are they from? How long have they been in the United States? What holidays do they observe? Ask questions with interest, face to face, and at the beginning of conversations. A few cultures, such as many Native American groups, may find direct inquiries about personal matters intrusive. Other sources, such as job application forms or personnel records, may provide some information in these situations. Most cultural groups, however, will welcome polite questions about family and background. Avoid interrogations.

2. *Learn about general differences in communication styles* (see Table 12.3). Listen carefully, and proceed cautiously and respectfully whenever there is any uncertainty about conversational patterns.

3. *Understand employees' expectations about their relationship with management.* Many Latinos prefer a work environment that

is an extension of their families, with a supervisor who is warm, caring, and willing to give advice in personal matters. Latinos sometimes feel that they are inaccurately stereotyped as "lazy" and that managers have low expectations for them. Asians often assume that a manager is an expert in the field, someone who has solutions to problems. Asians may also expect managers to provide authoritative direction in a formal manner and may be unwilling to ask for clarication when questions arise. African Americans sometimes experience difficulties in proving competency in the workplace and may feel that they are oversupervised or undersupervised (Blank & Slipp, 1994). Many blacks prefer a direct, task-oriented approach that allows the individual to accomplish an assignment without micromanagement. Mutual respect is essential. People from the Middle East respect the powerful position of superiors and may become suspicious of managers who delegate their authority. At the same time, they assume personal responsibility and expect individual recognition for their job performance. Tactful, implicit direction is preferred.

4. *Treat all employees equitably and consistently, but do not treat them all the same.* Acknowledge differences in communication context, the role of the individual, uncertainty avoidance, power distance, and nonverbal practices. Try to meet the needs of each employee or group regarding these differences. An employee from India may work well independently with little supervision, while someone from France may prefer a more structured environment. A person from Puerto Rico may appreciate a hug in greeting and departing, whereas a Korean would be deeply offended by any form of touching.

5. *Encourage discussion of cultural differences and similarities that promotes understanding.* Do not single out a specific group when gathering information informally, in employee questionnaires, or in training sessions, which can be alienating and divisive.

6. *Provide diverse opportunities for employees to contribute to the organization.* Do not expect that everyone will verbally express their opinions during meetings or that individual recognition is desired. Some employees will provide input most effectively in one-on-one conversations or in writing. Others may be most productive when group feedback is requested.

7. *Do not tolerate discrimination or harassment in the workplace.* Know company policies and enforce them promptly and uniformly. Watch for negative remarks based on cultural background, race, or religion, which can be especially damaging to the workplace environment. Counsel employees who engage in stereotypical commentary that such behavior adversely impacts morale and is not acceptable.

8. *Finally, establish relationships.* Whenever possible, know employees individually, not as a group, and acknowledge each

employee as a composite of cultural upbringing, life experience, and personal preferences.

Intercultural Communication Skills

Beyond a supportive environment, managers can practice intercultural communication skills that increase employee morale and reduce conflict resulting from culturally based misunderstandings.

Name Traditions   First, determine how employees prefer to be addressed. White, majority Americans are among the most informal worldwide, frequently calling strangers and acquaintances by their given names. Nearly all other cultures expect a more respectful approach. This can include the use of title or prefixes (Mr., Mrs., Miss, Ms., Dr., Sir, Madam, etc.), use of surname, and proper pronunciation. Never use "Dear," "Honey," "Sweetie," "Fella," "Son," or other endearments or pejorative terms in place of proper names.

Name order is often different than the American pattern of title, given name, middle name, and surname. In many Latin American countries a married woman uses her given name and her maiden surname, followed by *de* (of) and her husband's family surname. Children typically use their given name, their father's surname, then their mother's family surname also. This causes confusion, because while most Latino men prefer to be addressed by their father's family surname, it is often the name that sequentially is placed on the "middle name" line of forms. Persons reading the form often assume the mother's family surname is a Latino's last name (Dresser, 1996).

Middle Easterners use their title, given name, and surname. They may also use *bin* (for men) or *bint* (for women) meaning "of" a place or "son/daughter of." It is not to be confused with the given name Ben (although it is pronounced similarly). If the grandparent of a Middle Easterner is well known, his or her last name may be added to the name order, following the surname, with another *bin.* The Vietnamese, Mein, Hmong, and Cambodians place the surname first, followed by the given name (although many make the switch to the American name order with acculturation). The Chinese and Koreans use a similar system, although they also include a generational name following the family name and before the given name (the generational name is sometimes hyphenated with the given name or the two names are run together). Married women in China and Korea do not take their husband's surname. In Japan the surname is followed by *san,* meaning Mr. or Ms. Given names are only used among close friends and intimates. Hindus in India do not traditionally use surnames. A man goes by his given name, preceded by the initial of his father's given name. A woman follows the same pattern, using her father's initial until marriage, at which time she uses her given name, followed by her husband's given name. Muslims in India use the Middle Eastern order, and Christian Indians use the American pattern

The given name Benjamin is derived from Middle Eastern tradition. It means "son of Jamin."

TABLE 12.3
Communication Style Differences

Native Americans	Asians	Latinos
Speak slowly and softly	Speak softly	Speak softly: may perceive normal white voice as yelling
Indirect gaze when speaking and listening	Avert eyes as sign of respect	Avert eyes as sign of respect
Seldom make responses to indicate listening or offer encouragement to continue, rarely interject	Rules similar to Native Americans'	Rules similar to Native Americans'
Delayed auditory (silence valued)	Mild delay (silence valued)	Mild delay
Expression restrained	Polite, restrained; articulation of feelings considered immature	Men restrained, women expressive
Prefer direct approach	Indirect approach: may appear indifferent	Indirect approach
Rarely ask questions; yes/no responses considered complete	Rarely ask questions	Will ask questions when encouraged
Smile, handshake (*not* vigorous) customary greeting	Touching between strangers inappropriate	Shake hands, embrace, kiss cheeks, pat backs; sit and stand closer

(Morrison, et al., 1994). There are numerous other name traditions and preferences of address. When in doubt, it is best to ask.

Appropriate Language Use unambiguous language when working with employees who are limited in English. Choose common terms (not necessarily simple words), avoiding those with multiple meanings, such as "to address," which may mean to talk to someone, to give a speech, to send an item, or to consider an issue. Vague verbs, such as "go," "get," "make," and "do," may cause confusion. Use specific verbs, such as "purchase," "retrieve," "complete," or "prepare" when directing employees.

Slang and idioms may have no meaning in another culture. Many new English speakers interpret words literally. "How's it going?" makes no sense if one doesn't understand the meaning of "it" (Dresser, 1996). Sports analogies, including "score" and "strike out," are indecipherable if the game is unfamiliar. Phrases that suggest a mental picture, such as "run that by me" or "easy as pie" or "dodge a bullet," are barriers to comprehension (Harris & Moran, 1987). Some persons with limited English skills are embarrassed to admit that they do not understand what is being said or to ask that something be repeated. When comprehension is critical, respectfully request

TABLE 12.3
Communication Style Differences—continued

Middle Easterners	Whites	African Americans
Speak softly	Speak loudly, fast; control of listener	Speak fast; with affect and rhythm
Direct gaze, man to man and woman to woman, but woman may avert eyes with man	Eye contact when speaking and listening; staring rude	Direct eye contact when speaking (may avert if prolonged), look away when listening
Facial gestures responsive	Head nodding, murmuring	Interject (turn taking) often
Mild delay	Quick response	Quicker response
Very expressive, emotional	Task-oriented, focused	Very expressive, demonstrative
Indirect approach	Direct approach, minimal small talk	Respectful, direct approach
Will ask polite questions	Ask direct questions	Assertive questioning
Numerous greeting rituals, mild handshake; sit or stand very close, frequent touching (but no backslapping), use hands while speaking	Firm handshake; smile greeting; moderate touching (shoulder patting, backslapping)	Firm handshake, smile, hugging, kissing greeting; reluctance to touch may be interpreted as personal rejection

Source: Adapted from Sue, D. W. & Sue, D. Counseling the Culturally Different: Theory and Practice (2nd Ed.). John Wiley & Sons. Copyright 1990. © Reprinted with permission.

employees to repeat instructions in their own words, or ask that they demonstrate how to use equipment, so that misunderstandings can be corrected.

Avoid asking questions that can be answered with a simple "yes" or "no." For example, "Do you understand?" will almost always prompt a positive response in supervisor–employee conversations, regardless of comprehension level. It is better to ask leading questions, for example, "What confuses you?" or "Tell me what you don't understand" (Dresser, 1996). In some Asian cultures, it is impossible to say "no" to a request. The Japanese, for instance, have developed many ways to avoid a negative response, such as answering "maybe," countering or criticizing the question, issuing an apology, silence, or leaving the room (Usunier, 1993).

The direct, explicit communication style of white, majority Americans is predicated on the assumption that each person is saying what he or she means. This can cause difficulties when conversing with persons for whom negotiation is standard practice. For example, a manager offers coffee and cookies to a Persian employee. She refuses, so he sits down and begins the discussion. The employee is upset, because she was being polite and had expected the supervisor to ask again, then insist that she have something to eat (Dresser, 1996).

Typically Americans not only believe what is said initially; they also consider answers absolute. In some cultures, it is acceptable to make a commitment, then decide later to change the terms of the agreement or cancel altogether. People from these groups assume that one cannot predict intervening events or future needs. Further, there can be differences in what is accepted as "truth." In the United States, truth is considered objective, supported by immutable facts. In many other cultures, truth is subjective, often based on emotions (Harris & Moran, 1987; Morrison et al., 1994). A Filipino American may report to his manager that his assignment is behind schedule. The manager looks at the data and realizes that the job will probably be completed early. When he asks the employee about the discrepancy, he replies that he is feeling frustrated today and that he hasn't made much progress on the task during the past few hours. Understanding that the definitions of truth vary culturally can help diffuse communication discord.

Finally, managers in the bilingual workplace should learn a few words or phrases in the foreign language that is spoken by employees. This demonstrates respect for the other culture and can enhance overall communication (Morrison et al., 1998).

Praise and Criticism   In the United States, praise is considered motivational. A compliment on a job well done improves morale and encourages productivity. Forms of praise are not universal, however. For instance, a kitchen supervisor has a new employee who has recently arrived from Ethiopia. She is pleased with how quickly the new employee is learning the job, and she compliments him on how beautiful the carrot and jicama julienne looks. The employee is offended. He is disturbed that the supervisor would comment on the food, but not compliment his skills, which he takes as a personal affront. The relationship of the employee to the supervisor is more important to him than the tangible outcomes of his job. A similar situation can occur when a person is promoted from within a peer group. A Guatemalan employee may be unhappy when asked to assume supervision of co-workers, because she values the social relationships more than increased pay or the status of a management position. Conflicts can arise when such promotions are made without consideration of employee desires about personal relationships with the group.

In many Asian cultures, personal praise in front of a group is embarrassing. First, it may be considered inappropriate to compliment the accomplishments of an individual instead of those of the group. Second, being singled out for praise may be considered a subtle form of criticism, suggesting that the employee was not performing the job well before (Dresser, 1996).

Criticism of persons from high-context cultures should always be tactful and indirect. Explicit reproach is considered exceptionally offensive and can damage future communication. In most cultures other than those of the United States and northern European nations, both praise and criticism are best presented personally, in private. Written appraisals are usually considered disrespectful of the relationship between the manager and employee.

Conflict Conflict is unavoidable in most relationships. It can be due to differences in goals or practices (*instrumental* conflict) or to emotional tension (*expressive* conflict). While most cultural groups describe conflict as negative, it is how conflict is confronted and resolved that affects relationships and the workplace environment, for better or for worse (Olsen, 1978; Gudykunst, 1994).

The Chinese "swallow" bitterness, frustration, hostility, and loss to avoid conflict and increase harmony (Moran & Harris, 1982).

Communication style reflects how conflict is managed in each culture. White, majority Americans typically prefer direct, restrained (low-context) discussion. The problem is usually considered instrumental in source. It is separate from the person involved; thus people can remain on friendly terms after there is agreement on a solution. There may be a need, however, to prove a point or make judgments about right or wrong in the process. The other person involved is frequently considered at fault for any acrimony.

In contrast, African Americans use an expressive, forceful approach (high-context). Voices are raised and opinions are freely stated: each person wants to hear what the other one thinks and feels. Unlike white Americans, blacks take personal responsibility for their emotions. They do not usually blame another person for their own anger during an argument (Kochman, 1983).

When the good of the group outweighs that of the individual in a culture, conflict is usually considered expressive and is rarely separated from the person involved. When disputes arise, the whole relationship is at stake. Latinos, people from the Middle East, and most Asians prefer avoiding conflict rather than confronting it. If problems reach the point where they must be discussed, the priority is preservation of the relationship. Indirect approaches to resolution are used, emphasizing kindness, courtesy, and obligation. Compromise is accepted, so that neither person loses status or position (Harris & Moran, 1987).

There are three steps to take in managing intercultural conflict (adapted from Harris & Moran, 1987):

1. *Describe the problem.* Each person may view a dispute differently, or, in some cases, what is a problem for one person may not be a problem for another. For example, a manager from a low-context culture thinks of lunch as a 60-minute break from work. Employees from a high-context culture view lunch as an opportunity to build the relationships necessary for productivity. They are frequently late returning from lunch. This is a problem from the

perspective of the manager, but not from the perspective of the employees (Moran & Harris, 1982).

2. *Analyze underlying values and assumptions.* It is important to understand the cultural factors involved in the dispute. The manager is monochronistic and single-minded. He values promptness and measurable achievements by individuals. He assumes that employees are abusing the 1-hour limit for personal socializing. He is offended that they are so disrespectful of his schedule. The employees are polychronistic, used to multitasking. Not only are they eating lunch, but they are also strengthening the bonds of their workplace team. The intangible benefits of relationships are more important than personal accomplishment. They assume that the manager approves of this process because it results in increased group productivity.

The manager initially blamed the employees for tardiness. After describing and analyzing the problem, he realized that there were two viewpoints of the situation and that a solution required flexibility on his part. The employees learned that the manager was not upset when they were occasionally late getting back from lunch, but that consistent tardiness was insulting. They were willing to make changes in order to repair their damaged relationship with him.

3. *Practice intercultural problem solving.* This is often the most difficult step due to differences in communication styles. When working with persons from a high-context culture, a person from a lower-context culture must first decide if a solution is worth pursuing. While confrontation of an issue is encouraged in low-context cultures, persons from high-context cultures prefer avoidance. If confrontation is necessary, it is helpful to do it in private (to avoid embarrassing the other person in public), when emotions have subsided, and when each person has time to discuss it. Be cooperative, suggesting that it is a mutual problem, instead of being competitive, attempting to control or dominate the conversation. Be empathetic to the other person's viewpoint, and build on similarities in perspective. Some disputes are best handled by an impartial mediator willing to work toward a solution that benefits both parties. Acknowledge that reconciliation and restoration of harmony may be the primary goals of a person from a high-context culture, and, conversely, attaining these objectives may not appease a person from a low-context culture if the substantive issues are ignored. A collaborative approach, working toward solutions that meet the needs and concerns of each person, is the most satisfactory intercultural communication style in conflict situations.

The manager with the long lunch employees set up a meeting. He served lunch, encouraged socializing, then leisurely summarized his viewpoint of the problem. He carefully avoided making accusations or placing blame, and asked for suggestions on what they could do together to resolve the issue. After much discussion, it was mutually decided that a 60-minute break would be observed Mondays through Thursdays, but that Friday lunches would be unstructured, taken whenever the employees wanted and for up to 1½ hours. Both the manager and employees recognized the value in meeting each other's needs.

Training Programs

Intercultural Training Needs

Successful training strategies for pluralistic groups are as dependent on intercultural communication as is effective management. To date, most organizations have focused on cultural awareness issues in their training programs dealing with pluralism. While awareness can contribute to better employee morale and a more supportive workplace environment, it is not enough to address recruitment, retention, and productivity issues (Gardenswartz & Rowe, 1998).

Further, so-called diversity training that promotes awareness has a reputation for failure. Inexperienced trainers and trainers with a hostile agenda have contributed to ineffectiveness; trainings that blamed certain groups for discrimination (particularly white males) or forced participants to reveal personal biases, then chided them for political incorrectness, resulted in disturbed, distrustful employees. So many people have negative associations with the phrase *diversity* that it is best to avoid calling any intercultural training programs by that title (Hemphill & Haines, 1998).

Researchers suggest that within each organization there is a need for staff development in intercultural communication skills, particularly in the areas of problem-solving and conflict resolution (Gardenswartz & Rowe, 1998). In addition, foodservice supervisors may require training in culturally sensitive hiring interviews, performance reviews, mentoring, and meeting management. Externally, foodservice employees can benefit from learning the intercultural communication skills necessary in successful cross-cultural sales, marketing, and customer service.

Many white men feel that they are victims of bias and bigotry in today's pluralistic workplace. They may hesitate to express opinions for fear that they are assumed to be racists (Blank & Slipp, 1994).

Culturally Sensitive Training Program Development

After a need for intercultural training is determined, program development can commence. Identification of the target audience in training efforts is an important first step in program planning. Knowing the cultural heritage of participants is imperative. Primary language should be identified, as well as gender, average age, socioeconomic

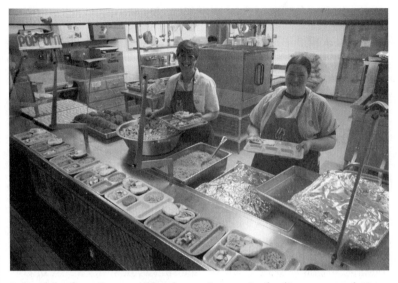

School foodservice provides for an increasingly diverse population. Intercultural communication skills between employees and students are important.

status, educational attainment, religious affiliation, and other "iceberg" factors in intercultural communication. Assessment of acculturation or bicultural adaptation is also useful. The more culturally homogeneous the participants, the easier it is to design a culturally appropriate program (Rabin, 1994). In some cases a larger, pluralistic audience can be stratified into smaller, segmented target groups for part of the training to take advantage of culturally specific educational materials.

The next step in intercultural program planning is to define goals and objectives that are clear and realistic within the cultural context of the target audience. Most trainers start with general goals for a group of participants, then modify and refine objectives as more information about the target audience is gathered. Ongoing feedback from company managers and involving employees in program planning are some of the best methods to determine the cultural orientation of participants. The role that community leaders or spokespersons can play in the planning process should not be overlooked. Seeking the respect, trust, and endorsement of influential persons within the target audience community for a particular training can open intercultural communication channels otherwise limited to the formal interactions reserved for strangers (Randall-David, 1989; Rabin, 1994).

After establishing goals for the program, appropriate materials must be chosen or developed to convey the training message. This is most effective when done simultaneously with planning learning activities and exercises. The training message must satisfy each individual's need to gain knowledge or offer a solution to a perceived problem before it is worth a person's time to process the information (Brown & Einsiedel, 1990). Messages should be as direct and explicit as allowed within cultural norms (Randall-David, 1989). The language relevant to the group as a whole should be used in the training, with supplementary materials in additional languages as needed (direct translation of existing materials should be avoided, however, to prevent inappropriate phrasing and terminology). Common words used by the target audience are effective, although it is important that they are not used in a way that is insincere or condescending. Written materials should be brief and prepared at the reading level of the training participants.

Marketing experts recognize that many cultural groups have high-context communicators who have greater abilities than the white American majority culture to send and receive messages through non-verbal modes (Rabin, 1994). Body language must be culturally congruent with the verbal message for successful communication to occur. The use of pictures, cartoons, and photographic images can symbolically enhance content meaning of a message in groups from high-context cultures, as well as aid participants with limited English language skills or reading abilities. Education messages are most effective when they are more personal than objective; the emotional dimension is as important as the content. Many researchers recommend the universally accepted format of storytelling to deliver the message (Esquivel & Keitel, 1990; Rabin, 1994). Stories can transcend many cultural boundaries; if a message is targeted toward one cultural group yet applicable to other participants, a spokesperson identified with the targeted audience may have broader appeal when using a narrative approach.

In conjunction with training material selection or development, learning activities and exercises should be planned for the program. The "action-learning" approach, based on "learning by doing," works well with adult participants (Harris & Moran, 1987). It gives responsibility for learning to the employee and uses a variety of teaching techniques. Action-learning in culturally sensitive training programs is:

1. *Situational.* Applies specifically to the workplace and is most effective with team or unit groups. It provides opportunities to practice new skills and internalize new information. One way to practice is role playing, in which a person plays himself or takes on the role of someone from another culture, then acts out incidents specific to the organization. In foodservice, such role playing might include manager–employee, employee–employee, or employee–client (e.g. student, hospital patient) intercultural communication episodes.

More than 20 percent of the U.S. population is considered functionally illiterate, reading below an eighth-grade level.

Marketing experts identify food habits as being among the strongest aspects of cultural identity.

2. *Experiential.* Data collected during the training draw on participant experience. It can be elicited directly from what occurs in program activities or from previous experience, but it should be voluntary, not mandatory (no one should be pressured into revealing personal information). Ample time is provided for sharing and examining what is learned. Self-awareness exercises are particularly useful.

3. *Plural.* Action-learning is concerned with both content and context; ideas and feelings are balanced. Simulation exercises that involve a task or game dependent on group dynamics, followed by debriefing and evaluation, are an example. Ideally the simulation mirrors organizational experiences, such as designing a menu for a cultural group not represented at the training or a chef–waiter/waitress–client simulation in which each person is provided with different communication rules, then asked to order, "prepare," and serve a meal.

4. *Problem-orientation.* Learning activities are focused on personal, group, and organizational problem-solving approaches, with opportunity to practice skills. Written, videotaped, or dramatized case studies work well when followed with group analysis. The emphasis should be on issues and concerns of persons in the organization, especially areas of existing or potential conflict (be certain that the identity of individuals or groups is disguised).

5. *Systematic.* The training effort does not exist in a vacuum. Employees in the program have opportunities for career growth and personal development in an organization that values both. Systems changes support intercultural training messages about new hires, performance reviews, mentoring, and promotions (Gardenswartz & Rowe, 1998).

6. *Personalized.* Learning needs and expectations of each participant are considered. Performance standards are set by each employee through goals and objectives, and self-assessment is encouraged. Followup activities are especially amenable to personalization. Computer-aided training on interactive programs allows employees to practice intercultural communication skills on a machine instead of on co-workers. While many people enjoy this type of one-on-one learning, it can be especially effective for persons with limited English proficiency or low literacy.

Training program assessment should include several forms of evaluation. Process evaluation, such as asking for employee input on session goals and objectives, can help keep track of progress throughout the duration of the program. It can identify group issues and concerns that may present obstacles to dissemination of the training message. Participant feedback and self-assessment are useful, as are pre/post tests administered immediately before and after the training. Summative evaluation is used after completion of the effort to assess program results. Followup questionnaires to participants and surveys of peers or supervisors are two methods of obtaining data (such methods are best repeated at 1-month, 6-month, and 1-year intervals to track short-term versus long-term change). As in most educational efforts, intercultural knowledge, awareness, and attitudes are relatively easy to ascertain. Changes in communication skills and behavior are much more difficult to verify. Intercultural communication competency takes time and practice.

Focus on Food Safety

It is estimated that there are between 24 and 81 million cases of foodborne illnesses annually in the United States, resulting in approximately 10,000 deaths. Nearly 80 percent of reported cases are traced to foodservice operations, defined as anyone preparing, serving, or dispensing food to the public—from restaurants, hotels, cafeterias, and grocery stores to correctional institutions, day care centers, country clubs, and festival vendors (Soukup, 1996). Human error is considered the leading cause of outbreaks (Costa, 1998).

Cultural background is one of many factors contributing to human error in foodservice organizations. Traditional preparation practices, beliefs and attitudes about food safety, and personal experience at home are significant factors in employee behavior that increases risk of microbial contamination or growth.

Some traditional customs are beneficial. For example, many cultural groups worldwide do not have access to food storage technology. Only enough food for a single meal is prepared and eaten. In other regions, people eat little raw food, with most dishes preferred thoroughly cooked and steaming hot (Foster & Käferstein, 1985). Some cuisines feature extensive spicing, which is believed to inhibit food spoilage, even when the food is stored at ambient temperatures for short periods (Billing & Sherman, 1998). Difficulties can arise, however, when practices like these are transferred to the foodservice setting. Immigrants to the United States may be inexperienced in preparing large volumes of food that require proper refrigeration (using small containers or frequent stirring of large quantities) to ensure adequate chilling throughout. They may not know that cooked foods can become contaminated by contact with raw items or insects. They may never have experienced any problems with saving spicy leftovers at room temperature.

Further, some cultural groups have preparation practices that can be harmful. A few cultural groups favor undercooked foods, or food aged with minimal preservation techniques applied. Raw beef and pork is often eaten in central Europe, in the dish called *steak Tartar,* for instance, and in certain sausages. The Inuits sometimes butcher seal meat on the ground, then bury it in plastic bags to ferment.

In Southeast Asia, large amounts of rice are often precooked, then stored at room temperature for use during the day. Some Asians still prefer this method in the United States, because refrigeration changes the texture of the rice.

Some Vietnamese and other immigrants believe that refrigeration is necessary only if the food is not fresh.

Alaska Natives have the highest rate of botulism poisoning in the world, mostly due to meat preparation techniques (Segal, 1992).

Items considered contaminants in the United States are often considered edible in other cultures, such as clay (some Africans), ashes (many Native Americans), even cockroaches (some native Australians and people from China, South America, and Louisiana).

Food safety experts report anecdotally that some group practices that appear dangerous do not have any adverse affects on the population, such as deer meat air-dried without preservatives by Native Americans or sandwiches that sit for many hours in the sun while Mexican farmworkers toil in fields. It is hypothesized that people may develop a tolerance for some microorganisms through repeated exposure.

Over 25 percent of participants in one survey did not use detergent or bleach to clean cutting boards after cutting raw meat or poultry (Klontz et al., 1995).

"Behavior scientists agree . . . human beings are not 'empty vessels' into which 'correct information' can simply be poured, which in turn, will eliminate undesirable customs" (Foster & Käferstein, 1985).

Hygiene also varies culturally. In areas with contaminated water, washing hands or food items and cleaning work surfaces can be dangerous practices. Cleanliness may not be directly associated with food safety. In some Latino cultures, health concerns about sudden changes in hot and cold temperatures may lead to hand-washing taboos (Foster & Käferstein, 1985). Many immigrant groups in the United States have poor access to health care, and hygiene is of special concern when ill or infected employees are handling food (Costa, 1998).

Conventionally it is thought that persons who attain educational levels above high school are more likely to engage in health-promoting activities than are persons with only a high school diploma or less. Recent research specifically measuring food safety behaviors has reported contradictory data (Klontz et al., 1995). Persons who continued their education beyond high school were more likely to eat foods with uncooked eggs (e.g., cookie dough, frosting, Caesar salad dressing, homemade mayonnaise), raw seafood (such as sushi or oysters), and rare meat. They were also more likely to clean a cutting board by simply wiping it. Assumptions about culture and educational level should be avoided when assessing risky food safety practices.

Employee training programs on food safety are thought to be effective in reducing the risk of foodborne disease (Costa, 1998). As in other foodservice trainings, intercultural communication differences must be addressed in planning food safety programs. Trainers should ascertain employee beliefs and practices regarding food preparation, hygiene, and foodborne illness prior to commencing education. Some traditional customs may be desirable and should be reinforced, such as peeling uncooked fruits and vegetables. Other customs may increase pathogenic contamination or growth and should be targeted for change. The three steps for managing intercultural conflict can be useful in planning an effective food safety training: describing the problem from all viewpoints, analyzing underlying beliefs and assumptions, then using collaborative problem-solving that benefits all participants. Opportunities for followup and practice of new food safety techniques are essential for behavioral change to take place.

Glossary of Ethnic Ingredients

Abalone: Large flat mollusk with finely textured sweet flesh in the broad muscular foot that holds it to rocks (must be pounded before use). It is common in the waters off Asia, California, Mexico, and New Zealand. Available fresh, frozen, canned, and dried.

Acerola Cherries: Caribbean berries resembling cherries that are exceptionally sour.

Achiote: See *Annatto*.

Adzuki Bean (aduki, azuki): Very small, dark red bean used primarily in Japanese cooking.

Ahipa: See *Jicama*.

Ajowan (ajwain, carom or lovage seeds): Similar to celery seeds in appearance and to thyme in flavor. Used in Asian Indian and Middle Eastern cooking.

Ajwain: See *Ajowan*.

Akee (ackee, achee): Red fruit with three segments containing large inedible seeds and flesh that looks like scrambled eggs. Available canned.

Alligator: Reptile native to rivers and swamps throughout the southern Gulf Coast region, from Florida to Texas. Mild white meat, with texture similar to veal. Tail and other parts eaten.

Almond Paste: Arab confection of ground almonds kneaded with sugar or cooked sugar syrup (some brands also contain egg white) used in many European and Middle Eastern desserts. Marzipan is a type of almond paste made with finely ground blanched almonds.

Amaranth (Chinese spinach, pigweed): Leafy, dark green vegetable similar to spinach. The high-protein seeds can be ground into flour and used in baked products, or boiled and eaten as cereal. Popular throughout Asia and Latin America.

Amchoor: Dried unripe mango slices or powder, with a sour flavor.

Angelica: Herb with a licorice flavor commonly used in European dishes. Usually available candied.

Annatto (achiote, atchuete): Seeds of the annatto tree used to color foods red or golden yellow. Used in Latin America, India, Spain, and the Philippines. In the United States, annatto is added to some baked goods, Cheddar-style cheeses, ice creams, margarines, and butter for color. May be cooked whole in oil or lard to produce the right hue or used as a ground spice.

Apios: See *Groundnuts*.

Apon Seeds (agonbono seeds): Seeds of the wild mango, commonly used in West Africa. Basis of the soup known as agonbono.

Areca Nuts: See *Betel*.

Arracacha (Peruvian carrot): Starchy white root of the carrot family used in South America, especially Colombia, Peru, and Venezuela.

Arrowroot: Many varieties of a bland, mealy tuber found in Asia and the Caribbean. When made into a powder, it is used to thicken sauces and stews.

Artichoke: Globelike vegetable member of the thistle family, with multiple edible bracts ("leaves") crowning the undeveloped edible flower (the "heart"). The flavor is slightly sweet. Popular in Middle Eastern and southern European dishes.

Arugula (rocket): Small member of the cabbage family native to the Mediterranean; the peppery leaves are popular in salads throughout Europe.

Asafetida: Dried resin with a pungent odor reminiscent of burnt rubber, which nonetheless imparts a delicate onion-like flavor. It is available as a lump or powder and is commonly used in Asian Indian dishes.

Asian Pear (apple pear): Round yellow fruit from Asia with the crispness of an apple and the flavor of a pear.

Avocado (alligator pear): Pear-shaped to round fruit with leathery skin (green to black) and light green buttery flesh. Native to Central America. Three varieties are often available. Eaten mostly as a vegetable, although considered a fruit in some cuisines.

Bacalao (bacalhau, baccala): Cod preserved by drying and salting. Must be soaked, drained, and boiled before use.

Bagoong: See *Fish Paste*.

Bagoong-Alamang: See *Shrimp Paste*.

Bambara Groundnut: Legume very similar to peanuts, native to Africa.

Bamboo Shoot: Crisp, cream-colored, conical shoot of the bamboo plant. Used fresh (stored in water) or available canned in brine (whole or sliced).

Bangus: See *Milkfish*.

Baobab (monkey bread, lalu powder): Slightly sweet seeds from the large fruit of the native African baobab tree. Used roasted or ground. Pulp of the fruit is also consumed.

Basmati Rice: See *Rice*.

Bean Curd (Cheong-po, tofu, tobu, tempeh): Custard-like, slightly rubbery white curd with a bland flavor made from soybean milk. Japanese bean curd (called tofu) tends to be softer than Chinese, which is preferred for stir-fried dishes. A chewier version common in Southeast Asia is called tempeh. Cheong-po, a Korean bean curd is made from mung beans.

Beans: See bean type.

Bean Sprouts: The young sprouts of mung beans or soybeans popular in Asian cooking (sprouts may also be grown from the tiny seeds of alfalfa, also a legume). The crisp 1- to 2-inch sprouts are eaten fresh or added to stir-fried dishes.

Berbere: Ethiopian spice paste (typically very hot) used to season many foods, usually including allspice, cardamom, cayenne, cinnamon, cloves, coriander, cumin, fenugreek, ginger, nutmeg, and black pepper.

Bergamot Orange: Pear-shaped orange with exceptionally tart flesh. Rind used to flavor dishes in the Mediterranean and North Africa; oil extracted from rind flavors Earl Grey tea.

Betel: The heart-shaped leaves of the betel vine (related to black pepper) are used to wrap areca nuts (from the Areca palm; the nuts are usually called betel nuts because of their use with betel leaves) and spices for paan in India. Betel nuts and leaves are chewed together in many Southeast Asian countries and in India to promote digestion. May stain the teeth red.

Bird's Nest: Swallows' nests from the cliffs of the South China Sea made from predigested seaweed; used in Chinese soups or sweetened for dessert.

Bitter Almond: An almond variety with an especially strong almond flavor, often used to make extracts, syrups, and liqueurs. Grown in the Mediterranean region, bitter almonds are used in European dishes. They contain prussic acid and are toxic when raw (they become edible when cooked) and are unavailable in the United States.

Bitter Melon (bitter gourd, foo-gwa): Bumpy-skinned Asian fruit similar in shape to a cucumber that is pale green when ripe. The flesh has melon-like seeds and an acrid taste due to high quinine content (flavor and odor become stronger the longer it ripens).

Bitter Orange: See *Seville Orange.*

Black Bean (turtle bean): Small (less than ½ inch) black bean (dried) used extensively in Central American, South American, and Caribbean cooking.

Black Beans, Fermented: Black soybeans salted and fermented to produce a piquant condiment. Used in Chinese cooking as a seasoning or combined with garlic, ginger, rice wine, and other ingredients to make black bean sauce.

Black-Eyed Pea (cow pea): Small legume (technically neither a pea nor a bean), white with a black spot, native to Africa and southern Asia.

Black Mushrooms: See *Mushrooms.*

Blood Orange: Old variety of orange with deep maroon–colored flesh, sometimes streaked with white. Intense sweet-tart flavor. Common in Spain and North Africa.

Blowfish (fugu, globefish): A popular Japanese specialty, blowfish contain a deadly toxin in the liver and sex organs. After careful cleaning the flesh reportedly has a slight tingle when eaten.

Bok Choy (Chinese chard): Vegetable of the cabbage family with long, white leaf stalks and smooth, dark green leaves.

Breadfruit: Large round tropical fruit with warty green skin and starchy white flesh. It must be cooked and is usually served as a vegetable. Available canned.

Buckwheat (kasha): Nutty-flavored cereal native to Russia (where it is called kasha), sold as whole seeds (groats) and ground seeds (grits if coarsely ground, flour if finely ground). It is common in Russian and Eastern European cooking.

Buffalo Berry: Scarlet berry of the *Sheperdia* genus, so called because it was usually eaten with buffalo meat by the Native Americans.

Bulgur (bulghur, burghul): Nutty-flavored cracked grains of whole wheat that have been precooked with steam. Available in coarse, medium, and fine grades.

Burdock Root (gobo): Long thin root with crisp white flesh and thin brown skin with an earthy, sweet flavor. Popular in Asian cooking.

Cactus: The paddles (nopales, or nopalitos, if cut into small pieces) and the juicy reddish fruit (tuna) of the prickly pear and Saguro cacti, eaten in the U.S. Southwest and Mexico. The paddles are used fresh, cooked, or pickled. Available canned.

Caimito: See *Star Apple.*

Calabash: Gourdlike fruit of a tropical tree native to the New World.

Calabaza: Round or oblong winter squash with yellow flesh and a flavor similar to pumpkin.

Calamansi: Small sour lime used to flavor foods in Filipino cooking.

Callaloo (cocoyam): Edible leaves of root vegetables, especially amaranth, malanga, and taro. Callaloo is sometimes the name of a dish made from these leaves.

Camass Root: Sweet bulb of the camass lily common in the U.S. Pacific Northwest.

Candlenut (kukui nut): Oily tropical nut sold only in roasted form (it is toxic when raw). Popular in Malaysia, Polynesia, and Southeast Asia.

Cannellini: See *Kidney Bean.*

Capers: Small gray-green flower buds from a bush native to the Mediterranean. They are commonly pickled.

Carambola: See *Star Fruit.*

Cardoon: Member of the artichoke family that looks like a spiny celery plant, popular in Italian cooking.

Cashew Apple: The fleshy "false fruit" to which the cashew nut is attached. Native to Brazil, it is eaten in the Caribbean and India as well.

Cassarep: Caribbean sauce made from the juice of the bitter variety of cassava cooked with raw sugar.

Cassava (manioc, yuca): Tropical Latin American tuber (now eaten in most tropical areas of the world) with rough brown skin and mild white flesh. Two types exist: bitter (poisonous unless leached and cooked) and sweet cassava. Flour used in Africa (gari), the Caribbean, and Brazil (farinha). Cassava starch is used to make the thickening agent tapioca.

Caviar: Fish roe classified by source and quality. Black or gray beluga caviar is harvested from large sturgeons and is considered best; sevruga and osetra caviar are obtained from smaller sturgeon and are therefore smaller and often darker colored. The large red eggs of salmon are commonly called red caviar. The choicest caviar is lightly salted and carefully sieved by hand. The poorer quality caviar is heavily salted and pressed into blocks.

Celeriac (celery root): Gnarled, bulbous root of one type of celery, with brown skin, tan flesh, and nutty flavor.

Cèpes: See *Mushrooms.*

Chanterelles: See *Mushrooms.*

Chayote (christophine, chocho, huisquil, mirliton, vegetable pear): Thin-skinned, green (light or dark), pear-shaped gourd. Native to Mexico, it is now common in Central America, the Caribbean, the southern United States, and parts of Asia.

Cheong-po: See *Bean Curd.*

Cherimoya (custard apple): Large, dimpled, light green fruit native to South America. White flesh is creamy in texture with a flavor reminiscent of strawberries, cherries, and pineapple.

Chicharrónes: Deep-fried pork skin, fried twice to produce puffy strips.

Chickpea (garbanzo bean): Pale yellow round legume popular in Middle Eastern, Spanish, Portuguese, and Latin American cooking. Can be purchased canned or dried.

Chicory: Bitter roasted root of the European chicory plant used as a substitute for coffee. Often added to dark coffee in Creole cooking.

Chile Pepper: Although chile peppers, or chiles, are often called hot peppers, the fruits are not related to Asian pepper (such as black pepper) but are pods of capsicum plants, native to Central and South America. More than 100 varieties are available, from less than ¼ inch in length to over 8 inches long. Used fresh or dried. The alkaloid *capsaicin,* found mostly in the ribs of the pods, is what makes chile peppers hot. In general, the smaller the chile, the hotter it is. Common types include mild Anaheim (also called California or New Mexico chile); Cayenne (used mostly dried and powdered as the spice cayenne); dark green, medium hot Jalapeño (often available canned—when smoked are known as *Chipolte*); spicy, rich green Poblano (used fresh, or ripened and dried, called *Ancho*); hot Serrano (small, bright green or red); and very hot Chile de Arbol, Japones, Péquin (tiny berry-like pepper, exceptionally hot, also known as *bird* or *bird's eye* peppers), and Tabasco (small, red chiles, often used dried).

Chili Powder: Ground, dried chile peppers, often with added spices such as oregano, cumin, and salt.

Chinese Date (dae-chu; jujube): Small Asian fruit (not actually belonging to the date family) usually sold dried. Red dates are the most popular, but black and white are also available.

Chinese Parsley: See *Coriander.*

Chitterlings (chitlins): Pork small intestines, prepared by boiling or frying.

Chokecherry: Tart, reddish black native American cherry (*Prunus virginiana*).

Chrysanthemum Greens ("chop suey" greens; *sook-gat*): Spicy leaves of a variety of chrysanthemum (not the American garden flower), popular in Asian stir-fried dishes, especially in Korea.

Cilantro: See *Coriander.*

Citron: Candied peel of a yellow-green, apple-size citrus fruit. Available crystallized and as preserves.

Citronella: See *Lemon Grass.*

Clotted Cream (Cornish cream, Devonshire cream): Very thick cream made by allowing cream to separate from milk, then heating it and cooling it so that it ferments slightly. Finally, the cream is skimmed from the milk (although Cornish cream is skimmed before heating and cooling). It is popular in southwest England, where it is spread on bread or used as a topping for desserts.

Cloud (Wood) Ears: See *Mushrooms.*

Coconut Cream: High-fat cream extracted from fresh grated coconut.

Coconut Milk: Liquid extracted with water from fresh grated coconut.

Cocoplum: Bland plum with white flesh

native to West Africa, found in the Caribbean and Central America. Eaten fresh or dried.

Cocoyam: See *Callaloo.*

Conch: Large, univalve mollusk found in waters off Florida and Caribbean (where it is sometimes called *lambi*). Chewy meat valued for its smoky flavor; can be bitter. Used especially in soups, stews.

Copra: Dried coconut kernels used in the extraction of coconut oil.

Coriander (cilantro, Chinese parsley): Fresh leaves of the coriander plant with a distinctive "soapy" flavor, common in Asian, Middle Eastern, Indian, and Latin American cooking. Seeds used as spice; root used in Thai cooking.

Corn Smut (huitlacoche): Fungus (*Ustilaginales*) that grows on corn ears. Prized in Chinese, Mexican and Native American cooking.

Couscous (cuscus, cuzcuz): Small granules of semolina flour used as a grain in African, Italian, Brazilian and Middle Eastern dishes.

Cow Pea: See *Black-Eyed Pea.*

Cracked Wheat: Cracked raw kernels of whole wheat used in Middle Eastern cooking.

Crawfish (crawdad, crayfish): Small freshwater crustacean, 4 to 6 inches long, that looks and tastes something like lobster. Found in Europe and the United States (California, Louisiana, Michigan, and the Pacific Northwest). The names crawfish and crayfish are also applied to the langostino, a saltwater crustacean that lacks large front claws.

Crème Fraîche: Slightly thickened, slightly fermented cream popular in France.

Curry Powder: The western version of the fresh Asian Indian spice mixture (garam masala) used to flavor curried dishes. Up to twenty spices are ground, then roasted, usually including black pepper, cayenne, cinnamon, coriander, cumin, fenugreek, ginger, cardamom, and turmeric for color.

Custard Apple: See *Cherimoya.*

Cuttlefish (inkfish): A mollusk that is similar to squid, but smaller. Available fresh or dried.

Daikon (icicle radish, white radish): Relatively mild white radish common in Asian cooking. The Japanese variety is the largest, often 12 inches long, and is shaped like an icicle. The Chinese variety tends to be smaller.

Dals: Indian term for hulled and split grains, legumes, or seeds. Many types are available, such as lentils or split peas.

Dashi: Japanese stock made from kelp and dried fish (bonita). *Dashi-no-moto* is the dried, powdered, instant mix.

Dilis (daing): Small silvery fish related to anchovies, dried and salted. Used in Filipino dishes.

Dragon's Eyes: See *Longan.*

Durian: Cantaloupe-size spiked fruit native to Malaysia, with a strong odor and sweet, creamy flesh.

Eggplant: Pear-shaped to round member of the nightshade family with smooth, thin skin (white or deep purple in color) and spongy, off-white flesh. Native to India, it has a mildly bitter flavor. Two types widely available are the small thin varieties known as Japanese and Chinese eggplant and the more common larger, rounder variety. The Thai type is small, round, white with green stripes.

Egusi: See *Watermelon Seeds.*

Elderberries: Small shrubs or trees up to 20 feet. Numerous species found throughout northern hemisphere. In the United States (genus *Sambucus*) produce edible, sweet berries used fresh and in preserves, pies, and wine. Blossoms fried as fritters.

Enoki: See *Mushrooms.*

Epazote (Mexican tea; pigweed): Pungent herb (*Chenopodium ambrosioides*) related to pigweed or goosefoot (and sometimes called by these names). Found in Mexico and parts of the United States. Often added to bean dishes to reduce gas.

Farinha: See *Cassava.*

Fava Bean (broad bean, horse bean, Windsor bean): Large green meaty bean sold fresh in the pod. Smaller white or tan fava beans are dried or canned and cannot be used interchangeably with the fresh beans. Common in Italian and Middle Eastern cooking.

Fennel: Light green plant with slightly bulbous end and stalks with feathery, dark green leaves, a little like celery. Used like a root vegetable. Delicate licorice or anise flavor.

Fenugreek: Tan seeds of the fenugreek plant, with a flavor similar to artificial maple flavoring. Essential in the preparation of Asian Indian spice mixtures.

Fiddlehead Ferns: Young unfurled fronds a specialty dish of the U.S. Northeast and southeastern Canada. Roots were eaten by Native Americans.

Filé Powder: See *Sassafras.*

Fish Paste (bagoong, pa dek, prahoc): Thick fermented paste made from fish, used as a condiment and seasoning in the Philippines and Southeast Asia.

Fish Sauce (nam pa, nuoc mam, patis, tuk-trey): Thin, salty, brown sauce made from fish fermented for several days. Asian fish sauces vary in taste from mild to very strong, depending on the country and the grade of sauce. Filipino patis is the mildest, Vietnamese nuoc mam is among the most flavorful. Nuoc cham is a sauce made from nuoc mam by the addition of garlic and chile peppers.

Five-Spice Powder: A pungent Chinese spice mixture of anise, cinnamon, cloves, fennel seeds, and Szechuan pepper.

Fufu: See *Yam.*

Fugu: See *Blowfish.*

Fuzzy Melon (hairy melon, mo gwa): Asian squash similar to zucchini with peach fuzz–like covering of the skin.

Garbanzo Bean: See *Chickpea.*

Gari: See *Cassava.*

Geoduck: Large (up to 15 pounds) clam native to U.S. Pacific Northwest, with "neck" or "siphon" as long as 3 feet. Neck used in soups, stews; body sliced for steaks.

Ghee: Clarified butter (*usli ghee*) used in India. The term *ghee* is also used for vegetable shortening.

Ginger Root: Knobby brown-skinned root with fibrous yellow-white pulp and a tangy flavor. Used sliced or grated in Asian dishes. Also available dried, ground, or candied.

Ginkgo Nut: Small pit of the fruit of the ginkgo tree (ancient species related to the pine tree), dried or preserved in brine, common in Japan.

Ginseng: Aromatic forked root with bitter, yellowish flesh, used in some Asian dishes and beverages; best known for therapeutic uses.

Glutinous Rice: See *Rice.*

Granadilla: See *Passion Fruit.*

Grape Leaves: Large leaves of grape vines preserved in brine, common in Middle Eastern cooking.

Gravlax: See *Salmon, Cured.*

Greens: Any of numerous cultivated or wild leaves, such as chard, collard greens, creases, cochan (coneflower), dandelion greens, dock, kale, milkweed, mustard greens, pokeweed, purslane, and spinach.

Grits: Coarsely ground grain, especially hominy, which is typically boiled into a thick porridge or fried as a side dish. Served often in the U.S. South.

Ground Cherries: Yellow fruit that looks like a tomato, from a bush native to Mexico.

Groundnuts (Apios, Indian potatoes): South American tuber (*Apios americana*) eaten by Native Americans, adopted by European settlers. Different from Africa groundnuts (referring to either peanuts or Bambara groundnuts).

Guanabana: See *Soursop.*

Guarana (Brazilian cocoa): Shrub indigenous to the Amazon. Dried leaves and seeds of the fruit are used to make a stimulating tea (containing caffeine) or mixed with cassava flour to form sun-dried sticks.

Guava: Small sweet fruit with an intense floral aroma, native to Brazil. Skin is yellow-green or yellow, and the grainy flesh ranges from white or yellow to pink and red. Many varieties are available, including strawberry guava and pineapple guava. Guava is popular as jelly, juice, or paste.

Head Cheese: Loaf of seasoned meat made from the hog's head and sometimes also feet and organs.

Heart of Palm: White or light green interior of the palm tree, especially popular in the Philippines. Available canned.

Hickory Nuts: Tree indigenous to North America (genus *Carya*), in same family as pecans. Eaten fresh, roasted, or ground into meal or pressed for a cream-like fluid by Native Americans; used in confections in the U.S. South.

Hog Peanut: A high-protein underground fruit that grows on the root of the vine *Falcata comosa* in the central and southern United States. The peanut has a leathery shell that can be removed by boiling or soaking. The nut meat can be eaten raw or cooked.

Hoisin Sauce: Popular Chinese paste or sauce, reddish brown in color, with a spicy sweet flavor. It is made from fermented soybeans, rice, sugar, garlic, ginger, and other spices.

Hominy (posole, pozole): Lime-soaked hulled corn kernels with the bran and germ removed.

Hot Pepper: See *Chile Pepper.*

Hot Pepper Sauce: Sauce made from fermented chile peppers, vinegar, and salt (Tabasco sauce is the best-known U.S. brand).

Huisquil: See *Chayote.*

Icicle Radish: See *Daikon.*

Indian Breadroot: Large white starchy root (*Psoralea esculenta*) indigenous to the western United States. It can be eaten raw, peeled and roasted, boiled, or dried and ground into a flour.

Indian Potato: See *Groundnuts.*

Jackfruit: Large (up to 100 pounds) fruit of the jack tree, related to breadfruit and figs, native to India. Two varieties are widely eaten, one sweeter than the other. Available dried or canned.

Jaggery: Unrefined sugar from the palmyra or sugar palm common in India.

Java Plum (rose apple, jambo, jaman): a small sour fruit grown in the Philippines.

Jerusalem Artichoke (sunchoke, sunroot): Small nubby-skinned tuber that is the root of a native American sunflower. It is neither from Jerusalem nor related to the artichoke, though the flavor when cooked is similar. It is used raw and cooked.

Jicama (Ahipa; yambean): Legume with medium to large tuber with light brown skin and crisp white flesh, indigenous to Brazil. Used raw in Latin American dishes, it has a sweet, bland flavor, similar to peas or water chestnuts.

Jujube: See *Chinese Date.*

Juniper Berry: Distinctively flavored dark blue berry of the juniper evergreen bush, native to Europe. Used to flavor gin.

Kaffir Lime: Aromatic citrus popular in Southeast Asia, especially in Thai cooking. Juice, rind, and leaves used to flavor curries, salad dressings, and sauces.

Kamis: Sour, cucumber-like vegetable native to the Philippines. Used to achieve a sour, cool flavor in Filipino cooking.

Kanpyo (kampyo): Ribbons of dried gourd used mostly for garnishing dishes in Japan.

Kaong: See *Palm Nuts.*

Kasha: See *Buckwheat.*

Kava: See *Pepper Plant.*

Kewra (pandanus): Perfumed essence of the screwpine flower used in Asian Indian Indonesian, Malaysian and Thai dishes.

Key Lime: Small, tart lime indigenous to the Caribbean. Popular in Florida Keys, known best as primary ingredient in Key Lime Pie.

Kidney Bean: Medium-size kidney-shaped bean light to dark red in color (a white variety is popular in Europe, especially Italy, where they are known as *cannellini*). The flavorful beans are common in Europe, Latin America, and the United States.

Kochujang: Korean fermented chile pepper paste added to many dishes.

Kohlrabi: Light green or purple bulbous vegetable that grows above the soil and produces stems bearing leaves on the upper part. A member of the cabbage family, it can be eaten raw or cooked.

Kola Nut: Bitter nut of the African kola tree (extracts from this nut were used in the original recipe for Coca-Cola).

Kukui Nut: See *Candlenut*.

Kumquat: Small, bright orange, oval fruit with a spicy citrus flavor common in China and Japan. Also available in syrup and candied.

Laverbread: Thick puree of laver (see *Seaweed*) that is baked. Used in sauces and stuffings in Great Britain.

Lemon Grass (citronella root): Large dull-green stiff grass with lemony flavor common in Southeast Asian dishes. Available fresh, dried, or powdered.

Lily Buds (golden needles): The dehydrated buds of lily flowers used in the cooking of China.

Lingonberry: Small wild variety of the cranberry found in Canada and northern Europe. Usually available as preserves.

Litchi (lychee): Small Chinese fruit with translucent white flesh and a thin brown hull and single pit. The flavor is grape-like but less sweet. Available fresh and canned. Dried litchis, also called litchi nuts, have different flavor and texture.

Lobster: Ocean-dwelling crustacean valued for its sweet flesh. Two main species consumed in United States. American lobster *(Homarus americanus)* found from Labrador to North Carolina; meat from large claws and tail, premature eggs called "coral," and liver eaten. Spiny lobster *(Panulirus argus* and other species) looks similar to American lobster but is a different animal. Found in warm waters from North Carolina to Brazil; small claws, only tail meat eaten.

Longan (dragon's eyes): Fruit of an Asian Indian tree related to litchis. Used fresh, canned, or dried.

Long Bean (Chinese green bean, yard-long bean): Roundish Asian bean, 12 to 30 inches long. Similar in taste to string beans, long beans are more soft and chewy, less juicy and crunchy than string beans.

Long-Grain Rice: See *Rice*.

Loquat: Slightly fuzzy yellow Asian fruit about 2 inches across, with a tart peach flavor. Available dried and in syrup.

Lotus Root (water lily root): Tubular vegetable (holes, as in Swiss cheese, run the length of the root, producing a flower-like pattern when the root is sliced) with brownish skin and crisp, sweet, white flesh. Becomes starchy when overcooked or canned.

Lox: See *Salmon, Smoked*.

Luffa (cee gwa, Chinese okra, loofa): Long, thin-skinned Asian vegetable, a member of the cucumber family, with spongy flesh.

Lupine Seeds (tremecos): Bitter seeds of a legume used for fodder. Must be leached in water before eating.

Macadamia Nut: Round creamy nut native to Australia, now grown in Africa, South America, and Hawaii.

Mahimahi (dolphinfish): A saltwater finfish found off the coasts of Florida and Hawaii.

Mahleb: Middle Eastern spice made from ground black cherry kernels, which impart a fruity flavor to foods.

Malagueta Pepper (grains of paradise, guinea pepper): Small West African berries related to cardamom, with a hot, peppery flavor. In Brazil the term refers to a tiny Pequin chile pepper.

Malanga (yautia): Caribbean tuber with cream-colored, yellow, or pinkish flesh, dark brown skin, and nutty flavor.

Mamey: Medium-size egg-shaped fruit with brown skin and soft flesh ranging in color from orange to yellowish to reddish. It has a flavor similar to pumpkin.

Mango: Fruit native to India, yellow to red when ripe, averaging 1 pound in weight. The flesh is pale and sour when the fruit is unripe, bright orange and very sweet when it is ripe. Used unripe for pickles and chutneys, ripe as a fresh fruit.

Manioc: See *Cassava*.

Marzipan: See *Almond Paste*.

Masa: Dough used to make tortillas and tamales. Usually made fresh from dried corn kernels soaked in a lime solution, or from one of two instant "flours" available: masa harina (tortilla mix made from dehydrated fresh masa) or masa trigo (wheat flour tortilla mix).

Mastic: Resin from the lentisk bush that has a slightly piney flavor, used to flavor Middle Eastern foods. Available in crystal form.

Mate: Plant in holly family *(Ilex paraguariensis)* native to South America. Dried, powdered leaves, called *yerba*, are brewed to make a stimulating tea (containing caffeine) that is popular in Argentina, Brazil, and Paraguay.

Mayhaw: Type of hawthorne tree found in U.S. South. Fruit looks like cranberries with a tart apple flavor. Used in preserves, syrups and wines.

Mikan: Japanese citrus related to tangerines and mandarin oranges. Eaten fresh, frozen, and canned in syrup.

Milkfish (bangus): Silvery bony fish with oily flesh popular in Filipino cooking.

Millet: Cereal native to Africa, known for its high-protein, low-gluten content and ability to grow in arid areas. The variety common in Ethiopia is called *teff*.

Mirin: Sweet rice wine used in Japanese dishes.

Miso: Fermented soybean paste, white (mild flavored) or red (strongly flavored), common in Japanese cooking.

Morels: See *Mushrooms*.

Mullet: Finfish of two families that can be black, gray, or red. The flesh is a mix of dark, oily meat and light, nutty-tasting meat. The texture is firm but tender.

Mung Bean: Yellow-fleshed bean with olive or tan skin common in the cooking of China and India.

Mushrooms: Fresh or dried fungi used to flavor dishes throughout the world. Common Asian types include enoki (tiny yellow mushrooms with roundish caps), oyster mushrooms (large, delicately flavored grey-beige caps that grow on trees), shiitake (dark brown with wide flat caps, available dried as Chinese black mushrooms), straw mushrooms (creamy colored with bell-like caps), and cloud ears or wood ears (a large flat fungus with ruffled edges, available dried). Popular mushrooms in Europe, available both fresh and dried, include chanterelles (a golden mushroom with an inverted cap), morels (a delicately flavored mushroom with a dark brown wrinkled cap), and porcini or cèpes (large brown mushrooms with caps that are spongy underneath, also called *boletus*).

Nam pa: See *Fish Sauce.*

Nance: Small, yellow tropical fruit similar to cherries with a slightly tart flavor. Two varieties are available.

Napa Cabbage (celery cabbage, Chinese cabbage): Bland crunchy vegetable with broad white or light green stalks with ruffled leaves around the edges. Several types are available, similar in taste (do not confuse with bok choy).

Naranjilla (lulo): Walnut-size, orange-skinned, green-fleshed fruit indigenous to the Americas, used mostly for its juice. Particularly popular in Central America.

Nongus: Fruit of the palmyra palm, grown in India, Indonesia, and Malaysia as a source of sugar.

Nopales (nopalitos): See *Cactus.*

Nuoc Cham: See *Fish Sauce.*

Nuoc Mam: See *Fish Sauce.*

Okra: Small, green, torpedo-shaped pod with angular sides. A tropical African plant valued for the carbohydrates in it that are sticky and mucilaginous. It is used as a vegetable and to thicken soups and stews.

Olive: Fruit of a tree native to the Mediterranean. Green olives are preserved unripe and include the large, soft Greek olives. Kalamata olives are a medium-size, purplish Greek olive. Dark olives (such as Niçoise) are picked in autumn, often cured in salt, with a tannic flavor. Ripe, black olives are smooth-skinned and mild-flavored or wrinkled with a strong tannic flavor.

Olive Oil: Extracted from the olive flesh, it is labeled according to percent acidity, from *extra virgin* to *virgin* (or "pure"). U.S. labeling laws restrict the use of the term "virgin" to only olive oil made from the first press; virgin olive oils mixed with refined olive oils to reduce acidity are labeled "pure."

Ostiones: Oyster native to the Caribbean that grows on the roots of mangrove trees.

Oyster Mushrooms: See *Mushrooms.*

Oyster Sauce: Thick brown Chinese sauce made with soy sauce, oysters, and cornstarch.

Pacaya Bud: The bitter flower stalk of the pacaya palm found in Central America. The edible stalk is about 10 inches long and is encased in a tough green skin, which must be removed before cooking.

Pa dek: See *Fish Sauce.*

Palillo: Peruvian herb, used dried and powdered to provide a yellowish orange color to foods.

Palmetto Cabbage: See *Heart of Palm.*

Palm Nuts (*Kaong*): Seeds from palms; pounded into palm butter in West Africa. Also boiled and added to halo-halo mix in Philippines.

Palm Oil (dende oil): Oil from the African palm, unique for its red-orange color.

Pandanus: See *Kewra.*

Papaya: Thin-skinned green (under-ripe), yellow, or orange fruit with sweet flesh colored gold to light orange to pink. Mexican (large and round) and Hawaiian (smaller and pear shaped) varieties are available. The shiny round black seeds are edible. Unripe papaya is used in pickles; the ripe fruit is eaten fresh.

Paprika: Powdered red peppers especially popular in Hungarian cooking. Paprika is made from several types of *Capsicum annum,* related to bell and chile peppers. Paprika is usually designated "sweet" or "hot." Spanish paprika, used in Spanish and Middle Eastern dishes, is more flavorful.

Passion Fruit (granadilla): Small oval fruit with very sweet gelatinous pulp. Yellow- and purple-skinned varieties are available. Passion fruit is often made into juice.

Patis: See *Fish Sauce.*

Pawpaw (tree melon): Light orange fruit that tastes like a cross between a banana and a melon. Native to the Americas, it is approximately 6 inches long.

Peanuts (groundnuts, goobers, monkeynuts): Legume native to South America, introduced to Africa by the Portuguese, then brought to the United States in the seventeenth century by black slaves. Eaten raw, roasted, or pulverized into peanut butter. Popular in Africa and the United States; used in some Chinese, Southeast Asian, and Asian Indian dishes.

Pejibaye (peach palm): Fruit of a Central American palm, especially popular in Costa Rica.

Pepitas: Pumpkin or squash seeds common in Latin American cooking. May be hulled or unhulled, raw or roasted, salted or unsalted.

Pepper Plant (*Piper methysticum*): Leaves of the South Pacific plant used to produce the intoxicating beverage called *kava* or *awa.*

Peppers: Misnamed pods of the capsicum plants native to South and Central America (not actually related to Asian pepper plants, which produce black pepper). Peppers are divided into sweet and hot types (see *Chile Pepper*). Sweet peppers include bell peppers (green, red, yellow, and purple), pimentos, and peppers used to make paprika.

Perilla (shiso; beefsteak plant; quenneep): Aromatic herb with distinctive minty flavor; green or red. Available fresh or pickled. Used mostly as a seasoning or garnish in many Japanese and Korean dishes; sometimes served as a side dish or to wrap rice and other items.

Pigeon Pea: Small pea in a hairy pod (a member of the legume family, but not a true pea) common in the cooking of Africa, the Caribbean, and India. Yellow or tan when dried.

Pignoli: See *Pine Nut.*

Pigweed: See *Amaranth; Epazote.*

Pili-pili: Hot sauce used in West Africa made with the piri-piri chile pepper and other ingredients such as tomatoes, onions, garlic or horseradish.

Pili Nut: Almond-like nut of a tropical tree found in the Philippines.

Pine Nut (pignoli, piñon seed): Delicately flavored kernel from any of several species of pine tree. Pine nuts are found in Portugal (most expensive type), China (less costly, with a stronger taste), and the southwestern United States. Common in some Asian, European, Latin American, Middle Eastern, and Native American dishes.

Pink Bean (rosada): Small oval meaty bean that is a light tannish pink in color.

Piri-piri: Thin, fiery chile favored in West Africa. Used in sauces and marinades, and is the name of dishes that include some form of the pepper.

Plantain: Starchy type of banana with a thick skin, which can be green, red, or black. There are many varieties, ranging in size from 3 to 10 inches. The pulp is used as a vegetable and must be cooked. It is similar in taste to squash.

Poi: See *Taro.*

Porcini: See *Mushrooms.*

Posole, Pozole: See *Hominy.*

Prahoc: See *Fish Paste.*

Pulses: Term used especially in India for edible legume seeds, including peas, beans, lentils, and chickpeas.

Quinoa: Cereal native to the Andes, prepared like rice.

Radicchio: Magenta-colored, slightly bitter member of the chicory family used throughout southern and northern Europe.

Rambutan: Bristly, juicy, orange or bright red fruit used in Southeast Asian cooking; related to the litchi.

Ramp: Strong-flavored indigenous American onion that tastes somewhat like a leek. Both leaves and bulbs are edible.

Red Bean: Small, dark red bean native to Mexico and the southwestern United States.

Rice: Grain native to India. More than 2,500 varieties are available worldwide, including basmati rice (small grain with a flavor similar to popcorn, very popular in India and the Middle East); brown rice (unmilled rice with the bran layer intact; can be short-, medium-, or long-grain); glutinous rice (also called sweet or pearl rice, very short-grain and very sticky when cooked); long-grain rice (white, polished grains that flake when cooked); and short-grain rice (slightly sticky when cooked, popular in Japan).

Rose Apple (kopo): small, thin-skinned pink or red fruit native to Southeast Asia with somewhat spongy flesh that has slightly acidic flavor.

Roselle (Florida cranberry; karkadeh; red sorrel): Pods of a Hibiscus plant relative, common in Africa, the Caribbean, Southeast Asia, Australia, and Florida. Used to make a tart tea popular in Egypt and Senegal. Also used for chutneys and preserves.

Saewujeot: See *Shrimp Paste.*

Saffron: Dried stamens of the crocus flower. It has a delicate, slightly bitter flavor and bright red-orange color. Available as threads or powder.

Salal: Thick-skinned black berries of a native American plant in the heath family (*Gaultheria shallon*).

Salmon, Cured: Salmon fillets cured in a mixture of salt, sugar, and dill weed, common in Sweden (where it is known as gravlax), Finland, and Norway.

Salmon, Smoked: Raw, tender salmon slices lightly smoked and cured in salt produced in Norway, Nova Scotia, and Scotland. Smoked salmon soaked in a brine solution is called *lox*, a Jewish specialty.

Salmon Roe: See *Caviar.*

Salt Pork: White fat from the side of the hog, streaked with pork meat, cured in salt.

Saluyot ("okra leaves"): Leaves from Southeast Asian bush with slippery texture when cooked. Added to soups and stews in Filipino cooking.

Sapodilla: See *Zapote.*

Sassafras (filé powder): Native American herb used to thicken soups and stews.

Sea Cucumber (sea slug): Brown or black saltwater mollusk up to 1 foot in length. They lack a shell, but have a leathery skin and look something like smooth, dark cucumbers. Sold dried, they are rehydrated for Chinese dishes, becoming soft and jelly-like, with a mild flavor.

Sea Urchin Roe (uni): Small, delicate eggs of the spiny sea urchin, popular in Japan.

Seaweed (kim): Many types of dried seaweed are used in Chinese, Korean, and Japanese dishes, including *aonoriko* (powdered green seaweed), *kombu* (kelp sheets), *laver* (tissue-thin, dark purple sheets), and *nori* (paper-thin sheets of dark green seaweed). Also popular in the Pacific Islands. See also *Laverbread.*

Sesame Seeds (benne seeds): Seeds of a plant native to Indonesia. Two types are available: tan colored (white when hulled) and black (slightly bitter). Commonly grown for their oil. Light sesame oil is pressed from raw seeds, dark oil from toasted seeds; the dark oil has a strong taste and is used as a flavoring.

Seville Orange (bitter orange; naranja aria, sour orange): Orange with tough skin and dark flesh native to Mediterranean. Inedible raw; juice used in liqueurs (Grand Marnier, Cointreau, Curaçao) and in cooking of the Mediterranean, Caribbean, Central America, and Korea.

Shallot: Very small bulb covered with a reddish, papery skin, related to onions but with a milder, sweeter flavor.

Shea Nut: Nut from the African shea tree, grown for its thick oil, called *shea butter.*

Shiso: See *Perilla.*

Shiitake Mushrooms: See *Mushrooms.*

Short-Grain Rice: See *Rice.*

Shoyu: See *Soy Sauce.*

Shrimp Paste: Strongly flavored fermented Asian sauce or paste made from small dried shrimp or similar crustaceans. Many types are available (bagoong-alamang is the Filipino variety; saewujeot is the Korean type).

Snail (escargot): Small, edible land snail (a common variety of garden snail, cleansed with a commercial feed). Popular in France.

Snow Pea (Chinese pea pod, sugar pea): Flat, edible pod with small, immature peas.

Sorghum (guinea corn): Cereal common to tropical regions of Africa with seeds produced on a stalk. In the Appalachians, Ozarks, and the U.S. South, sorghum is often processed to make sweet syrup.

Sorrel (dock, sourgrass): Small, sour green.

Sour Orange: See *Seville Orange.*

Soursop (guanabana): Large (often 12 inches long), rough-skinned fruit with cottony, fluffy flesh that can be white, pink, or light orange. Often made into juice or conserves.

Soybean: Small high-protein bean common in Asia. Many varieties of different colors, including black, green, red, and yellow, are available. They are used fresh, dried, and sprouted, most often processed into sauces, condiments, and other products (see *Hoisin Sauce, Oyster Sauce, Miso, Soy Milk, Soy Sauce,* and *Bean Curd*).

Soy Milk: Soybeans that are boiled, pureed, then strained and boiled again to produce a white milklike drink.

Soy Sauce (shoyu): Thin, salty, brown sauce made from fermented soybeans. Several types are available. Chinese soy sauces tend to be lighter in flavor than the stronger, darker Japanese shoyu.

Spicebush: Shrub (*Lindera benzoin*) with spicy-smelling bark and leaves; red berries. Used to make Native American teas.

Spiny Lobster: See *Lobster.*

Star Anise: Eight-armed pods from a plant in the magnolia family, with an anise-like flavor. Native to China.

Star Apple (caimito): Purple, apple-size fruit with mild, gelantinous, lavender-colored flesh native to the Caribbean. Seeds form a star around the center.

Star Fruit (carambola): Small, deeply ribbed, oval fruit with thin skin that is shaped like a star when sliced. Green and sour when unripe, yellow and slightly sweet (though still tart) when ripe. The unripe fruit is used in Indian and Chinese dishes; when ripe it is eaten fresh.

Straw Mushrooms: See *Mushrooms.*

Sumac: Sour red Middle Eastern spice made from the ground berries of a nontoxic variety of the sumac plant.

Sunflowers: Native to the United States (genus *Helianthus*); over sixty varieties. Seeds eaten by Native Americans raw, dried, and powdered (in breads). Unopened flower head can be cooked and eaten like an artichoke. Petals are used like saffron in Southwest, dried and powdered.

Sweet Peppers: See *Peppers.*

Szechwan Pepper (fagara): Aromatic berries with a hot flavor popular in some Chinese and Japanese dishes.

Tabasco Sauce: See *Hot Pepper Sauce.*

Tamarind: Tart pulp from the pod of the tamarind bean. Available in the pod, as a paste, in a brick, or as a liquid concentrate.

Tanier (tannia): See *Taro, Malanga;* both are referred to as tannier.

Tapioca: See *Cassava.*

Taro (eddo, dasheen): Starchy underground vegetable similar to cassava with brown hairy skin and white to grayish flesh, common in the Caribbean and Polynesia. In Hawaii the boiled, pounded taro paste called *poi* is a staple in the traditional diet. The large leaves are also eaten (see *Callaloo*).

Tarpon: Large silver fish of the herring family found off the coasts of Mexico and Central America.

Teff: See *Millet.*

Tempeh: See *Bean Curd.*

Tepary Beans: Small, high-protein bean with wrinkled skin. Grows wild in the southwest United States.

Ti: Tropical plant popular in Polynesia (not related to tea). Ti leaves are used to wrap food packets, and the root is eaten and brewed for a beverage.

Tilapia: Small freshwater fish with sweet, firm, white flesh.

Tobu, Tofu: See *Bean Curd.*

Tomatillo: Small, light green, tomato-like fruit surrounded by a green or tan papery husk, common in Mexico. The flesh is slightly tart and is eaten cooked, usually in sauces and condiments. Available fresh or canned.

Tremecos: See *Lupine Seeds.*

Truffle: Black (French) or white (Italian) fungus found underground. Truffles vary from the size of small marbles to as large as tennis balls and are distinctively flavored, similar to a wild mushroom. Available fresh or canned.

Tuk-trey: See *Fish Paste.*

Tuna: See *Cactus.*

Turtle: Popular in Carribean, Central America, and U.S. South. Diamondback terrapin (*Malaclemys terrapin*) is the primary ingredient in turtle soups of the Atlantic states. Green turtle (*Chelonia mydas*) is a sea turtle, commonly eaten as steaks or stews Other turtles eaten occasionally (including eggs) are alligator snapping turtle, common snapping turtle, and loggerhead turtle.

Ugli Fruit: Citrus fruit that is a cross between an orange and a grapefruit, with a very bumpy yellow-orange skin and a sweet orange-like flavor. Especially popular in Jamaica.

Uni: See *Sea Urchin Roe.*

Usli Ghee: See *Ghee.*

Verjuice: Juice of unripe lemons used in Middle Eastern fare to give a tang to dishes.

Wasabi: Light green Japanese condiment from root of plant similar to horseradish with a powerful pungency. Available fresh or powdered; green-dyed horseradish often sold as wasabi.

Water Chestnut: Aquatic, walnut-size tuber with fibrous brown peel and crunchy, sweet, ivory-colored flesh. Available fresh or canned.

Watermelon Seeds: Seeds often eaten in Africa (called *egusi,* toasted, ground or pounded into meal or paste for thickening soups and stews) and in Asia (toasted as a snack; sometimes flavored or dyed red).

Wax Gourd: White, oblong fruit of a vine with starchy flesh, common in Southeast Asia.

White Bean: Three types of white bean are widely used: cannellini (see *Kidney Bean*); Great Northern beans, which are large, soft, and mild tasting; and the smaller, firmer navy beans.

White Radish: See *Daikon.*

Wild Rice: Seeds of a native American grass.

Winged Bean: Edible legume (*Psophocarpus tetragonolobus*) called the "soy-bean of the tropics." All parts of the plant are consumed, including the shoots, leaves, flowers, pods and seeds, and tuberous root. The pods are large, from 12 to 24 inches long, and feature winglike flanges.

Winter Melon (dong gwa, wax melon): Round green-skinned member of the squash family with a waxy white coating and translucent white green or pink flesh. Similar in taste to zucchini, it is used cooked in Chinese dishes.

Worcestershire Sauce: Sauce developed by the British firm of Lea and Perrins including anchovies, garlic, onions, molasses, sugar or corn sweetener, tamarind, and vinegar, among other ingredients.

Yam (ñame; yampi; cush-cush; mapuey): Tuber with rough brown skin and starchy white flesh (not related to the orange sweet potato called *yam* in the United States). Numerous varieties; may grow quite large, up to 100 pounds. Found in all tropical regions. Yam paste called *fufu* in West Africa.

Yambean: See *Jicama.*

Yautia: See *Malanga.*

Yerba Buena: A variety of mint used in some Native American teas.

Yuca: See *Cassava.*

Yucca (Navajo banana): Spiky-leaved desert plant (*Yucca baccata*) with large, pulpy fruit that ripens in summer. Eaten fresh, boiled, baked, or dried into fruit leather.

Zapote (sapodilla, black sapote, naseberry): Drab-colored fruit of the sapodilla tree (which is the source of chicle used in chewing gum). It has granular, mildly sweet flesh, which can be yellow, red, or black. The zapote is a member of the persimmon family.

Resources

In many ways a book like this poses more questions than it answers. Knowledge of cultural foods is neither balanced nor complete. Many interested readers are undoubtedly asking why there is so little research on adaptations of food habits in the United States or why there are such limited data available on certain cultural groups. As stated in the preface, only the major American cultural groups are presented in this book. Although the authors reviewed many resources, the resulting text is undeniably inadequate in some areas. Thus the most urgent question is, "Where to go from here?"

Classes, seminars, association memberships, research, client interaction, and community involvement are all useful ways to learn more about cultural foods. In the nutrition field, many departments of dietetics and home economics offer courses in food and culture. Culinary schools often offer similar classes. Nutrition, dietetic, and food service organizations occasionally sponsor seminars on general topics in food habits, as well as on culturally specific diets. Of special note, the Multi Cultural Foodservice and Hospitality Alliance (MFHA) promotes business solutions through diversity.

Research on foods and food habits is published in a limited number of journals. *American Journal of Clinical Nutrition, American Journal of Public Health, Ecology of Food and Nutrition, Food and Foodways, Journal of the American Dietetic Association, Journal of Nutrition Education,* and *Social Science and Medicine* are a few that frequently feature articles on diet, nutrition, and culture. Food service, hospitality, and restaurant journals sometimes address cultural food issues. Anthropology, folklore, history, home economics, human resources, geography, management, medicine, nursing, psychology, and sociology publications are occasionally good resources as well.

There are numerous books that have contributed to research on foods and food habits. Cookbooks and other popular literature often include anecdotal information of interest. On-line web sites are an additional source of data. Some of the many resources available follow.

Observation and participation in the community, at markets, at festivals and fairs, and at public religious events are also good ways to learn about a population. Community leaders, traditional healers, restauranteurs, and grocers can all contribute to cultural knowledge about foods and food habits. Accumulated experience with a minority population can be an important adjunct to printed research.

The authors encourage food professionals to undertake and publish studies on cultural foods to expand the limited information on the topic. We also hope that all professionals share their diversity experiences through associations and journals. In addition, you may contact our web site at www.eatethnic.com to discuss these issues on line. Such research and communication help us to become more culturally competent and thus become more effective health care providers and educators.

General Bibliography

Barer-Stein, T. 1979. *You Eat What You Are.* Toronto: McClelland and Stewart.

Brown, L. K., & Mussell, K. (Eds.). 1984. *Ethnic and Regional Foodways in the United States.* Knoxville: University of Tennessee Press.

Bryant, C. A., Courtney, A., Markesbery, B. A., & Dewalt, K. M. 1985. *The Cultural Feast: An Introduction to Food and Society.* St. Paul, MN: West.

Carlson, B. 1997. *Food Festivals.* Detroit, MI: Visible Ink.

Claiborne, C. 1985. *Craig Claiborne's The New York Times Food Encyclopedia.* New York: Times Books.

Cole, K. W. 1985. *Minority Organizations: A National Directory.* Garrett Park, MD: Garrett Park Press.

Counihan, C., & Van Esterik, P. (Eds.). 1997. *Food and Culture: A Reader.* New York: Routledge.

Cunningham, S. 1991. *The Magic of Food: Legends, Lore and Spellwork.* St. Paul, MN: Ilewellyn.

Farb, P., & Armelagos, G. 1980. *Consuming Passions: The Anthropology of Eating.* New York: Washington Square Press.

Fieldhouse, P. 1995. *Food and Nutrition: Customs and Culture* (2nd ed.). London: Chapman & Hall.

Fitzgerald, T. K. (Ed.). 1977. *Nutrition and Anthropology in Action.* Amsterdam: Van Gorcum.

Freedman, R. L. 1981. *Human Food Uses: A Cross-Cultural Comprehensive Annotated Bibliography.* Westport, CT: Greenwood Press.

Harris, M. 1985. *Good to Eat: Riddles of Food and Culture.* New York: Simon & Schuster.

Jacobs, J. 1995. *The Eaten Word: The Language of Food, Food in Our Language.* New York: Birch Lane Press.

Jerome, N. W., Kandel, R. F., & Pelto, G. H. (Eds.). 1980. *Nutritional Anthropology: Contemporary Approaches to Diet and Culture.* Pleasantville, NY: Redgrave.

Jones, E. 1981. *American Food: The Gastronomic Story* (2nd ed.). New York: Vintage Books.

Lankevich, F. J. 1981. *Ethnic America.* London: Oceana.

Lee, H. G. 1992. *Taste of the States: A Food History of America.* Charlottesville, VA: Howell Press.

Levenstein, H. 1993. *Paradox of Plenty: A Social History of Eating in Modern America.* New York: Oxford University Press.

Lowenberg, M. E., Todhunter, E. M., Wilson, E. D., Feeney, M. C., Savage, J. R., & Lubawski, J. L. 1979. *Food and People* (3rd ed.). New York: Wiley.

MacClancy, J. 1992. *Consuming Culture: Why You Eat What You Eat.* New York: Holt.

Macdonald, D. 1983. *Resources on Food, Nutrition and Culture.* Toronto. Nutrition Information Service, Ryerson Polytechnic Institute Library.

Mariani, J. F. 1983. *Dictionary of American Food and Drink.* New Haven, CT: Tichnor & Fields.

McClelland, D. A. 1991. *Good as Gold—Foods America Gave the World.* Washington, DC: National Museum of History/Smithsonian Institution.

McGee, H. 1984. *On Food and Cooking: Science and Lore of the Kitchen.* New York: Scribner.

Menzel, P. & D'Alusio, F. 1998. *Man Eating Bugs: The Art and Science of Eating Insects.* Berkeley, CA: Ten Speed Press.

Montagne, P. 1977. *The New Larousse Gastronomique.* New York: Crown.

National Agricultural Library. 1988. *Diet, Race & Ethnicity in the US: Research and Reference Material.* 1979–1987 (NALBIBL. QB 88–29), Beltsville, MD.

National Research Council. 1945. *The Problem of Changing Food Habits.* Washington, DC: National Research Council Bulletin 108.

Newman, J. M. 1993. *Melting Pot: An Annotated Bibliography and Guide to Food and Nutrition Information for Ethnic Groups in America* (2nd ed.). New York: Garland.

Nichter, M., & Nichter, M. 1981. *An Anthropological Approach to Nutrition Education.* Newton, MA: International Nutrition Communication Service.

Powers, J. M., & Stewart, A. (Eds.). 1995. *Our Northern Bounty: A Celebration of Canadian Cuisine.* Toronto: Random House of Canada.

Roberts, C. 1992. *Cultural Perspectives on Food and Nutrition.* Beltsville, MD: National Agricultural Library.

Root, W. 1980. *Food.* New York: Simon & Schuster.

Root, W., & de Rochemont, R. 1976. *Eating in America.* New York: Ecco Press.

Sanjur, D. 1982. *Social and Cultural Perspective in Nutrition.* Englewood Cliffs, NJ: Prentice-Hall.

Schivelbusch, W. 1992. *Taste of Paradise: A Social History of Spices, Stimulants and Intoxicants.* New York: Pantheon Books.

Schwabe, C. W. 1979. *Unmentionable Cuisine.* Charlottesville: University Press of Virginia.

Shortridge, B. G., & Shortridge, J. R. 1995. Cultural geography of American foodways: An annotated bibliography. *Journal of Cultural Geography, 15,* 79–107.

Shortridge, B. G., & Shortridge, J. R. (Eds.). 1998. *The Taste of American Place.* Lanham, MD: Rowman & Littlefield.

Simoons, F. J. 1994. *Eat Not This Flesh: Food Avoidances from Prehistory to the Present* (2nd ed.). Madison: University of Wisconsin Press.

Tannahill, R. 1989. *Food in History.* New York: Crown.

Thernstrom, S., Orlov, A., & Handlin, O. (Eds.). 1980. *Harvard Encyclopedia of American Ethnic Groups.* Cambridge, MA: The Belknap Press of Harvard University Press.

Trager, J. 1995. *The Food Chronology.* New York: Holt.

USDA/USDHHS. 1986. *Cross-Cultural Counseling: A Guide for Nutrition and Health Counselors.* United States Department of Agriculture FNS-250, U.S. Government Printing Office, 1987-720- 484-1302/60133.

Vissar, M. 1991. *The Rituals of Dinner: The Origins, Evolution, Eccentricities and Meaning of Table Manners.* New York: Grove Weidenfeld.

Von Welanetz, D., & Von Welanetz, P. 1982. *The Von Welanetz Guide to Ethnic Ingredients.* Los Angeles: Tarcher.

Wilson, C. S. (Ed.). 1979. Food: Custom and nurture. An annotated bibliography on sociocultural and biocultural aspects of nutrition. *Journal of Nutrition Education, 11* (Suppl. 1), 212–261.

Wood, R. C. 1995. *The Sociology of the Meal.* Edinburgh, Scotland: Edinburgh University Press.

Cookbooks

African

Clark, L. (Ed.). 1991. *The Black Reunion Cookbook.* Memphis, TN: Wimmery House.

Copage, E. V. 1991. *Kwanzaa.* New York: Morrow.

DeWitt, D., Wilan, M. J., & Stock, M. J. 1998. *Flavors of Africa Cookbook.* Rocklin, CA: Prima.

Hafner, D. 1993. *A Taste of Africa.* Berkeley, CA: Ten Speed Press.

Harris, J. B. 1998. *The Africa Cookbook: Tastes of a Continent.* New York: Simon & Schuster.

Van der Post, L. (Ed.). 1970. *African Cooking.* New York: Time-Life Books.

American

Adams, M. 1997. *New Recipes from Quilt Country: More Food and Folklore from the Amish and Mennonites.* New York: Clarkson Potter.

Anderson, J. 1997. *The American Century Cookbook.* New York: Clarkson Potter.

Belk, S. 1991. *Around the Southern Table.* New York: Simon

& Schuster.

Brown, D. 1968. *American Cooking.* New York: Time-Life Books.

Brown, D. 1971. *American Cooking: The Northwest.* New York: Time-Life Books.

Chateau Ste. Michells. 1985. *Taste of Liberty: A Celebration of Our Great Ethnic Cooking.* Woodinville, WA: Documentary Book Publisher.

Claiborne, C. 1987. *Craig Claiborne's Southern Cooking.* New York: Times Books.

Cox. B. 1996. *Spirit of the West: Cooking from Ranch House and Range.* New York: Artisan.

Dedominic, L. M. 1997. *Rocky Mountain Gourmet Cookbook.* Helena, MT: Falcon.

Dupree, 1993. *Southern Memories.* New York: Clarkson Potter.

Feibleman, P. S. 1971. *American Cooking: Creole and Acadian.* New York: Time-Life Books.

Hafner, D. 1997. United Tastes of America: *Recipes and Cultural Origins of Your Favorite Dishes.* New York: Ballantine Publishing Group.

Hibler, J. 1996. *Dungeness Crabs and Blackberry Cobblers: The Northwest Heritage Cookbook.* New York: Knopf.

Jamison, C. A., & Jamison, B. 1995. *The Border Cookbook: Authentic Home Cooking of the American Southwest and Northern Mexico.* Cambridge, MA: Harvard Common Press.

Jones, E. 1981. *American Food: The Gastronomic Story* (2nd ed.). New York: Vintage Books.

Kirlin, K. S., & Kirlin, T. M. 1991. *Smithsonian Folklife Cookbook.* Washington, DC: Smithsonian Institution Press.

Landen, R. 1996. *The Food of Paradise: Exploring Hawaii's Culinary Heritage.* Honolulu: University of Hawaii Press.

Leonard, J. N. 1971. *American Cooking: New England.* New York: Time-Life Books.

Leonard, J. N. 1971. *American Cooking: The Great West.* New York: Time-Life Books.

Mandel, A. 1996. *Celebrating the Midwestern Table.* New York: Doubleday.

Murphy, M. D., & Richardson, H. W. 1996. *The Boston Globe Cookbook: A Collection of Classic New England Recipes.* Old Saybrook, CN: Globe Pequot Press.

Page, L. G., & Wigginton, E. 1984. *The Foxfire Book of Appalachian Cookery.* New York: Dutton.

Shenton, J. P., Pellegrini, A. M., Brown, D., & Shender, I. 1971. *American Cooking: The Melting Pot.* New York: Time-Life Books.

Smith, J. 1990. *The Frugal Gourmet on Our Immigrant Ancestors.* New York: Morrow.

Walter, E. 1971. *American Cooking: Southern Style.* New York: Time-Life Books.

Weaver, W. W. 1983. *Sauerkraut Yankees: Pennsylvania German Foods and Foodways.* Philadelphia: University of Pennsylvania Press.

Wilson, J. 1971. *American Cooking: The Eastern Heartland.* New York: Time-Life Books.

Asian Indian

Jaffrey, M. 1995. *Madhur Jaffrey's Indian Cooking.* Woodbury, NY: Barron's.

Rau, S. R. 1969. *The Cooking of India.* New York: Time-Life Books.

Ray, S. 1986. *Indian Regional Cooking.* London: Macdonald.

Caribbean

Creen, L. H. 1991. *A Taste of Cuba.* New York: Dutton.

Harris, J. B. 1991. *Sky Juice and Flying Fish.* New York: Simon & Schuster.

Kaufman, W. I. (Ed.). 1964. *Recipes from the Caribbean and Latin America.* New York: Dell.

Ortiz, E. L. 1986. *The Complete Book of Caribbean Cooking.* New York: Ballantine Books.

Rivera, O. 1993. *Puerto Rican Cooking in America: Nuyorican and Bodega Recipes.* New York: Four Walls Eight Windows.

Wolfe, L. 1970. *Cooking of the Caribbean Islands.* New York: Time-Life Books.

Central American

Marks, C. 1985. *False Tongues and Sunday Bread: A Guatemalan and Mayan Cookbook.* New York: Evans.

Central European and Russian

Hazelton, N. S. 1969. *The Cooking of Germany.* New York: Time-Life Books.

Martin, P. 1981. *The Czech Book: Recipes and Traditions.* Iowa City: Penfield Press.

Papashvily, H., & Papashvily, G. 1969. *Russian Cooking.* New York: Time-Life Books.

Visson, L. 1982. *The Complete Russian Cookbook.* Ann Arbor, MI: Ardis.

Wechsberg, J. I. 1968. *The Cooking of Vienna's Empire.* New York: Time-Life Books.

Won Bremzen, A., & Welchman, I. 1990. *Please to the Table: The Russian Cookbook.* New York: Workingman.

Zermuska, A. 1981. *The Art of Polish Cooking.* Gretna, LA: Pelican.

Chinese

Chang, W. W. 1973. *An Encyclopedia of Chinese Food and Cooking.* New York: Crown.

Chen, P. K., Chen, T. C., & Tseng, R. 1983. *Everything You Want to Know about Chinese Cooking.* Woodbury, NY: Barron's.

Hahn, E. 1968. *The Cooking of China.* New York: Time-Life Books.

Horn, K. 1990. *The Taste of China.* New York: Simon & Schuster.

Simonds, N. 1983. *Classic Chinese Cuisine.* Boston: Houghton Mifflin.

Japanese

Omae, K., & Tachibana, Y. 1981. *The Book of Sushi*. Tokyo: Kodansha International USA.

Ortis, E. L., & Endo, M. 1976. *The Complete Book of Japanese Cooking*. New York: Evans.

Steinberg, R. 1969. *The Cooking of Japan*. New York: Time-Life Books.

Tokimasa, E. C. 1982. *Japanese Foods*. Honolulu: Temmy.

Jewish

Levy, F. 1991. *International Jewish Cookbook*. New York: Warner Books.

Nathan, J. 1998. *The Jewish Holiday Kitchen*. New York: Schocken Books.

Roden, C. 1996. *The Book of Jewish Food: An Odyssey from Samarkand to New York*. New York: Knopf.

Sogolow, R. 1996. *Memories from a Russian Kitchen—From Shtetl to Golden Land*. Santa Barbara, CA: Fithian Press.

Korean

Cho, J. O. 1981. *Home-Style Korean Cooking in Pictures*. New York: Kodansha International USA (distributed through Harper and Row).

Kwak, J. 1998. *Dok Suni: Recipes from My Mother's Kitchen*. New York: St. Martin's Press.

Millon, M., & Millon, K. 1991. *Flavours of Korea*. London: Deutsch.

Mexican

Bayless, R. 1987. *Authentic Mexican*. New York: Morrow.

Hamman, C. 1998. *Mayan Cooking: Recipes from the Sun Kingdoms of Mexico*. New York: Hippocrene Books.

Kennedy, D. 1989. *The Cuisines of Mexico*. New York: Harper Collins.

Leonard, J. N. 1970. *Latin American Cooking*. New York: Time-Life Books.

Long, K. 1992. *Mexican Light Cooking*. New York: Perigee Books.

Rexach, N. L. 1985. *The Hispanic American Cookbook*. Secaucus, NJ: Stuart.

Middle Eastern

Abdennour, S. 1998. *Egyptian Cooking: A Practical Guide*. New York: Hippocrene Books.

Baron, R. 1991. *Flavors of Greece*. New York: Morrow.

Corey, H. 1962. *The Art of Syrian Cooking*. Garden City, NY: Doubleday.

Davies, G. 1991. *The Taste of Cyprus*. Lancaster, England: Gazelle.

Day, I. F. 1975. *The Moroccan Cookbook*. New York: Perigee Books.

Dosti, R. 1982. *Middle Eastern Cooking*. Tucson: HP Books.

Helou, A. 1994. *Lebanese Cuisine*. New York: St. Martin's Press.

Khalil, N. E. 1980. *Egyptian Cuisine*. Washington, DC: Worldwide Graphics.

Najmieh, B. 1986. *Food of Life: A Book of Ancient Persian and Modern Iranian Cooking and Ceremonies*. Washington, DC: Mage.

Nickles, H. G. 1969. *Middle Eastern Cooking*. New York: Time-Life Books.

Rodin, C. 1968. *A Book of Middle Eastern Food*. New York: Vintage Books.

Uvezian, S. 1974. *The Cuisine of Armenia*. New York: Harper and Row.

Vassilian, H. B. (Ed.). 1991. *Ethnic Cookbooks and Food Marketplace*. Glendale, CA: Armenian Reference Books.

Yianilos, T. K. 1970. *The Complete Greek Cookbook*. New York: Funk and Wagnalls.

Multicultural

Albya, C. A., & Webb, L. S. 1993. *The Multicultural Cookbook for Students*. Phoenix, AZ: Oryx Press.

Claiborne, C. 1971. *The New York Times International Cookbook*. New York: Harper and Row.

Foods of the World. (A series of 27 volumes on individual countries or regions). New York: Time-Life Books.

Gordon, E. 1965. *Cuisines of the Western World*. New York: Golden Press.

Laas, W. 1967. *Cuisines of the Eastern World*. New York: Golden Press.

Smith, J. 1992. *The Frugal Gourmet on Our Immigrant Ancestors: Recipes You Should Have Gotten from Your Grandmother*. New York: Avon.

Native American

Cox, B., & Jacobs, M. 1991. *Spirit of the Harvest*. New York: Stewart, Tabori & Chang.

Kavasch, E. B. 1995. *Enduring Harvests*. Old Saybrook, CN: Globe Pequot Press.

Keegan, M. 1977. *Pueblo and Navajo Cookers*. Dobbs Ferry, NY: Earth Books.

Keegan, M. 1987. *Southwest Indian Cookbook*. Weehawken, NJ: Clear Light.

Kimball, Y., & Anderson, J. 1986. *The Art of American Indian Cooking*. Garden City, NY: Doubleday.

Neithammer, C. 1974. *American Indian Food and Lore*. New York: A Fireside Book, Simon & Schuster.

Northern European

Bailey, A. 1969. *The Cooking of the British Isles*. New York: Time-Life Books.

Child, J., & Beck, S. 1970. *Mastering the Art of French Cooking* (vol. 2). New York: Knopf.

Child, J. Bertholle, L., & Beck, S. 1961. *Mastering the Art of French Cooking* (vol. 1). New York: Knopf.

Claiborne, C. 1970. *Classic French Cooking*. New York: Time-Life Books.

Fisher, M. F. K. 1969. *The Cooking of Provincial France.* New York: Time-Life Books.

FitzGibbon, T. 1983. *Irish Traditional Food.* New York: St. Martin's Press.

Pacific Islander

Bazore, K. 1947. *Hawaiian and Pacific Foods: A Cook Book of Culinary Customs and Recipes Adapted for the American Hostess.* New York: Barrows.

Corum, A. K. 1983. *Ethnic Foods of Hawai'i.* Honolulu: The Bess Press.

Steinberg, R. 1970. *Pacific and Southeast Asian Cooking.* New York: Time-Life Books.

Scandinavian

Brown, D. 1968. *The Cooking of Scandinavia.* New York: Time-Life Books.

Hazelton, N. S. 1987. *Classic Scandinavian Cooking.* New York: Scribner.

Ojakangas, B. 1992. *Scandinavian Feasts.* New York: Stewart, Tabori & Chang.

South American

Harris, J. B. 1992. *Tasting Brazil: Regional Recipes and Reminiscences.* New York: Macmillan.

Rojas-Lombardi, F. 1991. *The Art of South American Cooking.* New York: HarperCollins.

Umaña-Murray, M. 1996. *Three Generations of Chilean Cuisine.* Los Angeles: Lowell House.

Southeast Asian

Alejandro, R. 1982. *The Philippine Cookbook.* New York: Coward-McCann.

Duong, B. 1991. *Simple Art of Vietnamese Cooking.* New York: Prentice-Hall.

Gelle, G. G. 1997. *Filipino Cuisine.* Santa Fe, NM: Red Crane Books.

Law, R. 1990. *The Southeast Asian Cookbook.* New York: Perigee Books.

Loha-Unchit, K. 1995. *It Rains Fishes: Legends, Traditions, and the Joys of Thai Cooking.* Rohnert Park, CA: Pomegranate.

Sananikone, K. 1999. *Keo's Thai Cuisine.* Berkeley, CA: Ten Speed Press.

Sing, P. 1981. *Traditional Recipes of Laos.* London: Prospect Books.

Steinberg, R. 1970. *Pacific and Southeast Asian Cooking.* New York: Time-Life Books.

Southern European

Anderson, J. 1994. *The Food of Portugal.* New York: Morrow.

Bugialli, G. 1982. *Classic Techniques of Italian Cooking.* New York: Simon & Schuster.

Casas, P. 1983. *The Foods and Wines of Spain.* New York: Knopf.

Casas, P. 1996. *Delisioso! The Regional Cooking of Spain.* New York: Knopf.

Feibleman, P. S. 1969. *The Cooking of Spain and Portugal.* New York: Time-Life Books.

Field, C. 1997. *Celebrating Italy: The Tastes and Traditions of Italy as Revealed through Its Feasts, Festivals, and Sumptuous Foods.* New York: HarperCollins.

Rogers, A. 1968. *A Basque Story Cookbook.* New York: Scribner.

Root, W. 1968. *The Cooking of Italy.* New York: Time-Life Books.

Food Composition Tables

Some of these tables are now out of print but may be available through university and college libraries. Foreign food composition tables may be difficult to use for the following reasons: (1) A given food may have several names within a cultural region, and (2) several different foods used within a cultural region may have the same name.

Argon, G., & Gibson, R. 1969. *Food Composition Tables for Use in Ethiopia.* Stockholm, Sweden: Almqvist and Wiksell.

Caribbean Food and Nutrition Institute. 1974. *Food Composition Tables for Use in the English-Speaking Caribbean.* Kingston, Jamaica: University of the West Indies.

Department of Nutrition of the Chinese Academy of Sciences. 1981. *Table of Food Composition.* S. M. You (Ran.). Beijing: Department of Nutrition of the Chinese Academy of Sciences.

De Reguero, L. C., & De Santiago, S. M. R. 1981. *Tabla de Composicion de Alimentos de USA Corriente en Puerto Rico.* San Juan: University of Puerto Rico.

Food Research and Industry Development Institute. 1971. *Table of Taiwan Food Composition.* Hsinchu, Taiwan: FIRDI.

Four Winds Food Specialists. 1999. *Ethnic Foods Nutrient Database.* Ethnic food items, most from those listed in the glossary of this book. Supplement compatible with *Nutritionist Five* (First DataBank) or hardcopy available. Sunnyvale, CA: Four Winds Food Specialists.

Gopalan, C., Rama-Sastri, B. V., & Balasubramanian, S. C. 1971. *Nutritive Value of Indian Foods.* Hyderabad: National Institute of Nutrition.

Jardin, C. 1967. *List of Foods Used in Africa.* Rome: Nutrition Division of the FAO of the United Nations.

Leung, W. T. W., & Chang, F. H. 1972. *Food Composition Tables for Use in East Asia.* Bethesda, MD: National Institutes of Health.

Leung, W. T. W., Firsson, F., & Jardin, C. 1968. *Food Composition Table for Use in Africa.* Rome: Nutrition Division of the FAO of the United Nations.

Leung, W. T. W., & Flores, M. 1961. *Food Composition Table for Use in Latin America.* Rome: Nutrition Division of the FAO of the United Nations.

Leung, W. T. W., Pecot, R. K., & Watt, B. K. 1952. *Composition of Foods Used in Far Eastern Countries.* Washington, DC: USDA Handbook 32.

Louie, J., & Gee, R. 1982. *Sodium Values of Common Asian/Pacific Islander Foods.* San Francisco: Division of Outpatient and Community Services, San Francisco General Hospital.

National Institute of Science and Technology. 1968. *Food Composition Table Recommended for Use in the Philippines* (3rd ed.). Manila: National Institute of Science and Technology of the Philippines.

Pellett, P., & Shadarevian, S. 1970. *Food Composition Tables for Use in the Middle East.* Beirut: American University of Beirut.

On-Line Resources

EatEthnic (http://eatethnic.com): This site is maintained by Four Winds Food Specialists, a partnership of this book's authors. Information on ethnic ingredients and food habits, recipes, holiday food traditions, cultural foods resources, and links to other sites of interest.

Edibilia (http://www.ibmpcug.co.uk/~owls/edibilia.html): This links site has sections on European, African, Sub-Continental (Asian Indian and Bangladesh), Far Eastern, and cuisine of the Americas. Other resources for baking, drinks, etc.

Epicurus (http://www.epicurus.com): Sponsored by a leading food and hospitality industry consultant, this site features a monthly e-zine with short, informative articles on foods, beverages, herbs and spices, interviews with chefs and hoteliers, and breaking food news, as well as tantalizing recipes. Information on some ethnic ingredients and cultural food events.

Food Composition Resource List for Professionals (http://www.nal.usda.gov/fnic/pubs/bibs/gen/97fdcomp.htm): These food composition resources are all available from the National Agriculture Library, including books, U.S. government publications, software databases, and journals. There is also a contact for assistance with specific requests, and a bulletin board.

Mimi's Cyber Kitchen (www.cyber-kitchen.com): A premier links site with thousands of well-organized listings of cooking, food, and recipe sites. Recipe exchange, cookbook reviews, and more.

Nutrition and Food on the Web (http://sfu.ca/~jfremont): Canadian dietitian Jean Fremont has put together a very well-organized links site for both the health professional and the consumer, with an excellent listing of international food and nutrition pages.

Sally's Place (http://www.sallys-place.com): An overview of several international cuisines can be found at this site. Recipes, restaurants, and ingredient sources are listed in some. Another useful page on this site lists professional food organizations, including descriptions and addresses.

SOAR—Searchable Online Archive of Recipes (http://soar.berkeley.edu/recipes/): This site has catalogued over 45,000 recipes from throughout the world. Just enter the name of the dish you are searching for, and a definition appears, with links to actual recipes. Excellent for specific food inquiries.

The Web of Culture (http://www.webofculture.com): This site is sponsored by a cross-cultural communications consultant. It has information on everything from currencies, languages, gestures, holidays, and religions to embassies, with a small bookstore and a few recipes.

World Food Habits Bibliography (wwwilstu.edu/class/anth273-foodways/foodbib.html): An outstanding listing of research in the field of food and culture. Search by region or topic (such as eating attitudes, festivals and feasting, and taboos).

World in Your Kitchen (http://www.creative-homeliving.com/World-Kitchen/home.htm): This excellent links site includes international cooking sites, American cooking sites, a spice tour of sites, cookbooks, an interactive chat room, and a culinary tour.

References

CHAPTER 1

American Dietetic Association. 1993. *Survey of American Dietary Habits: Exective Summary.* Chicago: Author.

American School Foodservice Association. 1998. Diversity today. *School Foodservice & Nutrition, 52,* 64-72.

Anderson, E. N. 1987. Why is humoral medicine so popular? *Social Science and Medicine, 25,* 331-337.

Apfel, I. 1998. Diversity dollars and sense. *Restaurants USA, 18,* 22-26.

Axelson, M. L. 1986. The impact of culture on food-related behavior. *Annual Review of Nutrition, 6,* 345-363.

Banks, C. G. 1992. "Culture" in culture-bound syndrome: The case of anor-exia nervosa. *Social Science and Medicine, 34,* 867-884.

Brookins, G. K. 1993. Culture, ethnicity, and bicultural competence: Implications for children with chronic illness and disability. *Pediatrics, 91,* 1056-1062.

Camp, C. 1989. *American Foodways.* Little Rock, AR: August House.

Camp, C. 1991. More American than apple pie. In *Good as Gold: Foods the Americas Gave the World.* Smithsonian Institution Quincentenary Symposium Proceedings. Washington, DC: National Museum of History.

Cassell, J. A. 1995. Social anthropology and nutrition. A different look at obesity in America. *Journal of the American Dietetic Association, 95,* 424-427.

Cassidy, C. M. 1994. Walk a mile in my shoes: Culturally sensitive food-habit research. *American Journal of Clinical Nutrition, 59* (suppl.), 190S-197S.

Centers for Disease Control and Prevention. 1994. Prevalence of selected risk factors for chronic disease by education level in racial/ethnic populations—United States, 1991-1992. *Mortality and Morbidity Weekly Report, 43,* 894-899.

Chalmers, I., & Glaser, M. 1986. *Great American Food Almanac.* New York: Harper & Row.

Cunningham, S. 1990. *The Magic in Food: Legends, Lore, and Spellwork.* St. Paul, MN: Llewellyn.

Dagnelie, P. C., & van Stavern, W. A. 1994. Macrobiotic nutrition and child health: Results of a population-based, mixed longitudinal cohort study in the Netherlands. *American Journal of Clinical Nutrition, 59* (suppl.) 1187S-1196S.

Dewey, K. G., Strode, M. A., & Fitch, Y. R. 1984. Dietary change among migrant and nonmigrant Mexican-American families in Northern California. *Ecology of Food and Nutrition, 14,* 11-24.

Dougherty, D., Bankhead, R., Kushner, R., Mirtallo, J., & Winkler, M. 1995. Nutrition care given new importance in JCAHO standards. *Nutrition in Clinical Practice, 10,* 26-31.

Douglas, M. 1972. Deciphering a meal. *Daedalus, 101,* 61-81.

Dressler, W. W., Mata, A., Chavez, A., & Viteri, F. E. 1987. Arterial blood pressure and individual modernization in a Mexican community. *Social Science and Medicine, 24,* 679-687.

Ekoe, J. M. 1988. *Diabetes Mellitus: Aspects of the World-wide Epidemiology of Diabetes Mellitus and Its Long-term Complications.* Amsterdam: Elsevier.

Fewster, W. J., Bostian, L. R., & Powers, R. D. 1973. Measuring the connotative meanings of foods. *Home Economics Research Journal, 2,* 44-53.

Fitzgerald, P. 1998. Introducing . . . ethnic! *School Foodservice & Nutrition, 52,* 129-132.

Fong, A. K. H. 1991. Educating clients: Successful communication creates change. *Journal of the American Dietetic Association, 91,* 289-290.

Freimer, N., Echenberg, D., & Kretchmer, N. 1983. Cultural variation—Nutritional and clinical implications. *Western Journal of Medicine, 139,* 928-933.

Furnham, A., & Alibhai, N. 1983. Cross-cultural differences in the perception of female body shapes. *Psychological Medicine, 13,* 829-837.

Gofton, L. 1986. The rules of the table: Sociological factors influencing food choice. In C. Ritson, L. Gofton, & J. McKenzie (Eds.), *The Food Consumer.* New York: Wiley.

Gryder, S. D. 1998. Lunchtime in the Tower of Babel. *School Foodservice & Nutrition, 52,* 54-62.

Gudykunst, W. B., & Nishida, T. 1994. *Bridging Japanese/North American Differences.* Thousand Oaks, CA: Sage.

Hahn, R. A. 1992. The state of federal health statistics on racial and ethnic groups. *Journal of the American Medical Association, 267,* 232-268.

Harnack, L., Story, M., Martinson, B., Neumark-Sztainer, D., & Stang, J. 1998. Guess who's cooking? The role of men in meal planning, shopping, and preparation in U.S. families. *Journal of the American Dietetic Association, 98,* 995-1000.

Harwood, A. 1981. *Ethnicity and Medical Care.* Cambridge, MA: Harvard University Press.

Henderson, G., & Primeaux, M. 1981. Health care. In G. Henderson & M. Primeaux (Eds.), *Transcultural Health Care.* Menlo Park, CA: Addison-Wesley.

Henry, J. P., & Cassel, J. C. 1969. Psychosocial factors in essential hypertension: Recent epidemiologic and animal experimental evidence. *American Journal of Epidemiology, 90,* 171-200.

Hertzler, A. A., Wenkam, N., & Standal, B. 1982. Classifying cultural food habits and meanings. *Journal of the American Dietetic Association, 80,* 421-425.

Hull, D. 1979. Migration, adaptation, and illness: A review. *Social Science and Medicine, 131,* 25-36.

Jelliffe, D. B. 1967. Parallel food classifications in developing and industrialized countries. *American Journal of Clinical Nutrition, 20,* 279-281.

Jelliffe, D. B., & Bennett, F. J. 1961. Cultural and anthropological factors in infant and maternal nutrition. Proceedings of the Fifth International Congress of Nutrition. *Federation Proceedings, 20*, 185-188.

Josling, T., & Ritson, C. 1986. Food and the nation. In C. Ritson, L. Gofton, & J. McKenzie (Eds.), *The Food Consumer.* New York: Wiley.

Jouris, D. 1994. *All Over the Map: An Extraordinary Atlas of the United States.* Berkeley, CA: Ten Speed Press.

Kittler, P. G., Sucher, K., & Tseng, R. Y. 1986. Cultural foods education: An exploratory study of dietitians and Plan IV programs in California. *Journal of the American Dietetic Association, 86*, 1705-1708.

Land O'Lakes FoodWire. 1997. *FoodWire Ethnic Foods Survey.* Minneapolis, MN: FoodWire.

Lannon, J. 1986. How people choose food: The role of advertising and packagings. In C. Ritson, L. Gofton, & J. McKenzie (Eds.), *The Food Consumer.* New York: Wiley.

Levi-Straus, C. 1969. *The Raw and the Cooked.* New York: Harper & Row.

Livingston, A. D., & Livingston, H. 1993. *Edible Plants and Animals.* New York: Facts on File.

Lowenberg, M. E. 1970. Socio-cultural basis of food habits. *Food Technology, 24*, 27-32.

MacClancy, J. 1992. *Consuming Culture.* New York: Holt.

Marmot, M. G., & Syme, S. L. 1976. Acculturation and coronary heart disease in Japanese-Americans. *American Journal of Epidemiology, 104*, 225-247.

McComber, D. R., & Postel, R. T. 1992. The role of ethnic foods in the food and nutrition curriculum. *Journal of Home Economics, 84*, 52-54, 59.

McGarvey, S. T. 1991. Obesity in Samoans and a perspective on its etiology in Polynesians. *American Journal of Clinical Nutrition, 53*, 1586S-1594S.

McMurray, M. P., Ceriqueira, M. T., Conner, S. L., & Conner, W. E. 1991. Changes in lipid and lipoprotein levels and body weight in Tarahumara Indians after consumption of an affluent diet. *New England Journal of Medicine, 325*, 1704-1708.

Meleis, A. I., Lipson, J. G., & Paul, S. M. 1992. Ethnicity and health among five Middle Eastern immigrant groups. *Nursing Research, 42*, 98-103.

Miller, J. E., Porter, M., & Drummond, K. E. 1998. *Supervision in the Hospitality Industry.* New York: Wiley.

Mogelonsky, M. 1995. *Everybody Eats: Supermarket Consumers in the 1990s.* Ithaca, NY: American Demographics Books.

Mogelonsky, M. 1996. *Who's Buying Food and Drink.* Ithaca, NY: New Strategist Publications.

Monsen, E. R. 1992. Respecting diversity helps America eat right. *Journal of the American Dietetic Association, 92*, 282.

Murphy, N. J., Schraer, C. D., Thiele, M. C., Boyko, E. J., Bulkow, L. R., Doty, B. J., & Lanier, A. P. 1995. Dietary change and obesity associated with glucose intolerance in Alaska natives. *Journal of the American Dietetic Association, 95*, 676-682.

National Research Council. 1945. (Cited by M. E. Lowenberg.) Socio-cultural basis of food habits. *Food Technology, 24*, 27-32.

National Restaurant Association. 1998. 1997 menus: Old and new share the plate. *Restaurants* USA, *8*, 38-46.

Neuendorf, K. A. 1990. Health images in the mass media. In E. B. Ray & L. Donohew (Eds.), *Communication and Health: Systems and Applications.* Hillsdale, NJ: Lawrence Erlbaum Associates.

Ornish, D. 1990. *Dr. Dean Ornish's Program for Reversing Heart Disease.* New York: Random House.

Ots, T. 1990. The angry liver, the anxious heart and the melancholy spleen: The phenomenology of perceptions in Chinese culture. *Culture, Medicine, and Psychiatry, 14*, 21-58.

Palinkas, L. A., & Pickwell, S. M. 1995. Acculturation as a risk factor for chronic disease among Cambodian refugees in the United States. *Social Science and Medicine, 40*, 1643-1653.

Pangborn, R. M., & Bruhn, C. M. 1971. Concepts of food habits of "other" ethnic groups. *Journal of Nutrition Education, Winter*, 106-110.

Passariello, P. 1990. Anomalies, analogies and sacred profanities: Mary Douglas on food and culture 1957-1989. *Food and Foodways, 4*, 53-71.

Passim, H., & Bennett, J. W. 1943. Social process and dietary change. In *The Problem of Changing Food Habits.* Washington, DC: National Research Council Bulletin, p. 108.

Pelto, G. H. 1981. Anthropological contributions to nutrition education research. *Journal of Nutrition Education, 13* (suppl.), S2-S8.

Pelto, G. H., Pelto, P. J., & Lung'aho, M. S. 1981. "Modern" and "traditional" food use in West Finland: An example of quantitative pattern analysis. *Nutrition Research, 1*, 63-71.

Plawecki, H. 1992. Cultural considerations. *Journal of Holistic Nursing, 10*, 4-5.

Randall-David, E. 1989. *Strategies for Working with Culturally Diverse Communities and Clients.* Bethesda, MD: Association for the Care of Children's Health.

Raymond, C. A. 1986. Biology, culture, dietary changes conspire to increase incidence of obesity. *Journal of the American Medical Association, 256*, 2157-2158.

Root, W., & deRochemont, R. 1976. *Eating in America: A History.* New York: Ecco Press.

Rozin, P. 1991. The promise of plenty: Food in American history. In *Good as Gold: Foods the Americas Gave the World.* Smithsonian Institution Quincentenary Symposium Proceedings. Washington, DC: National Museum of History.

Rozin, P., Fallon, A., & Augustoni-Ziskind, M. 1985. The child's conception of food: The development of contamination sensitivity to "disgusting" substances. *Developmental Psychology, 21*, 1075-1079.

Sadella, E., & Burroughs, J. 1981. Profiles in eating: Sexy vegetarians and other diet-based stereotypes. *Psychology Today, October*, 51-57.

Schilling, B., & Brannon, E. 1986. *Cross-cultural Counseling: A Guide for Nutrition and Health Counselors.* Alexandria, VA: U.S. Department of Agriculture/U.S. Department of Health and Human Services, FNS #250.

Sodowsky, G. R., & Carey, J. C. 1988. Relationships between acculturation-related demographics and cultural attitudes of an Asian-Indian immigrant group. *Journal of Multicultural Counseling and Development, 16*, 117-136.

Sorlie, P. D., Backlund, E., & Keller, J. B. 1995. U.S. mortality by economic, demographic, and social characteristics: The National Longitudinal Study. *American Journal of Public Health, 85*, 949-956.

Spector, R. E. 1996. *Cultural Diversity in Health and Illness* (4th ed.). Norwalk, CT: Appleton & Lange.

Stein, R. I., & Nemeroff, C. J. 1995. Moral overtones of food: Judgments of others based on what they eat. *Personality and Social Psychology Bulletin, 21*, 480-490.

Sucher, K. P., & Kittler, P. G. 1991. Nutrition isn't colorblind. *Journal of the American Dietetic Association, 91*, 297-298.

Swartz, L. 1987. Illness negotiation: The case of eating disorders. *Social Science and Medicine, 24*, 613-618.

Swinburn, B. A., Bergman, V. L., Howard, B. V., & Bogardus, C. 1991. Deterioration in carbohydrate metabolism and lipoprotein changes induced by modern, high fat diet in Pima Indians and caucasians. *Journal of Clinical Endocrinology and Metabolism, 73*, 156-165.

Szathmary, E. J. E., Ritenbaugh, C., & Goodby, C. S. M. 1987. Dietary change and plasma glucose levels in an Amerindian population undergoing cultural transition. *Social Science and Medicine, 24*, 791-804.

Terry, R. D. 1994. Needed: A new appreciation of culture and food behavior. *Journal of the American Dietetic Association, 94*, 501-503.

Tsunehara, C. H., Leonetti, D. L., & Fujimoto, W. Y. 1990. Diet of second-generation Japanese-American men with and without non-insulin-dependent diabetes. *American Journal of Clinical Nutrition, 52*, 731-738.

Ward, M. 1998. Dare to be different? *School Foodservice & Nutrition, 52*, 38-50.

Wenkam, N. S., & Wolff, R. J. 1970. A half century of changing food habits among Japanese in Hawaii. *Journal of the American Dietetic Association, 57*, 29-32.

Whittemore, A. S., Wu-Williams, A. J., Lee, M., Shu, Z., Gallagher, R. P., Deng-ao, J., Lun, Z., Xianghui, W., Kun, C., Jung, D., Teh, C. Z., Chengde, L., Yao, X. J., Paffenbarger, R. S., & Henderson, B. E. 1990. Diet, physical activity, and colorectal cancer among Chinese in North America and China. *Journal of the National Cancer Institute, 82*, 915-926.

Wilson, C. S. 1985. Nutritionally beneficial cultural practices. *World Review of Nutrition and Diet, 45*, 68-96.

Wong, E. I. L., McProud, L. M., & Giampaoli, J. M. 1995. Hospital foodservice and ethnic foods: A survey of hospitals in two counties of northern California. *Journal of Foodservice Systems, 8*, 257-272.

Wood, R. C. 1995. *The Sociology of the Meal.* Edinburgh: Edinburgh University Press.

Wray, L. A. 1992. Health policy and ethnic diversity in older Americans: Dissonance or harmony? *Western Journal of Medicine, 157*, 357-361.

Zelinsky, W. 1987. You are where you eat. *American Demographics, 9*, 30-33.

CHAPTER 2

Anonymous. 1957. *The World's Great Religions.* New York: Time.

Bar-David, M. L., & Lewinski, Y.-T. 1972. Food. In *Encyclopedia Judaica.* Jerusalem: Keter.

Chaudry, M. M. 1992. Islamic food laws: Philosophical basis and practical implications. *Food Technology, 46*, 92-93, 104.

Cole, W. O., & Singh, S. P. 1978. *The Sikhs.* Boston: Routledge & Kegan Paul.

Dresser, N. 1996. *Multicultural Manners.* New York: Wiley.

Greenberg, B. 1989. *How to Run a Traditional Jewish Household.* Northvale, NJ: Aronson.

Higgins, C., & Warshaw, H. S. 1989. *Jewish Food Practices, Customs, and Holidays.* Chicago: American Dietetic Association/American Diabetes Association.

Hussaini, M. M. 1993. *Islamic Dietary Concepts and Practices.* Bedford Park, IL: Islamic Food and Nutrition Council of America.

Kilara, A., & Iya, K. K. 1992. Food and dietary practices of the Hindu. *Food Technology, 46*, 94-102, 104.

Lowenberg, M. E., Todhunter, E. N., Wilson, E. D., Savage, J. R., & Lubawski, J. L. 1979. *Food and People* (3rd ed.). New York: Wiley.

Marsh, C. E. 1984. *From Black Muslims to Muslims: The Transition from Separatism to Islam, 1930-1980.* Metuchen, NJ: Scarecrow Press.

Natow, A. B., Heslin, J., & Raven, B. C. 1975. Integrating the Jewish dietary laws into a dietetic program. *Journal of the American Dietetic Association, 67*, 13-16.

Nelson, M. S., & Javanovic, L. 1987. Pregnancy, diabetes, and Jewish dietary law: The challenge for the pregnant diabetic women who keep kosher. *Journal of the American Dietetic Association, 87*, 1054-1058.

Rau, S. R. 1969. *The Cooking of India.* New York: Time-Life Books.

Regenstein, J. M., & Regenstein, C. E. 1992. The kosher food market in the 1990s—A legal view. *Food Technology, 46*, 122-124, 126.

Robinson, R. H., & Johnson, W. L. 1982. *The Buddhist Religion.* Belmont, CA: Wadsworth.

Roth, C. 1972. Dietary habits. In *Encyclopedia Judaica.* Jerusalem: Keter.

Sakr, A. H. 1971. Dietary regulations and food habits of Muslims. *Journal of the American Dietetic Association, 58*, 123-126.

Sakr, A. H. 1975. Fasting in Islam. *Journal of the American Dietetic Association, 67*, 17-21.

Sarma, D. S. 1953. The nature and history of Hinduism. In K. W. Morgon (Ed.), *The Religion of the Hindus.* New York: Ronald Press.

Spence, H. 1960. *The Story of America's Religions.* New York: Holt, Rinehart & Winston.

van Straalen, A. 1986. *The Book of Holidays Around the World.* New York: Dutton.

CHAPTER 3

Bass, M. A., & Wakefield, L. M. 1974. Nutrient intake and food patterns of Indians on Standing Rock Reservation. *Journal of the American Dietetic Association, 64*, 36-41.

Bernardo, S. 1981. *The Ethnic Almanac.* Garden City, NY: Doubleday.

Birchfield, D. L. 1995. Apaches. In R. J. Vecoli, J. Galens, A. Sheets, & R. V. Young (Eds.), *Gale Encyclopedia of Multicultural America.* New York: Gale Research.

Brown, A. C., & Brenton, B. 1994. Dietary survey of Hopi Native American elementary students. *Journal of the American Dietetic Association, 94*, 517-522.

Christensen, N. K., Sorenson, A. W., Hendricks, D. G., & Munger, R. 1998. Juniper ash as a source of calcium in the Navajo diet. *Journal of the American Dietetic Association, 98*, 333-334.

Conley, R. J. 1995. Cherokees. In R. J. Vecoli, J. Galens, A. Sheets, & R. V. Young (Eds.), *Gale Encyclopedia of Multicultural America.* New York: Gale Research.

Davis, M. B. (Ed.). 1994. *Native Americans in the Twentieth Century, An Encyclopedia.* New York: Garland.

Emboden, W. A. 1976. Plant hypnotics among North American Indians. In W. D. Hand (Ed.), *American Folk Medicine.* Los Angeles: University of California Press.

Farkas, C. S. 1986. Ethno-specific communication patterns: Implications for nutrition education. *Journal of Nutrition Education, 18*, 99-103.

Garrett, J. T. 1990. Indian health: Values, beliefs, and practices. In M. S. Harper (Ed.), *Minority Aging: Essential Curricula Content for Selected Health and Allied Health Professions.* Health Resources and Services Administration, Department of Health and Human Services. DHHS Publication No. HRS (P-DV-90-4). Washington, DC: U.S. Government Printing Office.

Halderson, K. 1993. *Alaska Native Food Practices, Customs, and Holidays.* Chicago: American Dietetic Association/American Diabetes Association.

Ikeda, J., Dugan, S., Feldman, R., & Mitchell, R. 1993. Native Americans in California surveyed on diets, nutrition needs. *California Agriculture, 47,* 8–10.

Jackson, M. Y. 1986. Nutrition in American Indian health: Past, present, and future. *Journal of the American Dietetic Association, 86,* 1561–1565.

Joos, S. K. 1980. Diet, obesity, and diabetes mellitus among the Florida Seminole Indians. *Florida Science, 43,* 148–152.

Kavasch, E. B. 1977. *Native Harvests.* New York: Random House.

Kavasch, E. B. 1995. *Enduring Harvests.* Old Saybrook, CN: Globe Pequot Press.

Keegan, M. 1977. *Pueblo and Navajo Cookery.* Dobbs Ferry, NY: Earth Books.

Kimball, Y., & Anderson, J. 1986. *The Art of American Indian Cooking.* New York: Simon & Schuster.

Kuhnlein, H. V. 1995. Benefits and risks of traditional food for indigenous peoples: Focus on dietary intakes of Arctic men. *Canadian Journal of Physiological Pharmacology, 73,* 765–771.

Kunitz, S. J., & Levy, J. E. 1981. Navajos. In A. Harwood (Ed.), *Ethnicity and Medical Care.* Cambridge, MA: Harvard University Press.

McClelland, D. A. 1992. *Good as Gold: Foods the Americas Gave the World.* Washington, DC: A Smithsonian Quincentenary Publication.

Mermelstein, N. H. 1992. Seeds of change: The Smithsonian Institution's Columbus Quincentenary Exhibition. *Food Technology, 46,* 86–89.

Nabhan, G. P. 1997. *Gathering the Desert.* Tucson, AZ: University of Arizona Press.

Niethammer, C. 1974. *American Indian Food and Lore.* New York: Macmillan.

Pelican, S., & Bachman-Carter, K. 1991. *Navajo Food Practices, Customs, and Holidays.* Chicago: American Dietetic Association/American Diabetes Association.

Perl, L. 1965. *Red-Flannel Hash and Shoo-fly Pie.* Cleveland: World.

Primeaux, M., & Henderson, G. 1981. American Indian patient care. In G. Henderson & M. Primeaux (Eds.), *Transcultural Health Care.* Menlo Park, CA: Addison-Wesley.

Reddy, M. A. (Ed.). 1993. *Statistical Record of Native North Americans.* Washington, DC: Gale Research.

Schilling, B., & Brannon, E. 1986. *Cross-Cultural Counseling: A Guide for Nutrition and Health Counselors.* Alexandria, VA: U.S. Department of Agriculture/U.S. Department of Health and Human Services, FNS #250.

Smith, C. J., Nelson, R. G., Hardy, S. A., Manahan, E. M., Bennett, P. H., & Knowler, W. C. 1996. Survey of the diet of Pima Indians using quantitative food frequency assessment and 24-hour recall. *Journal of the American Dietetic Association, 96,* 778–784.

Spicer, E. H. 1980. American Indians. In S. Thernstrom, A. Orlov, & O. Handlin (Eds.), *Harvard Encyclopedia of American Ethnic Groups.* Cambridge, MA: The Belknap Press of Harvard University Press.

Storey, M., Bass, M. A., & Wakefield, L. M. 1986. Food preferences of Cherokee teenagers in Cherokee, North Carolina. *Ecology of Food and Nutrition, 19,* 51–59.

Terry, R. D., & Bass, M. A. 1984. Food practices in an eastern Cherokee township. *Ecology of Food and Nutrition, 14,* 63–70.

Teufel, N. I., & Dufour, D. L. 1990. Patterns of food use and nutrient intake of obese and non-obese Hualapai Indian women in Arizona. *Journal of the American Dietetic Association, 90,* 1229–1235.

Thernstrom, S., Orlov, A., & Handin, O. (Eds.). 1980. *Harvard Encyclopedia of American Ethnic Groups.* Cambridge, MA: The Belknap Press of Harvard University Press.

Vaughn, I. A., Benyshek, D. C., & Martin, J. F. 1997. Food acquisition habits, nutrient intakes, and anthropometric data of Havasupai adults. *Journal of the American Dietetic Association, 97,* 1275.

Vogel, V. J. 1981. American Indian medicine. In G. Henderson & M. Primeaux (Eds.), *Transcultural Health Care.* Menlo Park, CA: Addison-Wesley.

Wilson, U. M. 1983. Nursing care of American Indian patients. In M. S. Orque, B. Bloch, & L. S. A. Monrroy (Eds.), *Ethnic Nursing Care: A Multicultural Approach.* St. Louis: Mosby.

Wolfe, W. S., & Sanjur, D. 1988. Contemporary diet and body weight of Navajo women receiving food assistance: An ethnographic and nutritional investigation. *Journal of the American Dietetic Association, 88,* 822–827.

Wolfe, W. S., Weber, C. W., & Arviso, K. D. 1985. Use and nutrient composition of traditional Navajo foods. *Ecology of Food and Nutrition, 17,* 323–326.

CHAPTER 4

Alexander, J. G. 1995. Slovak Americans. In R. J. Vecoli, J. Galens, A. Sheets, & R. V. Young (Eds.), *Gale Encyclopedia of Multicultural America.* New York: Gale Research.

Anderson, J. 1986. *The Food of Portugal.* New York: Morrow.

Andrews, C. 1988. *Catalan Cuisine.* New York: Atheneum.

Axtell, R. E. 1991. *Gestures: The Do's and Taboos of Body Language around the World.* New York: Wiley.

Bailey, A. 1969. *The Cooking of the British Isles.* New York: Time-Life Books.

Barer-Stein, T. 1981. *You Eat What You Are: A Study of Ethnic Food Traditions.* Toronto: McClelland & Stewart.

Barron, E. R. 1980. French Canadians. In S. Thernstrom, A. Orlov, & O. Handlin (Eds.), *Harvard Encyclopedia of American Ethnic Groups.* Cambridge, MA: The Belknap Press of Harvard University Press.

Beijborn, U. 1980. Swedes. In S. Thernstrom, A. Orlov, & O. Handlin (Eds.), *Harvard Encyclopedia of American Ethnic Groups.* Cambridge, MA: The Belknap Press of Harvard University Press.

Benkart, P. 1980. Hungarians. In S. Thernstrom, A. Orlov, & O. Handlin (Eds.), *Harvard Encyclopedia of American Ethnic Groups.* Cambridge, MA: The Belknap Press of Harvard University Press.

Berthoff, R. 1980. Welsh. In S. Thernstrom, A. Orlov, & O. Handlin (Eds.), *Harvard Encyclopedia of American Ethnic Groups.* Cambridge, MA: The Belknap Press of Harvard University Press.

Boyd, L. 1979. *British Cookery.* Woodstock, NY: Overlook Press.

Brandon, E. 1976. Folk medicine in French Louisiana. In W. D. Hand (Ed.), *American Folk Medicine*. Berkeley: University of California Press.

Brown, D. 1968. *The Cooking of Scandinavia*. New York: Time-Life Books.

Bugialli, G. 1984. *Guiliano Bugialli's Foods of Italy*. New York: Stewart, Tabori & Chang.

Casas, P. 1983. *The Foods and Wines of Spain*. New York: Knopf.

Chance, J. L. D. 1985. *Ma Chance's French Caribbean Creole Cooking*. New York: Putnam.

Colahan, C. 1995. Spanish Americans. In R. J. Vecoli, J. Galens, A. Sheets, & R. V. Young (Eds.), *Gale Encyclopedia of Multicultural America*. New York: Gale Research.

Conzen, K. N. 1980. Germans. In S. Thernstrom, A. Orlov, & O. Handlin (Eds.), *Harvard Encyclopedia of American Ethnic Groups*. Cambridge, MA: The Belknap Press of Harvard University Press.

Derecskey, S. 1972. *The Hungarian Cookbook*. New York: Harper & Row.

Donaldson, G. 1980. Scots. In S. Thernstrom, A. Orlov, & O. Handlin (Eds.), *Harvard Encyclopedia of American Ethnic Groups*. Cambridge, MA: The Belknap Press of Harvard University Press.

Douglass, W. A. 1980. Basques. In S. Thernstrom, A. Orlov, & O. Handlin (Eds.), *Harvard Encyclopedia of American Ethnic Groups*. Cambridge, MA: The Belknap Press of Harvard University Press.

Eckstein, E. F. 1983. *Menu Planning* (3rd ed.). Westport, CT: AVI.

Erickson, C. J. 1980. English. In S. Thernstrom, A. Orlov, & O. Handlin (Eds.), *Harvard Encyclopedia of American Ethnic Groups*. Cambridge, MA: The Belknap Press of Harvard University Press.

Feibleman, P. S. 1969. *The Cooking of Spain and Portugal*. New York: Time-Life Books.

Feibleman, P. S. 1971. *American Cooking: Creole and Acadian*. New York: Time-Life Books.

Ferro-Luzzi, A., & Branca, F. 1995. Mediterranean diet, Italian-style: Prototype of a healthy diet. *American Journal of Clinical Nutrition, 61* (suppl.), 1338S–1354S.

Field, M., & Field, F. 1970. *A Quintet of Cuisines*. New York: Time-Life Books.

Fisher, M. F. K. 1969. *The Cooking of Provincial France*. New York: Time-Life Books.

FitzGibbon, T. 1968. *A Taste of Ireland: Irish Traditional Food*. New York: Avenal Books.

Freeze, K. J. 1980. Czechs. In S. Thernstrom, A. Orlov, & O. Handlin (Eds.), *Harvard Encyclopedia of American Ethnic Groups*. Cambridge, MA: The Belknap Press of Harvard University Press.

Geissler, E. M. 1998. *Pocket Guide to Cultural Assessment* (2nd ed.). St. Louis, MO: Mosby.

Granquist, M. A. 1995. Swedish Americans. In R. J. Vecoli, J. Galens, A. Sheets, & R. V. Young (Eds.), *Gale Encyclopedia of Multicultural America*. New York: Gale Research.

Greeley, A. M. 1972. *That Most Distressful Nation: The Taming of the American Irish*. Chicago: Quadrangle Books.

Greene, V. 1980. Poles. In S. Thernstrom, A. Orlov, & O. Handlin (Eds.), *Harvard Encyclopedia of American Ethnic Groups*. Cambridge, MA: The Belknap Press of Harvard University Press.

Hall, E. T., & Hall, M. R. 1990. *Understanding Cultural Differences: Germans, French, and Americans*. Yarmouth, ME: Intercultural Press.

Hancock, I. 1991. Romani food ways: Gypsy culinary culture. *World and I, June*, 666–677.

Hanft, S. 1995. English Americans. In R. J. Vecoli, J. Galens, A. Sheets, & R. V. Young (Eds.), *Gale Encyclopedia of Multicultural America*. New York: Gale Research.

Harwood, A. 1981. *Ethnicity and Medical Care*. Cambridge, MA: Harvard University Press.

Hazelton, N. S. 1969. *The Cooking of Germany*. New York: Time-Life Books.

Hazelton, N. S. 1987. *Classic Scandinavian Cooking*. New York: Scribner's.

Heberle, M. O. 1985. *Polish Cooking*. Tucson, AZ: HP Books.

Heimlich, E. 1995a. Acadian Americans. In R. J. Vecoli, J. Galens, A. Sheets, & R. V. Young (Eds.), *Gale Encyclopedia of Multicultural America*. New York: Gale Research.

Heimlich, E. 1995b. Gypsy Americans. In R. J. Vecoli, J. Galens, A. Sheets, & R. V. Young (Eds.), *Gale Encyclopedia of Multicultural America*. New York: Gale Research.

Higonnet, P. L. R. 1980. French. In S. Thernstrom, A. Orlov, & O. Handlin (Eds.), *Harvard Encyclopedia of American Ethnic Groups*. Cambridge, MA: The Belknap Press of Harvard University Press.

Hillstrom, L. C. 1995. French Americans. In R. J. Vecoli, J. Galens, A. Sheets, & R. V. Young (Eds.), *Gale Encyclopedia of Multicultural America*. New York: Gale Research.

Hoglund, A. W. 1980. Finns. In S. Thernstrom, A. Orlov, & O. Handlin (Eds.), *Harvard Encyclopedia of American Ethnic Groups*. Cambridge, MA: The Belknap Press of Harvard University Press.

Hostetler, J. A. 1976. Folk medicine and sympathy healing among the Amish. In W. D. Hand (Ed.), *American Folk Medicine*. Berkeley: University of California Press.

Jones, M. A. 1980. Scotch-Irish. In S. Thernstrom, A. Orlov, & O. Handlin (Eds.), *Harvard Encyclopedia of American Ethnic Groups*. Cambridge, MA: The Belknap Press of Harvard University Press.

Jones, S. 1995a. Austrian Americans. In R. J. Vecoli, J. Galens, A. Sheets, & R. V. Young (Eds.), *Gale Encyclopedia of Multicultural America*. New York: Gale Research.

Jones, S. 1995b. Polish Americans. In R. J. Vecoli, J. Galens, A. Sheets, & R. V. Young (Eds.), *Gale Encyclopedia of Multicultural America*. New York: Gale Research.

Kinsella, M. 1983. *An Irish Farmhouse Cookbook*. Belfast: Appletree Press.

Kraybill, D. B. 1995. Amish Americans. In R. J. Vecoli, J. Galens, A. Sheets, & R. V. Young (Eds.), *Gale Encyclopedia of Multicultural America*. New York: Gale Research.

LeBreton, M. M. 1980. Acadians. In S. Thernstrom, A. Orlov, & O. Handlin (Eds.), *Harvard Encyclopedia of American Ethnic Groups,* Cambridge, MA: The Belknap Press of Harvard University Press.

Leistner, C. G. 1996. *Cajun and Creole Food Practices, Customs, and Holidays*. Chicago: American Dietetic Association/American Diabetes Association.

Leonard, J. N. 1971. *American Cooking: New England*. New York: Time-Life Books.

Lockwood, Y. R., & Lockwood, W. G. 1991. Pasties in Michigan's Upper Peninsula. In S. Stern & J. A. Cicala (Eds.), *Creative Ethnicity: Symbols and Strategies of Contemporary Ethnic Life*. Logan: Utah State University Press.

Lovoll, O. S. 1995. Norwegian Americans. In R. J. Vecoli, J. Galens, A. Sheets, & R. V. Young (Eds.), *Gale Encyclopedia of Multicultural America*. New York: Gale Research.

Magocsi, P. R. 1980. Russians. In S. Thernstrom, A. Orlov, & O. Handlin (Eds.), *Harvard Encyclopedia of American Ethnic Groups.* Cambridge, MA: The Belknap Press of Harvard University Press.

Magocsi, P. R. 1995. Russian Americans. In R. J. Vecoli, J. Galens, A. Sheets, & R. V. Young (Eds.), *Gale Encyclopedia of Multicultural America.* New York: Gale Research.

Martin, P. 1981. *The Czech Book: Recipes and Traditions.* Iowa City, IA: Penfield Press.

Molinari, C. 1995. Czech Americans. In R. J. Vecoli, J. Galens, A. Sheets, & R. V. Young (Eds.), *Gale Encyclopedia of Multicultural America.* New York: Gale Research.

Morrison, T., Conaway, W. A. & Borden, G. A. 1994. *Kiss, Bow, or Shake Hands.* Holbrook, MA: Adams.

Munch, P. 1980. Norwegians. In S. Thernstrom, A. Orlov, & O. Handlin (Eds.), *Harvard Encyclopedia of American Ethnic Groups.* Cambridge, MA: The Belknap Press of Harvard University Press.

Nelli, H. S. 1980. Italians. In S. Thernstrom, A. Orlov, & O. Handlin (Eds.), *Harvard Encyclopedia of American Ethnic Groups.* Cambridge, MA: The Belknap Press of Harvard University Press.

Nelli, H. S. 1983. *From Immigrants to Ethnics: The Italian American.* Oxford: Oxford University Press.

Nielsen, M., & Peterson, P. L. 1995. Danish Americans. In R. J. Vecoli, J. Galens, A. Sheets, & R. V. Young (Eds.), *Gale Encyclopedia of Multicultural America.* New York: Gale Research.

Norden, E. E. 1995. Portuguese Americans. In R. J. Vecoli, J. Galens, A. Sheets, & R. V. Young (Eds.), *Gale Encyclopedia of Multicultural America.* New York: Gale Research.

Ojakangas, B. 1992. *Scandinavian Feasts.* New York: Stewart, Tabori & Chang.

Pap, L. 1981. *The Portuguese-American.* Boston: Twayne.

Papashvily, H., & Papashvily, G. 1969. *Russian Cooking.* New York: Time-Life Books.

Parker, A. 1980. Austrians. In S. Thernstrom, A. Orlov, & O. Handlin (Eds.), *Harvard Encyclopedia of American Ethnic Groups.* Cambridge, MA: The Belknap Press of Harvard University Press.

Perl, L. 1965. *Red-Flannel Hash and Shoo-fly Pie.* Cleveland: World.

Pozzetta, G. 1995. Italian Americans. In R. J. Vecoli, J. Galens, A. Sheets, & R. V. Young (Eds.), *Gale Encyclopedia of Multicultural America.* New York: Gale Research.

Ragucci, A. T. 1981. Italian Americans. In A. Harwood (Ed.), *Ethnicity and Medical Care.* Cambridge, MA: Harvard University Press.

Rapple, B. A. 1995. Irish Americans. In R. J. Vecoli, J. Galens, A. Sheets, & R. V. Young (Eds.), *Gale Encyclopedia of Multicultural America.* New York: Gale Research.

Rippley, L. J. 1980. Germans from Russia. In S. Thernstrom, A. Orlov, & O. Handlin (Eds.), *Harvard Encyclopedia of American Ethnic Groups.* Cambridge, MA: The Belknap Press of Harvard University Press.

Rippley, L. J. 1995. German Americans. In R. J. Vecoli, J. Galens, A. Sheets, & R. V. Young (Eds.), *Gale Encyclopedia of Multicultural America.* New York: Gale Research.

Roden, C. 1987. *Mediterranean Cookery.* New York: Knopf.

Rogers, A. 1968. *A Basque Story Cook Book.* New York: Scribner's.

Rogers, M. R. 1980. Portuguese. In S. Thernstrom, A. Orlov, & O. Handlin (Eds.), *Harvard Encyclopedia of American Eth-*

nic Groups. Cambridge, MA: The Belknap Press of Harvard University Press.

Root, W. 1966. *Foods of France.* New York: Vintage Press.

Root, W., & DeRochemont, R. 1976. *Eating in America.* New York: Ecco Press.

Schelbert, L. 1995. Swiss Americans. In R. J. Vecoli, J. Galens, A. Sheets, & R. V. Young (Eds.), *Gale Encyclopedia of Multicultural America.* New York: Gale Research.

Shenton, J. P., Pellegrini, A. M., Brown, D., & Shenker, I. 1971. *American Cooking: The Melting Pot.* New York: Time-Life Books.

Skardel, D. B. 1974. *The Divided Heart.* Lincoln: University of Nebraska Press.

Skardel, D. B. 1980. Danes. In S. Thernstrom, A. Orlov, & O. Handlin (Eds.), *Harvard Encyclopedia of American Ethnic Groups.* Cambridge, MA: The Belknap Press of Harvard University Press.

Spector, R. E. 1991. *Cultural Diversity in Health and Illness* (3rd ed.). Norwalk, CT: Appleton & Lange.

Stolarik, M. M. 1980. Slovaks. In S. Thernstrom, A. Orlov, & O. Handlin (Eds.), *Harvard Encyclopedia of American Ethnic Groups.* Cambridge, MA: The Belknap Press of Harvard University Press.

Sutherland, A. 1992. Gypsies and health care. *Western Journal of Medicine, 157,* 276–280.

Várdy, S. B., & Szendrey, T. 1995. Hungarian Americans. In R. J. Vecoli, J. Galens, A. Sheets, & R. V. Young (Eds.), *Gale Encyclopedia of Multicultural America.* New York: Gale Research.

Visson, L. 1982. *The Complete Russian Cookbook.* Ann Arbor, MI: Ardis.

Wargelin, M. 1995. Finnish Americans. In R. J. Vecoli, J. Galens, A. Sheets, & R. V. Young (Eds.), *Gale Encyclopedia of Multicultural America.* New York: Gale Research.

Weaver, W. W. 1982. *Sauerkraut Yankees: Pennsylvania-German Foods and Foodways.* Philadelphia: University of Philadelphia Press.

Wechsberg, J. 1968. *The Cooking of Vienna's Empire.* New York: Time-Life Books.

Willet, W. C., Sacks, F., Trichopoulou, A., Drescher, G., Ferro-Luzzi, A., Helsing, E., & Trichopoulos, D. 1995. Mediterranean diet pyramid: A cultural model for healthy eating. *American Journal of Clinical Nutrition, 61* (suppl.), 1402S–1406S.

Wilson, J. 1971. *American Cooking: The Eastern Heartland.* New York: Time-Life Books.

Yoder, D. 1976. Hohman and Romanus: Origins and diffusion of Pennsylvania German powwow manual. In W. D. Hand (Ed.), *American Folk Medicine.* Berkeley: University of California Press.

Zeranska, A. 1989. *The Art of Polish Cooking.* Gretna, LA: Pelican.

CHAPTER 5

Bigelow, B. C. 1995. African Americans. In R. J. Vecoli, J. Galens, A. Sheets, & R. V. Young (Eds.), *Gale Encyclopedia of Multicultural America.* New York: Gale Research.

Byars, D. 1996. Traditional African American foods and African Americans. *Agriculture and Human Values, 13,* 74–78.

Brandon, E. 1976. Folk medicine in French Louisiana. In W. D. Hand (Ed.), *American Folk Medicine.* Los Angeles: University of California Press.

Burke, C. B., & Raia, S. P. 1995. *Soul and Traditional Southern*

Food Practices, Customs, and Holidays. Chicago: American Dietetic Association/American Diabetes Association.

Cussler, M., & DeGive, M. L. 1952. *'Twixt the Cup and the Lip.* New York: Twayne.

DeWitt, D., Wilan, M. J., & Stock, M. 1998. *Flavors of Africa Cookbook.* Rocklin, CA: Prima.

Eckstein, E. F. 1983. Foodways of blacks. In *Menu Planning* (3rd ed.). Westport, CT: AVI.

Emmons, L. 1986. Food procurement and the nutritional adequacy of diets in low-income families. *Journal of the American Dietetic Association, 86,* 1684-1693.

Fitzgerald, T. K. 1979. Southern folks' eating habits ain't what they used to be . . . if they ever were. *Nutrition Today, 14,* 16-21.

Gladney, V. M. 1972. *Food Practices of Some Black Americans in Los Angeles County.* Los Angeles: County of Los Angeles Department of Health Services.

Hafner, D. 1993. *A Taste of Africa.* Berkeley, CA: Ten Speed Press.

Harris, J. B. 1998. The *Africa Cookbook: Tastes of a Continent.* New York: Simon & Schuster.

Holt, T. 1980. Afro-Americans. In S. Thernstrom, A. Orlov, & O. Handlin (Eds.), *Harvard Encyclopedia of Ethnic Groups.* Cambridge, MA: The Belknap Press of the Harvard University Press.

Horner, R. D., Lackey, C. J., Kolasa, K., & Warren, K. 1991. Pica practices of pregnant women. *Journal of the American Dietetic Association, 91,* 34-38.

Hunter, J. M. 1973. Geophagy in Africa and the United States. *Geographical Review, 63,* 170-195.

Jackson, B. 1976. The other kind of doctor: Conjure and magic in black American folk medicine. In W. D. Hand (Ed.), *American Folk Medicine.* Los Angeles: University of California Press.

Jackson, J. J. 1981. Urban black Americans. In A. Harwood (Ed.), *Ethnicity and Medical Care.* Cambridge, MA: Harvard University Press.

Jerome, N. W. 1969. Northern urbanization and food consumption of Southern- born Negroes. *American Journal of Clinical Nutrition, 22,* 1667-1669.

Kant, A. K., Block, G., Schatzkin, A., Ziegler, R. G., & Nestle, M. 1991. Dietary diversity in the U.S. population NHANES II, 1976-1980. *Journal of the American Dietetic Association, 91,* 34-38.

Lackey, C. J. 1982. Pica—pregnancy's etiological mystery. In *Alternative Dietary Practices and Nutritional Abuses in Pregnancy.* Washington, DC: National Academy Press.

Mbiti, J. S. 1970. *African Religions and Philosophy.* Garden City, NY: Doubleday Anchor.

Mendes, H. 1971. *African Heritage Cookbook.* New York: Macmillan.

Newman, J. M. 1984. *The Melting Pot.* New York: Garland.

Randall-David, E. 1989. *Strategies for Working with Culturally Diverse Communities and Clients.* Bethesda, MD: Association for the Care of Children's Health.

Rotberg, R. I. 1996. African history. In *The 1996 Grolier Multimedia Encyclopedia.* Danbury, CT: Grolier Electronic Publishing.

Snow, L. F. 1983. Traditional health beliefs and practices among lower-class black Americans. *Western Journal of Medicine, 139,* 820-828.

Spector, R. E. 1991. *Cultural Diversity in Health and Illness* (3rd ed.). Norwalk, CT: Appleton & Lange.

Spindler, A. A., & Akosionu, N. 1985. Gross composition and crude and dietary fiber content of soups made with African mango seeds. *Nutrition Reports International, 31,* 1165-1169.

Thomas, D. N. 1981. Black American patient care. In G. Henderson & M. Primeaux (Eds.), *Transcultural Health Care.* Menlo Park, CA: Addison-Wesley.

Van der Post, L. 1970. *African Cooking.* New York: Time-Life Books.

Van der Post, L. 1978. *First Catch Your Eland.* New York: Morrow.

Walter, E. 1971. The South's great gift of soul food. In *American Cooking: Southern Style.* New York: Time-Life Books.

Wheeler, M., & Haider, S. Q. 1979. Buying and food preparation patterns of ghetto blacks and Hispanics in Brooklyn. *Journal of the American Dietetic Association, 75,* 560-563.

Wilson, E. G. 1971. *A West African Cookbook.* New York: Avon Books.

Wyant, K. W., & Meiselman, H. L. 1984. Sex and race differences in food preferences of military personnel. *Journal of the American Dietetic Association, 84,* 169-175.

CHAPTER 6

Algert, S. J., & Ellison, T. H. 1989. *Mexican American Food Practices, Customs, and Holidays. Ethnic and Regional Food Practices* (Series). Chicago: American Dietetic Association/American Diabetes Association.

Axtell, R. E. 1991. *Gestures: The Do's and Taboos of Body Language Around the World.* New York: Wiley.

Barer-Stein, T. 1979. *You Are What You Eat.* Toronto: McClelland & Stewart.

Barrett, B. 1995. Ethnomedical interactions: Health and identity on Nicaragua's Atlantic coast. *Social Science and Medicine, 40,* 1611-1621.

Boyle, J. S. 1989. Constructs of health promotion and wellness in a Salvadoran population. *Public Health Nursing, 6,* 129-134.

Boyle, J. S. 1991. Transcultural nursing care of Central American refugees. *National Student Nurses Association, Inc./Imprint, April/May,* 73-77.

Bruhn, C. M., & Pangborn, R. M. 1971. Food habits of migrant workers in California. *Journal of the American Dietetic Association, 59,* 347-355.

Buffington, S. T. 1995a. Cuban Americans. In R. J. Vecoli, J. Galens, A. Sheets, & R. V. Young (Eds.), *Gale Encyclopedia of Multicultural America.* New York: Gale Research.

Buffington, S. T. 1995b. Dominicans. In R. J. Vecoli, J. Galens, A. Sheets, R. V. Young (Eds.), *Gale Encyclopedia of Multicultural America.* New York: Gale Research.

Bullough, V., & Bullough, B. 1981. The Spanish-speaking minority groups. In *Health Care for the Other Americans.* New York: Springer.

Chase, C. S. 1995. Costa Rican Americans. In R. J. Vecoli, J. Galens, A. Sheets, & R. V. Young (Eds.), *Gale Encyclopedia of Multicultural America.* New York: Gale Research.

Chávez, N., Sha, L., Persky, V., Langenberg, P., & Pestano-Binghay, E. 1994. Effect of length of stay on food group intake in Mexican and Puerto Rican women. *Journal of Nutrition Education, 26,* 79-86.

Cortez, C. E. 1980. Mexicans. In S. Thernstrom, A. Orlov, & O. Handlin (Eds.), *Harvard Encyclopedia of American Ethnic Groups.* Cambridge, MA: The Belknap Press of Harvard University Press.

Cravioto, R., Lockhart, E. E., Anderson, R. K., Miranda, F., & Harris, R. S. 1945. Composition of typical Mexican foods. *Journal of Nutrition, 29,* 317-329.

Dewey, K. G., Strode, M. A., & Ruiz Fitch, Y. 1984. Dietary change among migrant and nonmigrant Mexican-American families in northern California. *Ecology of Food and Nutrition, 14,* 11-24.

DiSogra, L., Abrams, B., & Hudes, M. 1994. Low prevalence of healthful dietary behaviors in a California agricultural county: Emphasis on white and Mexican-American adults. *Journal of the American Dietetic Association, 94,* 544-546.

Duyff, R. L., Sanjur, D., & Nelson, H. V. 1975. Food behavior and related factors of Puerto Rican teenagers. *Journal of Nutrition Education, 7,* 99-103.

Eckstein, E. F. 1983a. Foodways of Chicanos. In *Menu Planning* (3rd ed.). Westport, CT: AVI.

Eckstein, E. F. 1983b. Foodways of Puerto Ricans and Cubans living in the United States. In *Menu Planning* (3rd ed.). Westport, CT: AVI.

Fitzpatrick, J. P. 1980. Puerto Ricans. In S. Thernstrom, A. Orlov, & O. Handlin (Eds.), *Harvard Encyclopedia of American Ethnic Groups.* Cambridge, MA: The Belknap Press of Harvard University Press.

Geissler, E. M. 1998. *Pocket Guide to Cultural Assessment* (2nd ed.). St. Louis, MO: Mosby.

Gladney, V. M. 1966. *Food Practices of Mexican Americans in Los Angeles County.* Los Angeles: Los Angeles County Health Department.

Graham, J. S. 1976. The role of the *curandero* in the Mexican American folk medicine system in west Texas. In W. D. Hand (Ed.), *American Folk Medicine.* Los Angeles: University of California Press.

Granger, B. H. 1976. Some aspects of folk medicine among Spanish-speaking people in southern Arizona. In W. D. Hand (Ed.), *American Folk Medicine.* Los Angeles: University of California Press.

Green, D. 1995. Puerto Ricans. In R. J. Vecoli, J. Galens, A. Sheets, & R. V. Young (Eds.), *Gale Encyclopedia of Multicultural America.* New York: Gale Research.

Guendelman, S., & Abrams, B. 1995. Dietary intake among Mexican-American women: Generational differences and a comparison with white non-Hispanic women. *American Journal of Public Health, 85,* 20-25.

Haider, S. Q., & Wheeler, M. 1979. Nutritive intake of black and Hispanic mothers in a Brooklyn ghetto. *Journal of the American Dietetic Association, 75,* 670-673.

Harris, M. 1985. *Good to Eat: Riddles of Food and Culture.* New York: Simon & Schuster.

Harris, J. B. 1992. *Tasting Brazil: Regional Recipes and Reminiscences.* New York: Macmillan.

Harwood, A. 1981. Mainland Puerto Ricans. In A. Harwood (Ed.), *Ethnicity and Medical Care.* Cambridge, MA: Harvard University Press.

Hong, M. 1995. Guatemalan Americans. In R. J. Vecoli, J. Galens, A. Sheets, & R. V. Young (Eds.), *Gale Encyclopedia of Multicultural America.* New York: Gale Research.

Ikeda, J., & Gonzales, M. M. 1986. *Food Habits of Hispanics Newly Immigrated to the San Francisco Bay Area* (abstract). Oakland, CA: California Dietetic Association annual meeting.

Immink, M. D. C., Sanjur, D., & Burgos, M. 1983. Nutritional consequences of U.S. migration patterns among Puerto Rican women. *Ecology of Food and Nutrition, 13,* 139-148.

Ingham, J. M. 1970. On Mexican folk medicine. *American Anthropologist, 72,* 76-87.

Kay, M. A. 1977. Health and illness in a Mexican American barrio. In E. H. Spicer (Ed.), *Ethnic Medicine in the Southwest.* Tucson: University of Arizona Press.

Laguerre, M. S. 1981. Haitian Americans. In A. Harwood (Ed.), *Ethnicity and Medical Care.* Cambridge. MA: Harvard University Press.

Leonard, J. N. 1968. *Latin American Cooking.* New York: Time-Life Books.

Maduro, R. 1983. *Curanderismo* and Latin views of disease and curing. *Western Journal of Medicine, 139,* 868-874.

Marks, C. 1985. *False Tongues and Sunday Bread: A Guatemalan and Mayan Cookbook.* New York: Evans.

Maxwell, W. 1995. Honduran Americans. In R. J. Vecoli, J. Galens, A. Sheets, & R. V. Young (Eds.), *Gale Encyclopedia of Multicultural America.* New York: Gale Research.

McGee, H. 1984. *On Food and Cooking: The Science and Lore of the Kitchen.* New York: Scribner.

Melville, M. B. 1985. Salvadorans and Guatemalans. In D. W. Haines (Ed.), *Refugees in the United States.* Westport, CT: Greenwood Press.

Messer, E. 1981. Hot/cold classification: Theoretical and practical implications of a Mexican study. *Social Science and Medicine, 158,* 133-145.

Miller, M. E. 1996. Mayans. In *The 1996 Grolier Multimedia Encyclopedia.* Danbury, CT: Grolier Electronic Publishing.

Miller, R. 1996. Central America. In *The 1996 Grolier Multimedia Encyclopedia.* Danbury, CT: Grolier Electronic Publishing.

Miralles, M. A. 1989. *A Matter of Life and Death: Health-Seeking Behavior of Guatemalan Refugees in South Florida.* New York: AMS Press.

Monrroy, L. S. 1983. Nursing care of Raza/Latina patients. In M. S. Orque, B. Bloch, & L. S. A. Monrroy (Eds.), *Ethnic Nursing Care: A Multicultural Approach.* St. Louis: Mosby.

Morrison, T., Conaway, W. A., & Borden, G. A. 1994. *Kiss, Bow, or Shake Hands.* Holbrook, MA: Bob Adams.

Mumford, J. 1995. Salvadoran Americans. In R. J. Vecoli, J. Galens, A. Sheets, & R. V. Young (Eds.), *Gale Encyclopedia of Multicultural America.* New York: Gale Research.

Murphy, S. P., Castillo, R. O., Martorell, R., & Mendoza, F. S. 1990. An evaluation of food group intakes by Mexican-American children. *Journal of the American Dietetic Association, 90,* 388-393.

Orlov, A., & Ueda, R. 1980. Central and South Americans. In S. Thernstrom, A. Orlov, & O. Handlin (Eds.), *Harvard Encyclopedia of American Ethnic Groups.* Cambridge, MA: The Belknap Press of Harvard University Press.

Ortiz, E. L. 1979. *The Book of Latin American Cooking.* New York: Vintage Books.

Pasquali, E. A. 1985. The impact of acculturation on the eating habits of elderly immigrants: A Cuban example. *Journal of Nutrition for the Elderly, 5,* 27-36.

Pasquali, E. A. 1994. Santeria. *Journal of Holistic Nursing, 12,* 380-390.

Perez, L. 1980. Cubans. In S. Thernstrom, A. Orlov, & O. Handlin (Eds.), *Harvard Encyclopedia of American Ethnic Groups.* Cambridge, MA: The Belknap Press of Harvard University Press.

Peterson, D., & Peterson, J. 1995. *Eat Smart in Brazil.* Madison, WI: Gingko Press.

Randall-David, E. 1989. *Strategies for Working with Culturally Diverse Communities and Clients.* Bethesda, MD: Association for the Care of Children's Health.

Risser, A., & Mazur, L. J. 1995. Use of folk remedies in a Hispanic population. *Archives of Pediatric and Adolescent Medicine, 149,* 978-981.

Rodriguez, J. 1995. Argentinean Americans. In R. J. Vecoli, J. Galens, A. Sheets, & R. V. Young (Eds.), *Gale Encyclopedia of Multicultural America.* New York: Gale Research.

Rojas-Lombardi, F. 1991. *The Art of South American Cooking.* New York: HarperCollins.

Romero-Gwynn, E., Gwynn, D., Grivetti, L., McDonald, R., Stanford, G., Turner, B., West, E., & Williamson, E. 1993. Dietary acculturation among Latinos of Mexican descent. *Nutrition Today, 28,* 6-12.

Sanjur, D. 1982. *Social and Cultural Perspectives in Nutrition.* Englewood Cliffs, NJ: Prentice-Hall.

Sanjur, D. 1995. *Hispanic Foodways, Nutrition, and Health.* Boston: Allyn & Bacon.

Smagula, S. 1995. Nicaraguan Americans. In R. J. Vecoli, J. Galens, A. Sheets, & R. V. Young (Eds.), *Gale Encyclopedia of Multicultural America.* New York: Gale Research.

Smith, L. 1979. Mexican-American views of Anglo medical and dietetic practices. *Journal of the American Dietetic Association, 74,* 463-464.

Spector, R. E. 1991. *Cultural Diversity in Health and Illness* (3rd ed.). Norwalk, CT: Appleton & Lange.

Umaña-Murray, M. 1996. *Three Generations of Chilean Cuisine.* Los Angeles: Lowell House.

Unaeze, F. E., & Perrin, R. E. 1995. Haitians. In R. J. Vecoli, J. Galens, A. Sheets, & R. V. Young (Eds.), *Gale Encyclopedia of Multicultural America.* New York: Gale Research.

Valle, V. M., & Valle, M. L. 1995. *Recipe of Memory: Five Generations of Mexican Cuisine.* New York: The New Press.

Wallendorf, M., & Reilly, M. D. 1983. Ethnic migration, assimilation, and consumption. *Journal of Consumer Research, 10,* 292-302.

Wheeler, M., & Haider, S. Q. 1979. Buying and food preparation patterns of ghetto blacks and Hispanics in Brooklyn. *Journal of the American Dietetic Association, 75,* 560-563.

Wolfe, L. 1970. *The Cooking of the Caribbean Islands.* New York: Time-Life Books.

CHAPTER 7

Anderson, E. N. 1987. Why is humoral medicine so popular? *Social Science and Medicine, 25,* 331-337.

Axtell, R. E. 1991. *Gestures: The Do's and Taboos of Body Language Around the World.* New York: Wiley.

Barer-Stein, T. 1981. *You Eat What You Are: A Study of Ethnic Food Traditions* (2nd ed.). Toronto: McClelland & Stewart.

Campbell, T., & Chang, B. 1981. Health care of the Chinese in America. In G. Henderson & M. Primeaux (Eds.), *Transcultural Health Care.* Menlo Park, CA: Addison-Wesley.

Chang, K. C. (Ed.). 1977. *Food in Chinese Culture: Anthropological and Historical Perspectives.* New Haven, CT: Yale University Press.

Chau, P., & Lee, H. S. 1987. *Dietary Habits, Health Beliefs, and Related Food Practices of Female Chinese Elderly.* Master's project, California State University, San Jose.

Chau, P., Lee, H., Tseng, R., & Downes, N. J. 1990. Dietary habits, health beliefs, and food practices of elderly Chinese women. *Journal of the American Dietetic Association, 90,* 579-580.

Chen, P. K., Chen, T. C., & Tseng, R. 1983. *Everything You Want to Know about Chinese Cooking.* Woodbury, NY: Barron's.

Chen-Louie, T. 1983. Nursing care of Chinese American Patients.

In M. S. Orque, B. Bloch, & L. S. A. Monrroy (Eds.), *Ethnic Nursing Care: A Multicultural Approach.* St. Louis: Mosby.

Chin, S. Y. 1992. This, that, and the other: Managing illness in a first-generation Korean-American family. *Western Journal of Medicine, 157,* 305-309.

Cho, J. O. 1981. *Home-style Korean Cooking in Pictures.* New York: Kodansha International.

Crews, D. E. 1994. Obesity and diabetes. In N. W. S. Zane, D. T. Takeuchi, & K. N. J. Young (Eds.), *Confronting Critical Health Issues of Asian and Pacific Islander Americans.* Thousand Oaks, CA: Sage.

Easton, S. E., & Ellington, L. 1995. Japanese Americans. In R. J. Vecoli, J. Galens, A. Sheets, & R. V. Young (Eds.), *Gale Encyclopedia of Multicultural America.* New York: Gale Research.

Eckstein, E. F. 1983. *Menu Planning* (3rd ed.). Westport, CT: AVI.

Erdman, J. W., & Fordyce, E. J. 1989. Soy products and the human diet. *American Journal of Clinical Nutrition, 49,* 725-737.

Geissler, E. M. 1998. *Pocket Guide to Cultural Assessment* (2nd ed.). St. Louis: Mosby.

Gould-Martin, K., & Ngin, C. 1981. Chinese Americans. In A. Harwood (Ed.), *Ethnicity and Medical Care.* Cambridge, MA: Harvard University Press.

Grivetti, L. E., & Paquette, B. 1978. Nontraditional ethnic food choices among first-generation Chinese in California. *Journal of Nutrition Education, 10,* 109-112.

Hahn, E. 1968. *The Cooking of China.* New York: Time-Life Books.

Hall, R. B. 1996a. North Korea. In *The 1996 Grolier Multimedia Encyclopedia.* Danbury, CT: Grolier Electronic Publishing.

Hall, R. B. 1996b. South Korea. In *The 1996 Grolier Multimedia Encyclopedia.* Danbury, CT: Grolier Electronic Publishing.

Hashizume, S., & Takano, J. 1983. Nursing care of Japanese-American patients. In M. S. Orque, B. Bloch, & L. S. A. Monrroy (Eds.), *Ethnic Nursing Care: A Multicultural Approach.* St. Louis: Mosby.

Hosokawa, B. 1969. *Nisei: The Quiet American.* New York: Morrow.

Ichiro, H., Fujio, I., Tsuneya, W., & Keiichi, Y. 1972. *Japanese Religion.* Palo Alto, CA: Kodansha International.

Kim, H. C. 1980. Koreans. In S. Thernstrom, A. Orlov, & O. Handlin (Eds.), *Harvard Encyclopedia of American Ethnic Groups.* Cambridge, MA: The Belknap Press of Harvard University Press.

Kitano, H. H. 1976. *Japanese-Americans: The Evolution of a Subculture* (2nd ed.). Englewood Cliffs, NJ: Prentice-Hall.

Koh, F. M. 1985. *Creative Korean Cooking.* Minneapolis, MN: East-West Press.

Koo, L. C. 1984. The use of food to treat and prevent disease in Chinese culture. *Social Science and Medicine, 18,* 757-766.

Kwak, J. 1998. *Dok Suni: Recipes from My Mother's Korean Kitchen.* New York: St. Martin's Press.

Lands, E. M., Hamazaki, T., Yamazaki, K., Okuyama, H., Sakai, K., Goto, Y., & Hubbard, V. S. 1990. Changing dietary patterns. *American Journal of Clinical Nutrition, 51,* 991-993.

Latourette, K. S. 1964. *The Chinese: Their History and Culture* (4th ed.). New York: Macmillan.

Lee, C. 1965. *Chinatown, U.S.A.* New York: Doubleday.

Lee, R. H. 1960. *The Chinese in the United States of America.* Hong Kong: Hong Kong University Press.

Lock, M. 1990. Rationalization of Japanese herbal medication: The hegemony of orchestrated pluralism. *Human Organization, 49,* 41-47.

Ludman, E. K., Kang, K. J., & Lynn, L. L. 1992. Food beliefs and diets of pregnant Korean-American women. *Journal of the*

American Dietetic Association, 92, 1519-1520.

Ludman, E. K., & Newman, J. M. 1984. Yin and yang in the health-related food practices of three Chinese groups. *Journal of Nutrition Education, 16,* 3-5.

Ludman, E. K., Newman, J. M., & Lynn, L. L. 1989. Blood-building foods in contemporary Chinese populations. *Journal of the American Dietetic Association, 89,* 1122-1124.

Marks, C., & Kim, M. 1993. *The Korean Kitchen.* San Francisco: Chronicle Books.

Morrison, T., Conaway, W. A., & Borden, G. A. 1994. *Kiss, Bow, or Shake Hands.* Holbrook, MA: Adams.

Nash, A. 1995. Korean Americans. In R. J. Vecoli, J. Galens, A. Sheets, & R. V. Young (Eds.), *Gale Encyclopedia of Multicultural America.* New York: Gale Research.

Newman, J. M. 1998a. China: Transformations of its cuisine, a prelude to understanding its people. *Journal for the Study of Food and Society 2,* 5-6.

Newman, J. M. 1998b. Chinese ingredients: Both usual and unusual. In J. M. Powers (Ed.), *From Cathay to Canada: Chinese Cuisine in Transition.* Willowdale, Ontario: Ontario Historical Society.

Ots, T. 1990. The angry liver, the anxious heart and the melancholy spleen: The phenomenology of perceptions in Chinese culture. *Culture, Medicine, and Psychiatry, 14,* 21-58.

Pang, K. Y. 1989. The practice of traditional Korean medicine in Washington, DC. *Social Science and Medicine, 28,* 875-884.

Pang, K. Y. C. 1991. *Korean Elderly Women in America: Everyday Life, Health, and Illness.* New York: AMS Press.

Pang, K. Y. C. 1994. Understanding depression among elderly Korean immigrants through their folk illnesses. *Medical Anthropology Quarterly, 8,* 209-216.

Randall-David, E. 1989. *Strategies for Working with Culturally Diverse Communities and Clients.* Bethesda, MD: Association for the Care of Children's Health.

Reischauer, E. O. 1974. *Japan: The Story of a Nation.* New York: Knopf.

Schultz, J. D., Spindler, A. A., & Josephson, R. V. 1994. Diet and acculturation in Chinese women. *Journal of Nutrition Education, 26,* 266-272.

Sheikh, A. A., & Sheikh, K. S. (Eds.). 1989. *Eastern and Western Approaches to Healing: Ancient Wisdom and Modern Knowledge.* New York: Wiley.

Spector, R. E. 1991. *Cultural Diversity in Health and Illness* (3rd ed.). Norwalk, CT: Appleton & Lange.

Spindler, A. A., & Schultz, J. D. 1996. Comparison of dietary variety and ethnic food consumption among Chinese, Chinese American, and white women. *Journal of Agriculture and Human Values, 131,* 64-73.

Steinberg, R. 1969. *The Cooking of Japan.* New York: Time-Life Books.

Sun, H. P. 1996. *Dietary Habits, Health Beliefs, and Food Practices of Chinese Americans Living in the San Francisco Bay Area.* Master's thesis, California State University, San Jose.

Wang, L. L. 1995. Chinese Americans. In R. J. Vecoli, J. Galens, A. Sheets, & R. V. Young (Eds.), *Gale Encyclopedia of Multicultural America.* New York: Gale Research.

Yom, M. S., Gordon, B. H. J., & Sucher, K. P. 1995. Korean dietary habits and health beliefs in the San Francisco Bay area. *Journal of the American Dietetic Association, 95* (suppl.), A-98.

Zhou, Y. D., & Britten, H. C. 1994. Increased iron content of some Chinese foods due to cooking in steel woks. *Journal of the American Dietetic Association, 94,* 1153-1154.

CHAPTER 8

Adler, S. R. 1995. Refugee stress and folk belief: Hmong sudden deaths. *Social Science and Medicine, 40,* 1623-1629.

Alejandro, R. 1982. *The Philippine Cookbook.* New York: Coward McCann.

Anderson, J. N. 1983. Health and illness in Filipino immigrants. *Western Journal of Medicine, 139,* 811-819.

Axtell, R. E. 1991. *Gestures: The Do's and Taboos of Body Language around the World.* New York: Wiley.

Bankston, C. L. 1995a. Cambodian Americans. In R. J. Vecoli, J. Galens, A. Sheets, & R. V. Young (Eds.), *Gale Encyclopedia of Multicultural America.* New York: Gale Research.

Bankston, C. L. 1995b. Hmong Americans. In R. J. Vecoli, J. Galens, A. Sheets, & R. V. Young (Eds.), *Gale Encyclopedia of MulticulturalAmerica.* New York: Gale Research.

Bankston, C. L. 1995c. Laotian Americans. In R. J. Vecoli, J. Galens, A. Sheets, & R. V. Young (Eds.), *Gale Encyclopedia of Multicultural America.* New York: Gale Research.

Bankston, C. L. 1995d. Vietnamese Americans. In R. J. Vecoli, J. Galens, A. Sheets, & R. V. Young (Eds.), *Gale Encyclopedia of Multicultural America.* New York: Gale Research.

Bazore, K. 1947. *Hawaiian and Pacific Foods: A Cook Book of Culinary Customs and Recipes Adapted for the American Hostess.* New York: Barrows.

Brennan, J. 1981. *The Original Thai Cookbook.* New York: Perigee Books.

Brennan, J. 1984. *The Cuisines of Asia: Nine Great Oriental Cuisines by Technique.* New York: St. Martin's/Marek.

Brissendan, R. 1970. *Joys and Subtleties: South East Asian Cooking.* New York: Pantheon Books.

Claudio, V. S. 1994. *Filipino American Food Practices, Customs, and Holidays.* Chicago: American Dietetic Association.

Corum, A. K. 1983. *Ethnic Foods of Hawai'i.* Honolulu: Bess Press.

Cox, P. 1995. Samoan Americans. In R. J. Vecoli, J. Galens, A. Sheets, & R. V. Young (Eds.), *Gale Encyclopedia of Multicultural America.* New York: Gale Research.

Crane, N. T., & Green, N. R. 1980. Food habits and food preferences of Vietnamese refugees living in northern Florida. *Journal of the American Dietetic Association, 76,* 591-593.

Cushner, N. P. 1966. Philippines. In *The 1996 Grolier Multimedia Encyclopedia.* Danbury, CT: Grolier Electronic Publishing.

Dirige, O. V. 1995. Filipino-American diet and foods. *The Asian American Business Journal, Feb. 28,* 11-17.

Eckstein, E. F. 1983. *Menu Planning* (3rd ed.). Westport, CT: AVI.

Fitzpatrick-Nietschmann, J. 1983. Pacific Islanders—Migration and health. *Western Journal of Medicine, 139,* 848-853.

Geissler, E. M. 1998. *Pocket Guide to Cultural Assessment.* St. Louis: Mosby.

Gelle, G. G. 1997. *Filipino Cuisine.* Santa Fe, NM: Red Crane Books.

Gilman, S. C., Justice, J., Saepharn, K., & Charles, G. 1992. Use of traditional and modern health services by Laotian refugees. *Western Journal of Medicine, 157,* 310-315.

Hanna, J. M., Pelletier, D. L., & Brown, V. J. 1986. The diet and nutrition of contemporary Samoans. In P. T. Baker, J. M. Hanna, & T. S. Baker (Eds.), *The Changing Samoans: Behavior and Health in Transition.* New York: Oxford University Press.

Hart, D. V. 1981. Bisayan Filipino and Malayan folk medicine. In G. Henderson & M. Primeaux (Eds.), *Transcultural Health Care.* Menlo Park, CA: Addison-Wesley.

Hart, D. V. 1996. Guam. In *The 1996 Grolier Multimedia Encyclopedia*. Danbury, CT: Grolier Electronic Publishing.

Healy, J. R. 1996. Hawaii. In *The 1996 Grolier Multimedia Encyclopedia*. Danbury, CT: Grolier Electronic Publishing.

Howard, A. 1980. Hawaiians. In S. Thernstrom, A. Orlov, & O. Handlin (Eds.), *Harvard Encyclopedia of American Ethnic Groups*. Cambridge, MA: The Belknap Press of Harvard University Press.

Howard, A. 1986. Samoan coping behavior. In P. T. Baker, J. M. Hanna, & T. S. Baker (Eds.), *The Changing Samoans: Behavior and Health in Transition*. New York: Oxford University Press.

Ikeda, J. P. 1992. *Hmong American Food Practices, Customs, and Holidays*. Chicago: American Dietetic Association.

Ikeda, J. P., Ceja, D. R., Glass, R. S., Harwood, J. O., Lucke, K. A., & Sutherlin, J. M. 1991. Food habits of the Hmong living in central California. *Journal of Nutrition Education, 23,* 168-175.

Janes, C. R. 1990. *Migration, Social Change, and Health: A Samoan Community in California*. Stanford, CA: Stanford University Press.

Kinloch, P. 1985. *Talking Health But Doing Sickness: Studies in Samoan Health*. Wellington, New Zealand: Victoria University Press.

Law, R. 1990. *The Southeast Asia Cookbook*. New York: Fine.

Leonelli, L. 1987. *We Eat What We Are: Food Use Patterns of Hmong and Mien in Sacramento, California*. Master's thesis, California State University, Sacramento.

Lewis, J. S., & Glaspy, M. F. 1975. Food habits and nutrient intakes of Filipino women in Los Angeles. *Journal of the American Dietetic Association, 67,* 122-125.

Melendy, H. B. 1995. Filipino Americans. In R. J. Vecoli, J. Galens, A. Sheets, & R. V. Young (Eds.), *Gale Encyclopedia of Multicultural America*. New York: Gale Research.

Montepio, S. N. 1986-87. Folk medicine in the Filipino American experience. *Amerasia Journal, 13,* 151-162.

Morrison, T., Conaway, W. A., & Borden, G. A. 1994. *Kiss, Bow, or Shake Hands*. Holbrook, MA: Adams.

Muecke, M. A. 1983a. Caring for Southeast Asian patients in the USA. *American Journal of Public Health, 73,* 431-438.

Muecke, M. A. 1983b. In search of healers—Southeast Asian refugees in the American health care system. *Western Journal of Medicine, 139,* 835-840.

Nguyen, M. D. 1985. Culture shock: A review of Vietnamese culture and its concepts of health and disease. *Western Journal of Medicine, 142,* 409-412.

Orque, M. S. 1983a. Nursing care of Filipino American patients. In M. S. Orque, B. Bloch, & L. S. A. Monrroy (Eds.), *Ethnic Nursing Care: A Multicultural Approach*. St. Louis: Mosby.

Orque, M. S. 1983b. Nursing care of South Vietnamese patients. In M. S. Orque, B. Bloch, & L. S. A. Monrroy (Eds.), *Ethnic Nursing Care: A Multicultural Approach*. St. Louis: Mosby.

Palinkas, L. A. 1995. Health under stress: Asian and Central American refugees and those left behind. *Social Science and Medicine, 40,* 1591-1596.

Pobocik, R. S., & Shovic, A. C. 1996. Development of a nutrition exchange booklet for Guam using culturally accepted foods. *Journal of the American Dietetic Association, 96,* 285-287.

Pouesi, D. 1994. *An Illustrated History of Samoans in California*. Carson, CA: KIN Publications.

Rairdan, B., & Higgs, Z. R. 1992. When your patient is a Hmong refugee. *American Journal of Nursing, March,* 52-55.

Ratner, M. 1995. Thai Americans. In R. J. Vecoli, J. Galens, A. Sheets, & R. V. Young (Eds.), *Gale Encyclopedia of Multicultural America*. New York: Gale Research.

Schindler, R., & Schindler, G. 1970. *Hawaii Kai Cookbook*. New York: Hearthside Press.

Shore, B. 1980. Pacific Islanders. In S. Thernstrom, A. Orlov, & O. Handlin (Eds.), *Harvard Encyclopedia of American Ethnic Groups*. Cambridge, MA: The Belknap Press of Harvard University Press.

Shovic, A. C. 1994. Development of a Samoan nutrition exchange list using culturally accepted foods. *Journal of the American Dietetic Association, 94,* 541-543.

Snaden, J. W. 1996. Tonga. In *The 1996 Grolier Multimedia Encyclopedia*. Danbury, CT: Grolier Electronic Publishing.

Snyder, P. 1981. Ethnicity and folk healing in Honolulu, Hawaii. *Social Science and Medicine, 15B,* 125-132.

Snyder, P. 1984. Health service implications of folk healing among older Asian Americans and Hawaiians in Honolulu. *Gerontologist, 24,* 471-476.

Steinberg, R. 1970. *Pacific and Southeast Asian Cooking*. New York: Time-Life Books.

Stephenson, P. H. 1995. Vietnamese refugees in Victoria BC: An overview of immigrant and refugee health care in a medium-sized Canadian urban centre. *Social Science and Medicine, 40,* 1631-1642.

Story, M., & Harris, L. J. 1988. Food preferences, beliefs, and practices of Southeast Asian refugee adolescents. *Journal of School Health, 58,* 273-276.

Story, M., & Harris, L. J. 1989. Food habits and dietary change of Southeast Asian refugee families living in the United States. *Journal of the American Dietetic Association, 89,* 800-803.

Tate, D. J. M. 1979. *The Making of Modern South East Asia* (vols. 1 & 2). Oxford: Oxford University Press.

Tong, A. 1986. Food habits of Vietnamese immigrants. *Family Economic Review, 2,* 28-30.

U.S. Department of Agriculture, Food and Nutrition Service. 1980. *Southeast Asian American Food Habits*. Publication No. FNS-225. Washington, DC: U.S. Department of Agriculture.

Winters, E., & Swartz, M. 1995. Hawaiians. In R. J. Vecoli, J. Galens, A. Sheets, & R. V. Young (Eds.), *Gale Encyclopedia of Multicultural America*. New York: Gale Research.

Yardley, M. 1970. *Hawaii Cooks*. Tokyo: Tuttle.

Ziegler, V. S., Sucher, K. P., & Downes, N. J. 1989. Southeast Asian renal exchange list. *Journal of the American Dietetic Association, 89,* 85-92.

CHAPTER 9

Abraham, N. 1995. Arab Americans. In R. J. Vecoli, J. Galens, A. Sheets, & R. V. Young (Eds.), *Gale Encyclopedia of Multicultural America*. New York: Gale Research.

Altschiller, D. 1995. Turkish Americans. In R. J. Vecoli, J. Galens, A. Sheets, & R. V. Young (Eds.), *Gale Encyclopedia of Multicultural America*. New York: Gale Research.

Axtell, R. E. 1991. *Gestures: The Do's and Taboos of Body Language around the World*. New York: Wiley.

Gillis, M. 1995. Iranian Americans. In R. J. Vecoli, J. Galens, A. Sheets, & R. V. Young (Eds.), *Gale Encyclopedia of Multicultural America*. New York: Gale Research.

Gobetz, E. 1995. Slovenian Americans. In R. J. Vecoli, J. Galens, A. Sheets, & R. V. Young (Eds.), *Gale Encyclopedia of Multicultural America*. New York: Gale Research.

Hall, E. T. 1979. Learning the Arab's silent language. *Psychology Today, August*, 45-54.

Helman, C. G. 1990. *Culture, Health, and Illness: An Introduction for Health Professionals* (2nd ed.). London: Wright.

Hitti, P. K. 1961. *The Near East History.* New York: Van Nostrand.

Ifkovic, E. 1995. Croatian Americans. In R. J. Vecoli, J. Galens, A. Sheets, & R. V. Young (Eds.), *Gale Encyclopedia of Multicultural America.* New York: Gale Research.

Jurgens, J. 1995. Greek Americans. In R. J. Vecoli, J. Galens, A. Sheets, & R. V. Young (Eds.), *Gale Encyclopedia of Multicultural America.* New York: Gale Research.

Kromhout, D., Keys, A., Aravanis, C., Buzina, R., Fidanza, F., Giampaoli, S., Jansen, A., Menotti, A., Nedeljkovic, S., Pekkarinen, M., Simic, B. S., & Toshima, H. 1989. Food consumption patterns in the 1960s in seven countries. *American Journal of Clinical Nutrition, 49*, 889-894.

Kurson, K. 1995. Palestinian Americans. In R. J. Vecoli, J. Galens, A. Sheets, & R. V. Young (Eds.), *Gale Encyclopedia of Multicultural America.* New York: Gale Research.

Lipson, J. G., & Meleis, A. I. 1983. Issues in health care of Middle Eastern patients. *Western Journal of Medicine, 139*, 854-861.

Luna, L. 1994. Care and cultural context of Lebanese Muslim immigrants: Using Leininger's theory. *Journal of Transcultural Nursing, 5*, 12-20.

Meleis, A. I. 1981. The Arab-American in the health care system. *American Journal of Nursing, 81*, 1180-1183.

Meleis, A. I., Lipson, J. G., & Paul, S. M. 1992. Ethnicity and health among five Middle Eastern immigrant groups. *Nursing Research, 41*, 98-103.

Morrison, T., Conaway, W. A., & Borden, G. A. 1994. *Kiss, Bow, or Shake Hands.* Holbrook, MA: Adams.

Naff, A. 1980. Arabs. In S. Thernstrom, A. Orlov, & O. Handlin (Eds.), *Harvard Encyclopedia of American Ethnic Groups.* Cambridge, MA: The Belknap Press of Harvard University Press.

Nickles, H. G. *Middle Eastern Cooking.* New York: Time-Life Books.

Packard, D. P., & McWilliams, M. 1993. Cultural foods heritage of Middle Eastern immigrants. *Nutrition Today, May-June*, 6-12.

Packard, D. P., & McWilliams, M. 1994. Tips on counseling Middle Eastern clients. *Journal of the American Dietetic Association, 94*, 1254.

Perl, L. 1967. *Rice, Spice, and Bitter Oranges: Mediterranean Food Festivals.* New York: World.

Peterson, J., & Peterson, D. 1996. *Eat Smart in Turkey.* Madison, WI: Gingko Press.

Roden, C. 1974. *A Book of Middle Eastern Food.* New York: Vintage Books.

Scourby, A. 1984. *The Greek Americans.* Boston: Twayne.

Sheikh, A. A., & Sheikh, K. S. (Eds.). 1989. *Eastern and Western Approaches to Healing: Ancient Wisdom and Modern Knowledge.* New York: Wiley.

Spector, R. E. 1991. *Cultural Diversity in Health and Illness* (3rd ed.). Norwalk, CT: Appleton & Lange.

Stevanovic, B. 1995. Serbian Americans. In R. J. Vecoli, J. Galens, A. Sheets, & R. V. Young (Eds.), *Gale Encyclopedia of Multicultural America.* New York: Gale Research.

Takooshian, H. 1995. Armenian Americans. In R. J. Vecoli, J. Galens, A. Sheets, & R. V. Young (Eds.), *Gale Encyclopedia of Multicultural America.* New York: Gale Research.

Valassi, K. 1962. Food habits of Greek Americans. *American Journal of Clinical Nutrition, 11*, 240-248.

Waterlow, J. C. 1989. Diet of the classical period of Greece and Rome. *European Journal of Clinical Nutrition, 43* (suppl. 2), 3-12.

Wechsberg, J. 1974. *The Cooking of Vienna's Empire.* Alexandria, VA: Time-Life Books.

Yianilos, T. K. 1970. *The Complete Greek Cookbook.* New York: Funk & Wagnalls.

Zubaida, S. & Tapper, R. 1994. *Culinary Cultures of the Middle East.* New York: I. B. Taurus.

CHAPTER 10

Achaya, K. T. 1994. *Indian Food: A Historical Companion.* Delhi: Oxford University Press.

Axtell, R. E. 1991. *Gestures: The Do's and Taboos of Body Language around the World.* New York: Wiley.

Carstairs, G. M. 1979. *Daru* and *bhang:* Cultural factors in the choice of intoxicant. In M. Marshall (Ed.), *Beliefs, Behaviors, and Alcoholic Beverages.* Ann Arbor, MI: University of Michigan Press.

Chakravarty, I. 1972. *Saga of Indian Food: A Historical and Cultural Survey.* New Delhi: Sterling.

Devi Dasi, I., & Devi Dasi, S. 1973. *The Hari Krishna Cookbook.* Los Angeles: Bhaktivedanta Book Trust.

Eckstein, E. F. 1983. *Menu Planning* (3rd ed.). Westport, CT: AVI.

Freedman, A. D. 1996. Traditional medicine. In *The 1996 Grolier Multimedia Encyclopedia.* Danbury, CT: Grolier Electronic Publishing.

Goody, J. 1982. The high and low: Culinary culture in Asia and Europe. In *Cooking, Cuisine, and Class.* Cambridge, England: Cambridge University Press.

Gupta, S. P. 1976. Changes in food habits of Asian Indians in the United States: A case study. *Sociology and Social Research, 60*, 87-99.

Harris, M. 1972. *Cows, Pigs, Wars, and Witches.* New York: Random House.

Ho, G. P., Nolan, F. L., & Dodds, M. L. 1966. Adaptation to American dietary patterns by students from oriental countries. *Journal of Home Economics, 58*, 277-280.

Jaffrey, M. 1975. *Invitation to Indian Cooking.* New York: Vintage Books.

Jensen, J. M. 1980. East Indians. In S. Thernstrom, A. Orlov, & O. Handlin (Eds.), *Harvard Encyclopedia of American Ethnic Groups.* Cambridge, MA: The Belknap Press of Harvard University Press.

Kakarala, M., Song, W., Hoerr, S., & Bond, J. 1994. Computerized database of Indian foods. *American Journal of Clinical Nutrition, 59* (Suppl.), 291S.

Karim, N., Bloch, D. S., Falciglia, G., & Murthy, L. 1986. Modifications of food consumption patterns reported by people from India, living in Cincinnati, Ohio. *Ecology of Food and Nutrition, 19*, 11-18.

Katone-Apte, J. 1975. Dietary aspects of acculturation: Meals, feasts, and fasts in a minority community in South Asia. In M. L. Arnott (Ed.), *Gastronomy: The Anthropology of Food Habits.* The Hague: Mouton.

Khanna, G. 1986. *Herbal Remedies: A Handbook of Folk Medicine* (4th ed.). New Delhi: Tarang Paperbacks.

Khare, R. S. 1976. *The Hindu Hearth and Home.* Durham, NC: Carolina Academic Press.

Kilara, A., & Iya, K. K. 1992. Food and dietary practices of the Hindu. *Food Technology, 46,* 94-102, 104.

Larson-Presswalla, J. 1994. Insights into eastern health care: Some transcultural nursing perspectives. *Journal of Transcultural Nursing, 5,* 21-24.

Morrison, T., Conaway, W. A., & Borden, G. A. 1994. *Kiss, Bow, or Shake Hands.* Holbrook, MA: Adams.

Pavri, T. 1995a. Asian Indian Americans. In R. J. Vecoli, J. Galens, A. Sheets, & R. V. Young (Eds.), *Gale Encyclopedia of Multicultural America.* New York: Gale Research.

Pavri, T. 1995b. Pakistani Americans. In R. J. Vecoli, J. Galens, A. Sheets, & R. V. Young (Eds.), *Gale Encyclopedia of Multicultural America.* New York: Gale Research.

Ramakrishna, J., & Weiss, M. G. 1992. Health, illness, and immigration. East Indians in the United States. *Western Journal of Medicine, 157,* 265-270.

Rau, S. R. 1969. *The Cooking of India.* New York: Time-Life Books.

Sheikh, A. A., & Sheikh, K. S. 1989. *Eastern and Western Approaches to Healing: Ancient Wisdom and Modern Knowledge.* New York: Wiley.

Singer, E. A. 1984. Conversion through foodways acculturation: The meaning of eating in an American Hindu sect. In L. K. Brown & K. Mussels (Eds.), *Ethnic and Regional Foodways in the United States.* Knoxville, TN: University of Tennessee Press.

Sodowsky, G. R., & Carey, J. C. 1988. Relationships between acculturation-related demographics and cultural attitudes of an Asian-Indian immigrant group. *Journal of Multicultural Counseling and Development, 16,* 117-137.

Yagalla, M. V., Hoerr, S. L., Song, W. O., Enas, E., & Garg, A. 1996. Relationship of diet, abdominal obesity, and physical activity to plasma lipoprotein levels in Asian Indian physicians residing in the United States. *Journal of the American Dietetic Association, 96,* 257-261.

CHAPTER 11

Anderson, J. 1997. *The American Century Cookbook.* New York: Clarkson Potter.

Armstrong, J. 1995. A taste of Quebec. In J. M. Powers & A. Stewart (Eds.), *Our Northern Bounty: A Celebration of Canadian Cuisine.* Toronto: Random House of Canada.

Aspler, T. 1995. Icewine. In J. M. Powers & A. Stewart (Eds.), *Our Northern Bounty: A Celebration of Canadian Cuisine.* Toronto: Random House of Canada.

Baird, E. 1995. The future of Ontario's fruit industry. In J. M. Powers & A. Stewart (Eds.), *Our Northern Bounty: A Celebration of Canadian Cuisine.* Toronto: Random House of Canada.

Barss, B. 1995. The chuckwagon tradition in Prairie culture. In J. M. Powers & A. Stewart (Eds.), *Our Northern Bounty: A Celebration of Canadian Cuisine,* Toronto: Random House of Canada.

Belman, D. 1997. Regional cuisine: Puts American cooking on the map. *Restaurants, USA, 17,* 22-26.

Brown, D. 1968. *American Cooking.* New York: Time-Life Books.

Brown, D. 1971. *American Cooking: The Northwest.* New York: Time-Life Books.

Brown, L. K., & Mussell, K. 1984. Introduction. In *Ethnic and Regional Foodways in the United States.* Knoxville: University of Tennessee Press.

Burkhard, J. 1995. Quebec goes country. In J. M. Powers, & A. Stewart (Eds.), *Our Northern Bounty: A Celebration of Canadian Cuisine.* Toronto: Random House of Canada.

Carlson, B. 1997. *Food Festivals.* Detroit: Visible Ink.

Chau, P., Lee, H., Tseng, R., & Downes, N. J. 1990. Dietary habits, health beliefs, and food practices of elderly Chinese women. *Journal of the American Dietetic Association, 90,* 579-580.

Claiborne, C. 1987. *Southern Cooking.* New York: Times Books.

Colohan, C. 1995. Spanish Americans. In R. J. Vecoli, J. Galens, A. Sheets, & R. V. Young (Eds.), *Gale Encyclopedia of Multicultural America.* New York: Gale Research.

Comfort, J. 1995. Some good! The Maritime harvest. In J. M. Powers & A. Stewart (Eds.), *Our Northern Bounty: A Celebration of Canadian Cuisine.* Toronto: Random House of Canada.

de Wit, C. W. 1992. Food-place associations on American product labels. *Geographical Review, 83,* 323-330.

Duncan, D. 1995. Ontario cooking: Cuisines in transition. In J. M. Powers & A. Stewart (Eds.), *Our Northern Bounty: A Celebration of Canadian Cuisine.* Toronto: Random House of Canada.

Edmondson, B. 1998. The line between beer and wine. *American Demographics 1,* 8-19.

Feibleman, P. S. 1971. *American Cooking: Creole and Acadian.* New York: Time-Life Books.

Ferguson, C. 1995. Our northern bounty. In J. M. Powers & A. Stewart (Eds.), *Our Northern Bounty: A Celebration of Canadian Cuisine.* Toronto: Random House of Canada.

Fraser, M. 1995. Canada's breadbasket: Decades of change. In J. M. Powers & A. Stewart (Eds.), *Our Northern Bounty: A Celebration of Canadian Cuisine.* Toronto: Random House of Canada.

Gillespie, A. K. 1984. A wilderness in the megalopolis: Foodways in the Pine Barrens of New Jersey. In *Ethnic and Regional Foodways in the United States.* Knoxville: University of Tennessee Press.

Gutierrez, C. P. 1984. The social and symbolic uses of ethnic/regional foodways: Cajuns and crawfish in South Louisiana. In *Ethnic and Regional Foodways in the United States.* Knoxville: University of Tennessee Press.

Herter, G. L., & Herter, B. E. 1960. *Bull Cook and Authentic Recipes and Practices.* Waseca, MN: Herter's.

Hess, K. 1992. *The Carolina Rice Kitchen.* Columbia: University of South Carolina Press.

Hines, D. 1959. *Adventures in Good Eating.* Ithaca, NY: Duncan Hines Institute.

Isern, T. D. 1990. Bierocks. In J. Hoy & T. Isern, *Plains Folk: The Romance of the Landscape* (vol. 2). Norman: University of Oklahoma Press.

Johnson, E. 1995. Historical influences on West Coast cooking. In J. M. Powers & A. Stewart (Eds.), *Our Northern Bounty: A Celebration of Canadian Cuisine.* Toronto: Random House of Canada.

Jones, E. 1981. *American Food: The Gastronomic Story* (2nd ed.). New York: Vintage Books.

Kalčik, S. 1984. Ethnic foodways in America: Symbol and the performance of identity. In *Ethnic and Regional Foodways in the United States.* Knoxville: University of Tennessee Press.

Kavasch, E. B. 1995. *Enduring Harvests.* Old Saybrook, CN: Globe Pequot Press.

Kelly, J. L. 1983. Loco moco: A folk dish in the making. *Social Process in Hawaii, 30,* 59-64.

Kirlin, K. S., & Kirlin, T. M. 1991. *Smithsonian Folklife Cookbook.* Washington, DC: Smithsonian Institution Press.

Lee, H. G. 1992. *Taste of the States: A Food History of America.* Charlottesville, VA: Howell Press.

Leonard, J. N. 1970. *American Cooking: New England.* New York: Time-Life Books.

Leonard, J. N. 1971. *American Cooking: The Great West.* New York: Time-Life Books.

Lewis, G. H. 1989. The Maine lobster as regional icon: Competing images over time and social class. *Food and Foodways, 3,* 303-316.

Lloyd, T. C. 1981. The Cincinnati chili culinary complex. *Western Folklore, 40,* 28-40.

Lockwood, Y. R., & Lockwood, W. G. 1991. Pasties in Michigan's Upper Peninsula. In S. Stern & J. A. Cicala (Eds.), *Creative Ethnicity: Symbols and Strategies of Contemporary Ethnic Life.* Logan: Utah State University Press.

Luchetti, C. 1993. *Home on the Range.* New York: Villard Books.

Mandel, A. 1996. *Celebrating the Midwestern Table.* New York: Doubleday.

Mariani, J. F. 1983. *The Dictionary of American Food and Drink.* New Haven, CN: Ticknor & Fields.

Matson, M. 1994. *Food in Missouri.* Columbia: University of Missouri Press.

McWatters, H. 1995. British Columbia wines take on the world. In J. M. Powers & A. Stewart (Eds.), *Our Northern Bounty: A Celebration of Canadian Cuisine.* Toronto: Random House of Canada.

Milbauer, J. A. 1990. The geography of food in Eastern Oklahoma: A small restaurant study. *North American Culture, 6,* 37-52.

Mogelonsky, M. 1995. *Everybody Eats.* Ithaca, NY: American Demographic Books.

Mogelonsky, M. 1996. *Who's Buying Food and Drink.* Ithaca, NY: New Strategist Publications.

Nightingale, M. 1995. The enduring influences on today's East Coast cooking. In J. M. Powers & A. Stewart (Eds.), *Our Northern Bounty: A Celebration of Canadian Cuisine.* Toronto: Random House of Canada.

Page, L. G., & Wigginton, E. 1984. *The Foxfire Book of Appalachian Cookery.* New York: E. P. Dutton.

Raspa, R. 1984. Exotic foods among Italian-Americans in Mormon Utah: Food as nostalgic enactment of identity. In *Ethnic and Regional Foodways in the United States.* Knoxville: University of Tennessee Press.

Root, W., & de Rochemont, R. 1976. *Eating in America.* New York: Ecco Press.

Schultz, J. 1995. Development of the Prairie palate: The red-meat eaters. In J. M. Powers & A. Stewart (Eds.), *Our Northern Bounty: A Celebration of Canadian Cuisine.* Toronto: Random House of Canada.

Shortridge, B. G., & Shortridge, J. R. 1998. Introduction: Food and American culture. In B. G. Shortridge & J. R. Shortridge (Eds.), *The Taste of American Place.* Lanham, MD: Rowman & Littlefield.

Skye, B. 1995. Traditional Cree and Iroquois foods. In J. M. Powers & A. Stewart (Eds.), *Our Northern Bounty: A Celebration of Canadian Cuisine.* Toronto: Random House of Canada.

Solomon, J., & Solomon, O. P. 1979. *Cracklin Bread and Asfidity.* Tuscaloosa: University of Alabama Press.

Staebler, E. 1995. Faith, family, and food: The old-order Mennonites in Waterloo County. In J. M. Powers & A. Stewart (Eds.), *Our Northern Bounty: A Celebration of Canadian Cuisine.* Toronto: Random House of Canada.

Stewart, A., & Powers, J. M. 1995. Introduction. In J. M. Powers & A. Stewart (Eds.), *Our Northern Bounty: A Celebration of Canadian Cuisine.* Toronto: Random House of Canada.

Trager, J. 1995. *The Food Chronology.* New York: Holt.

Trillin, C. 1974. *American Fried.* New York: Doubleday.

Turner, N. J., Philip, S., & Turner, R. D. 1995. Traditional native plant foods in contemporary cuisine in British Columbia. In J. M. Powers & A. Stewart (Eds.), *Our Northern Bounty: A Celebration of Canadian Cuisine.* Toronto: Random House of Canada.

Walter, E. 1971. *American Cooking: Southern Style.* New York: Time-Life Books.

Wilson, J. 1971. *American Cooking: The Eastern Heartland.* New York: Time-Life Books.

Wong, S. 1995. Asian flavors. In J. M. Powers & A. Stewart (Eds.), *Our Northern Bounty: A Celebration of Canadian Cuisine.* Toronto: Random House of Canada.

Wyman, C. 1993. *I'm a Spam Fan.* Stamford, CN: Longmeadow Press.

Zelinsky, W. 1973. *The Cultural Geography of the United States.* Englewood Cliffs, NJ: Prentice-Hall.

Ziraldo, D. 1995. Founding the Vintners Quality Alliance (VQA). In J. M. Powers & A. Stewart (Eds.), *Our Northern Bounty: A Celebration of Canadian Cuisine.* Toronto: Random House of Canada.

CHAPTER 12

Ammerman, A. S., Kirkley, B. G., Dennis, B., Hohenstein, C., Allison, A., Strecher, V. J., & Bulger, D. 1994. A dietary assessment for individuals with low literacy skills using interactive touch-screen computer technology. *American Journal of Clinical Nutrition, 59* (suppl.), 289S.

Axtell, R. E. 1991. *Gestures.* New York: Wiley.

Beck, A. 1988. *Love Is Never Enough.* New York: Harper & Row.

Billing, J., & Sherman, P. W. 1998. Antimicrobial functions of spices: Why some like it hot. *Quarterly Review of Biology, 73,* 3-49.

Blank, R., & Slipp, S. 1994. *Voices of Diversity: Real People Talk about Problems and Solutions in a Workplace Where Everyone Is Not Alike.* New York: AMA COM.

Blank, R., & Slipp, S. 1994. The white male: An endangered species? *Management Review, September,* 27-32.

Blank, R., & Slipp, S. 1998. Manager's diversity workbook. *HR Focus, July,* S7-S8.

Brookins, G. K. 1993. Culture, ethnicity, and bicultural competence: Implications for children with chronic illness and disability. *Pediatrics, 91,* 1056-1062.

Brown, J. D., & Einsiedel, E. F. 1990. Public health campaigns: Mass media strategies. In E. B. Ray & L. Donohew (Eds.), *Communication and Health.* Hillsdale, NJ: Lawrence Erlbaum Associates.

Burner, O. Y., Cunningham, P., & Hattar, H. S. 1990. Managing a multicultural nurse staff in a multicultural environment. *Journal of Nursing Administration, 20,* 30-34.

Costa, R. E. 1998. Applying the behavioral sciences to risk assessment in food service establishments. *Florida Journal of Environmental Health, March,* 12-14.

Dresser, N. 1996. *Multicultural Manners.* New York: Wiley.

Esquivel, G. B., & Keitel, M. A. 1990. Counseling immigrant children in the schools. *Elementary School Guidance & Counseling, 24,* 213-221.

Foster, G. M., & Käferstein, F. K. 1985. Food safety and the behavioral sciences. *Social Science and Medicine, 21,* 1273-1277.

Gardenswartz, L., & Rowe, A. 1998. Why diversity matters. *HR Focus, July,* S1-S3.

Gardner, W. E. 1972. The differential effects of race, education and experience in helping. *Journal of Clinical Psychology, 28,* 87–89.

Gardner, W. E. 1994. Mortality. In N. W. S. Zane, D. T. Takeuchi, & K. N. J. Young (Eds.), *Confronting Critical Health Issues of Asian and Pacific Islander Americans.* Thousand Oaks, CA: Sage.

Gilbert, S. E., & Gay, G. 1989. Improving the success in school of poor black children. In B. J. Robinson Shade (Ed.), *Culture, Style, and the Educative Process.* Springfield, IL: Thomas.

Gudykunst, W. B. 1994. *Bridging Differences: Effective Intergroup Communication* (2nd ed.). Thousand Oaks, CA: Sage.

Gudykunst, W. B., & Nishida, T. 1994. *Bridging Japanese/ North American Differences.* Thousand Oaks, CA: Sage.

Hall, E. T. 1977. *Beyond Culture.* Garden City, NY: Anchor Press/Doubleday.

Hand, W. D. 1980. *Magical Medicine.* Berkeley: University of California Press.

Harris, P. R., & Moran, R. T. 1987. *Managing Cultural Differences* (2nd ed.). Houston, TX: Gulf.

Hemphill, H., & Haines, R. 1998. Confronting discrimination in your workplace. *HR Focus, July,* S6.

Howell, W. 1982. *The Emphatic Communicator.* Belmont, CA: Wadsworth.

Klontz, K. C., Timbo, B., Fein, S., & Levy, A. 1995. Prevalence of selected food consumption and preparation behaviors associated with increased risk of food-bourne disease. *Journal of Food Protection, 58,* 927–930.

Kochman, T. 1983. *Black and White Styles in Conflict.* Chicago: University of Chicago Press.

Kreps, G. L. 1990. Communication and health education. In E. B. Ray & L. Donohew (Eds.), *Communication and Health.* Hillsdale, N.J.: Lawrence Erlbaum Associates.

Kreps, G. L., & Kunimoto, E. N. 1994. *Effective Communication in Multicultural Health Care Settings.* Thousand Oaks, CA: Sage.

Loria, C., Arroyo, D., & Briefel, R. 1994. Cultural biases influencing dietary interviews with Mexican Americans: The Hanes experience. *American Journal of Clinical Nutrition, 59* (suppl.), 290S.

Loria, C. M., McDowell, M. A., Johnson, C. L., & Woteki, C. E. 1991. Nutrient data for Mexican-American foods: Are current data adequate? *Journal of the American Dietetic Association, 91,* 919–922.

Masi, R. 1989. Multicultural medicine: Fad or forgotten concept? *Canadian Medical Association Journal, 140,* 1086–1087.

Miller, J. E., Porter, M., & Drummond, K. E. 1998. *Supervision in the Hospitality Industry.* New York: Wiley.

Moran R. T., & Harris, P. R. 1981. *Managing Cultural Synergy.* Houston, TX: Gulf.

Morrison, T., Conaway, W. A., & Borden, G. A. 1994. *Kiss, Bow, or Shake Hands: How to Do Business in Sixty Countries.* Holbrook, MA: Adams.

Olsen, M. E. 1978. *The Process of Social Organization: Power in Social Systems* (2nd Ed.). New York: Holt, Rinehart, & Winston.

Rabin, S. 1994. How to sell across cultures. *American Demographics, 16,* 56–57.

Randall-David, E. 1989. *Strategies for Working with Culturally Diverse Communities and Clients.* Bethesda, MD: Association for the Care of Children's Health.

Ronen, S. 1986. *Comparative and Multinational Management.* New York: Wiley.

Scarborough, J. 1998. *The Origins of Cultural Differences and Their Impact on Management.* Westport, CN: Quorum Books.

Schilling, B., & Brannon, E. 1986. *Cross-Cultural Counseling: A Guide for Nutrition and Health Counselors.* Alexandria, VA: U.S. Department of Agriculture/U.S. Department of Health and Human Services, FNS #250.

Segal, M. 1992. Native food preparation fosters botulism. *FDA Consumer, January-February,* 23–27.

Soukup, J. J. 1996. Extension serves up food protection management training. Texas A & M Agricultural News, http://agnews.tamu.edu/stories/ NUTR/foodprot.htm.

Sue, D. W., & Sue, D. 1990. *Counseling the Culturally Different: Theory and Practice* (2nd ed.). New York: Wiley.

Swartz, L. 1987. Illness negotiation: The case of eating disorders. *Social Science and Medicine, 24,* 613–618.

Usunier, J. C. 1993. *International Marketing.* New York: Prentice-Hall.

Wood, J. B. 1989. Communicating with older adults in health care settings: Cultural and ethnic considerations. *Educational Gerontology, 15,* 351–362.

Index